To Sammy
a true friend
& colleague
J. Sowers
Dec 29, 2000

ENDOCRINOLOGY OF THE VASCULATURE

Contemporary Endocrinology

P. Michael Conn, Series Editor

1. ***Endocrinology of the Vasculature,*** edited by *James R. Sowers*, 1996

Endocrinology of the Vasculature

Edited by

James R. Sowers, MD

School of Medicine,
Wayne State University,
Detroit, Michigan

Humana Press
Totowa, New Jersey

999 Riverview Drive, Suite 208
Totowa, New Jersey 07512

For additional copies, pricing for bulk purchases, and/or information about other Humana titles, contact Humana at the above address or at any of the following numbers: Tel.: 201-256-1699; Fax: 201-256-8341; E-mail: humana@interramp.com

This publication is printed on acid-free paper. ∞
ANSI Z39.48-1984 (American National Standards Institute)
Permanence of Paper for Printed Library Materials.

Printed in the United States of America. 10 9 8 7 6 5 4 3 2 1

PREFACE

In contrast to previous concepts that blood vessels were inert conduits for the transfer of nutrients to tissues, over the last decade we have come to recognize that the cells of the vessel wall are exquisitely active in the production of hormonal factors that behave in an autocrine or paracrine fashion. This recognition has led to the development of the new scientific discipline of vascular medicine and biology. Scientists and clinicians in this discipline include endocrinologists, cardiologists, vascular surgeons, radiologists, nephrologists, and others interested in the metabolic abnormalities associated with hypertension and atherosclerosis. Additionally, state-of-the-art techniques in cell and molecular biology are being applied to the study of vascular physiology and diseases. *Endocrinology of the Vasculature* is the first book comprehensively to explore the recent developments in this major new field. In this context, the book thoroughly examines the two most biologically active cells, the endothelium and vascular smooth muscle cells (VSMCs).

The inner layer of the blood vessels—the tunica intima—with its lining of endothelial cells, serves as more than an interface between the blood and tissues. Accumulating evidence suggests that the endothelium has a substantial role in regulating vascular function through complex autocrine–paracrine interactions. The spectrum of signaling processes that activate endothelial cells ranges from mechanical forces (flow and pressure) to vasoactive hormones, cytokines, and inflammatory mediators. Indeed, a diverse array of receptors is necessary to the role of the endothelium as the sensory interface of the blood vessel with the microenvironment of vascular tissue. Under normal circumstances, substances released from the endothelium—such as endothelium-derived relaxing factor(s)/nitric oxide, prostaglandins/arachidonic acid metabolites, and peptides—modulate vascular tone, platelet aggregation, thrombosis, and vascular growth and remodeling.

VSMCs also regulate vascular function through complex autocrine–paracrine interactions. For example, insulin-like growth factor 1 (IGF-1) is synthesized constitutively by VSMCs and its production is regulated by both angiotensin II, insulin, and platelet-derived growth factor, agents known to regulate vascular tone, growth, and remodeling. The IGF-1 produced by VSMCs can, in turn, affect vascular tone and VSMC proliferation. Additionally, this autocrine–paracrine factor has been shown to modulate glucose and cation transport in VSMC as well as endothelial cells. Another example of the complexity of these interactions is the observation that angiotensin II causes VSMCs to grow by inducing the autocrine growth factors, IGF-1, platelet-derived growth factor, basic fibroblast growth factor, and transforming growth factor-β. Recent novel observations that peptides such as angiotensin II, classically considered to act through membrane receptors, have direct nuclear actions, and steroids, classically acting at the nucleus, have membrane effects will also be reviewed. Nitric oxide is synthesized by VSMCs as well as endothelial cells and regulates many of the functions of these cells. Indeed, many of the hormonally regulated metabolic processes that have been extensively reviewed for other tissues (i.e., liver, fat, and skeletal muscle) will be explored for VSMCs in this book.

Thus, the vessel wall is an active, integrated organ that includes endothelial cells and VSMCs coupled to each other in a complex, autocrine–paracrine set of interactions. The

sively reviewed for other tissues (i.e., liver, fat, and skeletal muscle) will be explored for VSMCs in this book.

Thus, the vessel wall is an active, integrated organ that includes endothelial cells and VSMCs coupled to each other in a complex, autocrine–paracrine set of interactions. The blood vessel has the ability to sense changes within its milieu, integrating these signals by intercellular communication and local production of mediators that influence structure and function. The renal glomerulus has many properties analogous to those of vascular tissue. Indeed, glomerular endothelial cells and mesangial cells (modified VSMCs) have many characteristics in common with their vascular counterparts. The processes of glomerulosclerosis and atherosclerosis also display many similarities. Thus, the analogy between glomerular and vascular biology will also be reviewed in this book.

Endocrinology of the Vasculature is the first treatise systematically to explore the vasculature as an endocrine organ. The future should lead to exciting endocrine investigation of the vasculature which, in turn, should lead to vascular biology becoming an integral part of endocrinology training.

I wish to offer my sincere appreciation to Paddy McGowan for her painstaking and capable efforts in assisting me in the preparation of this book.

James R. Sowers, MD

CONTENTS

CONTRIBUTORS

GEORGE L. BAKRIS, MD, *Department of Preventive Medicine, Rush University Hypertension Center, Rush-Presbyterian-St. Luke's Medical Center, Chicago, IL*
MARIO BARBAGALLO, MD, *University of Palermo, Italy*
ALAIN D. BARON, MD, *Department of Medicine, Indiana University Medical Center, Indianapolis, IN*
JACK D. BARRETT, PHD, *Vascular Pharmacology Laboratory, Veterans Affairs Medical Center, Sepulveda, CA and Department of Medicine, University of California at Los Angeles, CA*
DANIEL BATLLE, MD, *Division of Nephrology/Hypertension, Northwestern University, Chicago, IL*
WILLIAM H. BEIERWALTES, PHD, *Hypertension and Vascular Research Division, Henry Ford Hospital and Health Sciences Center, Detroit, MI*
BRADFORD C. BERK, MD, PHD, *Department of Medicine, Cardiology Division, University of Washington, Seattle, WA*
KENNETH E. BERNSTEIN, MD, *Department of Pathology, Emory University, Atlanta, GA*
RICHARD D. BUKOSKI, PHD, *Section of Hypertension and Vascular Research, Departments of Internal Medicine and Vascular Research, University of Texas Medical Branch, Galveston Island, TX*
JOHN C. BURNETT, MD, *Cardiovascular Diseases and Internal Medicine, Mayo Foundation, Rochester, MN*
YIU-FAI CHEN, PHD, *Department of Medicine, University of Alabama at Birmingham, AL*
JOHN A. COLWELL, MD, PHD, *Medical University of South Carolina, Charleston, SC*
JOHN P. COOKE, MD, *Division of Cardiovascular Medicine, Stanford University School of Medicine, Stanford, CA*
MARK A. CREAGER, MD, *Vascular Medicine and Atherosclerosis Unit, Cardiovascular Division, Brigham and Women's Hospital, Harvard Medical School, Boston, MA*
JAMIE DANANBERG, MD, *Division of Endocrinology and Metabolism, Department of Internal Medicine, The University of Michigan and VA Medical Center, Ann Arbor, MI*
LIGIA J. DOMINGUEZ, MD, *Division of Endocrinology, Metabolism and Hypertension, Wayne State University, Detroit, MI*
JENNIFER L. DUFF, PHD, *Department of Dermatology, Emory University, Atlanta, GA*
BRENT M. EGAN, MD, *Division of Clinical Pharmacology, Departments of Pharmacology and Medicine, Medical University of South Carolina, Charleston, SC*
PETER EGGENA, PHD, *Renin Biochemistry Laboratory, Veterans Affairs Medical Center, Sepulveda, CA and Department of Medicine, University of California at Los Angeles, CA*
MARIE D. GERHARD, MD, *Vascular Medicine and Atherosclerosis Unit Cardiovascular Division, Brigham and Women's Hospital, Harvard Medical School, Boston, MA*
MICHAEL S. GOLUB, MD, *University of California at Los Angeles Medical Center, Los Angeles, CA and Veterans Affairs Medical Center, Sepulveda, CA*
HERMANN HALLER, MD, *Franz Volhard Clinic, Humboldt University of Berlin, Germany*

Katherine Hein, MD, *Department of Vascular Surgery, Deaconess Hospital, Boston, MA*
Mark T. Hori, BS, *University of California at Los Angeles Medical Center, Los Angeles, CA and Veterans Affairs Medical Center, Sepulveda, CA*
Andrew M. Kahn, MD, *Division of Renal Diseases and Hypertension, Department of Medicine, University of Texas Medical School, Houston, TX*
Nancy L. Kanagy, PhD, *Department of Physiology, University of Michigan Medical School, Ann Arbor, MI*
George L. King, MD, *Research Division, Joslin Diabetes Center, Brigham and Women's Hospital, Harvard Medical School, Boston, MA*
R. L. Klein, PhD, *Charleston Veterans Affairs Medical Center, Charleston, SC*
Iftikhar J. Kullo, MD, *Cardiovascular Diseases and Internal Medicine, Mayo Foundation, Rochester, MN*
Michael S. LaPointe, PhD, *Division of Nephrology/Hypertension, Northwestern University, Chicago, IL*
Ellis R. Levin, MD, *Departments of Medicine and Pharmacology, University of California, Irvine and Endocrinology and Metabolism, Long Beach Veterans Affairs, Medical Center, Long Beach, CA*
Ronald L. Levine, MD, MS, *Department of Medicine, University of Alabama at Birmingham, AL*
Friedrich C. Luft, MD, *Franz Volhard Clinic, Humboldt University of Berlin, Germany*
Steven B. Magill, MD, PhD, *Division of Endocrinology and Metabolism, Department of Internal Medicine, The University of Michigan and VA Medical Center, Ann Arbor, MI*
Mario B. Marrero, PhD, *Department of Pathology, Emory University, Atlanta, GA*
Jerry Nadler, MD, *Department of Diabetes, Endocrinology and Metabolism, City of Hope National Medical Center, Duarte, CA*
Rama Natarajan, PhD, *Department of Diabetes, Endocrinology and Metabolism, City of Hope National Medical Center, Duarte, CA*
Suzanne Oparil, MD, *Department of Medicine, University of Alabama at Birmingham, AL*
Carlos E. Palant, MD, *Division of Nephrology, University of Nevada School of Medicine, Reno, NV*
Kailash N. Pandey, PhD, *Department of Biochemistry and Molecular Biology, School of Medicine, Medical College of Georgia, Augusta, GA*
Jacob D. Peuler, PhD, *Department of Pharmacology, Midwestern University, Downers Grove, IL*
Jeffrey L. Ram, PhD, *Department of Physiology, Wayne State University, Detroit, MI*
Lawrence M. Resnick, MD, *Division of Endocrinology, Metabolism and Hypertension, Wayne State University Medical Center, Detroit, MI*
Willis K. Samson, PhD, *Department of Physiology, University of North Dakota School of Medicine, Grand Forks, ND*
Rajabrata Sarkar, MD, PhD, *Department of Physiology, University of Michigan Medical School, Ann Arbor, MI*
David H. Sigmon, PhD, *Hypertension and Vascular Research Division, Henry Ford Hospital and Health Sciences Center, Detroit, MI*
Jianben Song, PhD, *Department of Physiology, Wayne State University, Detroit, MI*

Tom Song, BS, *Division of Renal Diseases and Hypertension, Department of Medicine, University of Texas Medical School, Houston, TX*
James R. Sowers, MD, *Division of Endocrinology, Metabolism and Hypertension, Wayne State University, Detroit, MI*
Paul R. Standley, PhD, *Division of Endocrinology, Metabolism and Hypertension, Wayne State University, Detroit, MI*
Helmut O. Steinberg, MD, *Department of Medicine, Indiana University Medical Center, Indianapolis, IN*
Konrad T. Stepniakowski, MD, PhD, *Division of Clinical Pharmacology, Departments of Pharmacology and Medicine, Medical University of South Carolina, Charleston, SC*
Naftali Stern, MD, *Institute of Endocrinology, Tel-Aviv University, Tel-Aviv, Israel*
Philip S. Tsao, PhD, *Division of Cardiovascular Medicine, Stanford University School of Medicine, Stanford, CA*
Michael L. Tuck, MD, *University of California at Los Angeles Medical Center, Los Angeles, CA and Veterans Affairs Medical Center, Sepulveda, CA*
Mary F. Walsh, PhD, *Division of Endocrinology, Metabolism and Hypertension, Wayne State University, Detroit, MI*
Stephanie W. Watts, PhD, *Department of Physiology, University of Michigan Medical School, Ann Arbor, MI*
R. Clinton Webb, PhD, *Department of Physiology, University of Michigan Medical School, Ann Arbor, MI*

I

The Endothelium

1 Endothelium-Derived Relaxing Factor

An Overview

John P. Cooke, MD *and Philip S. Tsao*, PhD

Contents

INTRODUCTION

The endothelium is a diaphanous film of tissue only one cell layer in thickness that forms the luminal surface of all blood vessels. Its apparent fragility belies its substantial role in regulating blood fluidity, lipoprotein metabolism, capillary transport, angiogenesis, interactions of the vessel wall with circulating blood elements, vasomotion, and vascular structure. The normal endothelium elaborates a panoply of proteins, prostanoids, and other paracrine substances to maintain a delicate balance between vasoconstriction and vasodilation, coagulation and blood fluidity, and inhibition and promotion of vascular growth. As an example of the balance between countervailing endothelial mechanisms, the endothelium synthesizes and releases the potent antiplatelet agent and prostaglandin (PG) vasodilator, prostacyclin (PGI_2), but is also capable of elaborating other prostanoids, such as thromboxane A_2, which are vasoconstrictors as well as agonists of platelet aggregation. The endothelium also exerts a profound influence on vasomotion by its ability to metabolize circulating vasoactive substances such as serotonin, epinephrine, bradykinin, and angiotensin I.

The endothelium elaborates tissue plasminogen activators, thrombomodulin and heparin sulfate, which lend antithrombogenic properties to the luminal lining *(1–3)*; however, the endothelium also synthesizes von Willebrand factor, plasminogen activator

From: *Contemporary Endocrinology: Endocrinology of the Vasculature*
Edited by: J. R. Sowers Humana Press Inc., Totowa, NJ

inhibitor, and, under certain conditions, adhesive glycoproteins that enhance vessel wall interactions with circulating cells *(4–6)*. This diversity of endothelial synthetic function permits this tissue to maintain blood fluidity, and provides for hemostatic mechanisms in the event of intimal injury. A similar complexity exists between the endothelium and the underlying vascular smooth muscle cells (VSMC). Proliferation of VSMC is abetted by growth factors released from the endothelium, such as platelet-derived growth factor, basic fibroblast growth factor, insulin-like growth factor, and other paracrine factors *(7–9)*. These influences are modulated by antimitogenic endothelial products such as transforming growth factor-β *(10,11)*. In addition, the endothelium releases a variety of vasoactive factors which, in addition to regulating vascular tone, are also capable of modulating cellular proliferation. In general, the vasoconstrictors released from the endothelium, such as endothelin and angiotensin II (AII), are growth promoters *(12,13)*. Endogenous vasodilators (prostacyclin- and endothelium-derived relaxing factor) suppress vascular growth *(14,15)*.

In sum, the endothelium exerts major control over vascular functions by its elaboration of a diverse array of paracrine substances. In general, synthetic functions of the endothelium that predominate are those that promote vasodilation, and that inhibit thrombosis and cellular proliferation. Under certain conditions, the balance shifts to favor vasoconstriction, thrombosis, and/or initiation of cell cycle, and these alterations in endothelial function participate in the pathogenesis of vascular disease. This chapter reviews the nature and function of one of the endothelial substances that plays a critical role in this vascular homeostasis. Endothelium-derived relaxing factor (EDRF) is a potent regulator of vascular tone and structure. Disturbances in its elaboration or activity play an important role in the initiation and progression of vascular disorders.

THE NATURE OF EDRF

The discovery of EDRF was reported in 1980 *(16)*. This vasodilator was unlike the other known endogenous vasodilator substance, PGI_2, in that its activity was not inhibited by indomethacin. Because of its short half-life, EDRF defied biochemical characterization for nearly a decade. In 1986, several investigators independently proposed that EDRF was nitric oxide (NO), or a NO-containing substance, based on their observations of its similarity to other nitrovasodilators in its biological and physical properties *(17,18)*. Subsequently, chemiluminescence and bioassay techniques were used to provide definitive evidence that NO was synthesized by endothelial cells *(19)*, and was responsible for the relaxing activity of EDRF.

NO induces vasodilation by stimulating soluble guanylate cyclase in VSMC to produce cyclic guanosine 3'5'-monophosphate (cGMP). NO has a very short half-life and interacts avidly with sulfhydryl-containing proteins, heme proteins, and oxygen-derived free radicals. By virtue of its ability to nitrosylate proteins, it may change their activity or behavior. Endogenous NO is derived from the metabolism of L-arginine, specifically oxidation of the terminal guanidino-nitrogen atoms of this amino acid *(20)*. The enzyme responsible for the synthesis of NO has been purified and the genes encoding the three isoforms of nitric oxide synthase (NOS) have been cloned and characterized *(21–24)*.

The isoforms of NOS can be differentiated by their intracellular location (cytosolic vs. membrane-associated) and whether they are constitutively active or induced (as by interleukin-1 or endotoxin) *(21)*. NOS is not only present in the endothelial cells, but has been localized to other cells as well, including VSMC, macrophages, neutrophils, platelets, and neural cells. The endothelial isoform is membrane-associated and is constitutively active, although regulated by intracellular calcium ($[Ca^{2+}]_i$) levels, and by exposure of the endothelial cells to increases in blood flow.

VASODILATOR ACTIONS OF EDRF (NO)

Endothelium-derived NO is the most potent endogenous vasodilator, and the physiological importance of this factor has been demonstrated in animals and humans. Inhibitors of NOS elevate blood pressure, owing to an increase in systemic vascular resistance *(25,26)*, indicating that EDRF plays a major role in modulating homeostatic vascular resistance. It is released from the endothelium in response to a wide variety of neurohormonal agents or physical forces. The vasoconstrictor effects of norepinephrine, serotonin, vasopressin, AII, and endothelin are opposed by the endothelial release of NO. There are specific receptors for these agents on the endothelium, which induce the release of NO, thereby mitigating the direct effect of the vasoconstrictors on VSMC *(27–29)*. The same phenomenon is observed with aggregating platelets *(30,31)*. Aggregating platelets release adenosine diphosphate and serotonin to induce vasoconstriction in the absence of the endothelium. However, when the endothelium is intact, these agents interact with purinergic and serotoninergic receptors on the endothelial surface to induce NO synthesis and release.

There is great heterogeneity from one vascular bed to another in the response of endothelium to neurohormonal agents. In the human renal artery, acetylcholine (ACh), thrombin, serotonin, and adenosine diphosphate all induce endothelium-dependent relaxations *(32)*. By contrast, in human limb arteries only ACh of the agents mentioned induces vasodilation. An even greater contrast is seen between arteries and veins. In general, endothelium-dependent relaxations are more prominent in arteries than in veins *(33)*. Human internal mammary arteries are capable of prominent endothelium-dependent relaxations, whereas the ability of human veins to respond with endothelium-dependent relaxation is limited *(34)*. Since NO is not only a vasodilator, but has antiplatelet and antimitogenic properties (*see* Antiplatelet Effects and Antiproliferative Effects sections), one might speculate that the improved patency of internal mammary artery bypass grafts for coronary artery disease is in part owing to the greater influence of NO in these vessels.

The endothelium also responds to hemodynamic forces. As blood flow increases through a conduit vessel, the vessel dilates (Fig. 1). The integrity of the endothelium is essential for this flow-mediated vasodilation *(35–37)*. Flow-mediated vasodilation is largely caused by the release of NO, although in some vascular beds prostacyclin, endothelium-derived hyperpolarizing factor, or direct activation of potassium channels may contribute *(38–41)*.

Disturbances of flow-mediated vasodilation have pathophysiological consequences. In patients with coronary artery disease and impairment of endothelial vasodilator function, increases in blood flow through the diseased coronary artery cause a paradoxical vasoconstriction, which can contribute to myocardial ischemia during exercise or mental stress *(42,43)*.

Long-term changes in flow induce remodeling of the vessel. With sustained increases in flow rate through a conduit artery, the vessel diameter increases, as in the arterial segment proximal to an arteriovenous fistula. The opposite effect is seen with chronic reductions in flow rate. This remodeling is dependent on the presence of the endothelium

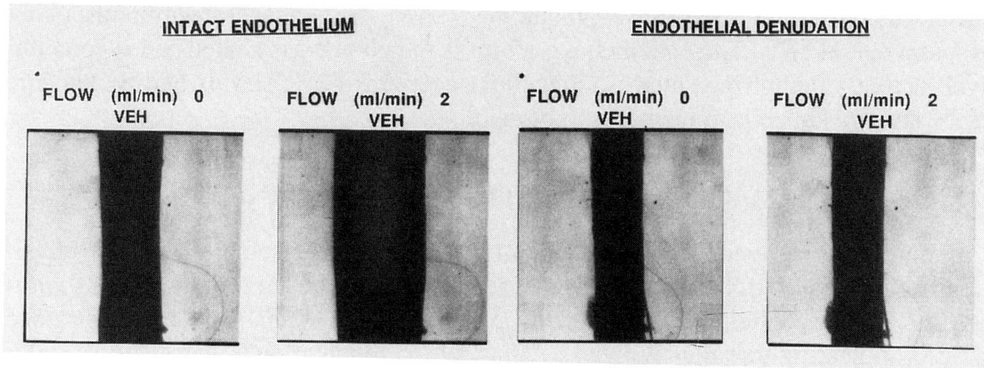

Fig. 1. Photographs of original records from one experiment, representative of five, demonstrating that flow-mediated vasodilation is endothelium-dependent. Intact endothelium: **(A)** Rabbit iliac artery segment contracted by norepinephrine $10^{-6}M$. Intraluminal perfusate flow is 0 mL/min. Intraluminal pressure is 60 mm Hg, and was held at this level throughout the experiment. **(B)** Immediately after recording the previous photograph, the flow of perfusate (physiological saline solution [VEH]) was increased to 2 mL/min for 2 min and this photograph recorded. The vessel has visibly dilated. After endothelial denudation: **(C)** After these observations were made, the endothelium of this vessel was removed using saponin. The vessel was again contracted by norepinephrine $10^{-6}M$, and this photograph was taken when the contraction had stabilized at an intraluminal flow of 0 mL/min and a pressure of 60 mm Hg. **(D)** Immediately after recording the previous photograph the flow of perfusate was increased to 2 mL/min for 2 min and this photograph taken. Flow-mediated vasodilation has been abolished. From ref. *38* with permission.

(44). NO is known to modulate VSMC; it is possible that changes in the release of NO may contribute to these structural alterations (*see* Antiproliferative Effects).

NO is a major regulator of vascular resistance, and under normal circumstances the major source of this vasodilator is the endothelium. However, the marked reduction in vascular resistance that is associated with septicemia is now known to be owing to NO derived from activated macrophages and VSMC *(45,46)*. Expression of NOS can be induced in monocytes and VSMC during sepsis. Subsequent production of NO by these activated cells greatly exceeds that of the endothelium, accounting in part for the hypotension observed in septic shock. In animal models of septic shock, administration of NOS antagonists reverses the drop in blood pressure, leading to increased survival *(46)*. However, the therapeutic dose range is narrow; administration of higher doses of the antagonists increases mortality (presumably owing to blockade of endothelial NOS attended by local vasoconstriction, tissue ischemia, and necrosis). Preliminary studies in humans indicate that NOS antagonists may reverse the hypotension associated with septic shock *(47)*. NO antagonists may become useful therapeutic adjuncts in septicemia; antagonists that are selective for the induced enzyme may avoid adverse effects on tissue perfusion and platelet aggregability.

ANTIPLATELET EFFECTS

The adherence of platelets to the vessel wall, and their aggregation, are suppressed by nitrovasodilators. These effects are associated with and mediated by an increase in intracellular cGMP. Therefore it is not surprising that NO has also been shown to have antiplatelet properties *(48–50)*. Like other nitrovasodilators, NO acts synergistically with

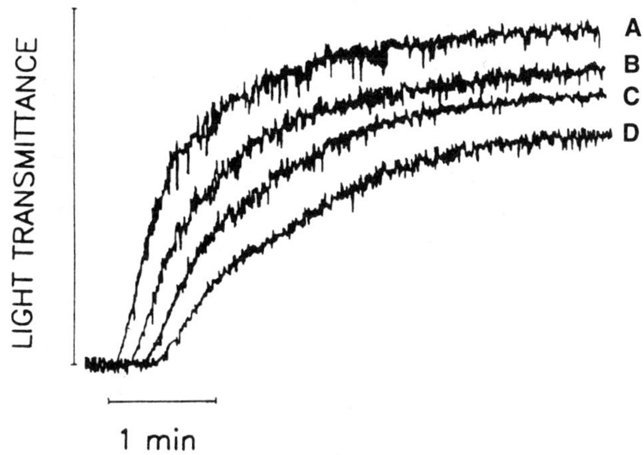

Fig. 2. Dose-dependent inhibition of platelet aggregation by aspirin-treated endothelial cells. Platelets were exposed to increasing concentrations of aspirin-treated aortic endothelial cells (A = 0, B = 4.4×10^5, C = 8.8×10^5, D = 1.3×10^6). This dose-dependent inhibition of platelet aggregation by endothelial cells is inhibited by methylene blue, the antagonist of EDRF action. From ref. *50* with permission.

PGI_2 to inhibit platelet aggregation and adherence, contributing in a major way to the antithrombogenic properties of the endothelium.

Adenosine diphosphate and serotonin released from aggregating platelets, as well as thrombin, act on specific endothelial receptors to induce the release of NO *(30,31)*. NO is an important component of the negative feedback loop that prevents the propagation of thrombus (Fig. 2). As previously mentioned, increases in flow rate also release NO. This phenomenon may be important in suppressing platelet adherence or aggregation favored by the rheologic changes induced by increases in blood flow. Indeed, NO inhibits the aggregation of circulating platelets. Platelets traversing the vascular bed of the perfused heart exhibit an elevation of intracellular cGMP, which leads to the phosphorylation of cGMP-dependent phosphoproteins (e.g., vasodilator-stimulated phosphoprotein), which suppress platelet reactivity. These effects on circulating platelets are blocked by antagonists of NO *(51,52)*.

ANTIPROLIFERATIVE EFFECTS

The endothelium plays an important role in maintaining the underlying VSMC in a quiescent state. Damage to the vessel wall with endothelial denudation occurs during balloon angioplasty. Loss of the endothelium, and injury to the VSMC, initiate a series of events that results in myointimal hyperplasia. This lesion is caused by the migration of VSMC into the intima, with proliferation of these cells and alteration in their phenotype from a "contractile" to a "secretory" form *(53)*. These altered VSMC elaborate extracellular matrix, which contributes to the thickness of the lesion. Platelets adhering to the vessel wall and injured VSMC release growth factors that play a major role to incite and to sustain this response to injury *(54)*. A number of endothelial products inhibit cell proliferation *(55)*. One of these antiproliferative agents is NO. Growth of VSMC in culture is inhibited by agents that release NO *(15)*. In addition, the stable analog of cGMP, 8-bromocyclic GMP, has the same effect *(15)*. Like NO, atrial natriuretic peptide increases

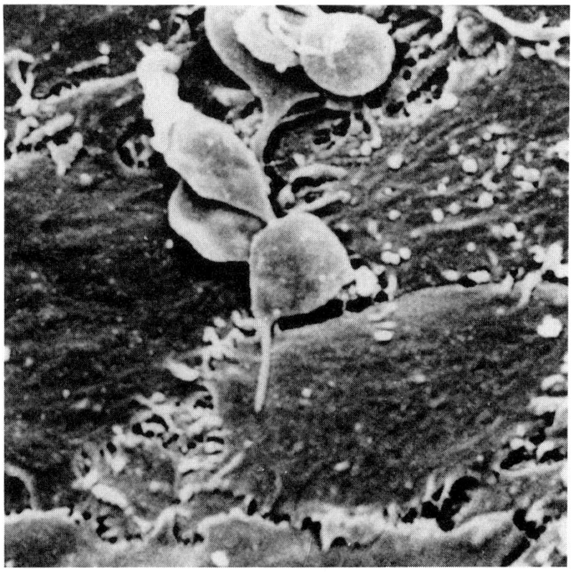

Fig. 3. Scanning electron micrograph of intimal surface from midportion of rabbit iliac artery 3 wk after angioplasty. The surface is covered by regenerated endothelial cells of irregular size and shape that are not aligned with blood flow. Interendothelial junctions are notable for the presence of interdigitating pseudopodia and the numerous intercellular gaps (large arrows). Adherent, activated platelets can be seen on the endothelial surface. Gold and palladium coated, original magnification, ×3000. From ref. *60* with permission.

levels of intracellular cGMP; this effect is associated with an inhibition of growth in cultured VSMC stimulated by AII *(56)*.

In animal models of myointimal hyperplasia, endogenous NO appears to inhibit myointimal hyperplasia. Although the endothelial source of NO synthesis is removed by angioplasty, the inducible isoform is expressed by VSMC in the vicinity of the injury. This may explain the observation that systemic administration of L-arginine (the NO precursor) can reduce the degree of myointimal hyperplasia after balloon angioplasty in animal models. The effect of arginine is blocked by coadministration of NOS antagonists *(57,58)*.

Further evidence that endogenous NO can act as a brake on proliferation of VSMC has been provided by our group. In the rat carotid artery we have successfully applied the technique of in vivo gene transfer to deliver the gene encoding NOS to the vessel wall. This has the effect of enhancing local release of NO and suppressing vascular lesion formation after balloon angioplasty *(59)*.

Proliferation of VSMC is seen in states of endothelial dysfunction that are characterized by reduced release of NO, providing further support for its role in regulating vascular structure. After balloon injury, the myointimal proliferation continues even after the vessel wall has been resurfaced by endothelium. Examination of this endothelium reveals that it is morphologically abnormal *(60)*. Cells are irregularly sized, polygonal, and not aligned with flow (Fig. 3). These cells appear to release less NO, as manifested by an attenuation of endothelium-dependent relaxations in these vessels. It is possible that this and other alterations in endothelial function are permissive in the sustained proliferation of VSMC. This endothelial dysregulation permits cellular proliferation in other disease states such as atherogenesis.

ENDOTHELIAL VASODILATOR DYSFUNCTION IN HYPERCHOLESTEROLEMIA AND ATHEROSCLEROSIS

In hypercholesterolemic animals and humans, endothelium-dependent relaxation is reduced and vasoconstriction is enhanced. This is largely the result of a reduction in NO activity *(61–64)* and not to denudation of the endothelium. The same effect of hypercholesterolemia is also observed in resistance vessels of atherosclerotic animals and humans *(64,65)*. Indeed, this abnormal vasoreactivity is seen well before any morphological changes of atherosclerosis. Coronary arteries isolated from pigs fed a high cholesterol diet for 8 wk exhibit an attenuation of endothelium-dependent relaxation without any significant pathology demonstrable by light microscopy *(66)*.

Endothelium-dependent vasodilation is reduced in hypercholesterolemic human epicardial coronary and resistance vessels *(63,67)*. These abnormalities likely contribute to angina during exertion or emotional stress. Indeed, human coronary arteries exhibiting an abnormal response to acetylcholine also vasoconstrict with mental stress *(42)*, exertion *(43)*, or the cold pressor test *(68)*. Improvement in endothelial function would likely be of clinical benefit in such patients: restoring normal vascular reactivity, preventing vasospasm, and inhibiting platelet adherence and aggregation. Cholesterol reduction has been shown to improve endothelial vasodilator function *(69)*. It is possible that this improvement in vascular function may explain in part some of the reduction in vascular events seen in patients receiving aggressive antilipid treatment. In addition, the administration of antioxidants *(70)*, estrogen *(71)*, and L-arginine *(67,72,73)* enhances endothelial vasodilator function in humans; their role in the treatment of coronary artery disease has not been defined, but may present alternative therapeutic strategies.

Vessels isolated from normal animals exhibit an endothelial dysfunction within minutes of exposure to cholesterol in vitro *(74,75)*. This abnormality appears to be owing to the low-density lipoprotein (LDL) component of cholesterol; especially the oxidized form of LDL cholesterol. The mechanism by which oxidized LDL inhibits endothelium-dependent relaxations is under investigation. Oxidized LDL or other oxygen-derived free radicals may chemically combine with and inactivate NO *(75,76)*. Controversy exists as to whether or not oxidized LDL can inhibit the activity of NOS. Hypercholesterolemia also induces the endothelium itself to generate superoxide anion *(77)*. This oxidative stress may play an important role in the pathogenesis of atherosclerosis by oxidizing lipoproteins and lipid membranes, as well as altering endothelial function. Specifically, alterations in redox state of the endothelium appear to enhance endothelial adhesiveness for monocytes *(78,79)*.

Endothelium-derived NO may act to oppose the hypercholesterolemia induced alterations in endothelial redox state. In normocholesterolemic rabbit thoracic aorta there is a basal production of superoxide anion by nonendothelial cells *(80)*. Exogenous NO donors significantly reduce the generation of superoxide anion. Administration of a NO precursor, benzoyl-L-arginine ethyl ester, decreases alloxan-stimulated superoxide production by rabbit aorta, an effect that is reversed by the NOS antagonist, L-N-monomethyl-arginine (L-NMMA) *(81)*.

The mechanism by which NO reduces oxidative stress remains undefined. It is possible that NO directly reacts with lipid peroxyl radicals, thereby disrupting the chain of autocatalytic reactions involved in the oxidation of intracellular lipid *(82)*. Indeed, NO donors inhibit copper catalyzed oxidation of LDL cholesterol in vitro *(83)*. Another mechanism by which NO may exert its effects is by inhibiting the generation of oxygen-derived free radicals by oxidative enzymes. When neutrophils are exposed to NO, their ability to generate superoxide anion is limited *(84)*. This appears to be the result of a direct effect of NO on the multimeric oxidative enzyme NADPH oxygenase. NO may interact with sulfhydryl or heme moieties within the membrane-bound component of this enzyme to prevent its activity. These observations are concordant with the observations that autocrine NO inhibits macrophage oxidation of LDL cholesterol *(85)*. This effect is reversed by an antagonist of NOS. In preliminary studies we have shown that the stimulation of endothelial cells by fluid flow reduces their generation of superoxide anion; this effect is NO dependent. Taken together, these studies indicate that NO reduces oxidant stress. The critical role of NO in modulating endothelial redox state has also been demonstrated by investigators who used intracellular fluorophores responsive to changes in redox state to demonstrate that antagonists of NOS precipitated oxidative stress *(86)*.

The effect of NO to reduce the generation of reactive oxygen species may explain its repression of NFκB-mediated gene expression. Antioxidants such as *n*-acetyl-cysteine and pyrolidine dithiocarbamate (PDTC) are known to inhibit the dissociation of NFκB from its inhibitor, IκBα *(78,87)*. In cultured human umbilical venous endothelial cells, interleukin-1 (IL-1)-induced expression of vascular cell adhesion molecule (VCAM-1) is selectively antagonized by exposure of the cells to the antioxidant PDTC *(78)*. NO donors mimic the effect of antioxidants to suppress NκB-mediated gene expression *(88)*. The activation of NFκB by tumor necrosis factor-α (TNF-α) in cultured human saphenous vein endothelial cells is blocked by exogenous NO, whereas NO donors have little effect on other nuclear binding proteins (AP-1 and GATA). Immunoprecipitation studies indicate that exogenous NO stabilizes the NFκB/IκBα complex. Moreover, exogenous NO enhances the transcription of IκBα, but not NFκB. These observations likely explain previous findings that exogenous NO donors inhibit IL-1 stimulated VCAM-1 expression and monocyte adhesion *(89)*.

Since fluid flow is a potent stimulus for the release of endothelium-derived NO, we speculated that the effects of flow to inhibit atherogenesis may be mediated in part by NO. In preliminary studies we have found that previous exposure to flow inhibited lipoprotein- or cytokine-mediated superoxide production, NFκB activation, VCAM-1 expression, and endothelial adhesiveness for monocytes. The effect of fluid flow appears to be caused by shear-induced release of NO since coincubation with L-nitro-arginine completely abolished, while an NO donor mimicked, these effects of flow (Fig. 4).

The tractive force exerted by fluid flow (shear stress) may directly influence gene expression by acting on shear stress-responsive elements (SSRE) in the promoter region of specific flow-responsive genes. One of these (GAGACC) was first defined in the 5' promoter region of the gene encoding platelet-derived growth factor (PDGF) B chain *(91)*. This SSRE is positively regulated by shear stress. This same SSRE is found in the promoter region of a number of genes regulated by flow. Six repeats of the SSRE are found in the 5' promoter region of the gene encoding endothelial NOS (ECNOS) *(24)*. Exposure of endothelial cells in vitro to fluid flow enhances the expression of ECNOS *(24,92)*.

Flow-stimulated NO has acute effects on monocyte-endothelial cell interaction, as well as the more chronic effects on redox regulation of gene expression. Monocyte adherence to endothelial cells in culture is inhibited by administration of NO with a time course that implies an effect on signal transduction of adhesion pathways *(93)*. We also have shown that the adherence of monocytoid cells to bovine aortic endothelial cells is

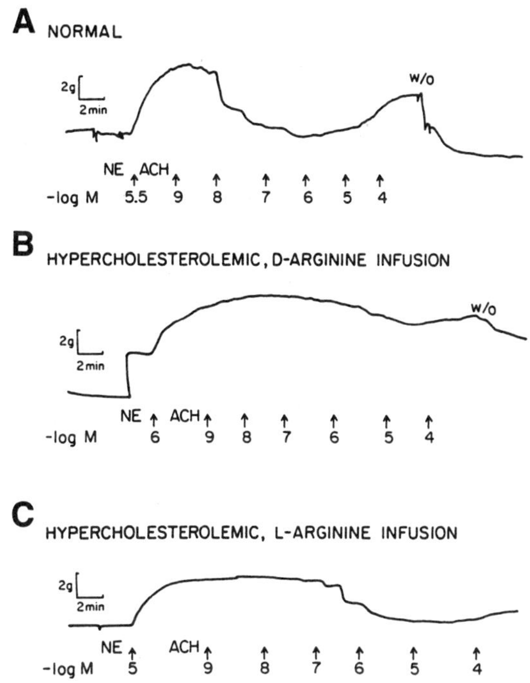

Fig. 4. Endothelium-dependent relaxation is inhibited by hypercholesterolemia and normalized by L-arginine. Tracings of original records showing endothelium-dependent relaxation in isolated thoracic aortas from normal and hypercholesterolemic rabbits. **(A)** Vascular ring from a normal rabbit is contracted by norepinephrine (NE) and then relaxed with increasing concentrations of acetylcholine (ACh) without washout (replacement of bathing solution with fresh physiological saline solution). **(B)** Vascular ring from a hypercholesterolemic rabbit that had received an intravenous infusion of D-arginine. Note impaired relaxation to ACh. **(C)** Vascular ring from a hypercholesterolemic rabbit that had received an iv infusion of L-arginine is exposed to protocol described in (A). Note normalized response to ACh. From ref. *90* with permission.

inhibited by brief (i.e., 15 min) exposure to flow in a NO-dependent manner, in the absence of any changes in the expression of endothelial molecules, indicating that, acutely, flow-released NO inhibits signal transduction of adhesion *(94)*. Longer term exposure to flow (e.g., 72 h) reduces monocyte adhesion in association with down-regulation of VCAM-1.

Acute and chronic effects of NO on endothelial adhesiveness may play an important role in atherogenesis. Effects of chronic exercise to inhibit atherosclerotic lesion formation *(95,96)* may be in part caused by the effect of exercise to enhance the vascular expression of ECNOS and the elaboration of NO *(97)*. Similarly, the predisposition for lesion formation at sites of branching may be in part the result of the reduced elaboration of NO at these sites *(98)*. We speculate that NO is an endogenous antiatherogenic molecule, which exerts its effects in part via its modulation of endothelial redox state.

We have tested this hypothesis in animal models. In hypercholesterolemic New Zealand white rabbits, NO-dependent relaxations can also be normalized by administration of the EDRF precursor, L-arginine *(90,99)*. Intravenous administration of L-arginine normalizes endothelium-dependent vasodilation in the hind limb resistance vessels as

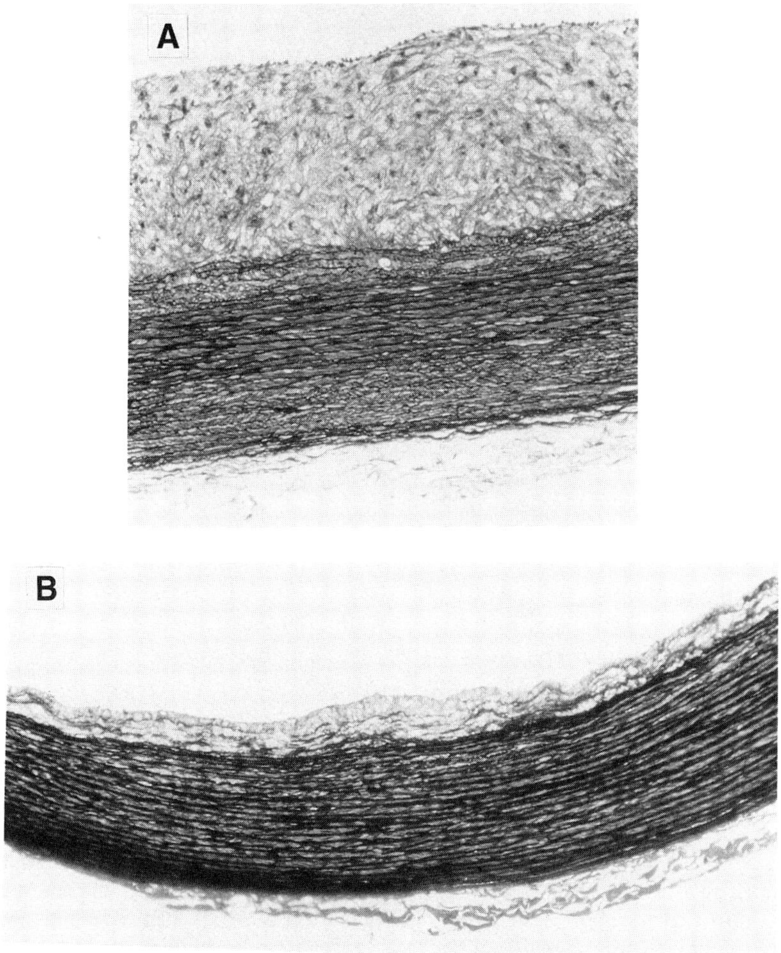

Fig. 5. New Zealand White rabbits were fed a 1% cholesterol diet, plus vehicle or 2.25% L-arginine in the drinking water. After 10 wk the thoracic aortae were harvested for histomorphometry. Arginine treatment significantly reduced intimal lesion formation. **(A)** Microphotograph of representative cross-section of 16 abdominal aortae taken from hypercholesterolemic animals and **(B)** arginine-treated animals. From ref. *100* with permission.

well as in the thoracic aorta (Fig. 4). This effect is likely caused by the metabolism of L-arginine, since its inactive enantiomer D-arginine does not mimic the beneficial effect. In humans, infusions of L-arginine normalize endothelium-dependent vasodilation to ACh in resistance vessels of the forearm and the coronary circulations *(67,73)*.

Chronic administration of L-arginine to hypercholesterolemic animals also improves endothelium-dependent relaxations. This improvement in vascular NO activity is associated with a striking inhibition of intimal lesion formation (Fig. 5) *(101)*. This appears to be the result of a direct effect of vascular NO on endothelial adhesiveness. In a separate study we used a functional binding assay to examine the adhesiveness of the endothelium for normal rabbit mononuclear cells or a monocytoid cell line *(102)*. After 2 wk of dietary interventions, the thoracic aorta was harvested, segments of the vessel were bisected longitudinally, and the endothelium exposed ex vivo to a solution containing mono-

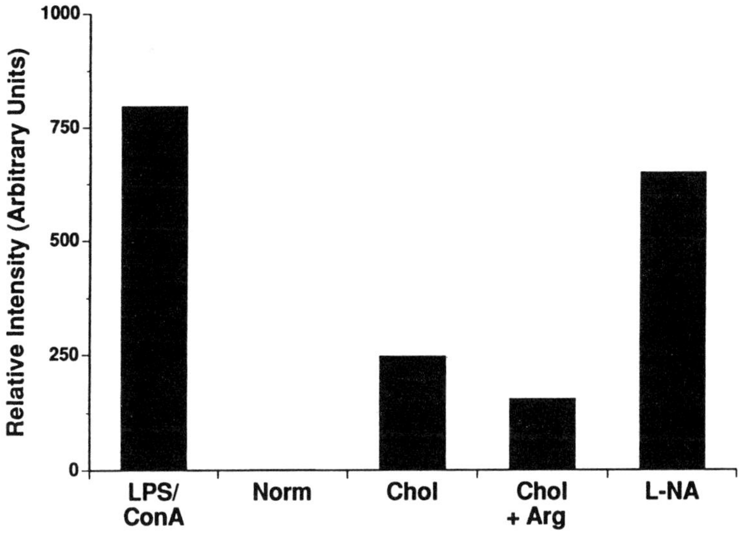

Fig. 6. Densitometry of Northern analysis of MCP-1 expression in hypercholesterolemic rabbit aortae. New Zealand White rabbits were fed normal or 0.5% cholesterol diet. Some rabbits received L-arginine or the NOS antagonist L-nitro-arginine in their drinking water to increase or decrease, respectively, NO release from the vessel wall. To perform quantitative analysis of whole-vessel mRNA, the following procedure was utilized. Thoracic aortae were harvested and snap-frozen in liquid nitrogen. Total RNA was isolated using acid guanidium thiocyanate lysis. MCP-1 mRNA expression was determined by Northern analysis using a full-length cDNA probe for rabbit MCP-1. Positive control was achieved by ex vivo exposure of normal aortae to lipopolysaccharide and concanavalin A (LPS/ConA) for 2 h.

nuclear or monocytoid cells. After ex vivo incubation for 30 min, nonadherent cells were removed with fresh media, and the preparations were fixed and bound cells counted. Thoracic aortae from hypercholesterolemic animals exhibited a threefold increase in adhesiveness for monocytes. By contrast, hypercholesterolemic animals receiving dietary arginine manifested a significant reduction in monocyte binding. Conversely, animals receiving normal chow with the addition of nitro-arginine (an antagonist of NOS) exhibited a 10-fold increase in cell binding (even more binding was observed than in hypercholesterolemic animals). mRNA was isolated from the thoracic aorta and probed for monocyte chemotactic protein-1 (MCP-1), a 76 amino acid chemokine thought to be a major chemotactic factor for monocytes in both inflammation and atherogenesis *(103)*. Expression of MCP-1 is induced by lipopolysaccharides (LPS), cytokines (TNF-α, IL-1 and -4), and phorbol esters. Human aortic endothelial and VSMC exposed to minimally modified LDL cholesterol express MCP-1; this protein accounts for virtually all of the chemotactic activity produced under these conditions *(104)*. Expression of MCP-1 could not be detected in aorta from normal animals, but was present in tissues from hypercholesterolemic rabbits. Administration of arginine attenuates the expression of MCP-1. Animals receiving normal chow, together with the endothelial antagonist nitroarginine, exhibit a dramatic increase in message for MCP-1 (Fig. 6). Recently, others also provided evidence that NO inhibits MCP-1 expression in cytokine-stimulated human umbilical venous endothelial cells (HUVECs), in a cGMP-independent fashion *(105)*.

These studies indicate that vascular NO is an important regulator of endothelial adhesiveness and monocytes in part by regulating the expression of MCP-1. Our findings are consistent with recent investigations revealing that chronic administration of NOS antagonists accelerates intimal lesion formation in hypercholesterolemic rabbits *(106,107)*.

ENDOTHELIAL VASODILATOR DYSFUNCTION IN HYPERTENSION

As previously discussed, NO plays a major role in the regulation of systemic vascular resistance. It is therefore conceivable that endothelial vasodilator dysfunction could precipitate hypertension. Indeed, an endothelial abnormality does appear to be associated with hypertension in animal models *(108–110)*. Depending on the experimental model, the reduction in endothelium-dependent relaxation is caused by an attenuation of NO activity or the augmented elaboration of an endothelium-derived contracting factor (possibly a prostanoid). Whether endothelial dysfunction is primary in the initiation of hypertension, or is merely an epiphenomenon, is not clear. Treatment of the elevated blood pressure normalizes endothelium-dependent relaxation, suggesting that the endothelial abnormality is secondary in the hypertensive process *(111,112)*. Conversely, infusions of NOS antagonists produce marked increases in blood pressure in experimental animals *(113)*. These inhibitors have been considered nonspecific and the effect on blood pressure could conceivably be the result of an effect on the neuronal NOS. However, more definitive data for a primary role of NO in the regulation of blood pressure was provided by the report that inactivation of the mouse endothelial NOS gene by homologous recombination produces mice that are significantly hypertensive *(114)*.

Two recent studies have provided evidence for endothelial vasodilator dysfunction in hypertensive humans *(115,116)*. In both studies, forearm blood flow was measured by strain-gage plethysmography in response to intra-arterial infusions of endothelium-dependent and endothelium-independent vasodilators. In these young patients with mild essential hypertension, endothelium-independent vasodilation was relatively undisturbed. By contrast, cholinergic vasodilation (presumably endothelium-dependent) was attenuated. Whether this is a primary or secondary phenomenon is not known. However, there is preliminary evidence that this endothelial deficit may precede the appearance of essential hypertension *(117)*. In young normotensive individuals with hypertensive parents cholinergic forearm vasodilation is impaired; by contrast, endothelium-independent vasodilation is normal.

SUMMARY

In conclusion, EDRF is NO (or a substance-releasing NO) derived from the metabolism of L-arginine. It is a potent vasodilator, and plays a key role in modulating conduit and resistance vessel tone. NO also has important effects on cell growth and interactions of circulatory blood cells with the vessel wall. As a consequence, disturbances of NO activity may initiate or contribute to diverse states such as septic shock, hypertension, vasospasm, toxemia, and atherosclerosis.

REFERENCES

1. Levin EG, Loskutoff DJ. Cultured bovine endothelial cells produce both urokinase and tissue type plasminogen activators. J Cell Biol 1982;94:631–636.
2. Marcum JA, McKenney JB, Rosenberg RD. Acceleration of thrombin–antithrombin complex formation in rat hindquarters via heparin-like molecules bound to the endothelium. J Clin Invest 1984;74:341–350.

3. Esmon C, Owen W. Identification of an endothelial cell cofactor for thrombin-catalyzed activation of protein C. Proc Natl Acad Sci USA 1981;78:2249–2251.
4. Jaffe EA, Hoyer LW, Nachmann RL. Synthesis of von Willebrand factor by cultured human endothelial cells. Proc Natl Acad Sci USA 1974;71:1906–1909.
5. Levin EG. Latent tissue plasminogen activator produced by human endothelial cells in culture: evidence for enzyme-inhibitor complex. Proc Natl Acad Sci USA 1983;80:6804–6808.
6. Butcher EC. Leukocyte-endothelial cell recognition: three (or more) steps to specificity and diversity. Cell 1991;67:1033–1036.
7. Fox PL, DiCorleto PE. Regulation of production of a platelet-derived growth factor-like protein by cultured bovine aortic endothelial cells. J Cell Physiol 1984;121:298–308.
8. Hansson H-A, Jennische E, Skottner A. Regenerating endothelial cells express insulin like growth factor-1 immunoreactivity after arterial injury. Cell Tissue Res 1987;250:499–505.
9. Vlodavsky I, Folkman J, Sullivan R, Fridman R, Ishai-Michaeli R, Sasse J, Klagsbrun M. Endothelial cell-derived basic fibroblast growth factor: synthesis and deposition into subendothelial extracellular matrix. Proc Natl Acad Sci USA 1987;84:2292–2296.
10. Antonelli-Orlidge A, Saunders KB, Smith S, D'Amore PA. An activated form of transforming growth factor-beta is produced by cocultures of endothelial cells and pericytes. Proc Natl Acad Sci USA 1989;86:4544–4548.
11. Owens GK, Geisterfer AAT, Yang YW-H, Komoriya A. Transforming growth factor β-induced growth inhibition and cellular hypertrophy in cultured vascular smooth muscle cell. J Cell Biol 1988;107:771–780.
12. Dubin D, Pratt RE, Cooke JP, Dzau VJ. Endothelin, a potent vasoconstrictor, is a vascular smooth muscle mitogen. J Vasc Med Biol 1989;1:150–154.
13. Naftilan AJ, Pratt RE, Dzau VJ. Induction of platelet-derived growth factor A-chain and c-myc gene expressions by angiotensin II in cultured rat vascular smooth muscle cells. J Clin Invest 1989;83:1419–1423.
14. Loesberg C, Wijk RV, Zandbergen J, van Aken WG, van Mourk JA, de Groot PG. Cell cycle-dependent inhibition of human vascular smooth muscle cell proliferation by prostaglandin E1. Exp Cell Res 1985;160:117–120.
15. Garg UC, Hassid A. Nitric oxide-generating vasodilators and 8-bromocyclic guanosine monophosphate inhibit mitogenesis and proliferation of cultured rat vascular smooth muscle cells. J Clin Invest 1989;83:1774–1777.
16. Furchgott RF, Zawadski JV. The obligatory role of endothelial cells in the relaxation of arterial smooth muscle by acetylcholine. Nature 1980;286:373–376.
17. Ignarro LJ, Byrns RE, Buga GM, Wood KS. Endothelium-derived relaxing factor from pulmonary artery and vein possesses pharmacologic and chemical properties identical to those of nitric oxide radical. Circ Res 1987;61:866–879.
18. Furchgott RF. Studies on relaxation of rabbit aorta by sodium nitrite: the basis for the proposal that the acid-activatable inhibitory factor from retractor penis is inorganic nitrite and the endothelium-derived relaxing factor is nitric oxide. In: Vanhoutte P, ed. Mechanisms of Vasodilation. Raven, New York, 1988, pp. 401–404.
19. Palmer RMJ, Ferrige AG, Moncada S. Nitric oxide release accounts for the biological activity of endothelium-derived relaxing factor. Nature 1987;327:524–526.
20. Palmer RMJ, Ashton DS, Moncada S. Vascular endothelial cells synthesize nitric oxide from L-arginine. Nature 1988;333:664–666.
21. Forstermann U, Schmidt HH, Pollock JS, Sheng H, Mitchell JA, Warner TD, Nakane M, Murad F. Isoforms of nitric oxide synthase: characterization and purification from different cell types. Biochem Pharmacol 1991;42:1849–1857.
22. Lamas S, Marsden PA, Li GK, Tempst P, Michel T. Endothelial nitric oxide synthase: molecular cloning and characterization of a distinct constitutive enzyme isoform. Proc Natl Acad Sci USA 1992;89:6348–6352.
23. Bredt DS, Hwang PM, Glatt CE, Lowenstein C, Reed RR, Snyder SH. Cloned and expressed nitric oxide synthase structurally resembles cytochrome P-450 reductase. Nature 1991;351:714–718.
24. Lowenstein CJ, Glatt CS, Bredt DS, Snyder SH. Cloned and expressed macrophage nitric oxide synthase contrasts with the brain enzyme. Proc Natl Acad Sci USA 1992;89:6711–6715.
25. Rees DD, Palmer RMJ, Moncada S. Role of endothelium-derived nitric oxide in the regulation of blood pressure. Proc Natl Acad Sci USA 1989;86:3375–3378.
26. Vallance P, Collier J, Moncada S. Effects of endothelium-derived nitric oxide on peripheral arteriolar tone in man. Lancet 1989;2:997–1000.

27. Cocks TM, Angus JA. Endothelium-dependent relaxation of coronary arteries by noradrenaline and serotonin. Nature 1983;305:627–630.
28. Katusic ZS, Shepherd JT, Vanhoutte PM. Vasopressin causes endothelium-dependent relaxations of the canine basilar artery. Circ Res 1984;55:575–579.
29. Anggard EE, Botting RM, Vane JR. Endothelin. Blood Vessels 1990;27:269–281.
30. Cohen RA, Shepherd TJ, Vanhoutte PM. Inhibitory role of the endothelium in the response of isolated coronary arteries to platelets. Science 1983;221:273,274.
31. Houston DS, Shepherd JT, Vanhoutte PM. Adenine nucleotides, serotonin, and endothelium-dependent relaxations to platelets. Am J Physiol 1985;248:H389–H395.
32. Lüscher TF, Cooke JP, Houston BS, Neves RJ, Vanhoutte PM. Endothelium-dependent relaxation in human arteries. Mayo Clinic Proc 1987;62:601–606.
33. DeMey JG, Vanhoutte PM. Heterogeneous behavior of the canine arterial and venous wall: importance of the endothelium. Circ Res 1982;51:439–447.
34. Lüscher TF, Diederich D, Siebenmann R, Lehmann K, Stulz P, von Segesser L, Yang Z, Turina M, Grädel E, Weber E, Bühler FR. Difference between endothelium-dependent relaxations in arterial and in venous coronary bypass grafts. N Engl J Med 1988;319:462–427.
35. Pohl V, Holtz J, Busse R, Bassenge E. Crucial role of the endothelium in the vasodilator response to increased flow in vivo. Hypertension 1986;8:37–44.
36. Yound MA, Vatner SF. Blood flow and endothelium-mediated vasomotion of iliac arteries in conscious dogs. Circ Res 1987;61(Suppl. II):88–93.
37. Cooke JP, Stamler J, Andon N, Davies PF, McKinley G, Loscalzo J. Flow stimulates endothelial cells to release a nitrovasodilator that is potentiated by reduced thiol. Am J Physiol 1990;259: H804–H812.
38. Cooke JP, Rossitch E Jr, Andon NA, Loscalzo J, Dzau VJ. Flow activates an endothelial potassium channel to release an endogenous nitrovasodilator. J Clin Invest 1991;88:1663–1671.
39. Koller A, Kaley G. Prostaglandins mediate arteriolar dilation to increased blood flow velocity in skeletal muscle microcirculation. Circ Res 1990;67:529–534.
40. Feletou M, Vanhoutte PM. Endothelium-dependent hyperpolarization of canine coronary smooth muscle. Br J Pharmacol 1988;93:515–524.
41. Olesen SP, Clapham DE, Davies PF. Haemodynamic shear stress activates a K^+ current in vascular endothelial cells. Nature 1988;331:168–170.
42. Yeung AC, Vekshtein VI, Krantz DS, Vita JA, Ryan TJ, Ganz P, Selwyn AP. The effect of atherosclerosis on the vasomotor response of coronary arteries to mental stress. N Engl J Med 1991;325:1551–1556.
43. Gordon JB, Ganz P, Nabel EG, Fish RD, Zebede J, Mudge GH, Alexander RW, Selwyn AP. Atherosclerosis influences the vasomotor response of epicardial coronary arteries to exercise. J Clin Invest 1989;83:1946–1952.
44. Langille BL, O'Donnell F. Reduction of arterial diameter produced by chronic decreases in blood flow are endothelium dependent. Science 1986;231:405–407.
45. Stuehr D, Gross S, Sakuma I, Levi R, Nathan C. Activated murine macrophages secrete a metabolite of arginine with the bioactivity of endothelium-derived relaxing factor and the chemical reactivity of nitric oxide. J Exp Med 1989;169:1011–1020.
46. Nava E, Palmer RMJ, Moncada S. Inhibition of nitric oxide synthesis in septic shock: how much is beneficial? Lancet 1991;338:1555–1557.
47. Petros A, Bennett D, Vallance P. Effect of nitric oxide synthase inhibitors on hypotension in patients with septic shock. Lancet 1991;338:1557,1558.
48. Forstermann U, Mugge A, Alheid U, Bode SM, Frolich JC. Endothelium-derived relaxing factor (EDRF). A defense mechanism against platelet aggregation and vasospasm in human coronary arteries. Eur Heart J 1989;10(Suppl. F):36–43.
49. Radomski MW, Palmer RM, Moncada S. An L-arginine/nitric oxide pathway present in human platelets regulates aggregation. Proc Natl Acad Sci USA 1990;87:5193–5197.
50. Stamler JS, Mendelsohn ME, Amarante P, Smick D, Andon N, Davies PF, Cooke JP, Loscalzo J. N-acetylcysteine potentiates platelet inhibition by endothelium-derived relaxing factor. Circ Res 1989;65:789–795.
51. Pohl U, Busse R. EDRF increases cyclic GMP in platelets during passage through the coronary vascular bed. Circ Res 1989;65:1798–1803.
52. Pohl U, Nolte C, Bunse A, Eigenthaler M, Walter U. Endothelium-dependent phosphorylation of vasodilator-stimulated protein in platelets during coronary passage. Am J Physiol 1994;266:H606–H612.

53. Schwartz SM, Heimark RL, Majesky MW. Developmental mechanisms underlying pathology of arteries. Physiol Rev 1990;70:1177–1209.
54. Fingerle J, Johnson R, Clowes AW, Majesky MW, Reidy MA. Role of platelets in smooth muscle cell proliferation and migration after vascular injury in rat carotid artery. Proc Natl Acad Sci USA 1989;86:8412–8416.
55. Dzau VJ, Gibbons GH. Endothelium and growth factors in vascular remodeling of hypertension. Hypertension 1991;18(Suppl. III): 115–121.
56. Itoh H, Pratt RE, Dzau VJ. Atrial natriuretic polypeptide inhibits hypertrophy of vascular smooth muscle cells. J Clin Invest 1990;86:1690–1697.
57. McNamara DB, Bedi B, Aurora H, Tena L, Ignarro LJ, Kadowitz PJ, Akers DL. L-arginine inhibits balloon catheter-induced intimal hyperplasia. Biochem Biophys Res Commun 1993;193:291–296.
58. Tarry JWC, Makhoul RG. L-arginine improves endothelium-dependent vasorelaxation and reduces intimal hyperplasia after balloon angioplasty. Arteriosclerosis Thromb 1994;6:938–943.
59. von der Leyen HE, Gibbons GH, Morishita R, Lewis NP, Zhang L, Nakajima M, Kaneda Y, Cooke JP, Dzau VJ. Gene therapy inhibiting neointimal vascular lesion: in vivo transfer of endothelial cell nitric oxide synthase gene. Proc Natl Acad Sci USA 1995;92:1137–1141.
60. Weidinger FF, McLenachan JM, Cybulsky M, Gordon JM, Rennke HA, Hollenberg NK, Ganz P, Cooke JP. Persistent dysfunction of regenerated endothelium following balloon angioplasty of rabbit iliac artery. Circulation 1990;81:1667–1679.
61. Verbeuren TH, Jordaens FH, Zonnekeyn LL, VanHove GE, Coene MC, Herman AG. Effect of hypercholesterolemia on vascular reactivity in the rabbit. Circ Res 1986;58:552–564.
62. Heistad DD, Armstrong MLI, Marcus ML, Piegors DJ, Mark AL. Augmented responses to vasoconstrictor stimuli in hypercholesterolemic and atherosclerotic monkeys. Circ Res 1984;54:711–718.
63. Ludmer PL, Selwyn AP, Shook TL, Wayne RS, Mudge GH, Alexander RW, Ganz P. Paradoxical vasoconstriction induced by acetylcholine in atherosclerotic coronary arteries. N Engl J Med 1986;315:1046–1051.
64. Creager MA, Cooke JP, Mendelsohn ME, Gallagher SJ, Coleman SM, Loscalzo J, Dzau VJ. Impaired vasodilation of forearm resistance vessels in hypercholesterolemic humans. J Clin Invest 1990;86:228–234.
65. Osborne JA, Lento PH, Siegfried MR, Stahl GL, Fusman B, Lefer AM. Cardiovascular effects of acute hypercholesterolemia in rabbits: reversal with lovastatin treatment. J Clin Invest 1989;83:465–473.
66. Cohen RA, Zitnay KM, Haudenschild CC, Cunningham LD. Loss of selective endothelial cell vasoactive functions in pig coronary arteries caused by hypercholesterolemia. Circ Res 1988;63:903–910.
67. Drexler H, Zeiher AM, Meinzer K, Just H. Correction of endothelial dysfunction in coronary microcirculation of hypercholesterolemic patients by L-arginine. Lancet 1991;338:1546–1550.
68. Zeiher AM, Drexler H, Wollschlaeger H, Saurbier B, Just H. Coronary vasomotion in response to sympathetic stimulation in humans: importance of the functional integrity of the endothelium. J Am Coll Cardiol 1989;14:1181–1190.
69. Harrison DG, Armstrong ML, Freiman P, Heistad DD. Restoration of endothelium-dependent relaxation by dietary treatment of atherosclerosis. J Clin Invest 1987;80:1808–1811.
70. Levine GN, Keaney JF Jr, Koulouris S, Gerhard MD, Frei B, Vita JA. Beneficial effect of ascorbic acid on endothelial vasomotor function. Circulation 1992;8:S456.
71. Tagawa H, Tagawa T, Shimokawa H. Estrogen acutey improves both nitric oxide-mediated and non nitric oxide-mediated endothelium-dependent vasodilation in postmenopausal women. Circulation 1992;8:S325.
72. Drexler H, Zeiher AM, Meinzer K, Just H. Correction of endothelial dysfunction in the coronary microcirculation of hypercholesterolemic patients by L-arginine. Lancet 1991;338:1546–1550.
73. Creager MA, Gallagher SJ, Girerd XJ, Coleman SM, Dzau VJ, Cooke JP. L-arginine improves endothelium-dependent vasodilation in hypercholesterolemic humans. J Clin Invest 1992;90:1248–1253.
74. Andrews HE, Bruckdorfer KR, Dunn RC, Jacobs M. Low-density lipoproteins inhibit endothelium-dependent relaxation in rabbit aorta. Nature 1987;327:237–239.
75. Chin JH, Azhar S, Hoffman BB. Inactivation of endothelial derived relaxing factor by oxidized lipoproteins. J Clin Invest 1992;89:10–18.
76. Minor RL, Myers PR, Guerra R, Bates JN, Harrison DG. Diet-induced atherosclerosis increases the release of nitrogen oxides from rabbit aorta. J Clin Invest 1990;86:2109–2116.
77. Ohara Y, Petersen TE, Harrison DG. Hypercholesterolemia increases endothelial superoxide anion production. J Clin Invest 1993;91:2546–2551.

78. Marui N, Offerman MK, Swerlick R, Kunsch C, Rosen CA, Ahmad M, Alexander RW, Medford RM. Vascular cell adhesion molecule-1 (VCAM-1) gene transcription and expression are regulated through an antioxidant-sensitive mechanism in human vascular endothelial cells. J Clin Invest 1993;92:1866–1874.
79. Faruqi R, de la Motte C, DiCorleto PE. Alpha-tocopherol inhibits agonist-induced monocytic cell adhesion to cultured human endothelial cells. J Clin Invest 1994;94:592–600.
80. Pagano PJ, Tornheim K, Cohen RA. Superoxide anion production by rabbit thoracic aorta: effect of endothelium-derived nitric oxide. Am J Physiol 1993;265:H707–H712.
81. Heim KF, Thomas G, Ramwell PW. Effect of substituted arginine compounds on superoxide production in the rabbit aorta. J Pharmacol Exp Therap 1991;257:1130–1135.
82. Rubbo H, Radi R, Trujillo M, Telleri R, Kalyanaraman B, Barnes S, Kirk M, Freeman BA. Nitric oxide regulation of superoxide and perosynitrite-dependent lipid peroxidation. Formation of novel nitrogen-containing oxidized lipid derivatives. J Biol Chem 1994;269:26,066–26,075.
83. Hogg N, Kalyanaraman B, Joseph J, Struck A, Parthasarathy S. Inhibition of low-density lipoprotein oxidation by nitric oxide. Potential role in atherogenesis. FEBS Lett 1993;34:170–174.
84. Clancy RM, Leszczynska P, Piziak J, Abramson SB. Nitric oxide, an endothelial cell relaxation factor, inhibits neutrophil superoxide anion production via a direct action on NADPH oxidase. J Clin Invest 1992;90:1116–1121.
85. Yates MT, Lambert LE, Whitten JP, McDonald I, Mano M, Ku G, Mao SJ. A protective role for nitric oxide in the oxidative modification of low density lipoproteins by mouse macrophages. FEBS Lett 1992;309:135–138.
86. Niu X-F, Smith CW, Kubes P. Intracellular oxidative stress induced by nitric oxide synthesis inhibition increases endothelial cell adhesion to neutrophils. Circ Res 1994;74:1133–1140.
87. Weber C, Erl W, Pietsch A, Strobel M, Ziegler-Heitbrock HWL, Weber PC. Antioxidants inhibit monocyte adhesion by suppressing nuclear factor-kb mobilization and induction of vascular cell adhesion molecule-1 in endothelial cells stimulated to generate radicals. Arteriosclerosis Throm 1994;14:1665–1673.
88. Peng HB, Libby P, Liao JK. Induction and stabilization of I kappa B alpha by nitric oxide mediates inhibition of NF-kappa B. J Biol Chem 1995;270:14,214–14,219.
89. DeCaterina R, Libby P, Peng H-B, Thannickal VJ, Rajavashisth TB, Gimbrone MA Jr, Shin WS, Liao JK. Nitric oxide decreases cytokine-induced endothelial activation. J Clin Invest 1995;96:60–68.
90. Cooke JP, Andon NA, Girerd XJ, Hirsch AT, Creager MA. Arginine restores cholinergic relaxation of hypercholesterolemic rabbit thoracic aorta. Circulation 1991;83:1057–1062.
91. Resnick N, Collins T, Atkins W, Bonthron DT, Dewey CF Jr, Gimbrone MA Jr. Platelet-derived growth factor B chain promoter contains a cis-acting fluid shear-stress-responsive element. Proc Natl Acad Sci USA 1993;90:4591–4595.
92. Noris M, Morigi M, Donadelli R, Aiello S, Foppolo M, Todeschini M, Orisio S, Remuzzi G, Remuzzi A. Nitric oxide synthesis by cultured endothelial cells is modulated by flow conditions. Circ Res 1995;76:536–543.
93. Bath PMW, Hassall DG, Gladwin A-M, Palmer RMJ, Martin JF. Nitric oxide and prostacyclin. Divergence of inhibitory effects on monocyte chemotaxis and adhesion to endothelium in vitro. Arteriosclerosis Thromb 1991;11:254–260.
94. Tsao PS, Lewis NP, Alpert SA, Cooke JP. Fluid flow decreases endothelial adhesiveness for monocytes: role of nitric oxide. Circulation 1995;92(12):3513–3519.
95. Richard MJ, Davis LD, Jacobson NL. The domestic goat: a useful model to determine effects of diet and exercise on cholesterol accumulation in the body. Comp Biochem Physiol 1990;95:275–280.
96. Jayo JM, Shively CA, Kaplan JR, Manuck SB. Effects of exercise and stress on body fat distribution in male cynomolgus monkeys. Int J Obes Rel Met Dis 1993;17:597–604.
97. Sessa WC, Pritchard K, Seyedi N, Wang J, Hintze TH. Chronic exercise in dogs increases coronary vascular nitric oxide production and endothelial cell nitric oxide synthase gene expression. Circ Res 1994;74:349–353.
98. Glagov S, Zarins C, Giddens DP, Ku DN. Hemodynamics and atherosclerosis. Insights and perspectives gained from studies of human arteries. Arch Pathol Lab Med 1988;112:1018–1031.
99. Girerd XJ, Hirsch AT, Cooke JP, Dzau VJ, Creager MA. L-arginine augments endothelium-dependent vasodilation in cholesterol-fed rabbits. Circ Res 1990;67:1301–1308.
100. Singer AH, Tsao PS, Wang B-Y, Bloch DA, Cooke JP. Discordant effects of dietary L-arginine on vascular structure and reactivity in hypercholesterolemic rabbits. J Cardiovasc Pharmacol 1995;25:710–716.

101. Cooke JP, Singer AH, Tsao PS, Zera P, Rowan RA, Billingham ME. Anti-atherogenic effects of L-arginine in the hypercholesterolemic rabbit. J Clin Invest 1992;90:1168–1172.
102. Tsao P, McEvoy LM, Drexler H, Butcher EC, Cooke JP. Enhanced endothelial adhesiveness in hypercholesterolemia is attenuated by L-arginine. Circulation 1994;89:2176–2182.
103. Cushing SD, Berliner JA, Valente AJ, Territo MC, Navab M, Perhami F, Gerrity R, Schwartz CJ, Fogelman AM. Minimally modified low density lipoprotein induces monocyte chemotactic protein 1 in human endothelial cells and smooth muscle cells. Proc Natl Acad Sci USA 1990;87:5134–5138.
104. Parhami F, Fang ZT, Fogelman AM, Andalibi A, Territo MC, Berliner JA. Minimally modified low density lipoprotein-induced inflammatory responses in endothelial cells are mediated by cyclic adenosine monophosphate. J Clin Invest 1993;92:471–478.
105. Zeiher AM, Fisslthaler B, Schray-Utz B, Busse R. Nitric oxide modulates the expression of monocyte chemoattractant protein 1 in cultured human endothelial cells. Circ Res 1995;76:980–986.
106. Cayette AJ, Palacino JJ, Horten K, Cohen RA. Chronic inhibition of nitric oxide production accelerates neointima formation and impairs endothelial function in hypercholesterolemic rabbits. Arterosclerosis Thrombo 1994;14:753–759.
107. Naruse K, Shimizu K, Muramatsu M, Toki Y, Miyazaki Y, Okumura K, Hashimoto H, Ito T. Long-term inhibition of NO synthesis promotes atherosclerosis in the hypercholesterolemic rabbit thoracic aorta. PGH2 does not contribute to impaired endothelium-dependent relaxation. Arteriosclerosis Thromb 1994;14:746–752.
108. Hirata Y, Hayakawa H, Suzuki E, Kimura K, Kikuchi K, Nagano T, Hirobe M, Omata M. Direct measurements of endothelium-derived nitric oxide release by stimulation of endothelin receptors in rat kidney and its alteration in salt-induced hypertension. Circulation 1995;91:1229–1235.
109. Lüscher TF, Raij L, Vanhoutte PM. Endothelium-dependent vascular responses in normotensive and hypertensive Dahl rats. Hypertension 1987;9:157–163.
110. Lockette WE, Otsuka Y, Carretero OA. Endothelium-dependent relaxation in hypertension. Hypertension 1986;8(Suppl. II):61–66.
111. Lüscher TF, Vanhoutte PM, Raij L. Antihypertensive treatment normalizes decreased endothelium-dependent relaxations in rats with salt-induced hypertension. Hypertension 1987;9(Suppl. III):193–197.
112. Shultz PJ, Raij L. Effects of antihypertensive agents on endothelium-dependent and endothelium-independent relaxations. Br J Clin Pharmacol 1989;28(Suppl. 2):151S–157S.
113. Ribeiro MO, Antunes E, de Nucci G, Lovisolo SM, Zatz R. Chronic inhibition of nitric oxide synthesis. A new model of arterial hypertension. Hypertension 1992;20:298–303.
114. Huang PL, Hyang Z, Mashimo H, Block KD, Moskowitz MA, Bevan JA, Fishman MC. Hypertension in mice lacking the gene for endothelial nitric oxide synthase. Nature 1995;377:239–242.
115. Panza J, Quyyumi AA, Brush JE Jr, Epstein SE. Abnormal endothelium-dependent vascular relaxation in patients with essential hypertension. N Engl J Med 1990;323:22–27.
116. Linder L, Kiowski W, Buhler FR, Luscher TF. Indirect evidence for release of endothelium-derived relaxing factor in human forearm circulation in vivo: blunted response in essential hypertension. Circulation 1990;81:1762–1767.
117. Taddei S, Mattei P, Virdis A, Sudano I, Ghiadoni L, Salvetti A. Forearm vasodilation in response to acetylcholine is increased by potassium in essential hypertensive patients. J Hypertens 1993;11(Suppl. 5):S144,S145.

2 Ionic Mechanisms of Peptide-Induced Responses in Vascular Endothelial Cells

Jianben Song, PHD *and Jeffrey L. Ram,* PHD

CONTENTS

INTRODUCTION

The single layer of endothelial cells (ECs) that lines the luminal side of blood vessels plays an important role in regulating blood vessel function. Underlying the EC layer are several layers of vascular smooth muscle cells (VSMC) (Fig. 1). Although the EC layer serves in part as a protective covering and permeability barrier to the movement of substances through the blood vessel wall, ECs also have an active role in mediating the effect of hormonal and locally produced substances that regulate VSMC tension and growth. There is evidence that relaxation or decreases in blood vessel contractility caused by steroid hormones *(1)*, acetyl choline *(2,3)*, and various peptides (described in Peptides and Vascular Responses) are mediated by the EC layer and do not occur in blood vessels in which the endothelial cell layer has been removed. There is a large body of evidence that shows that ECs release substances that cause blood vessels to dilate *(2–5)*. A major component of these endothelium-derived relaxing factors is nitric oxide (NO), the syn-

From: *Contemporary Endocrinology: Endocrinology of the Vasculature*
Edited by: J. R. Sowers Humana Press Inc., Totowa, NJ

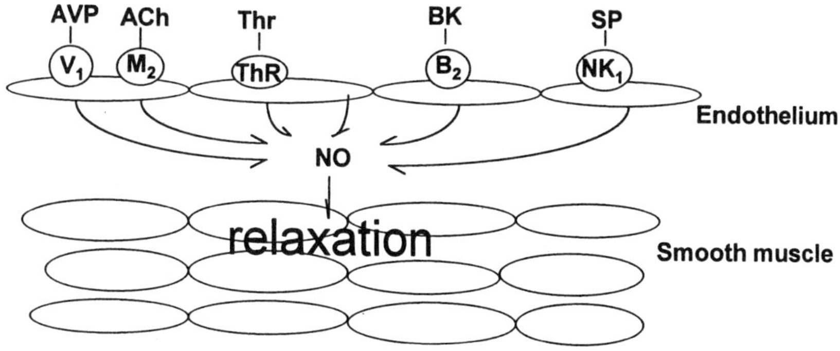

Fig. 1. Schematic illustration of a blood vessel wall, showing relationship between endothelium monolayer of cells and underlying smooth muscle cells. Like the neurotransmitter acetyl choline (ACh), which also causes vasodilatation, peptides from various sources act on their specific receptors to activate the synthesis of NO, which causes smooth muscle cells to relax. The peptides discussed in this review and their respective receptors are AVP, V_1; thrombin (Thr), thrombin receptor (ThR); BK, B_2; and SP, NK-1. ACh acts on muscarinic (M_2) receptors. Each endothelial cell can have more than one type of receptor.

thesis of which has been shown to be regulated by peptides and other agonists that cause VSMC relaxation. These peptides may also act directly on the underlying VSMC, so that the final outcome is an integrated response of the VSMC to EC-mediated and direct actions of the peptides.

Peptides that activate EC-mediated relaxation of blood vessels include bradykinin (BK), substance P (SP), vasopressin (AVP), and thrombin. As reviewed briefly in the next section for these peptides, their origins are diverse and include hormonal, neuronal, paracrine, and autocrine sources; however, all appear to activate G-protein coupled receptors, which in turn regulate ion fluxes and other mechanisms that lead to the synthesis and secretion of NO. The major focus of this chapter is on the ionic fluxes activated by these peptides in EC and the roles that ionic mechanisms have in regulating the synthesis and secretion of NO.

PEPTIDES AND VASCULAR RESPONSES

Bradykinin

BK is a nonapeptide (Arg-Pro-Pro-Gly-Phe-Ser-Pro-Phe-Arg) that acts primarily as a vasodilator *(6)*. It is produced extracellularly as the result of the proteolytic action of kininogenases, such as kallikrein, on kininogens, the high-mol-wt precursors of BK *(7,8)*. BK is inactivated by kininases I and II. Kininase II is the major BK degradative enzyme in vascular tissues and is a dipeptidyl carboxypeptidase known in the context of angiotensin metabolism as angiotensin-converting enzyme (ACE) *(7,9)*. BK acts on endothelial cells through B-2 receptors *(10)*, for which icatibant (HOE140) is an effective selective antagonist *(10–13)*. B-2 receptors have been cloned and belong to the family of seven transmembrane domain G-protein coupled receptors *(14,15)*.

Since BK is rapidly degraded in the circulation *(16–18)*, most BK probably originates locally in the vascular bed in which it acts. One source of BK acting on endothelial cells is the endothelial cells themselves, and it has been has shown that kininogen binds to the surface of endothelial cells *(19)*. Kallikrein causes rings of isolated arteries to relax, an effect that is dependent on the presence of intact endothelium, potentiated by ACE inhibitors (which would be expected to prevent the degradation of locally produced BK), and blocked by a kallikrein inhibitor *(20)*. BK has been found in the supernatant of endothelial cell cultures and is increased when ACE is inhibited *(21)*.

One of the stimuli that activates endothelial production of BK may be shear stress, since it has been shown that the endothelial-dependent relaxation caused by shear stress can be blocked by the selective BK receptor antagonist HOE140 *(22)*. Another potent activator of the local kallikrein–kinin system is ischemia. Kinin levels in peripheral blood have been shown to increase in humans after myocardial infarction *(23)*. Cardioprotective effects of ACE inhibitors following myocardial infarction have been shown to be reversed by simultaneous administration of HOE140 *(24)*. BK appears to be released, though at much lower rates, under physiological conditions.

Endothelial B-2 receptors activate phospholipase C and phospholipase A_2 and increase the synthesis of 1,4,5-inositol trisphosphate (IP_3) and arachidonic acid *(25)*. These mechanisms, and possibly others, result in an increase in intracellular calcium concentration ($[Ca^{2+}]_i$) and increased synthesis of NO and prostacyclin *(13)*. The vasorelaxant effect of BK is mediated in part through activation of NO synthesis in the endothelial cells, the mechanisms of which are discussed in the following sections. Numerous studies *(26,27)* have shown that relaxation of blood vessels in vitro by BK can be reduced by blocking NO synthesis with NO-synthase inhibitors. In addition, prostacyclin may also partly mediate BK's relaxant effects. BK also has direct actions on VSMC, including stimulation of IP_3 synthesis and increase in $[Ca^{2+}]_i$, which can cause VSMC contraction in the absence of endothelium *(28,29)*. However, in normal blood vessels the endothelial-mediated relaxing effects of BK are predominant.

Substance P

SP is a hendecapeptide (Arg-Pro-Lys-Pro-Gln-Gln-Phe-Phe-Gly-Leu-Met-NH_2) belonging to a family of biologically active peptides (tachykinins) having the carboxyl terminal structure of Phe-X-Gly-Leu-Met-NH_2 *(30,31)*. SP causes endothelium-dependent relaxation of blood vessels *(32,33)*. The source of SP appears to be both neurogenic and endothelial: Nerve fibers innervating coronary veins *(34)*, coronary arteries *(35)*, and superficial temporal artery *(32)* have been shown to contain SP, and the vasodilatation associated with antidromic activation of sensory nerves (known to use SP as a neurotransmitter *[36]*) may also be the result of release of substance P from collateral endings in the vicinity of blood vessels *(37)*. However, non-neuronal SP has also been demonstrated immunohistologically in endothelial cells of various blood vessels, including ovarian veins *(33)* and coronary and femoral arteries *(38)*, leading to the suggestion that SP of endothelial cell origin may also function in the local control of vascular tone.

The SP receptor, also known as the NK-1 receptor, is a seven transmembrane domain G-protein coupled receptor *(39,40)*. In transfected cells, as in endothelial cells, application of SP leads to activation of phospholipase C activity and IP_3 synthesis. SP-induced relaxation of blood vessels depends on endothelial synthesis of NO and can be reduced by either removal of endothelium or exposure of blood vessels to an NO-synthase inhibitor *(33,41,42)*.

Vasopressin

AVP, a nonapeptide (Cys-Tyr-Phe-Gln-Asn-Cys-Pro-Arg-Gly-NH_2) produced in the hypothalamus, can cause vasoconstriction of blood vessels. Under physiological conditions, AVP concentrations in the circulation are probably too low for these vasoconstrictive effects to be readily apparent. However, circulating AVP may have blood vessel regulatory effects under pathophysiologic conditions *(43–46)*. Although vasoconstrictive effects of AVP are usually most apparent, AVP also has relaxing effects mediated through the endothelium, so that the final effect of AVP is actually the integrated effect of contraction somewhat reduced by endothelial mechanisms *(47)*. In some blood vessels, such as the canine basilar artery *(48)* and the pulmonary artery *(49)*, the relaxing effects of AVP predominate.

AVP may also have a local vascular origin. Blood vessels have been shown to contain AVP of local origin *(50)*, and AVP has been demonstrated immunohistologically in EC of rat pulmonary artery *(51)*, human umbilical vein and artery *(52)*, rat coronary and femoral arteries *(38)*, and EC cultured from rabbit aorta *(53)*. As with similar observations described in the previous section for SP, further evidence is needed to demonstrate that these locally synthesized peptides have a functional role.

Endothelial-mediated relaxation effects of AVP on blood vessels are mediated in many cases by the V1 receptor *(49,54)*, a seven transmembrane domain G-protein coupled receptor whose mRNA has been demonstrated to be present in EC of brain blood vessels *(55)*. Activation of the V1 receptor in carotid artery ECs has been shown to increase IP_3 synthesis and $[Ca^{2+}]_i$ *(56)*. These actions probably result in an increase in NO synthesis since endothelial-mediated relaxation can be blocked by an NO-synthase inhibitor in pulmonary *(49)* and basilar arteries *(48)*. AVP may also mediate endothelial-dependent relaxation by an NO-synthase independent mechanism that can be reduced by indomethacin, a blocker of prostaglandin synthesis, as shown in mesenteric artery *(57)*.

Thrombin

Thrombin is an unusual peptide agonist of endothelial-mediated relaxation in that it is an enzyme (a serine protease) and is formed from a circulating precursor, prothrombin, during blood clot formation. Like the peptides already discussed, the receptor for thrombin is a seven transmembrane domain G-protein coupled receptor; however, it has the unusual property of being activated by proteolytic cleavage *(58)*. Thrombin cleaves a 41 amino acid peptide from the amino terminal portion of the receptor, leaving a new amino terminus whose sequence resembles peptides that are effective agonists for thrombin receptors. This thrombin receptor activating peptide (TRAP) sequence (in humans, Ser-Phe-Leu-Leu-Arg-Asn-Pro) has been suggested to act as a "tethered peptide ligand," that becomes available normally for activating the receptor only after thrombin proteolysis of the receptor *(59)*. Thus, although the physiological stimulus for the thrombin receptor is proteolysis, the receptor resembles other peptide receptors in being activated by a specific peptide sequence.

Both thrombin and TRAP cause endothelial-mediated relaxation, in part, through activation of NO synthesis. In pig coronary *(59)* and pulmonary *(60)* arteries and dog saphenous vein *(59)*, both thrombin and TRAP cause relaxation that can be blocked by an NO-synthase inhibitor. Thrombin has been shown to produce a marked increase in IP_3 synthesis in human umbilical artery ECs *(29)*, and both thrombin and TRAP have been shown to activate a large transient rise in $[Ca^{2+}]_i$, followed by a lower sustained level (plateau) of $[Ca^{2+}]_i$ in human umbilical vein ECs *(61,62)*. The plateau phase of Ca^{2+} influx, but not the transient phase, was inhibited by the tyrosine kinase inhibitor herbimycin *(62)*. In the absence of endothelium, thrombin and TRAP cause a concentration-dependent contraction, indicating that the overall response of intact blood vessels to thrombin may involve the integrated effect of thrombin on both EC and VSMC *(60)*.

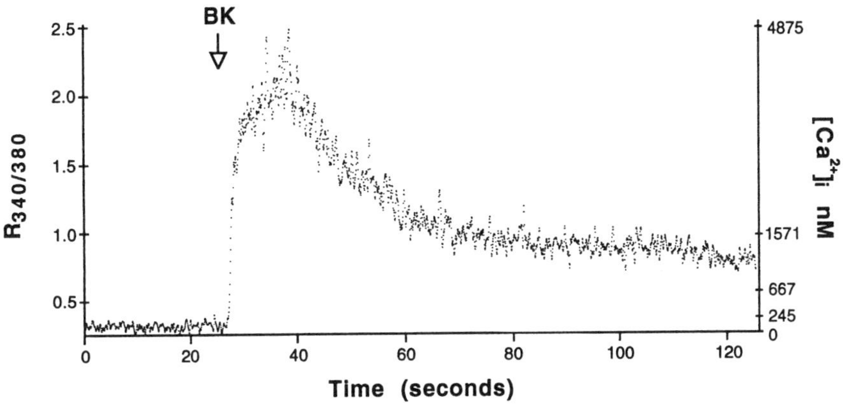

Fig. 2. BK elicited a biphasic increase in intracellular calcium concentration ($[Ca^{2+}]_i$) in a bovine coronary venule endothelial cell. About 3 s after BK reached the cell, a transient increase in $[Ca^{2+}]_i$ was observed first, reaching into the micromolar range within several seconds. The level of $[Ca^{2+}]_i$ declined quickly after reaching its peak, and a steady-state rise of $[Ca^{2+}]_i$ persisted for minutes. The ratio of fluorescence intensities at excitation wavelengths of 340 and 380 nm (left side of the vertical axis), measured by fura-2 microfluorimetry, were converted to $[Ca^{2+}]_i$ *(72)*. The extracellular medium is Tyrode's bath solution, containing 1 m*M* Ca^{2+} *(73)*.

THE ROLE OF CHANGES IN $[Ca^{2+}]_i$ IN PEPTIDE-INDUCED ENDOTHELIAL RESPONSES

All of the aforementioned peptides ultimately cause blood vessel relaxation by increasing the secretion of NO from ECs (Fig. 1). Changes in $[Ca^{2+}]_i$ underlie stimulus-secretion coupling in many cell types, and EC-dependent vasodilatation also requires a rise in $[Ca^{2+}]_i$ concentration. NO is synthesized from L-arginine via NO synthase *(63)*. Activation of NO synthase, which is the key step that links vasoactive peptides to endothelium-dependent vasodilatation, requires the rise of $[Ca^{2+}]_i$ above the resting level *(64–67)*. Thus, the synthesis of NO is a $[Ca^{2+}]_i$ dependent event, which can be triggered by a rise of $[Ca^{2+}]_i$ only above the resting level; at the resting level of $[Ca^{2+}]_i$, low Ca^{2+} even inhibits NO synthesis *(63,68)*.

In investigations of the mechanisms by which peptides induce the elevation of $[Ca^{2+}]_i$ in ECs, it has been found that peptides usually produce a biphasic increase in $[Ca^{2+}]_i$ when cells are bathed in a Ca^{2+}-containing medium *(69–71)*. A typical peptide-induced $[Ca^{2+}]_i$ response, illustrated for BK in Fig. 2, exhibits an initial transient rise of $[Ca^{2+}]_i$ followed by a somewhat lower sustained phase of $[Ca^{2+}]_i$ increase. Several seconds of delay are usually observed between agonist application and the onset of the $[Ca^{2+}]_i$ changes. This is believed to be the result of the involvement of a second messenger pathway *(69,70,73)*. The initial transient component of the $[Ca^{2+}]_i$ response has been shown to reflect IP_3-mediated release of Ca^{2+} from internal stores *(71,74)*, whereas the sustained component of the $[Ca^{2+}]_i$ increase depends on Ca^{2+} influx from the extracellular space *(70,75,76)*.

In general, the sequence of events in peptide-induced $[Ca^{2+}]_i$ increase in ECs can be described as follows:

1. The peptide binds to its specific receptor;
2. Receptor action is mediated through G-protein and phospholipase C, which generates IP_3 from phosphatidylinositol-bisphosphate (PIP_2);

3. IP_3 diffuses to bind to its receptor on endoplasmic reticulum (ER) membrane and triggers the release of Ca^{2+} from ER (transient $[Ca^{2+}]_i$ increase owing to the release of intracellular store).

IP_3 may further convert to 1,3,4,5-tetrakis-phosphate (IP_4). Together with Ca^{2+} and other unidentified substances, these intracellular messengers may activate the opening of plasma membrane ion channels, including those permeable to Ca^{2+} *(77,78)*.

Although the mechanisms involved in the release of Ca^{2+} from internal stores have been widely studied in a variety of nonexcitable cells, electrophysiological identification and characterization of the Ca^{2+}-influx pathway has been difficult. A commonly proposed explanation for peptide-induced Ca^{2+}-influx is that Ca^{2+}-activated outward K^+ currents hyperpolarize the EC and increase the driving force for Ca^{2+} to enter through leak pathways *(70)*. An alternative or supplementary explanation, suggested by the observation that BK and other agonists induce inward currents in ECs in the absence of voltage-gated Ca^{2+}-channels (*see* ref. *79* for an exception), is that Ca^{2+}-influx occurs through receptor- or second messenger-operated Ca^{2+} channels. Thus, the conductance of the membrane to Ca^{2+} (not only the driving force for Ca^{2+} entry) increases because of the stimulation by the agonist. Recent studies support the notion that peptides such as BK and SP increase EC membrane Ca^{2+} conductance through a second messenger-mediated pathway, which therefore contributes substantially to Ca^{2+}-influx *(73,80–83)*.

PEPTIDE-INDUCED CHANGES IN ENDOTHELIAL CELL MEMBRANE POTENTIAL

Ionic currents across plasma membranes are usually accompanied by changes in membrane potential. An indication of which ionic currents may be affected by peptides relies on the careful observation of changes in membrane potential caused by peptides. Membrane hyperpolarizations induced by BK and SP have been observed in several types of ECs *(42,83–88)*. Potassium channel blockers, such as D-tubocurarine and apamin, inhibit the hyperpolarization induced by BK in a dose-dependent manner *(84)*, indicating that K^+ channels may be the cause of the hyperpolarization. Furthermore, for those ECs in which BK caused hyperpolarization, a BK-induced outward K^+ current with a reversal potential near the K^+ equilibrium potential was also recorded *(83)*. In addition, the hyperpolarization induced by BK or SP was a transient event that peaked in several seconds and declined quickly. In studies using simultaneous recording of $[Ca^{2+}]_i$ and membrane potential, the transient hyperpolarization was found to coincide with the onset of the increase in $[Ca^{2+}]_i$ *(83,88)*. In Ca^{2+}-free extracellular medium, the rise in $[Ca^{2+}]_i$ and the hyperpolarization still occurred. This indicates that the release of Ca^{2+} from intracellular stores is the source of the transient rise in $[Ca^{2+}]_i$ and may also cause the hyperpolarization. Investigations of whether the hyperpolarization was indeed caused by Ca^{2+}-activated K^+ channels (I_{KCa}), identification of the I_{KCa} channels, and determination of the role that the hyperpolarization induced by BK or SP plays in peptide-induced Ca^{2+}-influx, are questions that are discussed in the next several sections of this chapter.

There have also been reports of membrane depolarization induced by peptides in some ECs *(83)*. Under identical recording conditions and without any obvious morphological variations or differences in cell culture conditions, BK produces depolarization in many cells from the same population *(83)*. When an initial transient hyperpolarization is observed, the membrane potential of ECs sometimes later depolarizes above its resting

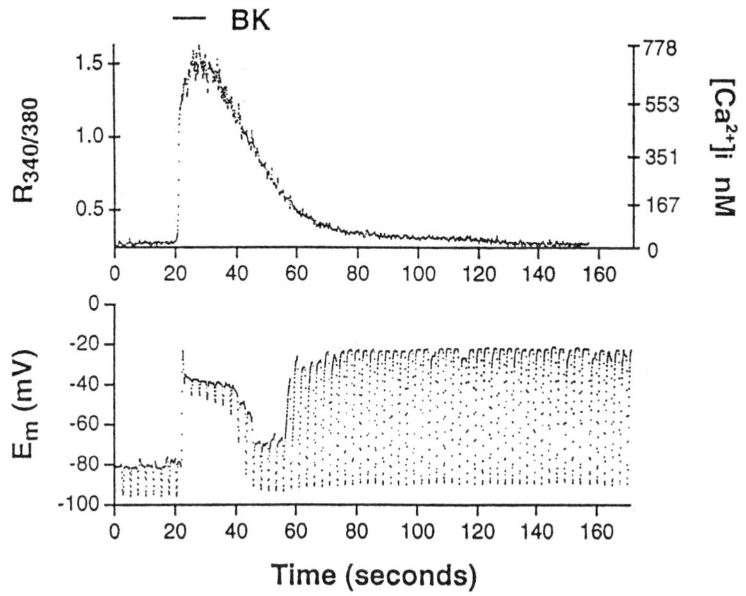

Fig. 3. Simultaneous recordings of BK-induced changes in $[Ca^{2+}]_i$ (upper graph) and membrane potential (lower graph) in a bovine coronary venule endothelial cell. $[Ca^{2+}]_i$ was measured as described in Fig. 2. Membrane potential was measured by whole-cell patch-clamp technique in current-clamp mode. BK caused a fast increase in $[Ca^{2+}]_i$ followed by a lower, but sustained level of $[Ca^{2+}]_i$. The transient rise in $[Ca^{2+}]_i$ was accompanied by a transient depolarization from –80 to –30 mV, followed by a transient hyperpolarization to –70 mV. During the sustained phase of $[Ca^{2+}]_i$ increase, the cell depolarized again to above –30 mV. To monitor whole-cell conductance changes, current pulses (–50 pA, 0.4-s duration) were injected into the cell at 2.5-s intervals, generating downward deflections of the membrane potential. BK caused an increase in conductance, indicating the opening of ion channels. Bath solution was Tyrode's solution and pipet solution contained 140 m*M* KCl. This figure is adapted from Fig. 1 of ref. *83*, with permission.

state *(83,84,87,88)*. In some cases, it is more complicated, as transient depolarization may be observed first, followed by a transient hyperpolarization and a long-lasting depolarization (Fig. 3). In this case, by examining the time-course of the change in membrane potential, it appears likely that three types of ionic currents are induced:

1. A transient inward current, which is responsible for the initial transient depolarization;
2. A transient outward current, which correlates with the hyperpolarization following the depolarization; and
3. A long-lasting inward current, which causes the membrane to depolarize slowly above its resting state *(83)*.

Characterization of the ion channels underlying each of these changes in membrane potential has been the focus of intensive research over the last few years.

POTASSIUM CHANNELS

Both voltage-dependent and Ca^{2+}-activated K^+ currents have been found in ECs. A hyperpolarization-activated, inwardly rectifying K^+ current has been described in cultured ECs from bovine aorta *(70,89–91)*, bovine pulmonary artery *(92–94)*, bovine coronary venules *(73)*, and porcine coronary artery *(88)*. Substitution of K^+ by Cs^+ in the pipet solution completely eliminates this inward rectifying current *(73,81)*, and the effect of peptides on the inwardly rectifying K^+ current is sometimes inhibitory. AVP inhibits this current in porcine cerebral capillary ECs *(95)*, but does not affect the inwardly rectifying K^+ current in all ECs.

At positive membrane potentials, a depolarization-activated transient outward K^+ current (A current) is observed in cultured ECs from bovine aorta *(89)* and pulmonary arteries *(94)*, and this current can be blocked by application of the A-channel blocker, 4-aminopyridine *(89)*. In one study *(89)*, one-third of the ECs exhibited A-current. In some ECs, the presence of both A-current and the inward rectifier current results in an "N" shaped I-V curve *(69)*. A role for the A-current in peptide responses has not been demonstrated. Under physiological resting condition, the A currents are not activated; however, they may provide negative feedback for maintaining resting membrane potential when membrane potential is changed by physiological stimuli. No evidence for voltage-gated inward Ca^{2+} or Na^+ current has been found at either the whole cell or single channel levels in patch-clamp studies on various types of ECs *(70,88–90,92–94)*. Thus, voltage-dependent K^+ channels are the only voltage-dependent cation channels present in ECs.

Several investigators have reported peptide-activated outward currents in ECs *(69,70,83,88,96,98)*. There appears to be a Ca^{2+}-activated K^+ channel that can be activated by BK *(97,99,100)* and SP *(88)*, and simultaneous recording of whole-cell current and $[Ca^{2+}]_i$ indicates that the outward K^+-current induced by BK or SP is correlated with the transient increase in $[Ca^{2+}]_i$ *(83,88,98)*. Furthermore, single channel recordings show a strong dependence of open probabilities of K^+-current on Ca^{2+} concentration *(88,97,101)*.

PEPTIDE-ACTIVATED INWARD CURRENTS

Investigators have also recorded peptide-activated inward currents. One group *(93)* recorded an inward current (at negative holding potentials) produced by the agonists thrombin and BK in 10% of the bovine aortic ECs (BAECs) they examined. At a holding potential (V_h) of –20 mV, investigators *(102)* found a histamine-activated inward current in 9% of human umbilical vein ECs. Others *(80)* have observed small net inward currents activated by BK in single cells when potassium channels were blocked. In BAECs, inward currents persisted in Ca^{2+}-free solution or in Na^+-free solutions and could be blocked by La^{3+} *(80)*. Collectively, these observations suggest that ECs contain nonselective cation channels permeable to both Ca^{2+} and Na^+ that can be activated by various agonists, including peptides.

In a recent study, BK activated two phases (fast and slow) of inward current when coronary venule ECs (CVECs) were recorded in physiological bath solution using a high K^+ pipet solution *(73)*. The amplitude of the fast current averaged -224 ± 20 pA (at $V_h = -70$) and the amplitude of the slow current averaged -81 ± 9 pA. The reversal potentials of the two currents were near 0 mV and were virtually identical. The two currents were characterized using La^{3+} (200 μM), a known blocker of the nonselective cation current and of Ca^{2+}-influx, and 4,4'-diisothiocyanatostilbene-2,2'-disulfonic acid (DIDS), a known Cl^--channel blocker *(73)*. La^{3+} did not significantly block the larger fast current, but attenuated both the slow current and the $[Ca^{2+}]_i$ increase during its plateau phase; DIDS blocked only the fast current. Furthermore, when cells were bathed in

Ca^{2+}-free/Na^+ solution, the fast current persisted but the slow current was reduced. Collectively, these results suggested that the fast-current was carried by Cl^- and the slow current by cations. The slow current was similar in time-course, magnitude, and La^{3+}-sensitivity to the inward current recorded by others *(80)*. An inward current in BAECs has been unmasked after blocking K^+ channels *(81)*. Other investigators *(102)* described a large, rapidly activating inward current, similar in magnitude and time-course to the fast inward current Song and Davis *(73)* recorded in CVECs. Although suggested to be a nonselective cation current *(103)*, the experiments do not rule out the possibility that it may be carried by Cl^-.

Slow inward currents are likely present in all ECs that have been studied, because even in cells that show a transient hyperpolarization, a slow depolarization is always observed (Fig. 3). The depolarization becomes evident during the plateau phase of the $[Ca^{2+}]_i$ increase, suggesting that the slow inward current may contribute to Ca^{2+}-influx. A small inward current recorded in bovine pulmonary artery ECs 30–60 s following the application of BK *(69)* is similar to the slow current in CVECs, and the current in both studies correlates with the plateau phase of the EC $[Ca^{2+}]_i$ increase. SP-induced inward current has been recorded while holding the membrane potential at the K^+ equilibrium potential to eliminate the outward K^+ current and unmask the inward current *(88)*. Evidence that this is a nonselective cation current is that La^{3+} blocks it, Na^+-free medium attenuates it, and high Ca^{2+}-medium potentiates it.

CHLORIDE CURRENTS

Large, voltage-sensitive endothelial Cl^- channels have been described by several groups. With inside-out patches or perforated patch outside-out vesicles of pig aortic ECs, Cl^- channels activate spontaneously with unitary conductance of 385 pS *(104)*. Similar Cl^- channels have been observed in BAECs with a conductance of 360 pS in symmetric Cl^- solutions *(105)*. Others *(106)* report that isoproterenol, a β-adrenergic agonist, activates BAEC voltage-dependent Cl^- channels via cyclic AMP-mediated phosphorylation. This voltage-dependent phosphorylation-regulated Cl^- channel also could be the target of peptide-activated events in ECs.

Chloride channels appear to contribute to whole cell peptide-induced currents of ECs. The fast current activated by BK was identified as a Cl^- current by its sensitivity to DIDS and the Cl^--dependence of its reversal potential *(73)*. When the equilibrium potential for Cl^- is changed by altering the intra- and extracellular Cl^- concentration, the reversal potential of the fast current varies linearly with the Cl^- equilibrium potential *(73)*. Application of BK to EC for several minutes increases the likelihood of observing Cl^- channels in cell-attached patches; however, a fast increase in opening of these channels is not observed when BK is applied while recording from on-cell patches *(104)*.

Since the fast Cl^- current is correlated with the rapid phase of the BK-elicited $[Ca^{2+}]_i$ increase, the Cl^- current may be the result of the opening of Ca^{2+}-activated Cl^--channels[72]. Ca^{2+}-activated Cl^--channels have been reported in other cell types *(107)*, and activation of anion fluxes of EC by thrombin is Ca^{2+}-dependent *(108)*. Furthermore, the opening probability of Cl^- channels in on-cell patches is increased by application of the Ca^{2+} ionophore A23187 in the presence of extracellular Ca^{2+} *(104)*. Nevertheless, the differences in time-course of the activation of EC Cl^- channels by Ca^{2+} *(105)* and by BK from the whole cell Cl^- current activated by BK *(73)* suggests that much remains to be learned about regulation of Cl^- currents in EC.

Ca^{2+} CURRENT ACTIVATED BY DEPLETION OF INTRACELLULAR Ca^{2+} STORES

As seen in other cells *(109,110)*, ECs also contain a Ca^{2+}-influx pathway activated by the depletion of IP_3-sensitive intracellular Ca^{2+}-stores. There is evidence from several groups that peptides can activate Ca^{2+} influx by this pathway. Both BK and 2,5-di-t-butylhydroquinone (BHQ), which inhibit the ER Ca-ATPase and thereby depletes IP_3-sensitive Ca^{2+} stores without causing an increase in IP_3 synthesis, activate a cation influx pathway that can carry either Ca^{2+} or Ba^{2+} *(111)*, and the influx activated by both chemicals is blocked by La^{3+}. Similar effects using thapsigargin (another chemical that depletes intracellular calcium stores) were observed in human umbilical vein ECs *(112)*. Using electrophysiological methods, investigators found that BHQ activated a nonspecific inward cation current that could be carried by Na^+, Ca^{2+}, or Ba^{2+}, and could be blocked by La^{3+} *(113)*. This BHQ-activated current is inactivated by conditions that refill Ca^{2+} stores. In single channel recordings, both BHQ and BK activate nonspecific cation channels in on-cell patches *(114)*. These channels have conductances of 5–11 pS (depending on ionic conditions), are closed by stimuli that refill Ca^{2+} stores, and are blocked by La^{3+}. SP has also been shown to activate a whole cell current in pig coronary ECs that has similar characteristics *(82)*. Thrombin activates a nonselective cation channel in bovine pulmonary ECs; however, the channel conductance is 30–40 pS, and no tests to determine whether it can be activated by maneuvers designed to deplete the Ca^{2+} store have been reported *(115)*. Although there are similarities between Ca^{2+}-depletion activated current and receptor-activated nonspecific cation currents, it is not clear at this time whether they represent the same or separate Ca^{2+} entry pathways.

The mechanism by which depletion of Ca^{2+} stores activates a nonspecific cation current has not yet been clearly delineated. It seems apparent, since BHQ and thapsigargin can activate the current without affecting IP_3 levels, that the current is not directly activated by IP_3. Investigators of a similar current in *Xenopus* oocytes suggest that emptying the Ca^{2+} store activates a yet-to-be-determined phosphatase-sensitive diffusible messenger *(116)*. A "calcium influx factor" released in response to emptying Ca^{2+} stores in Jurkat cells has also been suggested *(117)*.

SUMMARY AND CONCLUSIONS

ECs contain a heterogeneous set of ion channels that respond to activation by peptides (Fig. 4). The fact that peptides can stimulate either membrane hyperpolarization with net outward current, or depolarization with net inward current, suggests that in most ECs, K^+ channels, nonspecific cation (depletion-activated or receptor-operated) channels, and Cl^- channels coexist, and that the predominant channel type determines how an individual cell responds to peptides. The factors that determine which channel predominates are unknown, but several possibilities exist. Channels may vary with stage in the cell growth cycle, as has been shown for melanoma cells *(118)*. Another possible explanation for heterogenous cell responses is that the state of cell confluence determines, in part, the expression of a particular ion channel. There is some evidence to support this idea in VSMC *(119)*, but no information is available for ECs. Heterogeneity of EC responses to

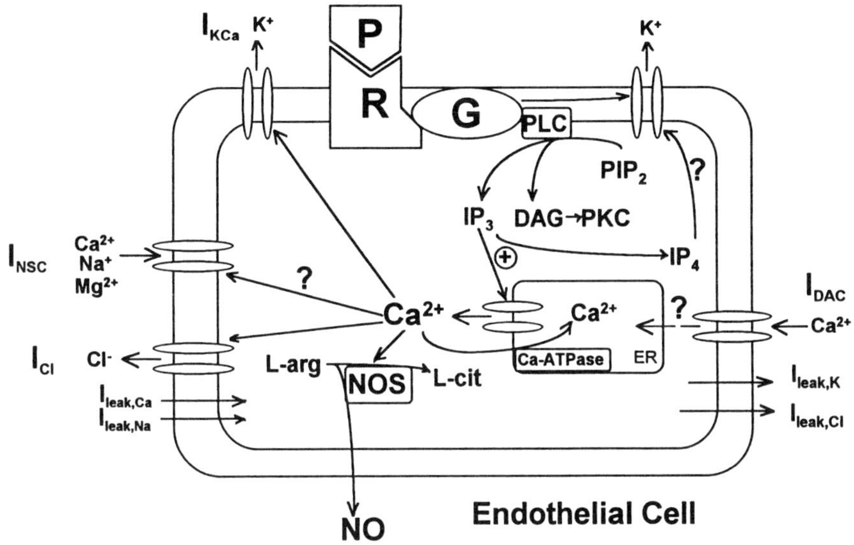

Fig. 4. Schematic illustration of peptide-regulated ionic mechanisms in endothelial cells. Abbreviations are as follows: DAG, diacylglycerol; ER, endoplasmic reticulum; G, g-protein; I_{DAC}, depletion-activated cation current; I_{NSC}, nonspecific cation current; I_{KCa}, Ca^{2+}-activated K^+ current; IP_3, inositol trisphosphate; IP_4, inositol tetrakisphosphate; L-arg, L-arginine; L-cit, L-citrulline; NO, nitric oxide; NOS, nitric oxide synthase; P, peptide; PIP_2, phosphatidylinositol bisphosphate; PLC, phospholipase C; PKC, protein kinase C; and R, receptor for peptide.

agonists and physical stimuli also appears to occur in vivo *(120)*, but the possible advantage this might confer to blood vessels is unknown.

In a "typical" peptide-induced EC response, activation of the Cl^--current and transient outward K+ currents usually precede the nonspecific cation current. The first two currents coincide with and may be activated by the transient $[Ca^{2+}]_i$ increase caused by release of Ca^{2+} from intracellular stores. The nonspecific cation current correlates with the plateau phase of $[Ca^{2+}]_i$ increase and may be triggered either by depletion of Ca^{2+} from endoplasmic reticulum or by other, as yet unknown, mechanisms. For an individual cell, if all three types of currents are present, an initial depolarization by inward Cl^--current would be observed, followed by a transient hyperpolarization (owing to the K^+ current), and then a prolonged depolarization (owing to inward cation current). Indeed, this is the pattern that is observed in many cells (Fig. 3, lower graph). If Cl^- and K^+ currents are activated simultaneously, the larger one would predominate, resulting in depolarization or hyperpolarization, respectively.

With respect to regulation of NO synthesis, the rise in $[Ca^{2+}]_i$ is critical to activate NO synthase. The initial events generating a rise in $[Ca^{2+}]_i$ involve release of Ca^{2+} from intracellular stores; however, for continued elevation of $[Ca^{2+}]_i$, influx of Ca^{2+} from outside the cell is necessary. The critical function of the nonspecific cation currents is not to produce depolarization, although this occurs as an epiphenomenon, but rather to provide an influx pathway for Ca^{2+}. In fact, both the Cl^- and K^+ channels counteract the depolarizing effect of the nonspecific cation channel, but in doing so they maintain a larger driving force for Ca^{2+} influx and hence provide more effective conditions for activating NO synthase.

REFERENCES

1. Bell DR, Rensberger HJ, Kortnik DR, Koshy A. Estrogen pretreatment directly potentiates endothelium-dependent vasorelaxation of porcine coronary arteries. Am J Physiol 1995;268:H377–H383.
2. Furchgott RF. Role of endothelium in responses of vascular smooth muscle. Circulation Res 1984;53:557–573.
3. Furchgott RF. Studies on relaxation of rabbit aorta by sodium nitrite: the basis for the proposal that the acid-activatable inhibitory factor from bovine retractor penis is inorganic nitrite and the endothelium-derived relaxing factor is nitric oxide. In: Vanhoutte, PM, ed. Vasodilatation: Vascular Smooth Muscle, Peptides, Autonomic Nerves and Endothelium. Raven, New York, 1988, pp. 401–414.
4. Vanhoutte PM, Rubanyi GM, Miller VM, Houston DS. Modulation of vascular smooth muscle contraction by endothelium. Annu Rev Physiol 1986;48:307–320.
5. Ignarro LJ, Buga GM, Wood KS, Byrns RE, Chadhuri G. Endothelium-derived relaxing factor produced and released from artery and vein is nitric oxide. Proc Natl Acad Sci USA 1987;84:9265–9269.
6. Cherry PD, Furchgott RF, Zawadski JV, Jonathidian D. Role of endothelial cells in relaxations of isolated arteries to bradykinin. Proc Natl Acad Sci USA 1982;79:2106–2110.
7. Linz W, Wiemer G, Gohlke P, Unger T, Scholkens BA. Contribution of kinins to the cardiovascular actions of angiotensin-converting enzyme inhibitors. Pharm Rev 1995;47:25–49.
8. Regoli D, Barabé J. Pharmacology of bradykinin and related kinins. Pharm Rev 1980;32:1–46.
9. Vanhoutte PM, Boulanger CM, Illiano SC, Nagao T, Vidal M, Mombouli J-V. Endothelium-dependent effects of converting-enzyme inhibitors. J Cardiovasc Pharmacol 1993;22(Suppl. 5):S10–S16.
10. Schini VB, Boulanger C, Regoli D, Vanhoutte PM. Bradykinin stimulates the production of cyclic GMP via activation of B2-kinin receptors in cultured porcine aortic endothelial cells. J Pharmacol Exp Ther 1990;252:581–585.
11. Regoli D, Jukic D, Gobeil F, Rhaleb N-E. Receptors for bradykinin and related kinins: a critical analysis. Can J Physiol Pharmacol 1993;71:556–567.
12. Cockcroft JR, Chowienczyk PJ, Brett SE, Bender N, Ritter JM. Inhibition of bradykinin-induced vasodilation in human forearm vasculature by icatibant, a potent B2-receptor antagonist. Br J Clin Pharmacol 1994;38:317–321.
13. Wiemer G, Popp R, Schölkens BA, Gogelein H. Enhancement of cytosolic calcium, prostacyclin and nitric oxide by bradykinin and the ACE inhibitor ramiprilat in porcine brain capillary endothelial cells. Brain Res 1994;638:261–266.
14. Hess JF, Borkowski JA, Young GS, Strader CD, Ransom RW. Cloning and pharmacological characterization of a bradykinin (BK-2) receptor. Biochem Biophys Res Commun 1992;184:260–268.
15. McEachern AE, Shelton ER, Bhakta S, Obernolte R, Bach C, Zuppan P, Fujisaki J, Aldrich RW, Jarnagin K. Expression cloning of a rat B_2 bradykinin receptor. Proc Natl Acad Sci USA 1991;88:7724–7728.
16. Pesquero JB, Jubilut GN, Lindsey CJ, Paiva ACM. Bradykinin metabolism pathway in the rat pulmonary circulation. J Hypertens 1992;10:1471–1478.
17. Ryan JW. Processing of the endogenous polypeptides by the lungs. Annu Rev Physiol 1982;44:241–255.
18. McCarthy DA, Potter DE, Nicolaides ED. An in vivo estimation of the potencies and half-lives of synthetic bradykinin and kallidin. J Pharmacol Exp Ther 1965;148:117–122.
19. Hasan AA, Cines DB, Ngaiza JR, Jaffe EA, Schmaier AH. High-molecular-weight kininogen is exclusively membrane bound on endothelial cells to influence activation of vascular endothelium. Blood 1995;85:3134–3143.
20. Mombouli JV, Vanhoutte PM. Kinins mediate kallikrein-induced endothelium-dependent relaxations in isolated canine coronary arteries. Biochem Biophys Res Commun 1992;185:693–697.
21. Wiemer G, Schölkens BA, Linz W. Endothelial protection by converting enzyme inhibitors. Cardiovasc Res 1994;28:166–172.
22. Mombouli JV, Vanhoutte PM. Kinins and endothelium-dependent relaxations to converting enzyme inhibitors in perfused canine arteries. J Cardiovasc Pharmacol 1991;18:926,927.
23. Hashimoto K, Hamamoto H, Honda Y, Hirose M, Furukawa S, Kumura E. Changes in components of kinin system and hemodynamics in acute myocardial infarction. Am Heart J 1978;95:619–626.
24. Linz W, Wiemer G, Schölkens BA. Contribution of bradykinin to the cardiovascular effects of ramipril. J Cardiovasc Pharmacol 1993;22(Suppl. 9):S1–S8.
25. Xu J, Qu ZX, Moore SA, Hsu CY, Hogan EL. Receptor-linked hydrolysis of phosphoinositides and production of prostacyclin in cerebral endothelial cells. J Neurochem 1992;58:1930–1935.
26. Hecker M, Bara T, Busse R. Relaxation of isolated coronary arteries by angiotensin-converting enzyme inhibitors: role of endothelium-derived kinins. J Vasc Res 1993;30:257–262.

27. Katusic ZS, Milde JH, Cosentino F, Mitrovic BS. Subarachnoid hemorrhage and endothelial L-arginine pathway in small brain stem arteries in dogs. Stroke 1993;24:392–399.
28. Briner VA, Tsai P, Schrier RW. Bradykinin: potential for vascular constriction in the presence of endothelial injury. Am J Physiol 1993;264:F322–F327.
29. Hawley J, Rubin PC, Hill SJ. Distribution of receptors mediating phosphoinositide hydrolysis in cultured human umbilical artery smooth muscle and endothelial cells. Biochem Pharmacol 1995;49:1005–1011.
30. Nakanishi S. Substance P precursor and kininogen: their structures, gene organizations, and regulation. Physiol Rev 1987;67:1117–1142.
31. Cascieri MA, Huang R-RC, Fong TM, Cheung AH, Sadowski S, Ber E, Strader CD. Determination of the amino acid residues in substance P conferring selectivity and specificity for the rat neurokinin receptors. Mol Pharm 1992;41:1096–1099.
32. Olesen IJ, Gulbenkian S, Valença A, Antunes JL, Wharton J, Polak JM, Edvinsson L. The peptidergic innervation of the human superficial temporal artery: immunohistochemistry, ultrastructure, and vasomotility. Peptides 1995;16:275–287.
33. Stones RW, Loesch A, Beard RW, Burnstock G. Substance P: endothelial localization and pharmacology in the human ovarian vein. Obstet Gynecol 1995;85:273–278.
34. Gulbenkian S, Opgaard OS, Barroso CP, Wharton J, Polak JM, Edvinsson L. The innervation of guinea pig epicardial coronary veins: immunohistochemistry, ultrastructure and vasomotility. J Auton Nerv Syst 1994;47:201–212.
35. Gulbenkian S, Edvinsson L, Opgaard OS, Wharton J, Polak JM, David-Ferreira JF. Peptide-containing nerve fibres in guinea-pig coronary arteries: immunohistochemistry, ultrastructure, and vasomotility. J Auton Nerv Syst 1990;31:153–168.
36. Cuello AC, Polak JM, Pearse AGE. Substance P: a naturally occurring transmitter in human spinal cord. Lancet 1976;11:1054–1056.
37. Lembeck F, Holzer P. Substance P as neurogenic mediator of antidromic vasodilation and neurogenic plasma extravasation. Naunyn-Schmiedeberg's Arch Pharmacol 1979;310:175–183.
38. Dikranian K, Loesch A, Burnstock G. Localization of nitric oxide synthase and its colocalization with vasoactive peptides in coronary and femoral arteries. An electron microscope study. J Anat 1994;184:583–590.
39. Gerard NP, Garraway LA, Eddy RL Jr, Shows TB, Iijima H, Paquet JL, Gerard C. Human Substance P receptor (NK-1): organization of the gene, chromosome localization, and functional expression of cDNA clones. Biochemistry 1991;30:10,640–10,646.
40. Takeda Y, Chou KB, Takeda J, Sachais BS, Krause JE. Molecular cloning, structural characterization and functional expression of the human Substance P receptor. Biochem Biophys Res Commun 1991;179:1232–1240.
41. Chester AH, O'Neil GS, Tadjkarimi S, Palmer RM, Moncada S, Yacoub MH. The role of nitric oxide in mediating endothelium dependent relaxations in the human epicardial coronary artery. Int J Cardiol 1990;29:305–309.
42. Von der Weid PY, Beny JL. Effect of Ca^{2+} ionophores on membrane potential of pig coronary artery endothelial cells. Am J Physiol 1992;262:H1823–H1831.
43. Cowley AW, Switzer SJ, Guinn MM. Evidence and quantification of the vasopressin arterial pressure control system in the dog. Circ Res 1980;46:58–67.
44. Rap ZM, Chwalbinska-Moneta J. Vasopressin concentration in the blood during acute short-term intracranial hypertension in cats. Adv Neurol 1978;20:381–388.
45. Wang BC, Share L, Guyton JT, Kumura T. Changes in vasopressin concentration in pressure and cerebrospinal fluid in response to hemorrhage in anesthetized dogs. Neuroendocrinology 1981;33:61–66.
46. Wilson MF, Brackett DJ, Hinshow LB, Tompkins P, Archer LT, Benjamin BA. Vasopressin release during sepsis and septic shock in baboons and dogs. Surg Gynecol Obstet 1981;153:869–872.
47. Stallone JN. Role of endothelium in sexual dimorphism in vasopressin-induced contraction of rat aorta. Am J Physiol 1993;265:H2073–H2080.
48. Cosentino F, Sill JC, Katusic ZS. Endothelial L-arginine pathway and relaxations to vasopressin in canine basilar artery. Am J Physiol 1993;264:H413–H418.
49. Evora PR, Pearson PJ, Schaff HV. Arginine vasopressin induces endothelium-dependent vasodilatation of the pulmonary artery. V1-receptor-mediated production of nitric oxide. Chest 1993;103:1241–1245.
50. Simon JS, Brody MJ, Kasson BG. Characterization of a vasopressin-like peptide in rat and bovine blood vessels. Am J Physiol 1992;262:H799–H804.

51. Loesch A, Tomlinson A, Burnstock G. Localization of arginine vasopressin in endothelial cells of rat pulmonary artery. Anat Embryol 1991;183:129–134.
52. Cai WQ, Bodin P, Loesch A, Sexton A, Burnstock G. Endothelium of human umbilical blood vessels: ultrastructural immunolocalization of neuropeptides. J Vasc Res 1993;30:340–355.
53. Loesch A, Bodin P, Burnstock G. Colocalization of endothelin, vasopressin, and serotonin in cultured endothelial cells of rabbit aorta. Peptides 1991;12:1095–1103.
54. Katusic ZS. Endothelial L-arginine pathway and regional cerebral reactivity to vasopressin. Am J Physiol 1992;262:H1557–H1563.
55. Ostrowski NL, Lolait SJ, Young WS 3rd. Cellular localization of vasopressin V1a receptor messenger ribonucleic acid in adult male rat brain, pineal, and brain vasculature. Endocrinology 1994;135:1511–1528.
56. Emori T, Hirata Y, Ohta K, Kanno K, Eguchi S, Imai T, Shichiri M, Marumo F. Cellular mechanism of endothelin-1 release by angiotensin and vasopressin. Hypertension 1991;18:165–170.
57. Martinez MC, Vila JM, Aldasoro M, Medina P, Flor B, Lluch S. Relaxation of human isolated mesenteric arteries by vasopressin and desmopressin. Br J Pharmacol 1994;113:419–424.
58. Thien-Khai HV, Hung DT, Wheaton VI, Coughlin SR. Molecular cloning of a functional thrombin receptor reveals a novel proteolytic mechanism of receptor activation. Cell 1991;64:1057–1068.
59. Tesfamariam B, Allen GT, Norman-Din D, Antonaccio MJ. Involvement of the "tethered ligand" receptor in thrombin-induced endothelium-mediated relaxations. Am J Physiol 1993;265:H1744–H1749.
60. Glusa E, Paintz M. Relaxant and contractile responses of porcine pulmonary arteries to a thrombin receptor activating peptide (TRAP). Naunyn-Schmiedeberg's Arch Pharm 1994;349:431–436.
61. Kruse H-J, Mayerhofer C, Siess W, Weber PC. Thrombin receptor-activating peptide sensitizes the human endothelial thrombin receptor. Am J Physiol 1995;268:C36–C44.
62. Kruse HJ, Negrescu EV, Weber PC, Siess W. Thrombin-induced Ca^{2+} influx and protein tyrosine phosphorylation in endothelial cells is inhibited by herbimycin A. Biochem Biophys Res Comm 1994;202:1651–1656.
63. Moncada S, Palmer RMJ, Higgs EA. Nitric oxide-physiology, pathophysiology, and pharmacology. Pharmacol Rev 1991;43:109–142.
64. Singer HA, Peach MJ. Calcium and endothelial-mediated vascular smooth muscle relaxation in rabbit aorta. Hypertension 1982;4(Suppl. 2):19–25.
65. Long CJ, Stone TW. The release of endothelium-derived relaxant factor is calcium dependent. Blood Vessels 1985;22:205–208.
66. Luckhoff A, Busse R. Increased free calcium in endothelial cells under stimulation with adenine nucleotides. J Cell Physiol 1986;126:414–420.
67. Peach MH, Singer HA, Izzo NJ, Loeb AL. Role of calcium in endothelium-dependent relaxation of arterial smooth muscle. Am J Cardiol 1987;59:35A–43A.
68. Knowles RG, Palacios M, Palmer RMJ, Moncada S. Formation of nitric oxide from L-arginine in the central nervous system: a transduction mechanism for stimulation of the soluble guanylate cyclase. Proc Natl Acad Sci USA 1989;86:5159–5162.
69. Cannell MB, Sage SO. Bradykinin-evoked changes in cytosolic calcium and membrane currents in cultured bovine pulmonary artery endothelial cells. J Physiol Lond 1989;419:555–568.
70. Colden-Stanfield M, Schilling WP, Ritchie AK, Eskin SG, Navarro LT, Kunze DL. Bradykinin-induced increases in cytosolic calcium and ionic currents in cultured aortic bovine endothelial cells. Circ Res 1987;61:632–640.
71. Luckhoff A, Zeh R, Busse R. Desensitization of the bradykinin-induced rise in intracellular free calcium in cultured endothelial cells. Pflugers Archiv Eur J Physiol 1988;412:654–658.
72. Grynkiewicz G, Poenie M, Tsien RY. A new generation of Ca^{2+} indicators with greatly improved fluorescence properties. J Biol Chem 1985;260:3440–3450.
73. Song J, Davis MJ. Chloride and cation currents activated by bradykinin in coronary venular endothelial cells. Am J Physiol 1994;267:H2508–H2515.
74. Dolor RJ, Hurwitz LM, Mirza Z, Strauss HC, Whorton AR. Regulation of extracellular calcium entry in endothelial cells: role of the intracellular calcium pool. Am J Physiol 1992;262:C171–C181.
75. Morgan-Boyd R, Stewart JM, Vavrek RJ, Hassid A. Effects of bradykinin and angiotensin II on intracellular Ca^{2+} dynamics in endothelial cells. Am J Physiol 1987;253:C588–C598.
76. Schilling WP. Effect of membrane potential on cytosolic calcium of bovine aortic endothelial cells. Am J Physiol 1989;257:H778–H784.
77. Luckhoff A, Clapham DE. Inositol 1,3,4,5-tetrakisphosphate activates an endothelial Ca^{2+}-permeable channel. Nature Lond 1992;355:356–358.

78. Merrit JE, Rink TJ. The effects of substance P and carbachol on inositol tris- and tetrakisphosphate formation and cytosolic free Ca^{2+} in rat parotid acinar cells. J Biol Chem 1987;262:14,912–14,916.
79. Bossu JL, Elhamdani A, Feltz A, Tanzi F, Aunis D, Thierse D. Voltage-gated Ca entry in isolated bovine capillary endothelial cells: instance of a new type of BAY K 8644-sensitive channel. Pflugers Archiv. Eur J Physiol 1992;420:200–207.
80. Mendelowitz D, Bacal K, Kunze D. Bradykinin-activated calcium influx pathway in bovine aortic endothelial cells. Am J Physiol 1992;262:H942–H948.
81. Himmel HM, Strauss HC. Agonist-induced changes in Ca^{2+} and membrane currents in bovine aortic endothelial cells (BAEC). Biophys J 1993;64:A391 (abstract).
82. Sharma NR, Davis MJ. Substance P-induced calcium entry in endothelial cells is secondary to depletion of intracellular stores. Am J Physiol 1995;268:H962–H973.
83. Song J, Zawieja DC, Granger HJ, Goodman A, Davis MJ. Multiple ionic mechanisms activated by bradykinin in coronary venular endothelial cells. Endothelium 1996;4:29–40.
84. Mehrke G, Daut J. The electrical response of cultured guinea-pig coronary endothelial cells to endothelium-dependent vasodilators. J Physiol Lond 1990;430:251–272.
85. Mehrke G, Pohl U, Daut J. Effects of vasoactive agonists on the membrane potential of cultured bovine aortic and guinea-pig coronary endothelium. J Physiol Lond 1991;439:277–299.
86. Bény JL. Effect of Substance P on the membrane potential of coronary arterial endothelial cells in situ. Agents Actions 1990;31:317–320.
87. Brunet PC, Bény JL. Substance P and bradykinin hyperpolarize pig coronary artery endothelial cells in primary culture. Blood Vessels 1989;26:228–234.
88. Sharma NR, Davis MJ. Mechanism of substance P-induced hyperpolarization of porcine coronary artery endothelial cells. Am J Physiol 1994;266:H156–H164.
89. Takeda K, Schini V, Stoeckel H. Voltage-activated potassium, but not calcium currents in cultured bovine aortic endothelial cells. Pflugers Arch 1987;410:385–393.
90. Olesen SP, Davies PF, Clapham DE. Muscarinic-activated K current in bovine aortic endothelial cells. Circ Res 1988;62:1059–1064.
91. Himmel HM, Whorton AR, Strauss HC. Intracellular calcium, currents, and stimulus-response coupling in endothelial cells. Hypertension 1993;21:112–127.
92. Lansman JB, Hallam TJ, Rink TJ. Single stretch-activated ion channels in vascular endothelial cells as mechanotransducers. Nature 1987;325:811–813.
93. Johns A, Lategan TW, Lodge NJ, Ryan US, van Breemen C, Adams DJ. Calcium entry through receptor-operated channels in bovine pulmonary artery endothelial cells. Tissue Cell 1987;19:733–745.
94. Bregestovski PD, Ryan US. Voltage-gated and receptor-mediated ionic currents in the membrane of endothelial cells. J Mol Cell Cardiol 1989;21(Suppl. 1):103–108.
95. Hoyer J, Popp R, Meyer J, Galla HJ, Gogelein H. Angiotensin II, vasopressin and GTP[gamma-S] inhibit inward-rectifying K^+ channels in porcine cerebral capillary endothelial cells. J Membr Biol 1991;123:55–62.
96. Adams DJ, Barakeh J, Laskey R, van Breemen C. Ion channels and regulation of intracellular calcium in vascular endothelial cells. FASEB J 1989;3:2389–2400.
97. Colden-Stanfield M, Schilling WP, Possani LD, Kunze DL. Bradykinin-induced potassium current in cultured bovine aortic endothelial cells. J Membr Biol 1990;116:227–238.
98. Himmel HM, Rasmusson RL, Strauss HC. Agonist-induced changes of and membrane currents in single bovine aortic endothelial cells. Am J Physiol 1994;267:C1338–C1350.
99. Sauve R, Chahine M, Tremblay J, Hamet P. Single-channel analysis of the electrical response of bovine aortic endothelial cells to bradykinin stimulation: contribution of a Ca^{2+}-dependent K^+ channel. J Hypertens 1990;8: suppl. 7, S193–S201.
100. Vaca L, Schilling WP, Kunze DL. G-protein mediated regulation of a Ca^{2+}-dependent K^+ channel in cultured vascular endothelial cells. Pflugers Archiv 1992;422:66–74.
101. Fichtner H, Frobe U, Busse R, Kohlhardt M. Single nonselective cation channels and Ca^{2+}-activated K^+ channels in aortic endothelial cells. J Membr Biol 1987;98:125–133.
102. Bregestovski P, Bakhramov A, Danilov S, Moldobaeva A, Takeda K. Histamine-induced inward currents in cultured endothelial cells from human umbilical vein. Br J Pharmacol 1988;95:429–436.
103. Takeda K, Klepper M. Voltage-dependent and agonist-activated ionic currents in vascular endothelial cells: a review. Blood Vessels 1990;27:169–183.
104. Groschner K, Kukovetz WR. Voltage-sensitive chloride channels of large conductance in the membrane of pig aortic endothelial cells. Pflugers Arch 1992;421:209–217.

105. Olesen SP, Bundgaard M. Chloride-selective channels of large conductance in bovine aortic endothelial cells. Acta Physiol Scand 1992;144:191–198.
106. Vaca L, Kunze DL. cAMP-dependent phosphorylation modulates voltage gating in an endothelial Cl^- channel. Am J Physiol 1993;264:C370–C375.
107. Klockner U. Intracellular calcium ions activate a low-conductance chloride channel in smooth-muscle cells isolated from human mesenteric artery. Pflugers Archiv Eur J Physiol 1993;424:231–237.
108. White CR, Brock TA. Calcium-mobilizing agonists stimulate anion fluxes in cultured endothelial cells from human umbilical vein. J Membr Biol 1994;142:171–179.
109. Mason MJ, Garcia-Rodriquez C, Grinstein S. Coupling between intracellular Ca^{2+} stores and the Ca^{2+} permeability of the plasma membrane. J Biol Chem 1991;266:20,856–20,862.
110. Hoth M, Penner R. Depletion of intracellular calcium stores activates a calcium current in mast cells. Nature Lond 1992;355:353–356.
111. Schilling WP, Cabello OA, Rajan L. Depletion of the inositol 1,4,5-trisphosphate-sensitive intracellular Ca^{2+} store in vascular endothelial cells activates the agonist-sensitive Ca^{2+}-influx pathway. Biochem J 1992;284:521–530.
112. Gericke M, Droogmans G, Nilius B. Thapsigargin discharges intracellular calcium stores and induces transmembrane currents in human endothelial cells. Pflugers Archiv 1993;422:552–557.
113. Vaca L, Kunze DL. Depletion and refilling of intracellular Ca^{2+} stores induce oscillations of Ca^{2+} current. Am J Physiol 1993;264:H1319–H1322.
114. Vaca L, Kunze DL. Depletion of intracellular Ca^{2+} stores activates a Ca^{2+}-selective channel in vascular endothelium. Am J Physiol 1994;267:C920–C925.
115. Adams DJ, Lategan TW, Lodge NJ, van Breemen C. Inward rectifying K^+ channels and thrombin-activated cation channels in cultured endothelial cells from bovine pulmonary artery. J Physiol Lond 1987;394:45P (abstract).
116. Parekh AB, Terlau H, Stuhmer W. Depletion of $InsP_3$ stores activates a Ca^{2+} and K^+ current by means of a phosphatase and a diffusible messenger. Nature Lond 1993;364:814–818.
117. Randriamampita C, Tsien RY. Emptying of intracellular Ca^{2+} stores releases a novel small messenger that stimulates Ca^{2+} influx. Nature Lond 1993;364:809–814.
118. Lepple-Wienhues A, Cahalan MD. Two different calcium-influx pathways in melanoma cells are cell cycle-dependent. Biophys J 1995;68:A122 (abstract).
119. Blennerhassett MG, Kannan MS, Garfield RE. Density-dependent hyperpolarization in cultured aortic smooth muscle cells. Am J Physiol 1989;256:(Heart and Circulatory Physiology 25) C644–C651.
120. Falcone JC, Kuo L, Meininger GA. Endothelial cell calcium increases during flow-induced dilation in isolated arterioles. Am J Physiol 1993;264:H653–H659.

3 Non-cGMP, Paracrine Effects of Nitric Oxide in the Vasculature

Nancy L. Kanagy, PHD,
Rajabrata Sarkar, MD, PHD,
Stephanie W. Watts, PHD,
and R. Clinton Webb, PHD

CONTENTS

REGULATION OF VASCULAR FUNCTION BY NITRIC OXIDE (NO)

Nitric oxide (NO) is as an important endogenous modulator of blood vessel function *(1,2)*. NO released from vascular endothelial cells acts in a paracrine fashion on adjacent vascular smooth muscle cells (VSMC) to activate soluble guanylyl cyclase and generate cyclic guanosine 3',5' monophosphate (cGMP) *(2)*. cGMP, in turn, mediates many of NO-mediated actions in VSMC. However, a number of cGMP-independent effects have been observed following NO stimulation, indicating that activation of guanylyl cyclase accounts for only a portion of the effects of NO.

cGMP-dependent effects are mediated by activation of cGMP-dependent protein kinase *(2)*. In contrast, cGMP-independent effects are mediated through nitrosylation *(3,4)* and/or adenosine diphosphate (ADP)-ribosylation *(5–7)* of proteins leading to altered signal transduction and attenuated VSMC contraction and proliferation. This chapter reviews a model of NO-induced modulation of VSMC function through acute cGMP-dependent effects and through chronic cGMP-independent effects. It is proposed that the combination of these two pathways constitutes the total antiproliferative and vasodilatory effects of NO. In this model, NO production acutely elevates cGMP levels, leading to vascular relaxation. By contrast, chronic elevation of NO production inhibits

From: *Contemporary Endocrinology: Endocrinology of the Vasculature*
Edited by: J. R. Sowers Humana Press Inc., Totowa, NJ

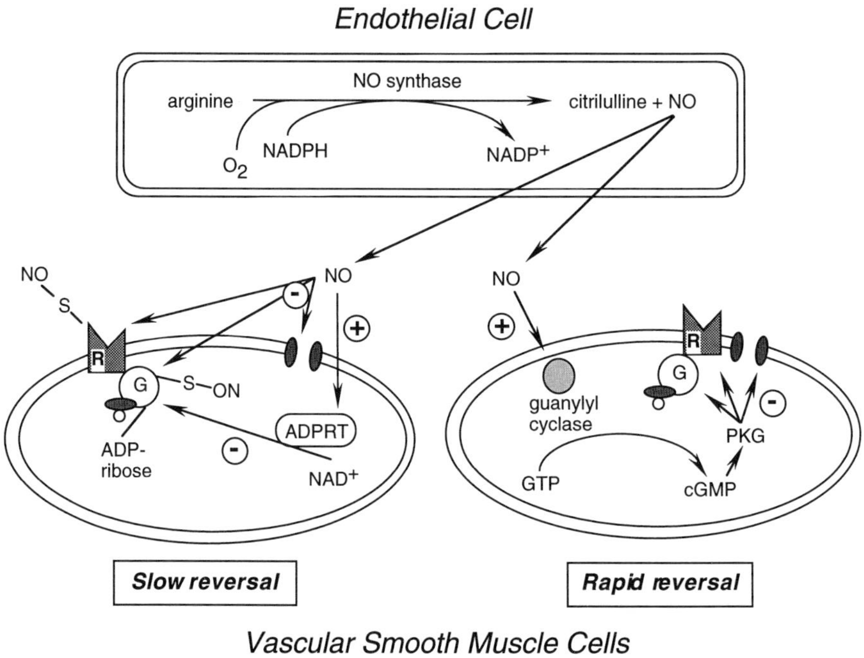

Fig. 1. Schematic depicting the possible ways NO can regulate vascular contractility. The left cell illustrates the possible cGMP-independent actions of NO that would result in decreased responsiveness to contractile agonists. These actions include the addition of a nitrosyl group to a thiol residue (*S*-nitrosylation) on receptor proteins (R), *S*-nitrosylation of G proteins (G), direct inhibition of channels proteins (*S*-nitrosylation), and activation of endogenous ADP-ribosyltransferases (ADPRT) to stimulate ADP-ribosylation and inhibition of G proteins. These covalent modifications are less slowly reversed than the modifications activated by cGMP and will persist in the absence of NO. The right cell depicts cGMP-dependent actions. These affects are mediated through activation of a cGMP-dependent protein kinase, which phosphorylates G proteins, receptors, and channel proteins.

protein expression, stimulates production of prostaglandins (PG), depresses G-protein activity, elevates K^+ channel activity, decreases Ca^{2+} channel activity, inhibits gap junctions, and suppresses cellular proliferation. Thus, acute NO production regulates moment-to-moment blood flow, whereas chronic NO generation leads to a generalized dampening of vascular reactivity through persistent covalent modifications of signal transduction proteins. Conversely, damage to endothelial cells or pharmacological inhibition of NO production elevates VSMC proliferation and reactivity. This hypothesis is depicted in Fig. 1 and is discussed as it relates to two general areas: receptor signaling resulting in vasodilation/vasoconstriction and VSMC proliferation. Specifically, this chapter discusses cGMP-independent effects defined as effects that occur under any of the following conditions:

1. In the absence of increased cGMP;
2. In the presence of guanylyl cyclase inhibitors;
3. In guanylyl cyclase-deficient cells;
4. In the presence of cGMP-dependent protein kinase inhibitors; or
5. Cannot be mimicked by cGMP analogs.

EFFECTS OF NO ON CONTRACTILITY AND FUNCTION

Nitrosylation of Intracellular Proteins

S-Nitrosylation by NO has been implicated in the regulation of several enzymes *(3)*. This posttranslational modification is initiated by oxidation of NO to form NO^+. NO^+ can then react with thiol residues to form RS-NOs. These RS-NOs are susceptible to the heterologous transfer of NO^+ to other sulfhydryl groups in target proteins and the formation of more stable covalent linkages *(4,8)*. This alteration is postulated to be the mechanism responsible for NO inhibition of N-methyl-D-aspartate (NMDA) receptors *(4)*, NO inhibition of adenylyl cyclase *(9)*, and NO inactivation of protein kinase C (PKC) *(10)*. The covalent linkage is reversible when NO levels are no longer elevated *(8)*.

Evidence indicates that this may be one way NO regulates cellular function. Incubation of isolated G proteins with NO stimulates guanosine triphosphatase (GTPase) activity in both heterotrimeric G proteins *(11)* and small intracellular G proteins *(12,13)*. This activation, in turn, leads to downregulation of G_i and eventual decreased GTPase activity *(11)*; this mechanism may mediate NO inhibition of Gi signaling pathways as NO treatment decreases mastoparan-stimulated Ca^{2+} transients and attenuates cellular response to endothelin *(14)*. These effects are cGMP-independent and appear to depend on *S*-nitrosylation and inactivation of G_i *(14)*. It is not clear if endogenous NO stimulates this pathway but in vitro observations indicate that a cGMP-independent modification of G proteins by NO can inhibit signal transduction in VSMC *(15)*.

NO activation of K_{Ca} *(16)* also appears to depend on cGMP-independent *S*-nitrosylation of a cysteine residue in the channel protein *(4)*, although the contribution of this mechanism to NO relaxation has not yet been described. In addition, NO nitrosylates several other proteins on both tyrosine and cysteine residues *(17)*. Nitrosylation can activate *(11)* or inhibit *(4)* enzyme activity and appears to contribute to the final cellular response in multiple tissues.

ADP-Ribosylation of Intracellular Proteins

Another cGMP-independent way that NO regulates enzyme function is through ADP-ribosylation. ADP-ribosylation involves the transfer of ADP-ribose from NAD^+ to an amino acid residue. Ribosylation of specific amino acid residues is primarily catalyzed by ribosyltransferases. Individual enzymes within this family have great specificity. For example, the enzyme present in pertussis toxin only ribosylates the thiol group of a cysteine residue of $G\alpha_i$ and some subtypes of $G\alpha_o$ *(18)*, whereas cholera toxin modifies only the arginine residue of $G\alpha_s$ *(19)*. Similar enzymes are also present in eukaryotic cells. These endogenous enzymes mono-ADP-ribosylate cellular proteins, including membrane-bound G proteins *(20,21)*, and may be endogenous regulators of G-protein activity *(20)*.

NO stimulates ADP-ribosylation of intracellular proteins by activating endogenous ADP-ribosyltransferases *(6)*. NO-modification of glyderaldehyde 3-phosphate dehydrogenase (GAPDH) is not true ADP-ribosylation, but involves the addition of NAD to a NO-nitrosylated cysteine residue *(3)*. Indeed, true ADP-ribosylation in both retinal *(21)* and neural *(22)* tissues has been reported. In addition, NO decreases the amount of pertussis toxin substrate in a variety of tissues *(22,23)*, suggesting that NO stimulates endogenous ADP-ribosylation and competes for substrate with pertussis toxin. Inhibitors of endogenous enzymes mediating ADP-ribosylation such as aminobenzamide or

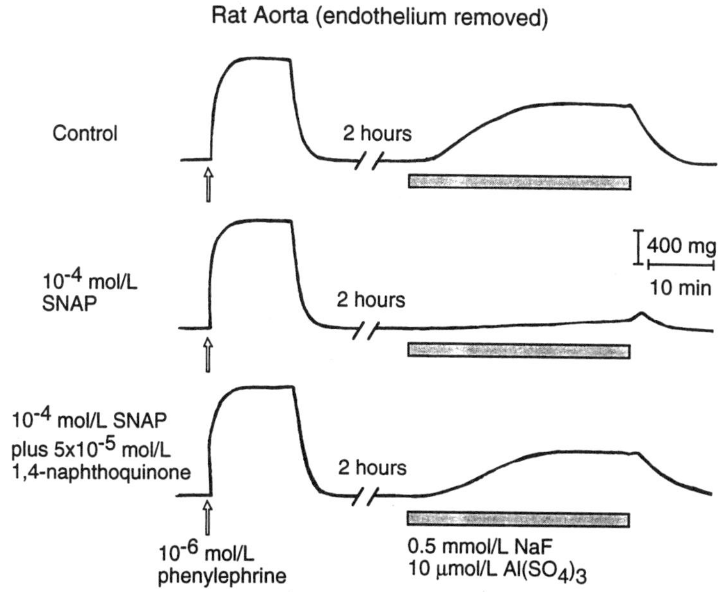

Fig. 2. Reversal of NO-induced inhibition of aluminum fluoride contractile response by an ADP-ribosyltransferase antagonist (1,4-naphthoquinone). Three strips of the same rat aorta (endothelium removed) were placed in separate muscle baths. Following equilibration, the strips were made to contract in response to 10^{-6} mol/L phenylephrine (concentration producing a maximal response). After washout of the alpha-adrenergic agonist, each strip was incubated for 2 h in buffer containing the indicated drugs (top: control; middle: 10^{-4} mol/L SNAP [*S*-nitroso-*N*-acetylpenicillamine]; bottom: 10^{-4} mol/L SNAP plus 5×10^{-5} mol/L 1,4-naphthoquinone). Following the 2-h incubation, the strips were rinsed with normal buffer and then stimulated with 5×10^{-4} mol/L NaF; 10^{-5} mol/L $Al(SO_4)_3$. Incubation with the ADP-ribosyltransferase inhibitor 1,4-naphthoquinone reversed the NO-induced attenuation of contractile responses to AlF_4^-. NO was derived from SNAP (*see* ref. *15* for additional details).

1,4-naphthoquinone, decrease NO-induced inhibition of contraction in vascular tissue (Fig. 2) *(15)*. In hippocampal cells, NO stimulates ADP-ribosylation and decreases pertussis toxin substrate, indicating G_i ADP-ribosylation by NO may be involved in long-term potentiation of neural transmission *(22)*. NO regulates protein synthesis *(11)* and inhibits G_i activation by ligand-bound receptors *(14)*. These observations indicate that activation of endogenous ADP-ribosyltransferases may mediate a portion of the effects of NO.

The most recent biochemical studies of ADP-ribosylation of GAPDH have found that the addition is actually the second step of an *S*-nitrosylation reaction. *S*-nitrosylation of a cysteine residue provides a target for auto-ADP-ribosylation and the R–S–NO linkage is an intermediate step in the covalent addition of ADP-ribose to a target protein *(4,5)*. NO has two ways of inhibiting contractility. First, acute decreases in NO lead to a loss of cGMP production and elevated tone. Over time, however, a reversal of NO-dependent covalent linkages to G proteins and other intracellular proteins leads to increased sensitivity to contractile agents and contributes to the elevated vascular tone apparent when NO is decreased. This is supported by the observation of increased sensitivity to receptor agonists and to direct G protein stimulation (mastoparan and AlF_4^-) in vascular tissue from hypertensive rats *(24)*. It is also supported by the observation that pertussis toxin-

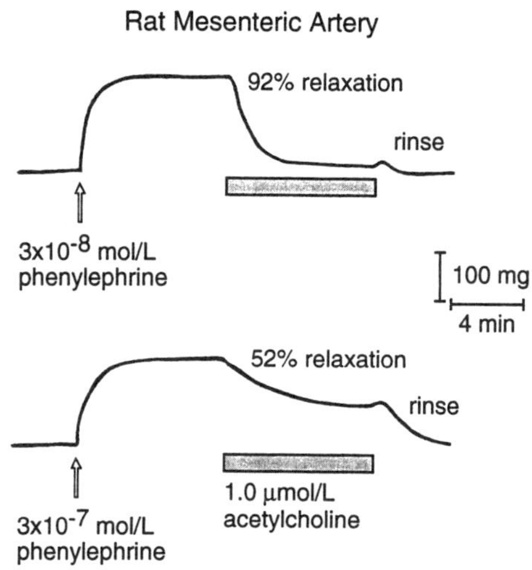

Fig. 3. Heptanol inhibits acetylcholine-induced relaxation in rat mesenteric artery. An isolated strip of rat mesenteric artery relaxed in response to Ach (10^{-6} mol/L) following contraction induced by phenylephrine (3×10^{-8} mol/L, a concentration producing a half-maximal response; top). Treatment with the gap junction inhibitor, heptanol (10^{-3} mol/L), attenuated the relaxation to Ach by approx 50% (bottom). Note that in the presence of heptanol, a higher concentration of phenylephrine was required to produce a response that was near the half-maximum effect. These observations suggest that gap junctional communication is essential for the dilator activity of acetylcholine (*see* ref. *33* for a more detailed explanation).

stimulated ADP-ribosylation in vivo selectively lowers blood pressure in spontaneously hypertensive rats (SHR) compared to Wistar-Kyoto (WKY) rats *(25,26)* and decreases the pressor responses to vasoconstrictors *(27–29)*.

Existing evidence therefore provides compelling support for the hypothesis that inhibition of NO production could cause increased vascular reactivity through long-lasting cGMP-independent modifications of signaling pathways. Conversely, these long-lasting modifications induced by NO may act in the normal individual as a balancing vasodilator force opposing vasoconstrictor stimuli.

Effects of NO on Gap Junction Conductance

An additional transduction mechanism that may be regulated by NO is signaling between cells. For NO to exert such a profound inhibitory effect on vascular contractility and yet be a short-lived and easily metabolized substance, NO may rely on cellular mechanisms that allow propagation of a message. Gap junctional communication is a likely explanation. Endothelial cell coupling has been demonstrated in the arterioles *(30)* and coronary arteries *(31)*, and there is bidirectional electrical communication between VSMC and endothelial cells *(31)*. Accordingly, cGMP stimulated by NO, which has a small effective diffusion radius, is able to traverse the gap junction and relay the message of VSMC relaxation *(32)*. Further, acetylcholine (ACh)-induced relaxation in the rat mesenteric artery is significantly reduced by the gap junctional inhibitor heptanol (Fig. 3) *(33)*. However, the dependence of NO on gap junctional communication is complicated by the ability of multiple second messengers (including cGMP) to modulate junctional conductance as well as to travel through gap junctions.

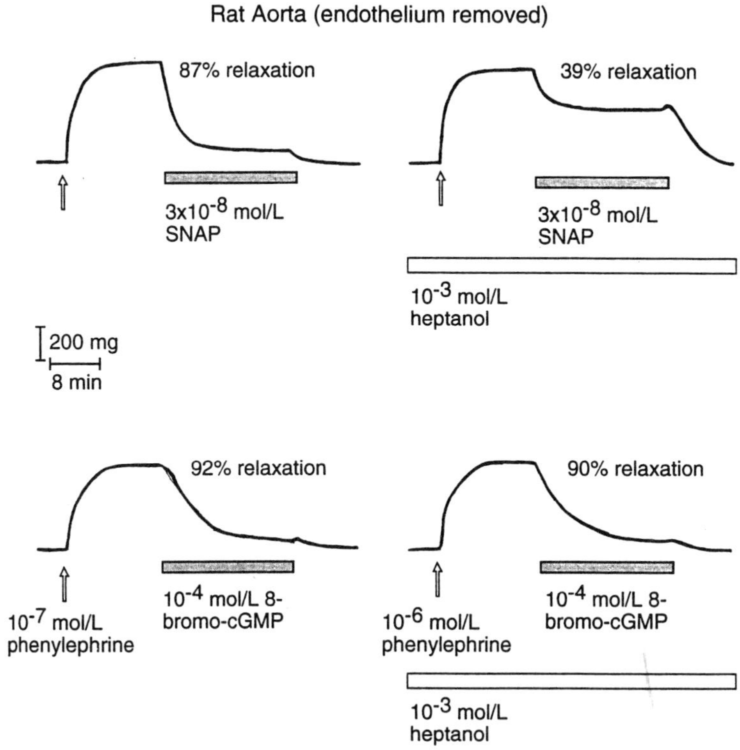

Fig. 4. Heptanol inhibits relaxation responses to SNAP but not 8-bromo-cGMP in rat aorta. Top: Following contraction induced by phenylephrine (10^{-7} mol/L; concentration producing a half-maximal response), SNAP (3×10^{-8} mol/L) induced a relaxation of approx 87% (left). Heptanol (10^{-3} mol/L) inhibited the relaxation response to SNAP (right). Note that a higher concentration of phenylephrine was used to produce a similar magnitude of force in the presence of heptanol compared to that in the absence of the inhibitor (control response). Bottom: Relaxation responses to 8-bromo-cGMP (10^{-4} mol/L) were not sensitive to the gap junction inhibitor, heptanol (compare left and right). These observations are consistent with the hypothesis that NO has inhibitory effects in vascular smooth muscle that are dependent on gap junctional communication and this inhibitory effect is not mediated by the second messenger, cGMP (*see* ref. *44* for additional details).

Connexins are the proteins that form gap junctions and several different connexins are known to exist *(34)*. In VSMC, connexin43 and connexin40 have been found *(34–36)*. The C-terminus of connexin43 contains a consensus sequence for cGMP-dependent kinase *(37)*. 8-Br-cGMP modestly decreased junctional conductance in cardiac myocytes containing connexin43 *(38–40)*. By contrast, 8-Br-cGMP did not alter junctional conductance in MDCK cells (connexin43) *(41)*, kidney cells (connexin45) *(42)*, axons *(43)*, and, importantly, A7r5 VSMC *(35)*. We found that 8-Br-cGMP-induced relaxation in the denuded rat aorta is minimally affected by octanol and heptanol (Fig. 4) *(44)*. Moreover, inhibition of SNAP-induced relaxation in the aorta by the gap junctional inhibitor sucrose is not affected by methylene blue, an inhibitor of soluble guanylate cyclase (Fig. 4). Thus, these studies suggest that NO depends on gap junctional communication to cause VSMC relaxation and this event is largely independent of cGMP production.

NO, Prostaglandins, and Membrane Hyperpolarization

ACh is often used as an agonist to stimulate the generation of NO from vascular preparations with intact endothelium. In addition to stimulating endothelial NO synthase, muscarinic agonist stimulates the release of endothelium-derived PGs and a factor that hyperpolarizes the VSMC *(45)*. To avoid complicated interpretations, an inhibitor of cyclooxygenase (CO) and depolarizing conditions (respectively) are used in experiments characterizing the vasodilator actions of NO in endothelium-intact preparations. Although these procedures allow for consistent observations about how NO acts, they interfere with at least two actions of NO that are independent of cGMP.

Membrane hyperpolarization in response to ACh in endothelium-intact vascular preparations may be caused either by NO or by an as yet unidentified endothelium-derived hyperpolarizing factor (EDHF). As mentioned, the effect of NO to cause membrane hyperpolarization has been reported in dispersed aortic VSMC *(16)*. This action of NO is mediated by activation of K_{Ca} and is not related to elevated cGMP levels. It appears to be a direct action of NO on the channel. This cGMP-independent action of NO, as well as the hyperpolarizing effect of EDHF, are not present in arterial preparations made to contract with a depolarizing stimulus.

Similarly, the practice of using CO inhibitors may mask an important effect of NO to stimulate the production of PGs by the endothelium *(45,46)*. Whether this effect of NO to stimulate PG production in the endothelium is important in the regulation of vascular tone is not readily apparent. Stimulation of PG synthesis in the endothelium by NO contributes to attenuated dilator and augmented constrictor responses in aortic segments from SHR *(45,47)*. In hypertensive humans *(48)*, the attenuated vasodilator activity to ACh is normalized by CO blockade with indomethacin. Using CO inhibitors masks this cGMP-independent effect of NO on PG synthesis and thus, the subsequent smooth muscle effects of the eicosinoids.

EFFECTS OF NO ON CELL PROLIFERATION AND MIGRATION

Augmentation of NO production in vivo inhibits the accumulation of VSMC in experimental arterial lesions in a number of models of vessel injury including balloon catheter injury *(49)*, hypercholesterolemia *(50)*, and arterial vein grafting *(51)*. These in vivo findings suggest that NO may inhibit VSMC proliferation and migration, two processes central to the development of neointimal hyperplasia after vessel injury.

NO activates guanylyl cyclase in both intact vessels and cultured VSMC, thereby elevating levels of intracellular cGMP, a second messenger implicated in relaxation of VSMC by NO. Pharmacologic donors of NO inhibit the proliferation of cultured VSMC, and similar inhibition is seen with analogs of cGMP, such as 8-bromo-cGMP, suggesting that intracellular cGMP may be responsible for the effects of NO *(52)*. However, there are other intracellular proteins that directly interact with NO, and several of these are involved in regulation of cell growth. NO binds to intracellular iron and this process can inactivate iron-containing enzymes, such as guanylyl cyclase, or it can inhibit iron-containing enzymes, such as ribonucleotide reductase or electron transport enzymes *(53)*.

The role of non-cGMP effects of NO on VSMC proliferation has been demonstrated by using a cell-cycle approach to characterize points in the cell cycle of VSMC where NO inhibits but cGMP does not. This approach has shown that exogenous NO added to cells in S phase inhibits ongoing DNA synthesis, an effect not seen with exogenous cGMP

(54). This cGMP-independent inhibition is consistent with inhibition of the enzyme ribonucleotide reductase, which is the rate-limiting enzyme during DNA synthesis and a known target of NO in other cell types such as macrophages and tumor cells *(53)*. That both NO and exogenous cGMP inhibit VSMC growth when added in G1 phase of the cell cycle does not prove that the inhibitory effects of NO are solely the result of activation of guanylyl cyclase. Ongoing protein synthesis is necessary during G1 phase of the cell cycle, and NO inhibits protein synthesis by directly binding and inhibiting iron-containing enzymes in the mitochondrial electron transport chain *(53)*. Since exogenous NO has been shown to decrease protein synthesis in VSMC *(55)*, it is possible that during the G1 phase NO inhibits growth by simultaneous activation of both cGMP-dependent and independent mechanisms.

NO is the first endogenous substance that inhibits growth in *S* phase—a process that may be important in regulation of proliferation of VSMC that have lost normal G1 mechanisms of growth control. This is particularly relevant to vasoproliferative disorders, as several phenotypes of VSMC have been identified in disease states that have lost normal growth inhibitory mechanisms in G1 phase. For example, smooth muscle cells from genetically hypertensive rats (stroke-prone SHR [SHRSP]) proliferate at an increased rate in culture in comparison to those from normotensive WKY rats and display a paradoxical mitogenic response when treated with the growth inhibitor transforming growth factor-beta (TGF-β), which inhibits mitogenesis in WKY cells *(56)*. Despite this differential response to a growth inhibitor that acts in G1 phase, proliferation and DNA synthesis of SHRSP and WKY cells are similarly inhibited by NO donors *(57)*. NO donors, which directly inhibit VSMC DNA synthesis in *S* phase, provide a mechanism that explains the disparate response to TGF-β and NO.

There is a consistent decrease in endothelial NO production in diabetes, cigaret smoking, hypercholesterolemia, and hypertension *(53)*, conditions known to accelerate both primary atherosclerosis and neointimal hyperplasia following interventions such as coronary bypass grafting. Development of VSMC phenotypes resistant to endogenous growth inhibitors that act in G1 phase, coupled with decreased production of NO, which can act in *S* phase, may contribute to this accelerated atherosclerosis.

Inhibition of VSMC migration may be another mechanism by which NO inhibits neointima formation under physiologic and pathologic conditions *(58)*. To test this hypothesis, the migration of cultured VSMC was examined in the presence of exogenous NO. NO donors inhibited the migration of VSMC in a concentration-dependent fashion. Migration was examined in the presence of hydroxyurea, which inhibits cell proliferation, to ensure that inhibition noted is not caused by inhibition of cell proliferation by NO. Although migration is partially inhibited by exogenous cGMP under similar conditions, non-cGMP mechanisms may also be active in mediating the inhibition of migration seen with NO. These findings delineate another potential mechanism to explain how NO limits development of neointimal hyperplasia following vessel injury, namely inhibition of VSMC migration from the media to the intimal lesion.

SUMMARY

NO has actions in the vasculature that are both cGMP-dependent and -independent. We hypothesize that acute stimulation of endothelium-derived NO above basal levels elevates VSMC cGMP levels, leading to vasodilation. By contrast, chronic elevation of

NO or concentrations of NO active in the basal, unstimulated state inhibit protein expression, stimulate PG production, depress G-protein activity, elevate K^+ channel activity, depress Ca^{2+} activity, inhibit gap junctions, and suppress cellular proliferation. Thus, acute NO production regulates moment-to-moment blood flow and many responses to endocrine and pharmacological agonists. Chronic NO generation leads to a generalized dampening of vascular reactivity through persistent covalent modification of signal transduction proteins.

ACKNOWLEDGMENTS

This work was supported by grants from the American Heart Association and the National Institutes of Health (HL-18575, HL-08892, HL-09099).

REFERENCES

1. Moncada S. Nitric oxide. J Hypertens 1994;12(Suppl. 10):S35–S39.
2. Murad F. The nitric oxide–cyclic GMP signal transduction system for intracellular and intercellular communication. Recent Prog Hormone Res 1994;49:239–248.
3. Mohr S, Stamler JS, Brune B. Mechanism of covalent modification of glyceraldehyde-3-phosphate dehydrogenase at its active site thiol by nitric oxide, peroxynitrite and related nitrosating agents. FEBS Lett 1994;348:223–227.
4. Stamler JS. Redox signaling: nitrosylation and related target interactions of nitric oxide. Cell 1994;78:931–936.
5. Brune B, Dimmeler S, Molina y Vedia L, Lapetina EG. Nitric oxide: a signal for ADP-ribosylation of proteins. Life Sci 1994;54:61–70.
6. Brune B, Lapetina EG. Activation of a cytosolic ADP-ribosyltransferase by nitric oxide-generating agents. J Biol Chem 1989;264:8455–8458.
7. Kanagy NL, Charpie JR, Webb RC. Nitric oxide regulation of ADP-ribosylation of G-proteins in hypertension. Med Hypoth 1995;44:159–164.
8. Lipton SA, Choi YB, Pan AH, Lei AZ, Chen JSV, Sucher NJ, Loscalzo J, Singel DJ, Stamler JS. A redox-based mechanism for the neuroprotective and neurodestructive effects of nitric oxide and related nitroso-compounds. Nature 1993;364:626–632.
9. Duhe RJ, Neilsen MD, Dittman AH, Villacres EC, Choi EJ, Storm JR. Oxidation of critical cysteine residues of type I adenylyl cyclase by o-iodosobenzoate or nitric oxide reversibly inhibits stimulation by calcium and calmodulin. J Biol Chem 1994;269:7290–7296.
10. Gopalakrichna R, Chen AH, Gundimeda U. Nitric oxide and nitric oxide-generating agents induce a reversible inactivation of protein kinase C activity and phorbol ester binding. J Biol Chem 1993;268:27,180–27,185.
11. Lander HM, Sehajpal PK, Novogrodsky A. Nitric oxide signaling: a possible role for G proteins. J Immunology 1993;151:7182–7187.
12. Lander HM, Ogiste JS, Frieda S, Pearce A, Levi R, Novogrodsky A. Nitric oxide-stimulated guanine nucleotide exchange on p21ras in T cells. FASEB J 1995;9:A672 (abstract).
13. Lander HM, Ogiste JS, Pearce SFA, Levi R, Novogrodsky A. Nitric oxide-stimulated guanine nucleotide exchange on p21*ras*. J Biol Chem 1995;270:7017–7020.
14. Goligorsky MS, Tsukahara H, Magazine H, Andersen TT, Malik AB, Bahou WF. Termination of endothelin signaling: role of nitric oxide. J Cell Physiol 1994;158:458–494.
15. Kanagy NL, Charpie JR, Dananberg J, Webb RC. Decreased sensitivity to G protein-mediated contraction in aortic rings after acute exposure to nitric oxide. Am J Physiol 1996; in press.
16. Bolotina VM, Najibi S, Palacino JJ, Pagano PJ, Cohen RA. Nitric oxide directly activates calcium-dependent potassium channels in vascular smooth muscle. Nature 1994;368:850–853.
17. Van der Vliet A, Eiserich JP, O'Neill CA, Halliwell B, Cross CE. Tyrosine modification by reactive nitrogen species: a closer look. Arch Biochem Biophys 1995;319:341–349.
18. Kopf GS, Woolkalis MJ. ADP-ribosylation of G proteins with pertussis toxin. In: Johnson RA, Corbin JD, eds. Adenylate cyclase, G proteins, and guanylyl cyclase. Academic, San Diego, CA, 1991, pp. 257–266.

19. Van Dop C, Tsubokasa M, Bourne HR, Ramachandran R. Amino acid sequence of retinal transducin at the site ADP-ribosylated by cholera toxin. J Biol Chem 1984;259:696–698.
20. Jacobson MK, Loflin PT, Aboul-Ela N, Mingmaung M, Moss J, Jobson EL. Modification of plasma membrane protein cysteine residues by ADP-ribose in vivo. J Biol Chem 1990;265:10,825–10,858.
21. Moss J, Stanley SJ, Nightingale MS, Murtagh JJ Jr., Monaco L, Mishima K, Chen GC, Bliziotes MM, Tsai SC. Molecular and immunological characterization of ADP-ribosylarginine hydrolases. In: Poirier GG, Moreau P, eds. ADP-Ribosylation Reactions. Springer-Verlag, New York, 1992, pp. 225–237.
22. Pozdnyakov N, Lloyd A, Reddy V, Sitaramayya A. Nitric oxide-regulated endogenous ADP-ribosylation of rod outer segment proteins. Biochem Biophys Res Comm 1993;192:610–615.
23. Schuman EM, Meffert MK, Schulman H, Madison DV. An ADP-ribosyltransferase as a potential target for nitric oxide action in hippocampal long-term potentiation. Proc Natl Acad Sci USA 1994;91:11,958–11,962.
24. Sheffler LA, Wink DA, Melillo G, Cox GW. Characterization of nitric oxide-stimulated ADP-ribosylation of various proteins from the mouse macrophage cell line ANA-1 using sodium nitroprusside and the novel nitric oxide- donating compound diethylamine dinitric oxide. J Leukocyte Biol 1995;57:152–159.
25. Kanagy NL, Webb RC. Enhanced vascular reactivity to mastoparan, a G protein activator, in genetically hypertensive rats. Hypertension 1994;23:946–950.
26. Anand-Srivastava MB, Picard S, Thibault C. Altered expression of inhibitory guanine nucleotide regulatory proteins (Gi alpha) in spontaneously hypertensive rats. Am J Hypertens 1991;4:840–843.
27. Tabrizchi R, Triggle CR. Pressor actions of arginine vasopressin in pithed Sprague Dawley, Wistar-Kyoto and spontaneously hypertensive rats before and after treatment with nifedipine or pertussis toxin. J Hypertens 1991;9:813–818.
28. Li XF, Triggle CR. Effects of pertussis and cholera toxins on alpha-adrenoceptor function in rat tail artery: differences in hypertension. Can J Physiol Pharmacol 1993;1:791–799.
29. Triggle CR, Tabrizchi R. Changes in vascular smooth muscle function in hypertension. Chin Med J 1993;106:250–257.
30. Segal, SS, Beny J-L. Intracellular recording and dye transfer in arterioles during blood flow control. Am J Physiol 1992;263:H1–H7.
31. Beny J-L, Pacicca C. Bidirectional electrical communication between smooth muscle and endothelial cells in the pig coronary artery. Am J Physiol 1994;266:H1465–H1472.
32. Christ GJ, Brink PR, Ramanan SV. Dynamic gap junctional communication: a delimiting model for tissue responses. Biophys J 1994;67:1335–1344.
33. Watts SW, Tsai M-L, Loch-Caruso R, Webb RC. Gap junctional communication and vascular smooth muscle reactivity: use of tretraethylammonium chloride. J Vasc Res 1994;31:307–313.
34. Bennett MVL, Barrio LC, Bargiello TA, Spray DC, Hertzberg E, Saez JC. Gap junctions: new tools, new answers, new questions. Neuron 1991;6:305–320.
35. Moore LK, Beyer EC, Burt JM. Characterization of gap junction channels in A7r5 vascular smooth muscle cells. Am J Physiol 1991;260:C975–C981.
36. Beyer EC, Reed KE, Westphale EM, Kanter HD, Larson DM. Molecular cloning and expression rat connexin40, a gap junction protein expressed in vascular smooth muscle. J Membr Biol 1992;127:69–76.
37. Beyer EC, Paul DL, Goodenough DA. Connexin43: a protein from rat heart homologous to a gap junction protein from liver. J Cell Biol 1987;105:2621–2629.
38. Burt JM, Spray DC. Iontropic agents modulate gap junctional conductance between cardiac myocytes. Am J Physiol 1988;254:H1206–H1210.
39. Spray DC, Burt JM. Structure–activity relations of the cardiac gap junction channel. Am J Physiol 1990;258:C195–C205.
40. Takens-Kwak BR, Jongsma HG. Cardiac gap junctions: three distinct single channel conductances and their modulation by phosphorylating treatments. Pflugers Arch 1992;422:198–200.
41. Berthoud VM, Ledbetter MLS, Hertzberg EL, Saez JC. Connexin43 in MDCK cells: regulation by a tumor-promoting phorbol ester and Ca^{2+}. Eur J Cell Biol 1992;57:40–50.
42. Butterweck A, Gergs U, Elfgang C, Willecke K, Traub O. Immunochemical characterization of the gap junction protein connexin45 in mouse kidney and transfected human HeLa cells. J Membr Biol 1994;141:247–256.
43. Perrachia C. Effects of the anesthetics heptanol, halothane and isoflurane on gap junction conductance in crayfish septate axons: a calcium- and hydrogen-independent phenomenon potentiated by caffeine and theophylline, and inhibited by 4-aminopyridine. J Membr Biol 1991;121:67–78.

44. Javid PJ, Watts SW, Webb RC. Inhibition of cGMP-dependent and -independent nitric oxide-induced vasodilation by gap junction inhibitors. J Vasc Res 1996; in press.
45. Vanhoutte PM, Boulanger CM. Endothelium-dependent responses in hypertension. Hypertens Res 1995;18:87–98.
46. Davidge ST, Baker PN, McLaughlin MK, Roberts JM. Nitric oxide produced by endothelial cells increases production of eicosanoids through activation of prostaglandin H synthase. Circ Res 1995;77:274–283.
47. Luscher TF, Vanhoutte PM. Endothelium-dependent contractions to acetylcholine in the aorta of the spontaneously hypertensive rat. Hypertension 1986;8:344–348.
48. Taddei S, Virdis A, Mattei P, Salvetti A. Vasodilatation to acetylcholine in primary and secondary forms of human hypertension. Hypertension 1993;21:929–933.
49. Tarry WC, Makhoul RG. L-Arginine improves endothelium-dependent vasorelaxation and reduces intimal hyperplasia after balloon angioplasty. Arteriosclerosis Thromb 1994;14:938–943.
50. Cooke JP, Singer AH, Tsao P, Zera P, Rowan RA, Billingham ME. Anti-atherogenic effects of L-arginine in the hypercholesterolemic rabbit. J Clin Invest 1992;90:1168–1172.
51. Davies MG, Kim JH, Dalen H, Makhoul RG, Svendsen E, Hagen PO. Reduction of experimental vein graft intimal hyperplasia and preservation of nitric oxide-mediated relaxation by the nitric oxide precursor L-arginine. Surgery 1994;116;557–568.
52. Garg UC, Hassid A. Nitric oxide-generating vasodilators and 8-bromo-cyclic guanosine monophosphate inhibit mitogenesis and proliferation of cultured rat vascular smooth muscle cells. J Clin Invest 1989;83:1774–1777.
53. Moncada S, Higgs A. The L-arginine-nitric oxide pathway. N Engl J Med 1993;329:2002–2012.
54. Sarkar R, Stanley JC, Webb RC. Nitric oxide inhibition of smooth muscle mitogenesis is independent of guanylate cyclase. Hypertension 1994;24:379.
55. Kolpakov V, Gordon D, Kulik TJ. Nitric-oxide generating compounds inhibit total protein and collagen synthesis in cultured vascular smooth muscle cells. Circ Res 1995;76:305–309.
56. Saltis J, Agrotis A, Bobik A. Differential regulation by transforming growth factor-b1 of platelet-derived growth factor-stimulated proliferation of vascular smooth muscle cells from SHR and WKY rats. Clin Exp Pharm Physiol 1992;19:396–399.
57. Shimizu S, Nara Y, Keiser HR. Differences in response between SHRSP and WKY vascular smooth muscle cells to inhibition of cell proliferation by sodium nitroprusside. Clin Exp Hypertens 1991;A13:787–795.
58. Sarkar RJ, Meinberg EG, Stanley JC, Gordon D, Webb RC. Nitric oxide reversibly inhibits the migration of cultured vascular smooth muscle cells. Circ Res 1996; in press.

4 The Endothelin Peptides

Roles in Physiology and Pathophysiology

Ellis R. Levin, MD

Contents

INTRODUCTION

Yanagisawa and colleagues *(1)* isolated a long sought endogenous vasoconstricting peptide family, in part from endothelial cells: This peptide family was named the endothelins (ET). Endothelin-1 (ET-1), ET-2, and ET-3 comprise those peptides produced in a variety of tissues, where they act as modulators of important cell processes. These peptides act through binding to two well-defined classes of transmembrane receptors, ET_A and ET_B, where the stimulation of several signaling pathways leads to their mitogenic, vasoconstricting, and developmental actions. In this chapter, the details of ET synthesis and regulation and action and defined physiologic and pathophysiologic roles are examined. In particular, there is an emphasis on defining the roles of ET-1 as an important vascular hormone.

CELL BIOLOGY OF ET

Isolation of the native ET peptides indicated that many cells can synthesize one or more members of the family, each of which is 21 amino acids in length. Endothelial cells synthesize only the ET-1, but ET-1 is also produced in vascular smooth muscle cells (VSMC), and hence may have a paracrine or autocrine role. ET-1 is also produced by cells in the central nervous system, uterus, liver, kidney, testis, and breast *(2,3)*. ET-1 is rapidly synthesized in response to important stimuli such as hypoxia, ischemia, or shear stress, and is not found in secretory granules within a storage pool in the endothelial cell *(4)*, as is often the situation with peptide hormones. The plasma half-life of ET-1 is about

From: *Contemporary Endocrinology: Endocrinology of the Vasculature*
Edited by: J. R. Sowers Humana Press Inc., Totowa, NJ

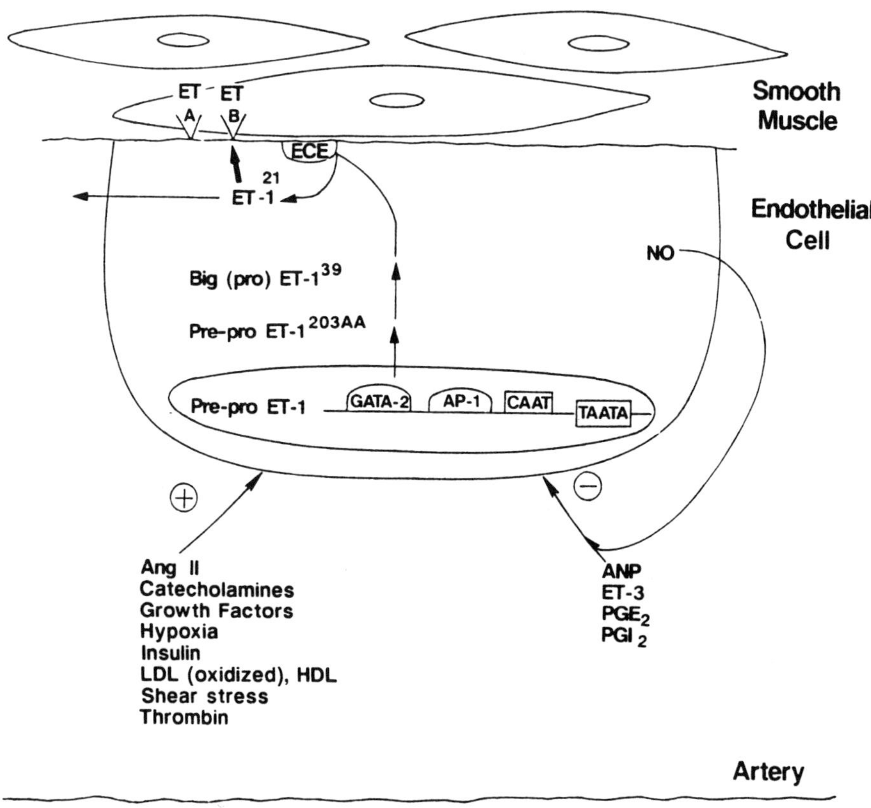

Fig. 1. The synthetic pathway and regulation of ET-1 related proteins produced in endothelial cells. The preproendothelin-1 messenger RNA is transcribed from the ET-1 gene, and is regulated by a variety of peptides and vasoactive substances, in part through GATA-2 and AP-1 protein binding to the ET-1 gene promoter. The 203 amino acid preproendothelin-1 protein is then processed to a 39 amino acid proendothelin-1 protein, Big endothelin-1, which is cleaved by an ECE to the 21 amino acid, ET-1 protein. ET-1 and some Big ET-1 are mainly secreted toward the adjacent smooth muscle layer, and smaller amounts of the peptides are secreted into the blood vessel lumen. CAAT and TAATA, nucleotide sequences essential for transcription; LDL, low-density lipoprotein; PGE2 and PGI2, are prostaglandin E2 and prostacyclin, respectively.

5 min, and the mRNA half-life is approx 15–20 min *(5)*. Because of the rapid turnover time, vascular cells can modulate the concentrations of ET-1 to meet the changing demands necessary for the regulation of vasomotor tone, depending on the stimulus. In the lungs, 80–90% of plasma ET is cleared after the first passage *(6)*, where it is inactivated through hydrolysis induced by the neutral endopeptidase 24.11 (enkephalinase) after the peptide is taken up by VSMC *(7)*.

Several in vitro studies have shown that endothelial cell-derived ET-1 secretion is directed toward the abluminal side, thereby contacting the VSMC layer (Fig. 1) *(8)*. Binding to specific receptors on the VSMC causes vasoconstriction. Because the majority of ET-1 enacts local effects at neighboring cells, ET-1 should be regarded more as a paracrine than an endocrine hormone. Abluminally secreted ET-1 probably does not contribute to the measured concentrations of plasma ET-1. Nevertheless, determining plasma ET-1 concentrations in certain situations is useful. For instance, plasma ET-1 concentrations correlate well with the severity of disease states, such as atherosclerosis *(9)* and congestive heart failure *(10)*.

ET-2 and ET-3

ET-2 is produced predominately within the kidney and intestine but it is also produced in the myocardium, placenta, and uterus; the cells of origin are not clear. ET-2 has no unique physiologic functions (as compared with ET-1), but is equipotent as a vasoconstrictor. Similarly to ET-1, ET-3 circulates in the plasma but its source of origin is not known. ET-3 may play a role as a vasodilator, but its precise role in vascular physiology is undefined. ET-3 has been found in high concentrations in the brain *(11)*, where it may regulate vasopressin production and secretion after an osmotic stimulus. ET-3 also may regulate neurotransmitter production/action and the proliferation and development of neurons and astrocytes. This peptide is also found throughout the gastrointestinal tract and in the lung and kidney.

Molecular Biology/Biochemistry

A separate gene codes for a large precursor protein messenger RNA for each of the ET peptides. The human ET-1 gene is on chromosome 6, and the mature peptide sequence is coded for in the second exon *(12)*. The promoter region has several cis elements that could provide regulatory sites for important stimuli regulating the transcription of ET-1. These include both typical CAAT and TATA sequences, and a site for the binding of the GATA-2 protein *(13)*, which is crucial to the basal or regulated production of ET-1 in endothelial cells. Several important vascular factors, including thrombin and transforming growth factor-beta (TGF-β), transactivate other genes through AP-1 sites and an AP-1 site where the c-*fos* and c-*jun* heterodimer protein can bind is present in the first 120 bases of 5' upstream ET-1 promoter segment (Fig. 1) *(5)*. It also has been found that vasoactive substances, such as the natriuretic peptides or high-density lipoproteins (HDL), can regulate the production of ET-1 at the level of translation *(14,15)*.

The 203 amino acid preprohormone, preproET-1 is processed to "Big" ET-1, a 39 amino acid prohormone which is secreted and has been found in plasma. Big ET-1 exhibits 1% of the potency of ET-1, and hence is felt to be biologically inactive. The plasma concentration of Big ET-1 is increased in moderate to severe heart failure, and could act as a substrate for the extracellular production of ET-1. Big ET-1 is converted to ET-1 by a processing enzyme termed endothelin converting enzyme (ECE). This glycoprotein enzyme preferentially acts against Big ET-1 at a Trp^{21}–Val^{22} linkage, yielding ET-1 as a cleavage product. ECE can be inhibited by phosphoramidon, and is a metallopeptidase, which is very similar to the neutral endopeptidase 24.11 (encephalinase) *(16)*.

ET Receptors

Two types of receptor classes (A and B) have been found expressed on the cells of many mammalian species, including humans. The receptors are members of the superfamily of seven transmembrane-spanning proteins, and are G protein linked. Depending on the tissue, they range from 45,000–50,000 Daltons. The two receptors are approx 50% identical in amino acid structure and each class is highly conserved between mammalian species (85–90%). Posttranslational modification of the ET receptor C-terminal is important for receptor function. Myristolation and palmitolation of this region of the receptors probably contribute to the membrane anchoring, stability of ligand binding, and recruitment of the *ras* protein to the membrane for signaling.

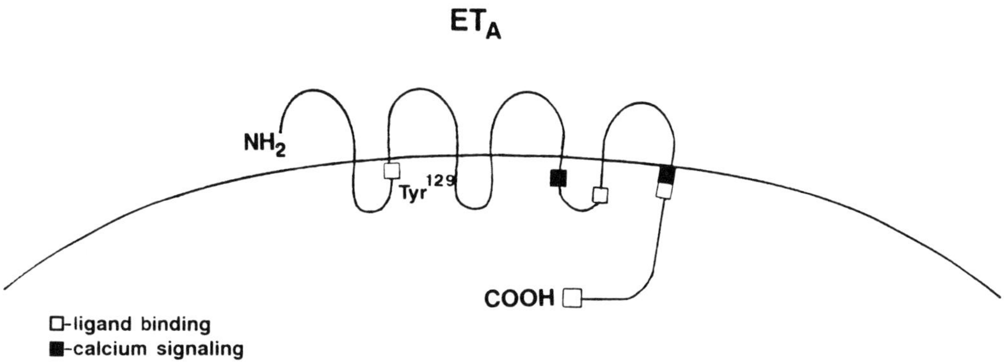

Fig. 2. Schematic representation of the ET_A receptor. The receptor is a seven transmembrane spanning, G-protein-linked protein, which, through discrete amino acids, binds ET-1 with the greatest affinity and transduces a series of signals that lead to biological actions.

ET_A Receptors

The ET_A receptors bind ET-1 (and ET-2) with a 10-fold greater affinity compared to ET-3 *(17)*. These receptors are expressed abundantly on VSMC and cardiac myocytes and mediate the vasoconstrictor action of ET-1. In some vascular beds, ET_B receptors also may cause vasoconstriction. The structure of the ET_A receptor is depicted in Fig. 2, and shows some of the critical residues that are necessary for the stability of ligand binding and cell signaling. The first extracellular loop is critical to ligand binding and, in addition, the tyrosine at position 129 within the second transmembrane spanning domain is important. The vasoconstriction induced by ET-1 is related to activated receptors signaling through phospholipase C (PLC) hydrolysis. This leads to the generation of inositol-1,4,5-triphosphate (IP_3), intracellular calcium $[Ca^{2+}]_i$ mobilization, and the opening of various Ca^{2+} channels in VSMC *(18)*. Importantly, the vasoconstriction persists after ET-1 is removed from the receptor, perhaps caused by persistent elevations in VSMC $[Ca^{2+}]_i$. Nitric oxide (NO) appears to shorten the duration of vasoconstriction by accelerating the return of $[Ca^{2+}]_i$ to basal levels *(19)*, and therefore in diseased blood vessels, the impairment of NO production or action prolongs the ET-1-induced vasoconstriction. It has also been appreciated that the ligated ET_A receptor cycles to the internal receptor pool, but ET-1 is not released or hydrolyzed for a prolonged period of time *(20)*. The result is prolonged ET-1 action, including vasoconstriction. Again, NO plays a role in the dissociation of ET-1 from its receptor *(19)*, and hence a lack of NO action can again enhance the action of ET-1. Another important signaling pathway involves protein kinase C (PKC) activation resulting from the hydrolysis of PLC, the generation of diacylglycerol, and Ca^{2+} mobilization (Fig. 3). Through the activation of PKC and cytosolic tyrosine kinases (like pp $60^{c\text{-}src}$), the mitogen-activated protein kinase (MAP) kinase (and possibly other kinases) cascade is activated. This probably involves stimulation of *ras* and c-*raf* kinase activity *(21)* directed against kinases immediately upstream of MAP-K, like MAP kinase kinase (also known as MEK). Translocation of the activated MAP kinase from the cytosol to the nucleus results in the increased transcription of c-*fos* and c-*jun*, immediate-early gene protein products that comprise the AP-1 heterodimeric proteins *(22,23)*. Through these mechanisms, the ET_A receptor/ET-1 peptide complex contributes to the mitogenic action of ET-1 *(2)*. However, ET-1 can also stimulate c-*myc*, *egr*-1, and other immediate-early

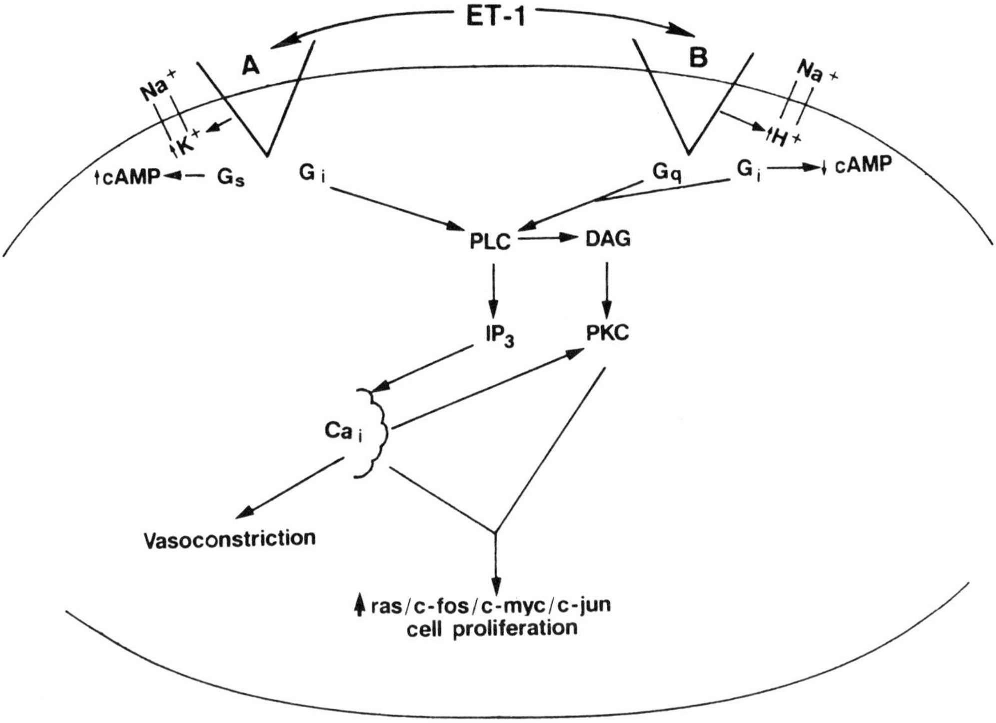

Fig. 3. The signaling pathways for ET_A and ET_B receptors in response to ET-1. ET-1 binds either receptor with equal affinity and triggers signaling involving several pathways, including inositol phosphate hydrolysis, G-protein-coupled changes in cyclic nucleotides, PKC activation, the mobilization of intracellular Ca^{2+}, and activation of ion exchange. These pathways account for the important actions of ET-1.

genes *(24,25)*. The stimulation of *egr*-1 in the heart leads to increased myocardial protein production *(26)*, and perhaps cardiac hypertrophy *(25)*. ET also activates the phospholipases D and A_2 *(27,28)*. ET stimulation of phospholipase A and the prostaglandin synthesis pathway is important for the regulation of vascular tone and may be involved in the development of pulmonary hypertension *(29)*.

ET-1 probably plays an important role to prevent ischemia-induced ventricular arrhythmia, following myocardial infarction. Catecholamines are released after the ischemic insult and induce a protein kinase A-related increase in chloride channels in the injured ventricular muscle. This shortens the action potential and can lead to ventricular arrhythmias. ET-1 inhibits the chloride channel activation and suppresses the pro-arrhythmic effects of the catecholamines *(30)*. This occurs through the peptide binding ET_A receptors, thereby activating a linked G protein. This also results in the inhibition of the activation of L-type Ca^{2+} channels. ET-1 also activates some cardiac potassium channels, which further decreases the electrical excitability of the heart.

ET_B Receptors

ET_B receptors are found mainly on endothelial cells throughout the body *(31)*, but they are also found to a much lesser extent on VSMC. The ET_B receptor binds ET-1 and ET-3 with comparable affinity in the low nanamolar range, and hence the actions of either

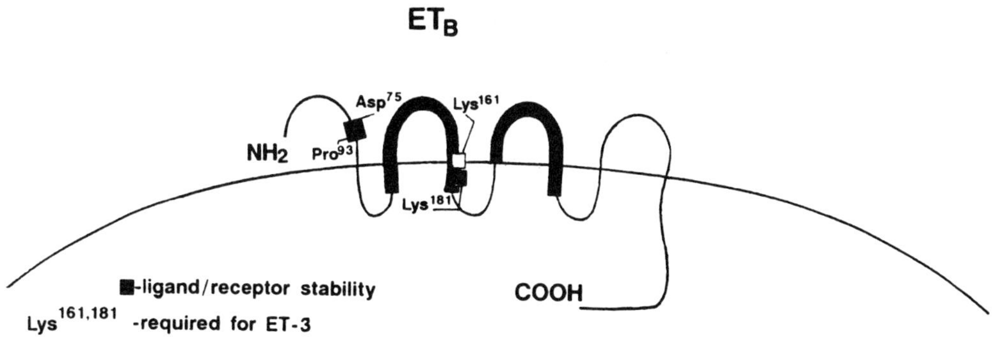

Fig. 4. Schematic representation of the ET_B receptor. This receptor binds ET-1 and ET-3 with equal affinity, and has been linked to the ability of ET-3 to stimulate NO production. Their critical determinants for ligand binding and stable insertion of the receptor into the cell membrane are emphasized.

peptide could be mediated through this receptor. The structure–functional arrangement of this receptor is seen in Fig. 4. ET_B and ET_A receptors signal similarly, in that PLC hydrolysis, IP_3 generation, and Ca^{2+} mobilization, all result following ligand binding. However, there must be some selectivity for a given cell that expresses both receptors and can respond to either peptide present in the cell environment. This may in part be related to the linkage of the two receptors with overlapping and distinct G proteins (Fig. 5). For instance, either ET_A or ET_B can activate PLC hydrolysis through activating Gq; this perhaps accounts for the fact that each receptor has been linked to activation of the MAP kinase pathway *(32)* and subsequent cell proliferation. However, the ET_B receptor also is linked to inhibitory G proteins (Gi), which, in some cells, leads to inhibition of the generation of adenosine 3',5'-cyclic monophosphate (cAMP) *(28)*, and activation of the Na^+–H^+ antiporter *(33)*. ET_A has been uniquely linked to Gs in several cell types, and this signaling mechanism is responsible for the generation of cAMP, leading to increased cathecholamine production. In the third transmembrane loop of both ET receptors, there is an Asp-Arg-Tyr sequence that is thought to contact the G protein and is found in the same location of many members of the superfamily of seven transmembrane spanning receptors. The two ET receptor genes have different nucleotides surrounding this critical sequence, and this may contribute to the specific linkage to unique G proteins for each of the receptors.

Binding of ET-3 to the ET_B receptor may result in the transient vasodilation that occurs when ET-3 is infused. The vasodilation is probably caused by increased NO production and the subsequent generation of guanine 3',5'-cyclic monophaste (cGMP), and prostacyclin production *(5,34,35)* or the activation of potassium (K) channels.

The ET_B receptor and its activation by ET-3 plays a critical role in the normal development and differentiation of cells derived from neural crest precursors *(36)*. Epidermal melanocytes and ganglionic neurons in the intestine do not develop when the ET_B receptor functions improperly, or when ET-3 is not produced *(36)*. ET_B or ET-3 "knockout" mice, or mice bearing naturally occurring inactivating mutations of the ET_B receptor gene have aganglionic megacolon and extensive white spotting of their coats *(37)*. A hereditary form of Hirschsprung's disease (aganglionic megacolon) in humans has been found to be associated with a mutation of the ET_B receptor gene; this mutation reduces ligand-induced Ca^{2+} mobilization *(38)*.

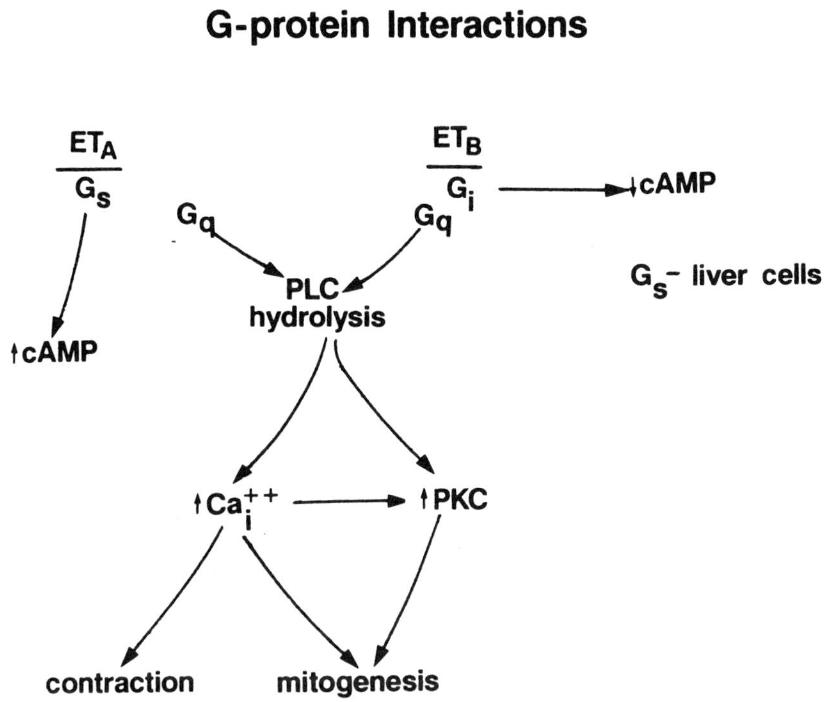

Fig. 5. Coupling of the ET receptors to G proteins. The ET_A and ET_B receptors activate several G-protein subtypes that lead to the intracellular signaling properties of the receptors. Both receptors contact Gq, but ET_A activates Gs and adenylate cyclase in many cell types, whereas ET_B contacts Gi, leading to the inhibition of cAMP and Gs only in the liver.

ET_C Receptors

There is some pharmacologic evidence that an ET-3 selective receptor (ET_C) exists in human tissue, but no such receptor has been isolated or cloned. Recent work has established a candidate ET_C receptor on frog melanophores; this receptor has three- to fourfold greater affinity and 500-fold greater biological response to ET-3 than to ET-1 *(39)*. This receptor is approx 50% homologous overall to ET_A or ET_B, on an amino acid basis, just as ET_A is 50% homologous to ET_B. The presence of a comparable receptor in mammals is presently unknown.

Regulation of ET Receptor Expression

Several substances stimulate the production of both the ET peptides and receptors. Hypoxia or cyclosporine stimulate ET-1 and ET_A receptor production in endothelial cells and VSMC, respectively *(2)*: This has the effect of augmenting ET-1 action. In response to hypoxia, the result is beneficial—an increase in local tissue perfusion, but the increased action of ET-1 probably contributes to the nephrotoxicity associated with cyclosporine *(40)*. Epidermal growth factor (EGF), basic fibroblast growth factor (bFGF), cAMP, and estrogen upregulate the ET_A receptor in some tissues (Fig. 6), whereas C-type natriuretic peptides, angiotensin II (AII) and perhaps bFGF upregulate the ET_B receptor expression. In contrast, ET peptides, AII, platelet-derived growth factor (PDGF), and TGF-β

Regulation of Receptor Numbers

A **Upregulation**

	ET_A	ET_B
c Amp	↑	
CNP		↑
Ang II		↑
b FGF	↑	↑
EGF	↑	
Estrogen	↑ (myometrium)	

B **Downregulation**

	ET_A	ET_B
ET-1	↓	
ET-3	↓	↓
Phorbol ester	↓ or ↑	↓
Ang II	↓	
c Amp		↓
Catecholamines		↓
PDGF	↓	
TGF-β	↓	

Fig. 6. The stimulation or inhibition of ET_A and ET_B receptor expression on the cell surface. Various vasoactive factors, cyclic nucleotides, and vascular cell growth-modulating proteins alter the expression of the endothelin receptors, often through effects on receptor synthesis. **(A)** Upregulation; **(B)** downregulation.

downregulate ET_A receptors, whereas cAMP and catecholamines inhibit ET_B receptor expression (Fig. 6).

Within a particular tissue, the distribution of ET_A and ET_B receptors varies and in this way contributes to the different actions of the various ET peptides. In the kidney, ET_A receptors are prominent in the vasa recta and arcuate arteries, whereas ET_B receptors are found predominantly in the collecting ducts, suggesting different roles in the modulation of salt and water reabsorption. Both receptors are found in glomeruli *(2)*. ET-1 reduces renal blood flow by dramatically increasing renal vascular resistance through constricting renal afferent and efferent arterioles, as well as arcuate and interlobular arteries. Systemic administration of ET-1 reduces the glomerular filtration rate, and can cause antinatriuresis (in part related to the stimulation of aldosterone production) *(41,42)*, probably through the ET_A receptor.

PHYSIOLOGY OF ET

ET and Other Vasoactive Factors Interactions

ET-1 production is regulated in vitro and in vivo by a variety of hormones, vasoactive substances, and vascular stress. AII, vasopressin, thrombin, high- and low-density lipoproteins, and insulin stimulate ET-1 production, as do growth factors, such as TGF-β, insulin-like growth factor-1, EGF, and bFGF. The effects of several vasoactive peptides and growth factors could be mediated through the stimulation of ET-1 production. For instance, AII stimulates cardiac hypertrophy *(43)* and, in some settings, vascular proliferation. Inhibition of either angiotensin-stimulated ET-1 production or the action of ET-1 can prevent the cardiac hypertrophic effects of the octapeptide *(44)*. In turn, ET-1 can stimulate the conversion of AI to AII, and potentiate AII-induced aldosterone production *(45)*. The interactions between these two hormones is potentially important in view of the strong evidence that angiotensin-converting enzyme inhibitors prolong survival in patients with left ventricular dysfunction after myocardial infarction *(46)*.

Production of ET-1 is regulated by the vasodilators NO and prostacyclin, inhibiting ET-1 via a common mechanism involving the generation of cGMP *(47,48)*. Atrial natriuretic peptide (ANP) inhibits basal and AII or thrombin-stimulated ET-1 production as well *(14,49)*. Vasodilator and antigrowth actions of NO, prostacyclin, or ANP in the vasculature may therefore be related in part to inhibiting both ET production and action. Interactions of these vasoactive substances could restrain VSMC growth in the setting of the early development of atherosclerosis, and could prevent the increased systemic vascular resistance owing to ET-1 production stimulated by the conditions of hypoxia or shear stress.

ET-3 probably stimulates NO production by endothelial cells via ET_B receptors *(34)*, and this interaction may be part of a paracrine/autocrine system of regulation. ET-1 (and ET-3) stimulates production of several prostaglandins; this could lead to inhibition of platelet aggregation *(50)* and transient vasodilation (both via prostacyclin) *(51)*, or contribute to pulmonary bronchoconstriction (thromboxane) *(52)*.

ET-1 Vascular and Circulatory Effects

Recent evidence has implicated ET-1 and the ET_A receptor as importantly contributing to the maintenance of basal vasomotor tone in humans. The infusion of a selective ET_A receptor antagonist, BQ-123, into the brachial artery of normal subjects caused a 64% increase in forearm blood flow after 1 h, because of progressive vasodilatation *(53)*. Although each ET is capable of producing vasoconstriction, ET-1 is the most potent endogenous constrictor yet identified and is the likely endogenous modulator of basal tone. For example, ET-1 is 100 times more potent as a vasoconstrictor than norepinephrine on a molar basis. This action is mediated mainly through signal transduction enacted after the peptide binds the ET_A receptors on VSMC *(17)*; but activation of ET_B receptors, expressed on coronary or other human VSMC, probably contributes to the vasoconstriction *(54)*. ET-1 and the catecholamines also potentiate the vasoconstriction caused by each other *(55)*. In the setting of acute vascular disease, the secretion of ET-1 and catecholamines, combined with the decreased production or action of NO in the diseased blood vessel, can create a potent vasoconstricting effect *(56)*. ET-1 also can stimulate ANP production from the heart via a Ca^{2+} dependent mechanism *(57)*, perhaps as a compensatory balance to oppose the vasoconstricting action of ET.

ROLE OF ETS IN CARDIOVASCULAR PATHOPHYSIOLOGY

Cardiovascular Disease

ET-1 is strongly implicated in the events leading to tissue damage after acute vascular insult and reperfusion of the myocardium. In animal models and humans *(58)*, plasma ET-1 concentrations are increased after myocardial infarction, whereas intravenous infusion of ET-1 markedly reduces coronary blood flow (>90%) *(59)*. This suggests that ET-1 released from hypoxic endothelial cells could contribute to the myocardial damage downstream of the thrombosed artery, in part through strong vasoconstriction.

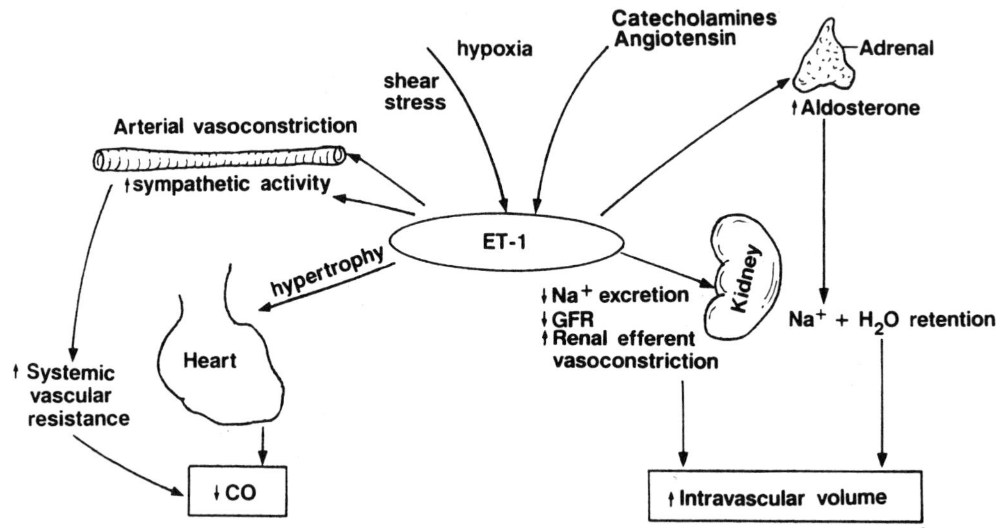

Fig. 7. Potential actions of ET-1 that may contribute to the manifestations or development of congestive heart failure. Hypoxia, shear stress, and hormones that are associated with evolving congestive heart failure stimulate ET production. ET-1 can stimulate aldosterone secretion, and decrease kidney function, thereby leading to sodium and water retention and increased intravascular volume. ET-1 also stimulates hypertrophy of the heart, and increases sympathetic activity and arterial vasoconstriction. Increased systemic vascular resistance decreases cardiac output. GFR, glomerular filtration rate; CO, cardiac output.

In a rat model, plasma ET-1 concentrations are markedly increased just distal to the site of ligation of a coronary artery; intracoronary infusion of ET-1 antibody before ligation reduces the extent of the resulting myocardial damage by 45% *(60)*. Similarly, in dogs, infusion of the ET_A receptor antagonist, BQ-123, reduced the extent of experimental myocardial infarction by 40% *(61)*. These studies point to a pathogenetic role for ET-1 in the myocardial damage after acute ischemia and suggest that ET antagonists may help salvage the injured myocardium. In rats with experimentally induced myocardial ischemia, ET-1 release is greatly augmented during reperfusion, suggesting a role for ET-1 in reperfusion injury *(62)*. Recent data, however, indicate that ET-1 probably does not play an important role in the reperfusion injury of experimental myocardial ischemia, since ET receptor antagonists have no significant effects on coronary flow or cardiac function in this setting *(63)*.

In humans with moderate to severe congestive heart failure, plasma ET concentrations are elevated two- to fourfold and closely correlate with the severity of this disorder, irrespective of the etiology *(10,64)*. ET levels may have prognostic significance in heart failure. The 1-yr mortality in patients who suffer a myocardial infarction strongly correlates to the plasma ET-1 concentrations determined 3 d after infarction *(65)*. Infusion of ET-1 into animals significantly increases systemic vascular resistance and depresses cardiac output *(66)*, indicating that ET-1 could importantly contribute to many of the manifestations of congestive heart failure (Fig. 7). ET-1 can induce the cellular and molecular steps leading to cardiac hypertrophy. These include initiation of the growth program involving immediate-early genes such as c-*fos* and *egr*-1, reactivation of embryonic genes, and stimulation of myosin light chain-2 into organized, contractile units *(25)*.

High plasma concentrations of ET-1 associated with severe heart failure could induce bronchospasm through ET_A receptors expressed on pulmonary bronchial smooth muscle cells *(52)*. In severe heart failure, a secondary hypersecretion of aldosterone leads to the retention of sodium and water. ET-1 augments both basal and angiotensin-stimulated adrenal aldosterone production *(67)*, thereby contributing to the state of aldosterone excess. The high concentrations of ET-1 can directly depress cardiac contractility, increase vascular tone in the kidney and blood vessels, and depress sodium excretion in the kidney, thereby further increasing intravascular volume and depress cardiac output from the failing heart. Support for these actions of ET come from studies in dogs with congestive heart failure, where infusion of the ET_A receptor antagonist, FR-139317, reduces peripheral vascular resistance and systemic blood pressure *(68)*.

ET-1 may have a role in the development of neointimal lesions after balloon angioplasty. Following experimental angioplasty of the common carotid artery, neointimal lesions could be reduced 50% in size by the administration of an ET receptor antagonist *(69)*. Stimulation of ET-1 production, and enhancement of its mitogenic action on smooth muscle by insulin may contribute to the accelerated vascular disease associated with hyperinsulinemia and diabetes mellitus *(70,71)*.

Hypertension

There is little support for the idea that the ETs play a role in the development or maintenance of human essential hypertension. Plasma ET-1 concentrations are normal in most patients with essential hypertension, but in isolated instances, ET-1 could contribute to hypertension. One patient with a hemangioendothelioma had hypertension and elevated plasma ET-1 concentrations that both disappeared after removal of the tumor *(72)*. In animal models, targeted disruption of the ET-1 gene resulted in mice in which one allele of the ET-1 gene was deleted. These mice had slightly elevated blood pressure (compared with normal littermates), suggesting that ET-1 is not important for the development of essential hypertension *(73)*. Rats with deletion of both alleles of the ET-1 gene have normal hearts at birth, indicating that ET-1 does not contribute to the development of the cardiovascular system. In a related but unclear association, the ET-2 gene may be an important marker for the genetic locus in rats with salt-sensitive hypertension *(74)*. What the important linkage involves is unknown. In women with preclampsia, plasma ET-1 concentrations are increased *(75)*, and ET-1 is known to be produced by amnionic and endometrial cells. In conjunction with decreased prostacyclin and NO production, ET-1 could contribute to the pregnancy-related hypertension.

Pulmonary Function and Disease

ET-1 induces pulmonary VSMC bronchoconstriction in vivo *(9,53)*, and therefore may contribute to the development of pulmonary hypertension. The bronchoconstriction is thought to be caused by the stimulation of thromboxane production and the subsequent activation of thromboxane receptors on pulmonary bronchial VSMC *(76)*. Human bronchial epithelial cells in culture secrete ET-1, and the peptide can act in paracrine fashion on neighboring VSMC *(77)*. The bronchoalveolar lavage fluids of patients with asthma have elevated ET-1 concentrations compared with fluid from normal subjects or patients with bronchitis; however, their plasma ET-1 concentrations are normal. In patients in remission after oral glucocorticoid and inhaled β-adrenergic drug treatment, brochoalveolar lavage fluid ET-1 concentrations decrease by 75% *(78)*. High levels of ET-1 mRNA and

ET-1 are present in the lungs of patients with cryptogenic fibrosing alveolitis *(79)* and vascular endothelial cells of patients with primary pulmonary hypertension *(80)*; peripheral plasma ET-1 concentrations are elevated sixfold in such patients.

Kidney Disease

ET-1 may contribute to several vascular-related diseases of the kidney. Cyclosporine nephrotoxicity is probably caused in part by increased ET-1 production *(81)*. In animal models, inhibiting ET-1 action prevents the vasoconstricting effects of cyclosporine in isolated arteries *(82)* and protects against drug-induced nephrotoxicity in vivo *(83)*. Similarly, postischemic renal failure in animals has been attributed to the release and action of ET-1 *(85)* and some forms of experimentally induced postischemic renal failure can largely be prevented by pretreatment with an ET receptor antagonist *(84,85)*.

Disorders of Development

Locally produced ET-1 has been implicated in causing closure of the ductus arteriosis at birth *(86)*. Inhibition of ET-1 production and action by prostacyclin or especially prostaglandin E_2 *(48)* may prevent premature closure of the ductus in the fetus. Persistent patency of the ductus arteriosis in newborn infants can be treated effectively with indomethacin; perhaps this is because indomethacin reverses the restraint on ET-1 production or action induced by endogenous prostanoids.

Homozygous ET-1-deficient mice have severe maldevelopment of craniofacial tissues derived from the first pharyngeal arch and die of respiratory failure at birth *(86)*. These findings indicate that ET-1 plays an important role in the differentiation and development of tissues derived from embryonic neural crest cells, an unanticipated finding. Abnormalities of cardiovascular development were seen in some of these mice, involving cells derived from neural crest lineage, which give rise to the great vessels and aortic arch, and septation of the ventricles *(87)*. Interestingly, similar phenotypes are seen in human diseases, such as the DiGeorge syndrome or Pierre-Robin syndrome. These disorders are often associated with deletions in chromosome 22q11, while the ET-1 receptor gene maps to chromosome 6. The ET_A receptor knockout mouse gives a similar phenotype to the ET-1 deficient mice, but the ET_A gene has been assigned to chromosome 4 in humans. It is possible that a member of the ECE family maps to 22q11, since deletion of ECE-1, preventing the processing of proET-1 to ET-1, gives an identical phenotype. ET-3 and ET_B receptors play a role in the development of the intestinal ganglionic neurons and melanocytes, perhaps in conjunction with the *RET* protooncogene. This has been previously discussed.

CENTRAL NERVOUS SYSTEM

Physiology

Both ET-1 and ET-3 and endothelin receptors are present in the brain and brain stem, although ET-3 is more abundant. Both peptides and their receptors are produced by neurons and astrocytes at a relatively early stage of fetal life in rats (d 14), and therefore may play a role in central and peripheral nervous system development *(88)*. The ET_B receptor is predominant at least on astrocytes, where it mediates the ability of the endothelins to stimulate DNA synthesis and to inhibit second messenger generation caused by other neurotransmitters *(89)*. ET-1 and ET-3 are the only peptides known to activate the Na^{+}-K^{+}-Cl^{-} transporter function of brain capillary endothelial cells. This important function of the microvascular cells that comprise the blood–brain barrier maintains a low potassium environment in the central nervous system *(90)*. This environment is important in allowing neuronal depolarization and the subsequent conduction of impulses between neurons.

ET increases blood pressure through the ligation of receptors expressed on discrete brainstem nuclei and circumventricular organs in the central nervous system. Stimulation of these areas within the central sympathetic nervous system leads to pressor effects, and these effects may be partly the result of ET-1 enhancing central vasopressin production and action *(91,92)*. ET-1 also exerts an antidipsogenic action by antagonizing the water-seeking behavior induced by AII *(93)*. ET is released during water deprivation and stimulates vasopressin secretion from the hypothalamus in vitro *(94)*. ET-1 has been found to stimulate growth hormone, thyroid-stimulating hormone, and luteinizing- and follicle-stimulating hormone from the anterior pituitary, and inhibit the secretion of prolactin *(95)*. Whether these actions of ET are physiologically important is not known.

Brain Ischemia

ET-1 may have a role in the events following ischemic infarction of the brain. Plasma ET concentrations increase markedly after acute ischemic cerebral infarction in humans *(96)*, and topical application of ET-1 to cerebral blood vessels in vitro induces vasospasm *(97)*. ET-1 could contribute to downstream ischemia after release from the damaged, hypoxic endothelium of cerebral vessels after cerebral thrombosis or infarction. This would further compromise the brain parenchyma, analogous to the situation in the heart or kidney.

Subarrachnoid Hemorrhage

ET-1 contributes to the vasospasm associated with subarrachnoid hemorrhage. In patients who develop vasospasm, cerebrospinal fluid concentrations of ET-1 are markedly increased, rising in coincidence with the onset of this complication *(98)*. Intracerebroventricular administration of ET-1 causes subarrachnoid hemorrhage followed by vasospasm in rabbits *(99)*. When rats are subjected to experimental subarrachnoid hemorrhage, the associated vasospasm is nearly completely prevented by pretreatment with ET receptor antagonists *(85,100)*. Because the extent of cerebral damage after subarrachnoid hemorrhage strongly correlates with the degree of vasospasm, one would like to prevent this complication, and ET receptor antagonists hold promise in this regard.

CONCLUSION

The application of specific ET receptor antagonists has rapidly followed advances in our understanding of the physiologic actions of this family of vasoactive peptides. Utilization of these antagonists has led to a clearer understanding of the important roles for ET in the physiology and pathology of the vasculature throughout the body (Table 1). Future work should provide definitive insight into the role of ET-1 in complex vascular diseases, such as atherosclerosis and cardiac hypertrophy. It may become possible to modulate the production or action of endothelin for the benefit of patients with these diseases, as is currently the situation with angiotensin.

Table 1
ET-1 in Vascular-Related Diseases

Probable
Myocardial damage caused by vascular insult
Heart failure manifestations
Cyclosporine-induced nephrotoxicity
Postischemic renal failure
Vasospasm secondary to subarachnoid hemorrhage
Possible
Pulmonary hypertension
Asthma
Patent ductus arteriosis
Vasospastic disorders (heart, peripheral circulation)
Acute cerebrovascular insufficiency

REFERENCES

1. Yanagisawa M, Kurihara H, Kimura S, Tomobe Y, Kokayash M, Mitsui Y, Yazaki, Goto K, Masaki T. A novel potent vasoconstrictor peptide produced by vascular endothelial cells. Nature 1988;332: 411–415.
2. Simonson MS. Endothelins: multifunctional renal peptides. Physiol Rev 1993;73:375–411.
3. Rubanyi GM, Polokoff MA. Endothelins: molecular biology, biochemistry, pharmacology, physiology, and pathophysiology. Pharmacol Rev 1994;46:328–415.
4. Nakamura S, Naruse M, Naruse K, Demura H, Uemura H. Immunocytochemical localization of endothelin in cultured bovine endothelial cells. Histochemistry 1990;94:475–477.
5. Inoue A, Yanagisawa M, Takuwa Y, Mitsui Y, Kobayashi M, Masaki T. The human preproendothelin-1 gene. J Biol Chem 1989;264:14,954–14,959.
6. DeNucci G, Thomas R, D'Orleans JP, Antunes E, Walder C, Warner TD, Vane JR. Pressor effects of circulating endothelin are limited by its removal in the pulmonary circulation and by the release of prostacyclin and endothelium derived relaxing factor. Proc Natl Acad Sci USA 1988;85:9797–9800.
7. Vijayayaraghavan J, Scicli AG, Carretero OA, Slaughter C, Moomaw C, Hersh LB. The hydrolysis of endothelins by neutral endopeptidase 24.11 (enkephalinase). J Biol Chem 1990:265:14,150–14,155.
8. Yoshimoto S, Ishizaki Y, Sasaki T, Murota S-I. Effect of carbon dioxide and oxygen on endothelin production by cultured porcine cerebral endothelial cells. Stroke 1991;22:378–383.
9. Lerman A, Edwards BS, Hallet JW, Heublein DM, Sandberg SM, Burnett JC Jr. Circulating and tissue endothelin immunoreactivity in advanced atherosclerosis. New Engl J Med 1991;325:997–1001.
10. Wei C-M, Lermin A, Rodeheffer RJ, McGregor CGA, Brandt RR, Wright S, Heublein DM, Kao PC, Edwards WD, Burnett JC Jr. Endothelin in human congestive heart failure. Circulation 1994;89: 1580–1586.
11. Shinmi O, Kimura S, Sawamura T, Sugita Y, Yoshizawa T, Uchiyama Y, Yanagisawa M, Goto K, Masaki T, Kanazawa I. Endothelin-3 is a novel neuropeptide: isolation and sequence determination of endothelin-1 and endothelin-3 in porcine brain. Biochem Biophys Res Commun 1989;164:587–593.
12. Lee M-E, Bloch KD, Clifford JA, Quertermous T. Functional analysis of the endothelin gene promoter. J Biol Chem 1990;265:10,446–10,450.
13. Wilson DB, Dorfman DM, Orkin SH. A nonerythroid GATA-binding protein is required for function of the human preproendothelin-1 promoter in endothelial cells. Mol Cell Biol 1990;10:4854–4862.
14. Hu R-M, Chuang E, Prins B, Kashyup M, Frank HJL, Levin ER. High density lipoproteins stimulate the production and secretion of endothelin-1 from cultured bovine aortic endothelial cells. J Clin Invest 1994;93:1056–1062.
15. Hu R-M, Levin ER, Pedram A, Frank HJL. Atrial natriuretic peptide inhibits the translation and secretion of endothelin from cultured bovine aortic endothelial cells: mediation through C receptors. J Biol Chem 1992;267:17,384–17,389.
16. Xu D, Emoto N, Giaid A, Slaughter C, Kaw S, Damiane D, Yanagasawa M. ECE-1: a membrane-bound metallopeptidase that catalyzes the proteolytic activation of big endothelin-1. Cell 1994;78:473–485.

17. Arai H, Hori S, Aramori I, Ohkubo H, Nakanishi S. Cloning and expression of a cDNA encoding an endothelin receptor. Nature 1990;348:730–732.
18. Simonsen MS, Dunn MJ. Cellular signalling by peptides of the endothelin gene family. FASEB J 1990;4:2989–3000.
19. Goligorsky MS, Tsukahara H, Magazine H, Andersen TT, Malik AB, Bahou WF. Termination of endothelin signaling: role of NO. J Cell Physiol 1994;158:485–494.
20. Chun M, Lin HL, Henis YI, Lodish HF. Endothelin-induced endocytosis of cell surface ETA receptors. J Biol Chem 1995;270:10,855–10,860.
21. Herman WH, Simonsen MS. Nuclear signalling by endothelin-1. J Biol Chem 1995;270(19):11,654–11,661.
22. Simonson MS, Herman WH. Protein kinase C and protein tyrosine kinase activity contribute to mitogenic signalling by endothelin-1. J Biol Chem 1993;268:9347–9357.
23. Koide M, Kawahara Y, Tsuda T, Ishida Y, Shii K, Yokoyama M. Endothelin stimulates tyrosine phosphorylation and the activities of two mitogen-activated protein kinases in cultured vascular smooth muscle cells. J Hypertens 1992;10:1173–1182.
24. Simonsen MS, Wann S, Mene P, Dubyak GR, Kester M, Nakazato Y, Sedor JR, Dunn MJ. Endothelin stimulates phospholipase C, Na^+/H^+ exchange, c-fos expression, and mitogenesis in rat mesangial cells. J Clin Invest 1989;83:708–712.
25. Shubeita HE, Harris HN, McDonough PM, Knowlton KU, Glembotski C, Brown JH, Chien KR. Endothelin induction of sarcomere assembly and cardiac gene expression in ventricular myocytes: a paracrine mechanism for myocardial cell hypertrophy. J Biol Chem 1990;265:20,555–20,562.
26. Neyses L, Nouskas J, Vetter H. Inhibition of endothelin-1 induced myocardial protein synthesis by an antisense oligonucleotide against the early response gene-1. Biochem Biophys Res Commun 1991;181:22–27.
27. Pai J-K, Dobeck EA, Bishop WR. Endothelin-1 activates phospholipase D and thymidine incorporation in fibroblasts overexpressing protein kinase $C_{\beta1}$. Cell Reg 1991;2:897–903.
28. Aramori I, Nakanishi S. Coupling of two endothelin receptor subtypes to differing signal transduction in transfected Chinese hamster ovary cells. J Biol Chem 1992;267:12,468–12,474.
29. Noveral JP, Rosenberg SM, Anbar RA, Pawlowski NA, Grunstein MM. Role of endothelin-1 in regulating proliferation of cultured rabbit airway smooth muscle cells. Am J Physiol 1992;263:L317–L324.
30. Ono K, Tsujimoto G, Sakamoto A, Eto K, Masaki T, Ozaki Y, Satake M. Endothelin-A receptor mediates cardiac inhibition by regulating Ca^{2+} and potassium currents. Nature 1994;370:301–304.
31. Sakurai T, Yanagagisawa M, Takuwa Y, Miyazaki H, Kimura S, Goto K, Masaki T. Cloning of a cDNA encoding a non-isopeptide-selective subtype of the endothelin receptor. Nature 1990;348:732–735.
32. Wang Y, Rose PM, Webb ML, Dunn MJ. Endothelins stimulate mitogen-activated protein kinase cascade through either ET_A or ET_B. Am J Physiol 1994;267:C1130–C1135.
33. Koh E, Morimoto S, Kim S, Nabata T, Miyashita Y, Ogihara T. Endothelin stimulates Na/H exchange in vascular smooth muscle cells. Biochem Int 1990;20:375–380.
34. Hirata Y, Emori T, Eguchi S, Kanno K, Imai T, Ohta K, Marumo F. Endothelin receptor subtype B mediates synthesis of NO by cultured bovine endothelial cells. J Clin Invest 1993;91:1367–1373.
35. Filep JG, Herman F, Battistini B, Chabrier PE, Braquet P, Sirois P. Antiaggregatory and hypotensive effects of endothelin 1 in beagle dogs: role for prostacyclin. J Cardiovasc Pharmacol 1991;17:S216–S218.
36. Baynash AG, Hosoda K, Giaid A, Richardson JA, Emoto N, Hammer RE, Yanagisawa M. Interaction of endothelin-3 with endothelin-B receptor is essential for development of epidermal melanocytes and enteric neurons. Cell 1994;79:1277–1285.
37. Hosoda K, Hammer RE, Richardson JA, Baynash AG, Cheung JC, Giaid A, Yanagisawa M. Targeted and natural (piebald-lethal) mutations of endothelin-B receptor gene produce megacolon associated with spotted coat color in mice. Cell 1994;79:1267–1276.
38. Puffenberger EG, Hosoda K, Washington SS, Nakao K, deWitt D, Yanagisawa M, Chakravarti A. A missense mutation of the endothelin-B receptor gene in multigenic Hirschsprung's Disease. Cell 1994;79:1257–1266.
39. Karne S, Jayawickreme J, Lerner MB. Cloning and characterization of an endothelin-3 specific receptor (ETc receptor) from Xenopus Laevis dermal melanophores. J Biol Chem 1993;268:19,126–19,133.
40. Kon V, Sugiura M, Inagami T, Harvie BR, Ichikawa I, Hoover RL. Role of endothelin in cyclosporine-induced glomerular dysfunction. Kidney Int 1990;37:1487–1491.
41. Ferrario RG, Foulkes R, Salvatti P, Patrono C. Hemodynamic and tubular effects of endothelin and thromboxane in the isolate perfused rat kidney. Eur J Pharmacol. 1989;171:127–134.
42. Goetz KL, Wang BC, Madwed JB, Zhu JL, Leadly RJ. Cardiovascular, renal, and endocrine responses to intravenous endothelin in conscious dogs. Am J Physiol 1988;255:R1064–R1068.

43. Sadoshima J-I, Xu Y, Slayter HS, Izumo S. Autocrine release of angiotensin II mediates stretch-induced hypertrophy of cardiac myocytes in vitro. Cell 1993;75:977–984.
44. Ito H, Hirata Y, Adachi S, Tanaka M, Tsujino M, Koike A, Nogami A, Marumo F, Hiroe M. Endothelin-1 is an autocrine/paracrine factor in the mechanism of angiotensin II-induced hypertrophy in cultured rat cardiomyocytes. J Clin Invest 1993;92:398–403.
45. Cozza EN, Chiou S, Gomez Sanchez CE. Endothelin-1 potentiation of angiotensin II. Stimulation of aldosterone production. Am J Physiol 1992;262:R85–R89.
46. Pfeffer MA, Braunwald E, Moye LA, Basta L, Brown EJ Jr, Cuddy TE, Davis BR, Geltman EM, Goldman S, Flaker GC, Klein M, Lamas GA, Packer M, Rouleau J, Rouleau JL, Rutherford J, Wertheimer JH, Hawkins CM. Effect of captopril on mortality and morbidity in patients with left ventricular dysfunction after myocardial infarction. Results of the survival and ventricular enlargement trial. N Engl J Med 1992;327:669–677.
47. Boulanger C, Luscher TF. Release of endothelin from the porcine aorta. Inhibition by endothelium-derived NO. J Clin Invest 1990;85:587–590.
48. Prins B, Hu R-M, Nazario B, Pedram A, Frank HJL, Weber MA, Levin ER. Prostaglandin E2 and prostacyclin inhibit the production and secretion of endothelin from cultured endothelial cells. J Biol Chem 1994;269:11,938–11,944.
49. Kohno M, Yasunari K, Yokokawa K, Murakawa K, Horio T, Takeda T. Inhibition by atrial and brain natriuretic peptides of endothelin-1 secretion after stimulation with angiotensin II and thrombin of cultured human endothelial cells. J Clin Invest 1991;87:1999–2004.
50. Thiemermann C, Lidbury PS, Thomas GR, Vane JR. Endothelin-1 releases prostacyclin and inhibits *ex vivo* platelet aggregation in the anesthetized rabbit. J Cardiovasc Pharm 1989;13:S138–S141.
51. Miura K, Yukimura T, Yamashita, Y, Shimmen T, Okumura M, Yamanaka S, Imanishi M, Yamamoto K. Renal and femoral vascular responses to endothelin-1 in dogs: role of prostaglandins J Pharmacol Exp Ther 1991;256:11–17.
52. Macquin-Mavier I, Levame M, Istin N, Harf A. Mechanism of endothelin-mediated bronchoconstriction in the guinea pig. J Pharmacol Exp Ther 1989;250:740–745.
53. Haynes WG, Webb DJ. Contribution of endogenous generation of endothelin-1 to basal vascular tone. Lancet 1994;344:852–854.
54. Seo B, Oemar BS, Siebenmann R, von Segesser L, Luscher T. Both ETA and ETB receptors mediate contraction to endothelin-1 in human blood vessels. Circulation 1994;89:1203–1208.
55. Tabuchi Y, Nakamuru M, Rakugi H, Nagano M, Mikami H, Ogihara T. Endothelin inhibits presynaptic adrenergic neurotransmission in rat mesenteric artery. Biochem Biophys Res Commun 1989;161:803–808.
56. Lopez JA, Armstrong ML, Piegors DJ, Heistad DD. Vascular responses to endothelin-1 in atherosclerotic primates. Arteriosclerosis 1990;10:1113–1118.
57. Scheibinger RJ, Gomez-Sanchez CE. Endothelin: a potent stimulus of atrial natriuretic peptide secretion by superfused rat atria and its dependency on Ca^{2+}. Endocrinology 1990;127:119–125.
58. Battistini B, D'Orleans-Juste P, Sirois P. Endothelins: circulating plasma levels and presence in other fluids. Lab Invest 1993;68:600–628.
59. Kurihara H, Yamaoki K, Nahai R, Yoshizumi M, Takaku F, Satoh H, Inui J, Yazaki Y. Endothelin: a potent vasoconstrictor associated with coronary vasospasm. Life Sci 1989;44:1937–1943.
60. Watanabe T, Suzuki N, Shimamoto N, Fujino M, Imada A. Endothelin in myocardial infarction. Nature 1990;344:114.
61. Grover GJ, Dzwonczk S, Parham CS. The endothelin-1 receptor antagonist BQ-123 reduced infarct size in a canine model of coronary occlusion and reperfusion. Cardiovasc Res 1993;27:1613–1618.
62. Brunner F, Du Toit EF, Opie LH. Endothelin release during ischaemia and reperfusion of isolated perfused rat hearts. J Mol Cell Cardiol 1992;24:1291–1305.
63. Daggassan PH, Breu V, Clozel M, and Clozel J-P. Role of endothelin during reperfusion after ischemia in isolated perfused rat heart. J Cardiovasc Pharmacol 1994;24:867–874.
64. Pacher R, Bergler-Klein J, Globits S, Teufelsbauer H, Schuller M, Krauter A, Ogris E, Rodler S, Wutte M, Hartter E. Plasma Big-endothelin-1 concentrations in congestive heart failure patients with or without systemic hypertension. Am J Cardiol 1993;71:1293–1299.
65. Omland T, Li RT, Aakvaag A, Aarsland T, Dickstein K. Plasma endothelin determination as a prognostic indicator of 1-year mortality after acute myocardial infarction. Circulation 1994;89: 1573–1579.
66. Lerman A, Hildebrand FL, Aarhus LL, Burnett JC. Endothelin has biological actions at physiologic concentrations. Circulation 1991;83:1808–1814.

67. Rosolowsky LJ, Campbell WB. Endothelin enhances adrenocorticotropin-stimulated aldosterone release from cultured bovine adrenal cells. Endocrinology 1990; 126:1860–1866.
68. Clavell AL, Wright RS, Thomas MR, Brandt RR, Opgenorth TJ, Burnett JC. Elevated endogenous endothelin mediates systemic vasoconstriction in experimental chronic congestive heart failure. J Am Coll Cardiol 1994;172A.
69. Douglas SA, Louden C, Vickery-Clark LM, Storer BL, Hart T, Feuerstein GZ, Elliott JD, Ohlstein EH. A role for endogenous endothelin-1 in neointimal formation after rat carotid artery balloon angioplasty. Circ Res 1994;75:190–197.
70. Oliver FJ, de laRubia G, Feener EP, Lee M-E, Loeken MR, Shiba T, Quertermous T, King GL. Stimulation of endothelin-1 gene expression by insulin in endothelial cells. J Biol Chem 1991;266: 23,251–23,256.
71. Frank HJL, Levin ER, Hu R-M, Pedram A. Insulin stimulates endothelin binding and action on cultured vascular smooth muscle. Endocrinology 1993;133:1092–1097.
72. Yokokawa K, Tahara H, Kohno M, Murakawa K-I, Yasunari K, Nakagawa K, Hamada T, Otani S, Yanagisawa M, Takeda T. Hypertension associated with endothelin-secreting malignant hemangioendothelioma. Ann Int Med 1991;114:213–215.
73. Kurihara Y, Kurihara H, Suzuki H, et al. Elevated blood pressure and craniofacial abnormalities in mice deficient in endothelin-1. Nature 1994;368:703–710.
74. Deng AY, Dene H, Pravenec M, Rapp JP. Genetic mapping of two new blood pressure quantitative trail loci in the rat by genotyping endothelin system genes. J Clin Invest 1994;93:2701–2709.
75. Branch DW, Dudley DJ, Mitchell MD. Preliminary evidence for homeostatic mechanism regulating endothelin production in pre-eclampsia. Lancet 1991; 337:943–945.
76. Schumacher WA, Steinbacher TE, Allen GT, Ogletree M. Role of thromboxane receptor activation in the bronchospastic response to endothelin. Prostaglandins 1990;40:71–79.
77. Mattoli S, Mezzetti M, Riva G, Allegra L, Fasoli A. Specific binding of endothelin on human bronchial smooth muscle cells in culture and secretion of endothelin like material from bronchial epithelial cells. Am J Resp Cell Mol Biol 1990;3:145–151.
78. Mattoli S, Soloperto M, Marinin M, Fasoli A. Levels of endothelin in the bronchoalveolar lavage fluid of patients with symptomatic asthma and reversible airflow obstruction. J Allergy Clin Immunol 1991;88:376–384.
79. Giaid A, Michel RP, Stewart DJ, Sheppard M, Corrin B, Hamid Q. Expression of endothelin-1 in lungs of patients with cryptogenic fibrosing alveolitis. Lancet 1993;341:1550–1554.
80. Giaid A, Yanagisawa M, Langleben D, Michel RP, Levy R, Shennib H, Kimura S, Masaki T, Duguid WP, Stewart DJ. Expression of endothelin-1 in the lungs of patients with primary pulmonary hypertension. New Engl J Med 1993;328:1732–1739.
81. Bouchman TE, Brookshire CA. Cyclosporine-induced synthesis of endothelin by cultured human endothelial cells. J Clin Invest 1991;88:310–314.
82. Lanese DM, Conger JD. Effects of endothelin receptor antagonist on cyclosporine-induced vasoconstriction in isolated rat renal arterioles. J Clin Invest 1993;93:2144–2149.
83. Fogo A, Hellings SE, Inagami T, Kon V. Endothelin receptor antagonism is protective in in vivo acute cyclosprorine toxicity. Kidney Int 1992;42:770–774.
84. Chan L, Chittinnandana J, Shapiro JI, Shanley PF, Schrier RW. Effect of an endothelin receptor antagonist on ischemic acute renal failure. Am J Physiol 1994;266:F135–F138.
85. Clozcl M, Breu V, Burri K, et al. Pathophysiological role of endothelin revealed by the first orally active endothelin receptor antagonist. Nature 1993;365:759–761.
86. Coceani F, Kelsey ZL. Endothelin-1 release from lamb ductus arteriosis: relevance to postnatal closure of the vessel. Can J Physiol Pharmacol 1991;69:218–221.
87. Kurihara K, Kurihara H, Oda K, Nagai R, Ishikawa T, Yazaki Y. Aortic arch malformations and ventriculae septal defect in mice deficient in endothelin-1. J Clin Invest 1995;96:293–300.
88. Levin ER. Atrial natriuretic peptide and endothelin: interactions in the central nervous system and periphery. Mol Cell Neurosci 1991;2:189–201.
89. Levin ER, Frank HJL, Pedram A. Endothelin receptor expression in fetal rat diencephalon. J Neurochem 1992;58:659–666.
90. Vigne P, Farre AL, Frelin C. Na^+-K^+-Cl^- cotransporter of brain capillary endothelial cells. J Biol Chem 1994;31:19,925–19,930.
91. Yamamoto T, Kimura T, Ota K, et al. Central effects of endothelin-1 on vasopressin release, blood pressure, and renal solute excretion. Am J Physiol 1992;262:E856–E862.

92. Ouchi Y, Nakamura S, Souza AC, et al. Central effects of endothelin on blood pressure in conscious rats. Am J Physiol 1989;256:H1747–H1751.
93. Samson WK, Murphy TC. Antidisogenic actions of endothelin are exerted via the endothelin-A receptor in the brain. Am J Physiol 1993;265:R1212–R1215.
94. Shichiri M, Hirata Y, Kanno K, Ohta K, Emori T, Marumo F. Effect of endothelin-1 on release of arginine-vasopressin from perifused rat hypothalamus. Biochem Biophys Res Commun 1989;163:1332–1337.
95. Kanyicksa B, Burris TP, Freeman ME. Endothelin-3 inhibits prolactin and stimulates LH, FSH, and TSH secretion from pituitary cell culture. Biochem Biophys Res Commun 1991;174:338–343.
96. Ziv I, Fleminger G, Djaldetti R, Achiron A, Melamed E, Sokolovsky M. Increased plasma endothelin-1 in acute ischemic stroke. Stroke 1992;23:1014–1016.
97. Encabo A, Ferrer M, Marin J, Villamor J, Bafagon G. Vasoconstrictive responses elicited by endothelin in bovine cerebral arteries. Gen Pharmacol 1992;23:263–267.
98. Suzuki R, Masaoka H, Hirata Y, Marumo F, Isotani E, Hirakawa K. The role of endothelin-1 in the origin of cerebral vasospasm in patients with aneurysmal subarrachnoid hemorrhage. J Neurosurg 1992;77:96–100.
99. Huneidi AHS, Thiemermann C, Lidbury PS, et al. ET-1 and big ET cause subarrachnoid hemorrhage in the anesthetized rabbit. J Cardiovasc Pharmacol 1991;17:S492–S495.
100. Willette RN, Zhang H, Mitchell MP, et al. Nonpeptide endothelin antagonist: cerebrovascular characterization and effects on delayed cerebral vasospasm. Stroke 1994;25:2450–2456.

5 Estrogen and Vascular Reactivity

Marie D. Gerhard, MD
and Mark A. Creager, MD

Contents

INTRODUCTION

Cardiovascular disease is the leading cause of death in American women, claiming more lives than cancer, diabetes, and accidents combined *(1,2)*. The risk of myocardial infarction and stroke increases dramatically in women after the menopause *(3)*. Of women ages 45–64 yr, one of nine have cardiovascular disease; yet after age 65, the ratio increases to one of three *(2)*. Loss of endogenous estrogens associated with menopause contributes to the increased cardiovascular risk. Conversely, in postmenopausal women taking estrogen replacement therapy, population-based studies indicate there are up to 50% fewer cardiovascular events *(4,5)*. These observations support an important role for estrogen replacement therapy in the prevention of cardiovascular disease.

The concept of a "cardioprotective" effect of estrogen was initially derived from retrospective evidence available in case control studies. In most of these studies, estrogen replacement therapy was associated with a decrease in the symptoms of coronary artery disease (CAD) *(6–14)*. This beneficial effect of estrogen is apparent despite small sample size and a duration of estrogen replacement therapy of less than 2 yr. Prospective, but nonrandomized trials, of estrogen replacement therapy (ERT) in postmenopausal women also have demonstrated a reduction in cardiovascular risk, particularly a lower rate of fatal myocardial infarction (Table 1) *(4,15–25)*. Among 16,638 women enrolled in the

From: *Contemporary Endocrinology: Endocrinology of the Vasculature*
Edited by: J. R. Sowers Humana Press Inc., Totowa, NJ

Table 1
Effect of Estrogen Replacement on Fatal and Nonfatal Myocardial Infarction[a]

Study	*Number in cohort*	*Number of cases*	*Relative risk*
Burch et al. (1974) *(15)*	737	9	0.4
Petitti et al. (1979) *(16)*	16,638	26	1.2
Hammond et al. (1979) *(17)*	610	58	0.3
Wilson et al. (1985) *(18)*	1234	116 (fatal)	1.9
		48 (nonfatal)	1.9
Stampfer et al. (1985) *(19)*	32,317	90	0.3
Petitti et al. (1986) *(20)*	16,638	294 (fatal and nonfatal)	0.5 (fatal) 1.0 (nonfatal)
Petitti et al. (1987) *(21)*	6593	34	0.5
Hunt et al. (1987) *(22)*	4544	20 (fatal)	0.5
Bush et al. (1987) *(23)*	2270	50 (fatal)	0.4
Henderson et al. (1988) *(24)*	8841	149 (fatal)	0.6
Criqui et al. (1988) *(25)*	1868	87 (fatal)	0.75
Stampfer et al. (1991) *(4)*	48,470	155 (nonfatal)	0.5
		21 (fatal)	0.5

[a]Adapted from ref. *14*. Reproduced with permission.

Table 2
Effect of Estrogen Replacement on Stroke

Study	*Number*	*Age*	*Events*	*Relative risk*
Boysen et al. (1988) *(26)*	13,088	55, median	295	1.0
Paganini-Hill et al. (1988) *(27)*	8807	73, median	63	0.5
Stampfer et al. (1991) *(4)*	48,470	30–63	123	1.0
Henderson et al. (1991) *(28)*	8881	73, median	436	0.6
Finucane et al. (1993) *(29)*	1910	55–74	250	0.7

Kaiser Permanente Health Plan, those receiving ERT had a relative risk of 0.5 for fatal myocardial infarction and 1.0 for nonfatal myocardial infarction *(17)*. Of the 48,870 postmenopausal women participating in the Nurses Health Study, those actively taking estrogen replacement had a risk of 0.5 for all clinical manifestations of CAD and 0.5 for fatal CAD *(4)*. Available epidemiologic evidence indicates that ERT in postmenopausal women is associated with up to a 50% reduction in the risk of clinical CAD.

ERT also may protect against stroke in older postmenopausal women (Table 2) *(27,29)*. Results from the National Health and Nutrition Examination Survey (NHANES) involving women ages 55–74 yr, suggest that postmenopausal ERT is associated with a decrease in both stroke incidence and mortality *(29)*. Also, a decrease in stroke incidence has been observed in postmenopausal women using a combination of estrogen and progesterone *(14,27)*. However, the Nurses Health Study, in which the population averaged 15 yr younger than NHANES, found no reduction in stroke incidence among women treated with estrogen *(4)*. In a population in Copenhagen, Denmark whose average age was younger than those studied in NHANES, there was no change in relative risk of stroke with ERT *(26)*.

EFFECT OF ESTROGEN ON ATHEROSCLEROSIS

Estrogen reduces the development of atherosclerosis in ovariectomized rabbits following balloon injury and cardiac transplantation *(30,31)*. Similar findings have been reported in nonhuman primates. Coronary artery atherosclerosis is more severe in cholesterol-fed ovariectomized cynomolgus monkeys compared to age-matched premenopausal monkeys *(32)*. Estrogen attenuates progression of atherosclerotic plaque in arteries of cholesterol-fed monkeys and rabbits *(33,34)*. When ovariectomized monkeys were randomly assigned to placebo, 17 β-estradiol or 17 β-estradiol plus progesterone *(35)*, the severity of coronary atherosclerosis detected at necropsy was reduced in both hormone replacement groups. Indeed, low-density lipoprotein (LDL) uptake is less in coronary arteries of ovariectomized monkeys treated with estrogen and progesterone than in hormone-deficient monkeys *(36)*. Also, estrogens have been shown to reduce the susceptibility of LDL to oxidation *(37–39)*. Despite observations that estrogen reduces progression of atherosclerosis, there is no evidence that estrogen is able to induce regression *(40)*.

EFFECT OF ESTROGEN ON LIPIDS

The mechanism by which estrogen exerts its cardioprotective effect includes modification of lipid profiles. When women enter menopause they develop a more atherogenic lipid profile that includes higher LDL cholesterol and lipoprotein (a) levels and lower high-density lipoprotein (HDL) cholesterol levels *(41–44)*. These lipoprotein profiles improve after ERT *(45–48)*. Commonly prescribed oral estrogens decrease plasma LDL cholesterol and increase levels of plasma HDL cholesterol including HDL_2 and HDL_3 and apolipoprotein A-1 by at least 15% *(45,49,50)*. Increased levels of endogenous apolipoprotein A-1 result primarily from increased production, whereas decreased levels of LDL cholesterol are largely a consequence of increased catabolism *(45,50)*. Transdermal estradiol preparations do not affect LDL or VLDL cholesterol *(45)*. The different effects on lipoprotein levels that occur may relate to the high concentrations of estradiol that reach the liver following intestinal absorption with oral, but not transdermal estradiol preparations.

Progesterone may attenuate the increase in HDL cholesterol level induced by estrogen, apparently by increasing hepatic lipase activity and thereby HDL_2 catabolism *(51)*. Progesterone does not affect LDL cholesterol concentration. The Postmenopausal Estrogen/Progestin Intervention (PEPI) trial compared conjugated estrogen therapy with progesterone to conjugated estrogen therapy without progesterone *(52)*. The increase in HDL cholesterol observed with estrogen alone was attenuated in the group receiving progesterone also. LDL cholesterol decreased comparably in both groups.

These beneficial changes in lipoprotein profile with oral ERT are likely to account for only 25–50% of the observed cardiovascular risk reduction *(23)*. This has been determined by multiple regression analysis of large epidemiological studies, utilizing inferences from decreased cardiovascular events in men in response to lipid profile modification. The presence of cardioprotective mechanisms of estrogen, which are unrelated to lipid lowering, are also evident in premenopausal women with heterozygous familial hypercholesterolemia *(53)*. These young women have higher LDL and total cholesterol levels than their age-matched male counterparts, but have significantly fewer manifestations of CAD *(53)*. Much of estrogen's beneficial cardiovascular effects may be mediated, in part, by its effect on vascular reactivity, specifically by modifying the functional state of the endothelium.

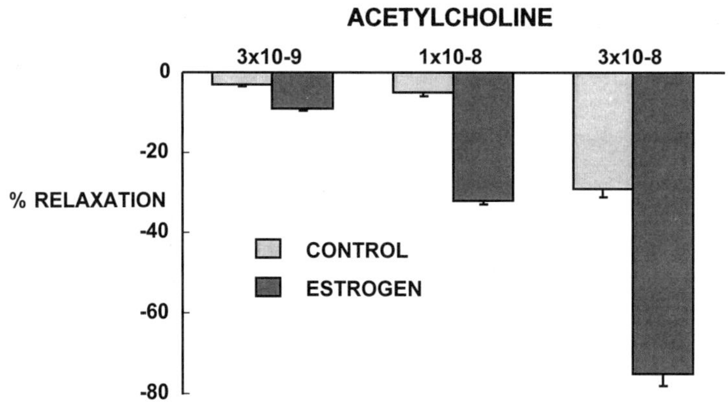

Fig. 1. Effect of estrogen on endothelium-dependent relaxation of rabbit femoral arteries in vitro. Ovariectomized rabbits were treated with estrogen prior to sacrifice. The vasorelaxant response to ACh was greater in the estrogen-treated group than the control group. Reproduced with permission from ref. *61*.

ESTROGEN AND VASCULAR REACTIVITY: EXPERIMENTAL MODELS

The vascular endothelium of healthy individuals provides a protective layer that has anticoagulant and vasodilatory properties, reduces adhesivity of leukocytes, and inhibits vascular smooth muscle cell (VSMC) proliferation *(54)*, partly through synthesis and release by the endothelium of endothelium-derived relaxing factor, identified as nitric oxide (NO). The characteristics of this molecule are described in detail in other chapters. NO may reduce vascular injury and retard atherogenesis by inhibiting monocyte chemotactic factors *(55)*, monocyte adhesion *(56)*, platelet aggregation *(57)*, and VSMC proliferation *(58)*.

Studies in a variety of experimental models have evaluated the effect of estrogen on endothelial function. Basal release of NO from endothelium-intact aortic rings is greater in female than male rabbits *(59)*. After ovariectomy, basal levels of NO are reduced to those detected in males. Moreover, ERT improves endothelium-dependent relaxation of rabbit, porcine, and canine coronary artery rings in vitro *(60,61)*. In female dogs after ovariectomy treated with estrogen, progesterone, or estrogen plus progesterone *(61)*, femoral artery endothelium-dependent relaxations are greatest among the estrogen-treated group (Fig. 1). Progesterone has minimal effects on endothelium-dependent responses. Treatment with estrogen for 16 wk improved endothelium-dependent relaxation of coronary artery rings in ovariectomized cholesterol-fed miniature swine *(39)*. Endothelium-dependent vasorelaxation in male and female porcine coronary arteries have been studied following treatment with 17β estradiol, tamoxifen plus 17β estradiol, 17 α-E_2 (inactive form), or estrogen vehicle *(62)*. Therapy with estrogen improved endothelium-dependent relaxation in the coronary arteries of both genders. Endothelial function did not improve with 17 α-E_2 or 17β estradiol plus tamoxifen, suggesting that estrogen receptors may mediate the response *(62)*.

Estrogen administration has been shown to improve endothelium-dependent vasodilation in vivo in nonhuman primates. Quantitative coronary angiography has been used to evaluate vasomotor responses of atherosclerotic coronary arteries in ovariectomized monkeys receiving chronic ERT *(33,63,64)*. There was a dramatic reduction in the vaso-

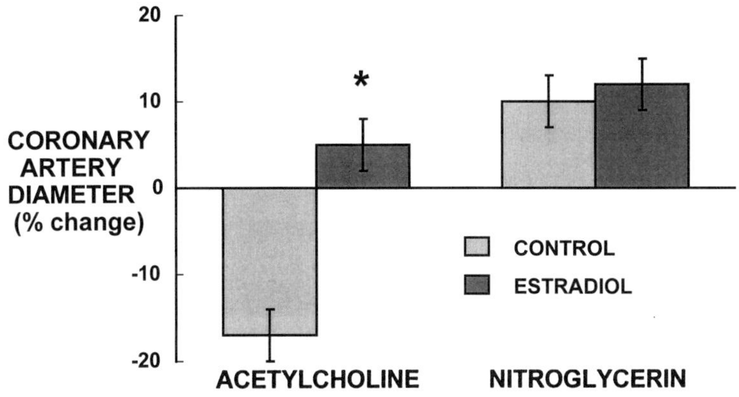

Fig. 2. Effect of acute administration of estrogen to cholesterol-fed ovariectomized cynomolgus monkeys on endothelium-dependent (ACh) and endothelium-independent (nitroglycerin) vasodilation in epicardial coronary arteries in vivo. Prior to estrogen, ACh caused coronary vasoconstriction. Following estrogen, ACh caused coronary vasodilation. Vasodilation to nitroglycerin was not affected by estrogen. Reproduced with permission from ref. *63*.

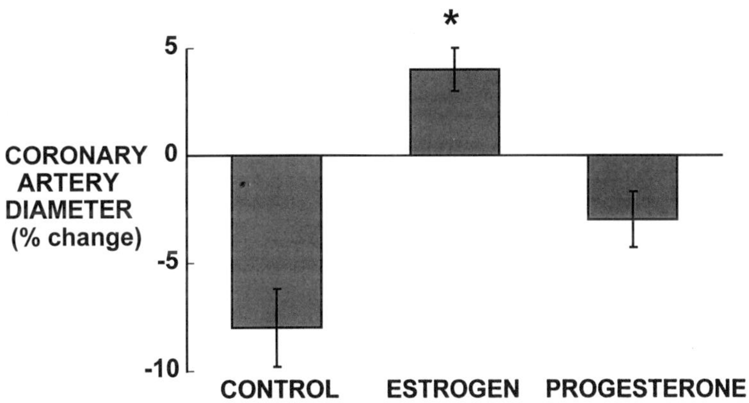

Fig. 3. Effect of chronic treatment with either estrogen or medroxyprogesterone on endothelium-dependent vasodilation of atherosclerotic coronary arteries of cholesterol-fed ovariectomized monkeys. Estrogen, but not medroxyprogesterone, treatment resulted in improved endothelium-dependent vasodilation. Reproduced with permission from ref. *64*.

constrictor response to acetylcholine (ACh) in those monkeys who received estrogen replacement compared to those monkeys who had not received estrogen replacement. This attenuated vasoconstrictive response to ACh is indicative of improvement in endothelial function. Subsequent histologic sectioning of the coronary arteries revealed less atherosclerotic plaque in the coronary arteries from those monkeys who received ERT. Further, acute administration of estrogen intravenously improved endothelium-dependent vasodilation in atherosclerotic coronary arteries (Fig. 2) *(63)*. This effect of acute estrogen treatment could not result from a change in plaque size or HDL cholesterol levels. These investigators also studied the effect of progestins, specifically medroxyprogesterone, on endothelial function in cholesterol-fed ovariectomized monkeys *(64)*, treated for 1 mo. In contrast to estrogen, medroxyprogesterone alone did not improve endothelium-dependent vasodilation (Fig. 3). When added to estrogen therapy,

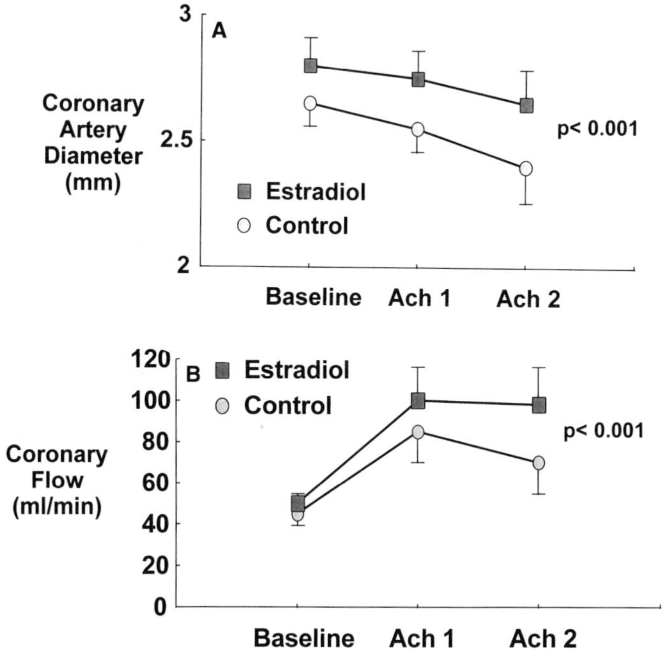

Fig. 4. Effect of the acute administration of estrogen on endothelium-dependent vasodilation of coronary conduit and resistance vessels in postmenopausal women. **(A)** Epicardial coronary vasodilation in response to ACh is increased following estrogen administration. **(B)** The coronary blood flow response to ACh increases significantly after estrogen administration. Reproduced with permission from ref. *65*.

medroxyprogesterone attenuated the favorable effects of estrogen on endothelium-dependent vasodilation.

EFFECT OF ESTROGEN ON VASCULAR REACTIVITY IN WOMEN

Estrogen compounds improve endothelium-dependent vasodilation in postmenopausal women. Ethinyl estradiol, administered acutely, improves endothelium-dependent vasodilation to ACh of atherosclerotic epicardial coronary arteries and coronary resistance vessels of postmenopausal women *(65)*. Endothelium-dependent vasomotion improves in both coronary conduit and resistance vessels following acute iv administration of physiologic doses of estrogen to postmenopausal women (Fig. 4) *(66)*. Intravenous administration of conjugated equine estrogen (Premarin) improves endothelium-dependent vasodilation of epicardial atherosclerotic coronary arteries of postmenopausal women *(67)*. Studies in both men and postmenopausal women with CAD have demonstrated that intracoronary administration of estrogen decreases the vasoconstrictor response to ACh in women but not in men *(68)*. The salutary effects of estrogen on coronary artery vasoreactivity may have direct clinical implications. Indeed, sublingual administration of estrogen to postmenopausal women undergoing treadmill exercise testing increased the time to ST segment depression and prolonged exercise duration *(69)*.

The beneficial effects of estrogen on vascular reactivity are not confined to atherosclerotic coronary arteries. Estrogen compounds also improve endothelium-dependent vasodilation in nonatheromatous peripheral vessels. Studies of the effects of conjugated

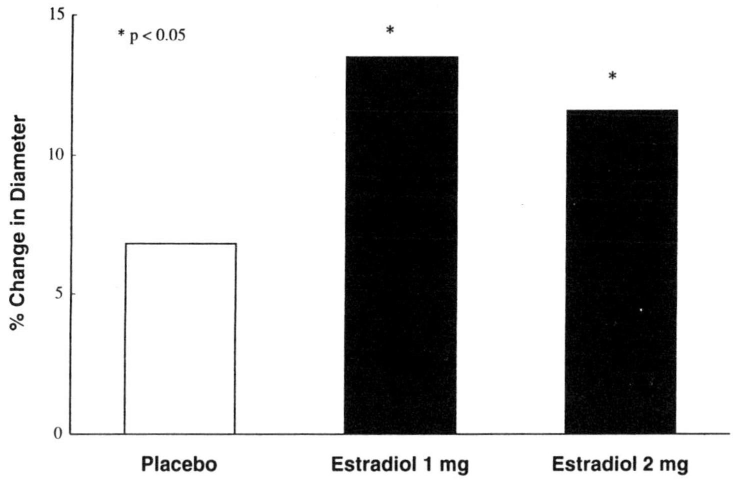

Fig. 5. Effect of estradiol on flow-mediated, endothelium-dependent vasodilation of the brachial artery in postmenopausal women. Oral estradiol at doses of 1 and 2 mg/d significantly increased the brachial artery diameter during a flow stimulus induced by reactive hyperemia ($*p < 0.05$ for each dose compared with placebo). Reproduced with permission from ref. *71*.

equine estrogen on forearm resistance vessels of healthy postmenopausal women *(70)* show that acute iv administration improves endothelium-dependent vasodilation to methacholine chloride, but not endothelium-independent vasodilation to nitroprusside. These data are consistent with other data showing that acute administration of estrogen improved endothelium-dependent vasodilation of forearm resistance vessels *(71)*. Vascular ultrasound has been used to assess flow-mediated endothelium-dependent vasodilation in the brachial arteries of postmenopausal women during chronic treatment with estrogen *(72)*. This double-blind placebo-controlled crossover trial evaluated two doses of estradiol, 1 and 2 mg compared to placebo. Endothelium-dependent responses were evaluated following 9 wk of treatment *(72)*. There was improvement in flow-mediated vasodilation in the women receiving both doses of estradiol (Fig. 5). Endothelium-independent vasodilation assessed after sublingual nitroglycerin did not change following estrogen therapy. Improvement in brachial artery responses could not be explained by changes in lipid profile.

MECHANISM OF ESTROGEN'S EFFECTS ON ENDOTHELIAL FUNCTION

Endothelium-derived NO can be inactivated by superoxide anion to form peroxynitrite *(73,74)*. Therefore, increased production of oxygen-derived free radicals may contribute to impairment of endothelium-dependent vasodilation that occurs in atherosclerosis *(75)*. One mechanism through which estrogen may restore endothelium-dependent relaxation is by acting as an antioxidant, thereby reducing the inactivation of NO. The antioxidant activity of estrogen may be related to the presence of the phenolic ring that is found in estriol and estrogen *(76)*. Endothelium-dependent vasorelaxation is restored and LDL oxidation is reduced in ovariectomized swine with dietary atherosclerosis following estradiol administration *(39)*. The susceptibility of LDL cholesterol to oxidation is also reduced in postmenopausal women receiving ERT *(77)*. Reduction of LDL oxidation does not explain the rapid benefits on endothelial function observed after acute administration of estrogen. Thus, a receptor-independent mechanism of antioxidation has been postulated to account for the ability of estrogen to rapidly restore endothelium-dependent vascular responses *(39)*.

Long-term effects of estrogen may involve more classic estrogen steroid receptor interaction. Typically, such steroid hormones bind to cytoplasmic receptors, and this complex translocates to the nucleus, where it binds to nonhistone proteins on the DNA. Once bound, this complex activates transcription of genes. Administration of estrogen upregulates the number of estrogen receptors *(78)*. Moreover, when guinea pigs are exposed to estrogen there is induction of calcium-dependent NO synthases (NOS), which occurs earlier in female guinea pigs than in male guinea pigs *(79)*. This estrogen-mediated increase in NOS in the vasculature could contribute to the cardioprotective effects of estrogen.

OTHER VASODILATOR EFFECTS OF ESTROGENS

Estrogen compounds may affect vascular reactivity by additional mechanisms. Estrogen has been shown to increase vasodilator prostaglandins (PG) *(80,81)*, and decrease vasoconstrictor prostanoids *(60,61)*. Estrogens also decrease α_2 adrenergic-mediated vasoconstriction *(82)*. Furthermore, estrogen may confer vascular relaxation via inhibition of Ca^{2+} flux in vascular smooth muscle *(83,84)*. Also, following estrogen treatment, VSMC contraction in response to Ca^{2+} channel agonist BAYK8644 or to endothelin-1 is inhibited *(84,85)*. In addition, estrogen enhances potassium conductance in VSMC, an effect likely to promote vasodilation *(86)*.

ESTROGEN AND VASCULAR STRUCTURE

In addition to the endothelium, estrogen causes changes in the vascular wall and extracellular matrix, and promotes collateral blood vessel formation. Production of collagen is decreased in the aortic VSMC cultured in the presence of estrogen *(87,88)*. The ratio of procollagen type I to procollagen type III is altered, which may reflect the production of a more soluble collagen *(89)*. Estrogen decreases synthesis of aortic collagen and elastin in rabbits with dietary atherosclerosis *(89)*. Together these data suggest that ERT may result in decreased vessel stiffness and less pathological accumulation of vascular connective tissue. Estrogen also enhances endothelial cell activities important for angiogenesis *(90)*. Specifically, estrogen increases attachment of human umbilical vein endothelial cells (HUVEC) to laminen, type I and IV collagen, and fibronectin *(90)* and increases the ability of endothelial cells to form tubular networks in vivo. Further, in vivo neovascularization is reduced in mice who have undergone ovariectomy, whereas following ERT the angiogenesis rate increases to levels similar to those observed in nonovariectomized mice *(90)*.

CONCLUSION

ERT reduces the risk of adverse cardiovascular events including fatal myocardial infarction and possibly stroke. Its beneficial effects are multifactorial and include improvement in lipoprotein levels and modification of vascular wall function and structure. Estrogen increases the bioavailability of endothelium-derived NO. In atherosclerotic vessels, preservation of endothelium-derived NO may attenuate myocardial ischemia, and lessen the chances of thrombus formation and consequently myocardial infarction. Other vasoactive properties of estrogen, including increased production of prostacyclin and decreased responsiveness to vasoconstrictive agonists also may have salutary effects. Whether or not progestins abrogate effects of estrogen on vasomotor function await the results of ongoing clinical investigations. Ultimately, understanding the precise mechanism underlying effects of estrogen on vascular disease will enable more targeted forms of therapy.

REFERENCES

1. Eaker ED, Chesebro JK, Sacks FM, Wenger NK, Whisnant JP, Winston M. Cardiovascular disease in women. Circulation 1993;88:1999–2009.
2. Sempos CT, Cleeman JI, Carroll MD, Johnson CI, Bachorik PS, Gordon DJ, Burt VI, Briefel RR, Brown CD, Lippel K, Rifkind BM. Prevalence of high blood pressure among US adults: an update based on guidelines from the second report of the National Cholesterol Education Program Adult Treatment Panel. JAMA 1993;269:3009–3014.
3. Barrett-Connor E, Bush TL. Estrogen and coronary heart disease in women. JAMA 1991;265: 1861–1867.
4. Stampfer MJ, Colditz GA, Willett WC, Manson JE, Rosner B, Speizer FE, Hennekens CH. Postmenopausal estrogen therapy and cardiovascular disease. Ten year follow-up from the Nurses Health Study. N Engl J Med 1991;325:756–762.
5. Grady D, Rubin SM, Petitti DB, Fox CS, Black D, Ettinger B, Ernster YL, Cumings SR. Hormone therapy to prevent disease and prolong life in postmenopausal women. Ann Int Med 1992;117:1016–1037.
6. Rosenberg L, Armstrong B, Jick H. Myocardial infarction and estrogen therapy in postmenopausal women. N Engl J Med 1976;294:1256–1259.
7. Pfeffer RI, Whipple GH, Kurosaki TT, Chapman JM. Coronary risk and estrogen use in postmenopausal women. Am J Epidemiol 1978;107:479–497.
8. Rosenberg L, Slone D, Shapiro S, Kaufman D, Stolley PD, Miettinen DS. Noncontraceptive estrogen use and myocardial infarction in young women. JAMA 1980;244:339–342.
9. Ross RK, Paganini-Hill A, Mack TM, Arthur M, Henderson BE. Menopausal oestrogen therapy and protection from death from ischaemic heart disease. Lancet 1981;1:858–860.
10. Bain C, Willet W, Henderson CH, Rosner B, Belanger C, Speizer PE. Use of postmenopausal hormones and risk of myocardial infarction. Circulation 1981;64:42–46.
11. Adam D, Williams V, Vessey MP. Cardiovascular disease and hormone replacement treatment. Br Med J 1981;282:1277,1278.
12. Szklo M, Tonascia J. Gordes L, Bloom I. Estrogen use and myocardial infarction: a case-control study. Prev Med 1984;13:510–516.
13. Thompson SG, Meade TW, Greenberg G. The use of hormonal replacement therapy and the risk of stroke and myocardial infarction in women. J Epidemiol Community Health 1989;43:173–178.
14. Belchetz PE. Hormonal treatment of postmenopausal women. N Engl J Med 1994;330:1062–1071.
15. Burch JC, Byrd BR Jr, Vaughn WK. The effects of long term estrogen use in hysterectomized women. Am J Obstet Gynecol 1974;188:778–782.
16. Petitti DB, Wingerd J, Pellegrin F, Ramcharan S. Risk of vascular disease in women: smoking, oral contraceptives, noncontraceptive estrogens and other factors. JAMA 1979;242:1150–1154.
17. Hammond CB, Jelovsek FR, Lee KL, Creesman WT, Parker RT. Effects of long term ERT. Am J Obstet Gynecol 1979;133:525–536.
18. Wilson PWF, Garrison RJ, Casselli WP. Postmenopausal estrogen use, cigarette smoking, and cardiovascular morbidity in women over 50: the Framingham Study. N Engl J Med 1985;313:1038–1043.
19. Stampfer MJ, Wille WC, Colditz GA, Rosner B, Speitzer FE, Hennekens CH. A prospective study of postmenopausal estrogen therapy and coronary heart disease. N Engl J Med 1985;313:1044–1049.
20. Petitti DB, Perlman JA, Sidney S. Postmenopausal estrogen use and heart disease. N Engl J Med 1986;315:131,132.
21. Petitti DB, Perlman JA, Sidney S. Noncontraceptive estrogens and mortality: long term follow up from the Walnut Creek Study. Obstet Gynecol 1987;70:289–293.

22. Hunt K, Vessey M, McPherson K, Coleman M. Long-term surveillance of mortality and cancer incidence in women receiving hormone replacement therapy. Br J Obstet Gynecol 1987;94:620–635.
23. Bush TL, Barrett-Connor E, Cowan LD, Criqui MH, Wallace RB, Suchindran CM, Tyroler HA, Rifkind BM. Cardiovascular mortality and noncontraceptive use of estrogen in women: results from the Lipid Research Clinics Program follow-up study. Circulation 1987;75:1102–1109.
24. Henderson BE, Paganini-Hill A, Ross RK. ERT and protection from acute myocardial infarction. Am J Obstet Gynecol 1988;159:312–317.
25. Criqui MH, Suarez L, Barrett-Connor E, McPhillips J. Wingerd DL, Garland C. Postmenopausal estrogen use and mortality: a prospective study in a defined homogenous community. Am J Epidemiol 1988;128:606–614.
26. Boysen G, Nyboe J, Appleyard M, Sorenson PS, Boas J, Somnier F. Stroke incidence and risk factors for stroke in Copenhagen, Denmark. Stroke 1988;18:1345–1353.
27. Paganini-Hill A, Ross RK, Henderson BE. Postmenopausal estrogen use and stroke: a prospective study. Br Med J 1988;297:519–522.
28. Henderson BE, Paganini-Hill A, Ross RK. Decreased mortality in users of estrogen replacement therapy. Arch Int Med 1991;151:75–78.
29. Finucane FF, Madans JH, Bush TL, Wolf PH, Kleinman JC. Decreased risk of stroke among postmenopausal hormone users. Arch Int Med 1993;153:73–79.
30. Foegh ML, Khirabadi BS, Nakanishi T, Vargas R, Ramwell PW. Estradiol protects against experimental cardiac transplant atherosclerosis. Transplant Proc 1987;19:90–95.
31. Weigensberg BI, Lough J, More RH, Katz E, Pugash E, Peniston C. Effects of estradiol on myointimal thickening from catheter injury and on organizing white mural non-occlusive thrombi. Atherosclerosis 1984;52:253–265.
32. Adams MR, Kaplan JR, Clarkson TB, Koritnik DR. Ovariectomy, social status, and atherosclerosis in cynomolgus monkeys. Arteriosclerosis 1985;5:192–200.
33. Williams JK, Adams MR, Klopfenstein HB. Estrogen modulates responses of atherosclerotic coronary arteries. Circulation 1990;81:1680–1687.
34. Kushwaha RS, Hazzard WR. Exogenous estrogens attenuate dietary hypercholesterolemia and atherosclerosis in the rabbit. Metabolism 1981;30:359–366.
35. Adams MR, Kaplan JR, Manuck SB, Koritnik DR, Parks JS, Wolfe MS, Clarkson TB. Inhibition of coronary artery atherosclerosis by estrogen in ovariectomized monkeys. Lack of an effect of added progesterone. Arteriosclerosis 1990;10:1051–1057.
36. Wagner JD, Clarkson TB, St. Clair RW, Schwenke DC, Shively CA, Adams MR. Estrogen and progesterone replacement therapy reduces low density lipoprotein accumulation in the coronary arteries of surgically postmenopausal cynomolgus monkeys. J Clin Invest 1991;88:1995–9002.
37. Maziere C, Auclair M, Ronveux MF, Salmon S, Santus R, Maziere JG. Estrogens inhibit copper and cell-mediated modification of low density lipoprotein. Atherosclerosis 1990;89:175–182.
38. Negre-Salvayre A, Pieraggi MT, Mabile L, Salvayre R. Protective effect of estrogen against the cytotoxicity of minimally oxidized LDL to cultured bovine aortic endothelial cells. Atherosclerosis 1993;99:207–217.
39. Keaney JF, Shwaery GT, Xu A, Nicolosi RJ, Loscalzo J, Foxall TL, Vita JA. 17 β-estradiol preserves endothelial vasodilator function and limits low-density lipoprotein oxidation in hypercholesterolemic swine. Circulation 1994;89:2251–2259.
40. Williams JK, Anthony MS, Honore EK, Herrington DM, Morgan TM, Register TC, Clarkson TB. Regression of atherosclerosis in female monkeys. Arterioscler Thromb Vasc Biol 1995;15:827–836.
41. Matthews KA, Meilahn E, Kuller LH, Kelsey ST, Caggiula AW, Wing RR. Menopause and risk factors for CAD. N Engl J Med 1989;321:641–646.
42. Stevenson JC, Crook D, Godsland IF. Influence of age and menopause on serum lipids and lipoproteins in healthy women. Atherosclerosis 1993;98:83–90.
43. Soma MR, Osnago-Gadda I, Paoletti R, Fumagalli R, Morrisett JD, Meschia M, Crosignani P. The lowering of lipoprotein [a] induced by estrogen plus progesterone replacement therapy in postmenopausal women. Arch Intern Med 1993;153:1462–1468.
44. Mendoza S, Velasquez E, Osona A, Hamer T, Glueck CJ. Postmenopausal cyclic estrogen-progestin therapy lowers lipoprotein [a]. J Lab Clin Med 1994;123:837–841.
45. Walsh BW, Schiff I, Rosner B, Greenberg L, Ravnikar V, Sacks FM. Effects of postmenopausal estrogen replacement on the concentrations and metabolism of plasma lipoproteins. N Engl J Med 1991;325: 1196–1204.

46. Lafferty FW, Fiske ME. Postmenopausal estrogen replacement: a long-term cohort study. Am J Med 1994;97:66–76.
47. Hong MK, Romm PA, Reagan K, Green CE, Rackley CE. Effects of ERT on serum lipid values and angiographically defined CAD in postmenopausal women. Am J Cardiol 1992;69:176–178.
48. Sacks FM, McPherson R, Walsh BW. Effect of postmenopausal estrogen replacement on plasma Lp(a) lipoprotein concentrations. Arch Intern Med 1994;154:1106–1110.
49. Nabulsi AA, Folsom AR, White A, Patsch W, Heiss G, Wu KK, Szklo M. Association of hormone-replacement therapy with various cardiovascular risk factors in postmenopausal women. The Atherosclerosis Risk in Communities Study Investigators. N Engl J Med 1993;328:1069–1075.
50. Walsh BW, Li H, Sacks FM. Effects of postmenopausal hormone replacement with oral and transdermal estrogen on HDL metabolism. J Lipid Res 1994;35:2083–2093.
51. Tikkanen MN, Nikkilä EA, Kuusic T, Sipiner S. Different effects of two progestins on plasma high density lipoprotein (HDL_2) and post-heparin plasma hepatic lipase activity. Atherosclerosis 1981;40:365–369.
52. The Writing Group for the PEPI Trial. Effects of estrogen or estrogen/progestin regimens on heart disease risk factors in postmenopausal women. JAMA 1994;273:199–208.
53. Hill JS, Hayden MR, Frolich J, Pritchard PH. Genetic and environmental factors affecting the incidence of CAD in heterozygous familial hypercholesterolemia. Arterioscler Thromb 1991;11:290–297.
54. Meredith IT, Yeung AC, Weidinger FF, Anderson TJ, Uehata A, Ryan TJ, Selwyn AP, Ganz P. Role of impaired endothelium-dependent vasodilation in ischemic manifestations of CAD. Circulation 1993;87:V56–V66.
55. Zeiher AM, Schray-Utz B, Busse R. NO modulates chemoattractant protein 1 in human endothelial cells: implications for the pathogenesis of atherosclerosis. Circulation 1993;88:I-367 (abstract).
56. Bath PM, Hassall DG, Gladwin AM, Palmer RM, Martin JF. NO and prostacyclin. Divergence of inhibitory effects on monocyte chemotaxis and adhesion to endothelium in vitro. Arterioscler Thromb 1991;11:254–260.
57. Hogan JC, Lewis MJ, Henderson AH. In vivo EDRF activity influences platelet function. Br J Pharmacol 1988;94:1020–1022.
58. Garg UC, Hassid A. NO generating vasodilators and 8-bromo-cyclic guanosine monophosphate inhibit mitogenesis and proliferation of cultured rat vascular smooth muscle cells. J Clin Invest 1989;83: 1774–1777.
59. Hayashi T, Fukoto JM, Ignarro LJ, Chaudhuri C. Basal release of NO from aortic rings is greater in female rabbits than in male rabbits: implications for atherosclerosis. Proc Natl Acad Sci 1992;89: 11,259–11,263.
60. Gisclard V, Miller VM, Vanhoutte PM. Effect of estrogen on endothelium-dependent responses in the rabbit. J Pharmacol Exp Ther 1988;244:19–22.
61. Miller VM, Vanhoutte PM. Progesterone and modulation of endothelium-dependent responses in canine coronary arteries. Am J Physiol 1991;261:1022–1027.
62. Bell DR, Rensberger HJ, Koritnik DR, Koshy A. Estrogen pretreatment directly potentiates endothelium-dependent vasorelaxation of porcine coronary arteries. Am J Physiol 1995;268: H377–H383.
63. Williams JK, Adams MR, Herrington DM, Clarkson TB. Short term administration of estrogen and vascular responses of atherosclerotic coronary arteries. J Am Coll Cardiol 1992;20:452–457.
64. Williams JK, Honore EK, Washburn SA, Clarkson TB. Effects of hormone replacement therapy on reactivity of atherosclerotic coronary arteries in cynomolgus monkeys. J Am Coll Cardiol 1994;24: 1757–1761.
65. Reis SE, Gloth ST, Blumenthal RS, Resar JR, Zacur HA, Gerstenblith G, Brinker JA. Ethinyl estradiol acutely attenuates abnormal coronary vasomotor responses to ACh in postmenopausal women. Circulation 1994;89:52–60.
66. Gilligan DM, Quyyumi AA, Cannon RO. Effects of physiological levels of estrogen on coronary vasomotor function in postmenopausal women. Circulation 1994;89:2545–2551.
67. Lieberman EH, Gerhard M, Yeung AC, Anderson TJ, Meredith IT, Ganz P, Selwyn AP. Estrogen improves coronary vasomotor responses to ACh in postmenopausal women. Circulation 1993;88:I-79 (abstract).
68. Collins P, Rosano GM, Sarrel PM, Ulrich L, Adamopoulos S, Beale CM, McNeill JG, Poole-Wilson PA. Estrogen attenuates ACh-induced coronary arterial constriction in women but not men with coronary heart disease. Circulation 1995;92:24–30.

69. Rosano GM, Sarrel PM, Poole-Wilson PA, Collins P. Beneficial effect of oestrogen on exercise-induced myocardial ischaemia in women with CAD. Lancet 1993;342:133–136.
70. Gerhard MD, Roddy MA, Knab ST, Creager SJ, Creager MA. Acute estrogen administration improves endothelium-dependent vasodilation in postmenopausal women. Circulation 1994;88:I-369 (abstract).
71. Gilligan DM, Badar DM, Panza JA, Quyyumi AA, Cannon RO. Acute vascular effects of estrogen in postmenopausal women. Circulation 1994;90:786–791.
72. Lieberman EH, Gerhard MD, Uehata A, Walsh BW, Selwyn AP, Ganz P, Yeung AC, Creager MA. Estrogen improves endothelium-dependent flow-mediated vasodilation in postmenopausal women. Ann Int Med 1994;121:936–941.
73. Gryglewski RJ, Palmer RM, Moncada S. Superoxide anion is involved in the breakdown of endothelium-derived vascular relaxing factor. Nature 1986;320:454–456.
74. Rubanyi GM, Vanhoutte PM. Hypoxia releases a vasoconstrictor substance from the canine vascular endothelium. J Physiol 1985:364:45–56.
75. Harrison DG, OHara Y. Physiologic consequences of increased vascular oxidant stresses in hypercholesterolemia and atherosclerosis: implications for impaired vasomotion. Am J Cardiol 1995;75:75B–81B.
76. Sugioka JM, Shimosegawa Y, Nakano MM. Estrogens as natural antioxidants of membrane lipid peroxidation. FEBS Lett 1987;210:37–39.
77. Sack MN, Rader DJ, Cannon RO. Oestrogen and inhibition of oxidation of low-density lipoproteins in postmenopausal women. Lancet 1994;343:269,270.
78. Rosser M, Chorich L, Howard E, Zamorano P, Mahesh VB. Changes in rat uterine receptor messenger ribonucleic acid levels during estrogen and progesterone induced estrogen receptor depletion and subsequent replenishment. Biol Reprod 1993;48:89–98.
79. Weiner CP, Lizasoain I, Baylis SA, Knowles RG, Charles IG, Moncada S. Induction of calcium-dependent NOSs by sex hormones. Proc Natl Acad Sci USA 1994;91:5212–5216.
80. Miller VM, Gisclard V, Vanhoutte PM. Modulation of endothelium-dependent and vascular smooth muscle responses by estrogens. Phlebology 1988;3:63–69.
81. Chang WC, Nakao J, Orimo H, Murota SI. Stimulation of prostacyclin activity in rat aorta smooth muscle cells in culture. Biochim Biophys Acta 1980;619:107–118.
82. Gisclard V, Flavahan NA, Vanhoutte PM. Alpha adrenergic responses, of blood vessels of rabbits after ovariectomy and administration of estrogen. J Pharmacol Exp Ther 1987;240:466–470.
83. Jiang C, Sarrel PM, Poole-Wilson PA, Collins P. Acute effect of 17β-estradiol on rabbit coronary artery contractile responses to endothelin-1. Am J Physiol 1992;263:H271–H275.
84. Zhang F. Ram JL, Standley PR, Sowers JR. 17β-estradiol attenuates voltage-dependent Ca^{2+} currents in vascular smooth muscle. Am J Physiol 1994;193:C975–C980.
85. Jiang C, Sarrel PM, Lindsey DC, Poole-Wilson PA, Collins P. Estrogen has calcium antagonistic properties in the rabbit coronary artery in vitro. Circulation 1991;84:II-272 (abstract).
86. Harder DR, Coulson PB. Estrogen receptors and effects of estrogen on membrane electrical properties of coronary vascular smooth muscle. J Cell Physiol 1979;100:375–382.
87. Beldekas JC, Smith B, Gerstenfeld LC, Sonenshein GE, Franzblau C. Effects of estrogen on the biosynthesis of collagen in cultured bovine aortic smooth muscle cells. Biochemistry 1981;20:2162–2167.
88. Fischer GM, Swain ML. Effects of estradiol and progesterone on the increased synthesis of collagen in atherosclerotic rabbit aortas. Atherosclerosis 1985;54:1770–1785.
89. Fischer GM, Cherian K, Swain ML. Increased synthesis of aortic collagen and elastin in experimental atherosclerosis. Atherosclerosis 1981;39:463–467.
90. Morales DE, McGowan KA, Grant DS, Maheshwari S, Bhartiya D, Cid MC, Kleinman HK, Schnaper HW. Estrogen promotes angiogenesis activity in human umbilical vein endothelial cells in vitro and in a murine model. Circulation 1995;91:755–763.

6 C-Type Natriuretic Peptide

The Vascular Component of the Natriuretic Peptide System

Iftikhar J. Kullo, MD
and John C. Burnett, Jr., MD

CONTENTS

INTRODUCTION

Atrial natriuretic peptide (ANP) is a 28 amino acid ringed structure peptide of myocardial cell origin *(1)*. ANP mediates natriuresis, renin-inhibiting, vasodilatory, and antimitogenic properties through actions of particulate guanylyl cyclase and the second messenger guanosine 3',5'-monophosphate (cGMP) *(2,3)*. Brain natriuretic peptide (BNP) shares similar biological actions with ANP, is structurally similar (but genetically distinct), and functions via activation of the same biologically active receptor *(3)*. ANP and BNP form a dual cardiac peptide endocrine system in which these two peptides function as circulating hormones in the control of intravascular volume and arterial pressure *(4)*.

CNP, a 22 amino acid peptide originally isolated in the brain *(5)*, is secreted by human, bovine, and canine vascular endothelial cells *(6,7)*. In human breast tissue *(6)*, immunostaining has been localized to vascular endothelial cells of small caliber arteries without immunoreactivity in veins or surrounding adventitial, stromal, or vascular smooth muscle cells (VSMC) (Fig. 1). CNP immunoreactivity is present in the conditioned

From: *Contemporary Endocrinology: Endocrinology of the Vasculature*
Edited by: J. R. Sowers Humana Press Inc., Totowa, NJ

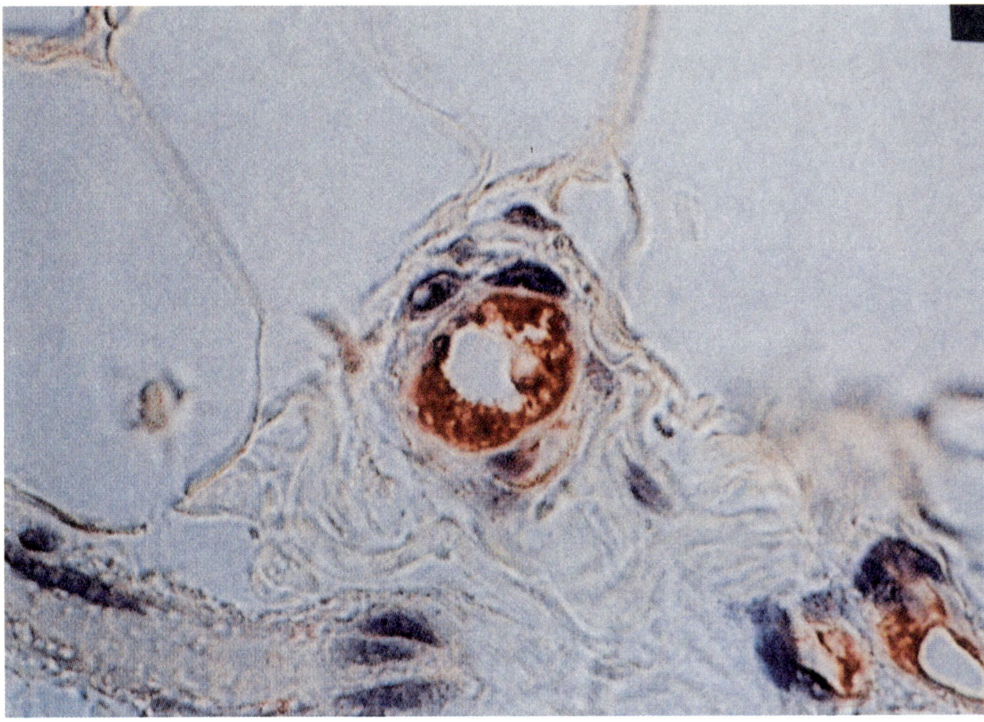

Fig. 1. Immunohistochemical staining for CNP in human breast tissue showing positive staining in the endothelium (magnification rate, ×100). Reprinted from ref. *6* with permission.

media of cultured bovine *(7)* and human *(8)* endothelial cells, and CNP is present in human plasma *(8)*. Expression of the CNP gene by endothelial cells *(7)*, the presence of CNP receptors on VSMC, and an antimitogenic effect of CNP on VSMC suggest that CNP is produced and released by the endothelium and acts on adjacent VSMC; thus serving as a component of an autocrine/paracrine endothelium-derived vasoregulatory system.

In this chapter, we review important details regarding the molecular biology and receptor system of CNP, the biological actions and interactions with other hormonal systems, the metabolism and degradation of CNP, the synthesis and release of CNP, and pathophysiological significance in cardiovascular disease.

CNP GENE AND RECEPTOR

CNP is a product of a gene that is separate from the ANP and BNP genes and is highly conserved among species with over 95% homology among rat, human, and porcine *(9,10)*. The human CNP gene contains two exons and one intron and the first exon codes for a 23 amino acid signal peptide and the first seven amino acids of the pro-CNP molecule (Fig. 2). The second exon codes for the remainder of the precursor including CNP-53 and CNP-22 *(10)*. The region upstream from exon-1 contains *cis* regulatory elements including a TATAAA sequence, two GC boxes, an inverted CCAAT box, and a cAMP response-like sequence *(10,11)*. The latter three sequences are not present in the ANP and BNP genes, suggesting differential regulation of the three genes *(11)*. The 126 amino acid prepro-CNP is processed by undefined proteases to a 103 amino acid pro-CNP peptide.

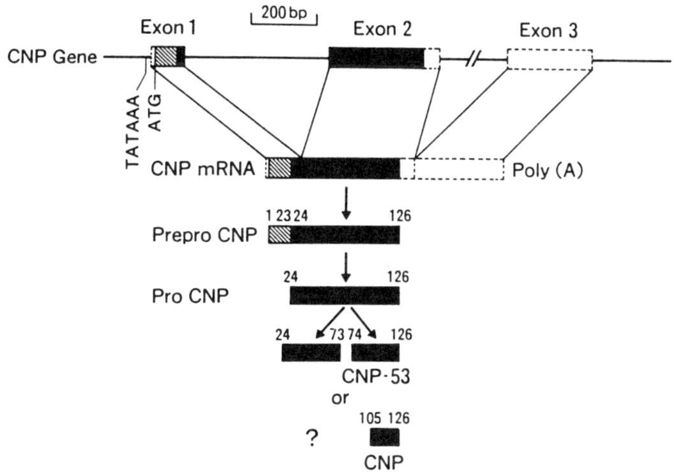

Fig. 2. Structure for the gene and biosynthetic pathway of human CNP. mRNA, messenger RNA; ▧, signal peptide sequence; ■, prohormone sequence; the putative transcriptional start site and exon 3 are indicated by dashed lines. Reprinted from ref. *9* with permission.

The biologically active form of CNP is contained in the C-terminal end of the pro-CNP molecule. Utilizing somatic hybrid cell methodology, the human CNP gene has been assigned to chromosome 2 *(12)*.

The mature biologically active form of CNP, CNP-22, possesses 22 amino acids with a 17-amino acid ring formed by a disulfide bond, and shares structural similarity to ANP and BNP. Unlike these two cardiac peptides, CNP lacks the C-terminal amino acid extension from the ring structure. An N-terminal extended form, CNP-53, is the major molecular form in the porcine brain *(13)*.

CNP Receptor

Natriuretic peptides are endogenous ligands for two well-characterized natriuretic peptide receptors (NPR) that are linked to particulate guanylyl cyclase and result in generation of intracellular cGMP. Importantly, the full biological actions of the natriuretic peptides are further dictated by activity of cGMP phosphodiesterases that modulate the magnitude of cGMP accumulation *(14)*. NPR-A and NPR-B receptors are structurally similar, having similar molecular weights, an extracellular peptide binding domain, and an intracellular protein kinase and guanylate cyclase domain *(15)*. Deletions of the protein kinase domain result in receptors that are constitutively active, indicating its suppressive influence on the guanylate cyclase activity *(16)*. The two biologically active receptors have been well characterized by molecular cloning studies and include the NPR-A receptor for which ANP and BNP are ligands, and the NPR-B receptor for which CNP is the endogenous ligand. Selectivity of these receptors for the three peptides has been studied in cell preparations expressing the cloned human receptors *(17)* by measuring binding affinities and production of cGMP. For the NPR-B receptor, the affinity is CNP>ANP>BNP, and for the NPR-A receptor, the affinity is ANP>BNP>>CNP *(18)*. The ring portion of the CNP molecule with the disulfide bond (CNP 6-22) is needed to stimulate cGMP production and also mediates the selectivity of the molecule for the NPR-B receptor.

A third natriuretic peptide receptor, the NPR-C receptor, has broad selectivity, binding all three peptides more or less equally *(19)*. The NPR-C receptor lacks the protein kinase and guanylate cyclase domains and thus does not mediate cGMP actions. NPR-C internalizes the bound peptide, delivering it to lysosomes for degradation, and the receptor itself is recycled *(20)*. Thus, this receptor is a "clearance receptor" limiting rapid increases in local and circulating natriuretic peptide concentrations and buffering against their excessive biological activity. However, the NPR-C receptor may not be simply a clearance receptor but may have additional biological actions unassociated with cGMP including stimulation of inositol triphosphate (IP_3) *(21)*, inhibition of cAMP production *(22)*, inhibition of neurotransmission in autonomic nerve terminals *(23)*, and inhibition of cell proliferation *(24,25)*.

Although the existence of three separate NPR supports unique and specific actions for the natriuretic peptides, distribution of these receptors is also important in determining biological actions. In the rat, NPR-B expression is present in nearly all tissues, including the brain, kidney, aorta, liver, lung, pituitary *(26)*, and the heart *(27)*. NPR-B receptors have been identified in human kidney *(28)*, but their function is unclear. Receptor expression also has been demonstrated in human aorta *(29)*, implying a role for CNP in the control of vascular function.

As discussed, receptor activation results in generation of cGMP in VSMC and the resulting vascular relaxation is associated with an increase in the activity of a cGMP-dependent kinase *(30)*. cGMP kinase decreases VSMC intracellular calcium $[Ca^{2+}]_i$ by several different mechanisms. These include phosphorylation of phospholamban leading to increased activity of the Ca^{2+}-ATPase localized in the sarcoplasmic reticulum *(31)* with Ca^{2+} extrusion from the cell, activation of Na^+/Ca^{2+} exchange *(32)*, and Na/K/Cl cotransport *(33)*; and inhibition of L-type Ca^{2+} channels *(34)*. cGMP also may inhibit Ca^{2+} release from intracellular stores *(35)* and inhibit IP_3 formation *(36)*. The drop in $[Ca^{2+}]_i$ decreases activity of myosin light-chain kinase and therefore attenuates myosin light-chain phosphorylation, which leads to relaxation *(37)*. cGMP also may have effects independent of activation of cGMP-dependent kinases. These include direct binding to ion channels with opening of K^+ channels and potentiation of cAMP levels in VSMC *(38)*.

CNP RELEASE AND PRESENCE IN THE CIRCULATION

Radioimmunoassays *(39)* have detected CNP-like immunoreactivity in cell extracts, cell supernatants, and in plasma. Utilizing high-performance liquid chromatography, studies suggest that CNP-53 is found intracellularly, whereas CNP-22 is the released form that is detectable in cell supernatant or in plasma. This supports the concept that CNP-53 is a precursor form because CNP-53 itself lacks significant biological action. Further, CNP mRNA has been detected in the thoracic aortic tissue of several species, including human *(26,29)*.

Synthesis of ANP and BNP is regulated by a variety of mechanical and humoral stimuli. Myocyte stretch has emerged as the most potent stimulus for ANP release and synthesis *(40)*. Humoral stimuli for ANP and BNP include angiotensin II (AII), endothelin-1 (ET-1), adrenergic agonists, thyroxine, and corticosteroids *(41)*. Thus, redundant systems participate in the regulation and release of these two cardiac hormones and support a highly integrated system for volume and pressure regulation.

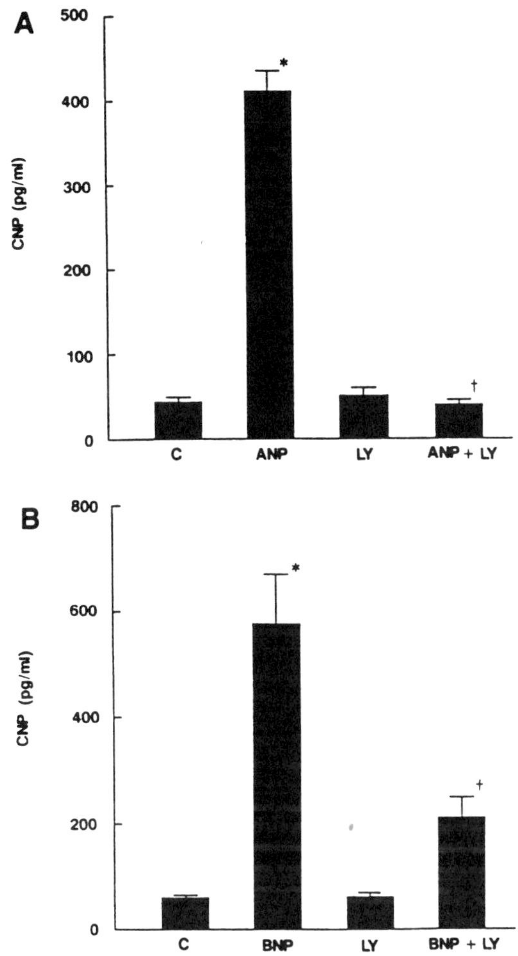

Fig. 3. Effects of ANP and BNP (100 n*M*) on the secretion of CNP from bovine aortic endothelial cell (BAEC). These effects are attenuated by LY 83583, an inhibitor of cGMP generation. Data are the mean ± SEM from two experiments combined ($n = 7$ wells/condition), and are representative of a third experiment. *$p < 0.05$ for ANP or BNP vs control; $^{+}p < 0.05$ for ANP or BNP vs the natriuretic peptide plus LY 83583 (modified from ref. *42*). Reprinted from ref. *42* with permission.

Stimuli for the release of CNP have not been completely elucidated, but the understanding of the autocrine and paracrine role of endothelial CNP in the control of VSMC growth and function may provide insight into possible mechanisms to be explored and defined. Release of other endothelial cell-derived vasoactive factors such as nitric oxide (NO) and ET-1 are sensitive to alterations in vascular wall shear stress as well as humoral stimuli. In contrast, no studies have conclusively demonstrated that alterations in endothelial cell shear stress and/or mechanical stretch results in increased CNP production or release.

In cultured bovine endothelial cells, the cardiac peptides ANP and BNP regulate CNP synthesis and secretion (Fig. 3) *(42)*. ANP and BNP strongly stimulate secretion of CNP from cultured aortic endothelial cells. BNP resulted in a 400-fold enhancement above basal secretion over a 24-h period, which is 20 times greater than the

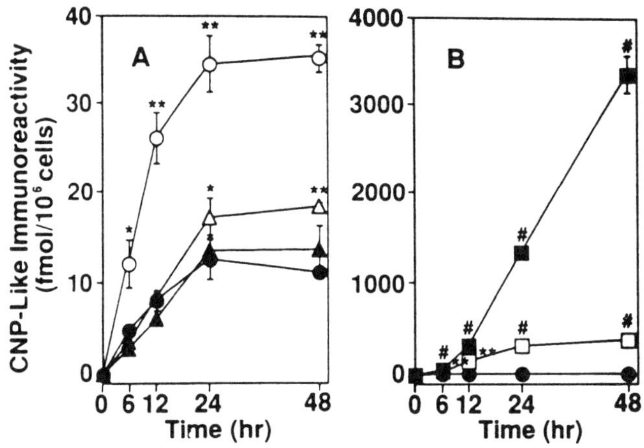

Fig. 4. Time-course of CNP concentrations in conditioned media of cultured endothelial cells stimulated by cytokines **(A)** and LPS (lipopolysaccharide) **(B)**. Cells were incubated with vehicle (●) or 100 ng/mL of IL-1α (○). IL-18 (Δ), IL-2 (Δ), TNF-α (■), or LPS (□). Each point represents mean ± SEM of three separate experiments. $*p < 0.05$; $**p < 0.01$; $^{\#}p < 0.001$ vs vehicle-treated cells. Reprinted from ref. *43* with permission.

action of ANP. In comparison, ET-1 and AII had little effect on CNP secretion. This action of BNP occurs via activation of particulate guanylyl cyclase and not through activation or binding to the NPR-C receptor. Thus, vasodilatory and antimitogenic effects of ANP and BNP may occur in the vasculature, through CNP production and subsequent action.

A potent stimulus to CNP production and release are cytokines and growth factors. Transforming growth factor-beta (TGF-β), a key molecule in vascular remodeling as well as in sepsis, induces more than a twofold increase in CNP secretion from vascular endothelial cells *(7)*. Other potent cytokines and/or growth factors that stimulate CNP release include tumor necrosis factor (TNF), interleukin-1 (IL-1), lipopolysaccharide, basic fibroblast growth factor, and thrombin (Fig. 4) *(43)*. Vascular actions of bradykinin are attenuated by an NPR antagonist *(44)*. This suggests that part of the effects of bradykinin on the vessel wall occur by the stimulation of CNP release *(44)*. Thus, major vascular components such as platelets, macrophages, endothelial cells, and VSMC secrete a number of factors that play a role in CNP synthesis and/or release and underscore an important role for CNP as a local paracrine and autocrine factor in the regulation of vascular wall biology.

CARDIOVASCULAR ACTIONS OF CNP

CNP and VSMC

CNP stimulates guanylate cyclase activity in the particulate fraction of cultured rat VSMC, thereby increasing intracellular levels of cGMP *(45)* fourfold higher than that by ANP. However, ANP was 4–16-fold stronger than CNP in vasorelaxant activity in the intact rat aorta. This is related to the preferential expression of NPR-B receptors in the cultured VSMC. CNP is also a potent inhibitor of VSMC proliferation *(46)*. CNP is 5–10-fold more potent than ANP in stimulating cGMP in bovine-cultured VSMC, and a low concentration of CNP ($2 \times 10^{-9} M$) inhibits up to 80% of the (^{3}H)-thymidine

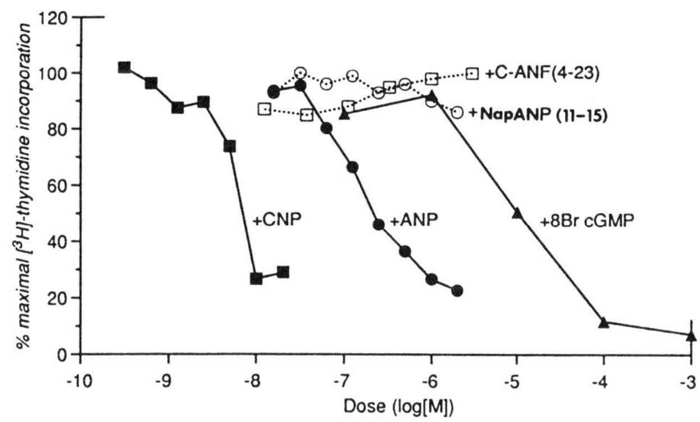

Fig. 5. Inhibition by ANP, CNP, and 8-bromo-cGMP of fibroblast growth factor-stimulated [^{3}H]-thymidine incorporation. Quiescent cultures of bovine aortic smooth muscle (BASM) cells are treated with growth factors for 24 h in absence or presence of indicated concentrations of rANP (99–126), hCNP (1–22), C-ANF (4–23), Nap ANP (11–15), or 8-bromo-cGMP. Data represents means of triplicate determinations *(47)*. Reprinted from ref. *47* with permission.

incorporation induced by basic fibroblast growth factor (Fig. 5) *(47)*. CNP may also be one of the endothelial-derived hyperpolarizing factors (EDHF), since part of the vasorelaxant activity on coronary arteries seems to be mediated through K^+ channel activation *(48)*.

Effects on Veins and Arteries

CNP has potent systemic cardiovascular actions that include reductions in cardiac filling pressures and output, secondary to vasorelaxation and decreases in venous return. Studies using CNP have been performed in isolated saphenous, femoral, and renal canine veins in the presence and absence of the endothelium *(49)* and actions of CNP compared to those of ANP. CNP as compared to ANP is a selective endothelium-independent venodilator as demonstrated by its potent ability to relax isolated precontracted veins (Fig. 6). Thus, CNP may be an endogenous "nitroglycerin type" venodilator that plays a regulatory role on cardiac output via control of venous return.

In contrast to marked actions on veins, CNP is less potent in relaxing peripheral arteries such as femoral and renal arteries. ANP, and not CNP, is a more selective arterial vasodilator supporting the concept that ANP and CNP have distinct vascular actions in the control of peripheral vascular tone. The differential action of ANP as compared to CNP in the control of vascular tone implies that the receptors, NPR-A and NPR-B, are also differentially localized to peripheral arteries and veins.

Although CNP may lack peripheral arterial vasorelaxation actions, it is a potent coronary vasodilator in preconstricted canine coronary arteries *(50)*. As in peripheral arteries and veins, this action of CNP is endothelium independent, and the high conductance Ca^{2+}-activated K^+ channel antagonist, charybtotoxin, as well as the ATP-sensitive K^+ channel antagonist, glibenclamide, attenuate the vasorelaxing action of CNP in these isolated coronary arteries.

Effects of CNP on whole-cell K^+ current and membrane potentials have been investigated utilizing single-cell patch-clamp electrophysiological studies in isolated porcine coronary VSMC. CNP increases whole-cell current in a dose-dependent fashion but has

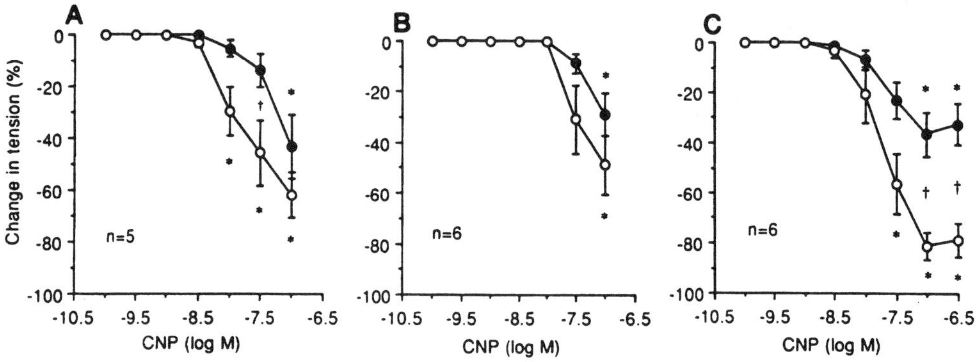

Fig. 6. Vasorelaxations to CNP in canine renal **(A)**, saphenous **(B)**, and femoral veins **(C)** with (●) and without (○) endothelium. Data are shown as mean ± SE and are expressed as a percent change in tension from a contraction to phenylphrine $10^{-6} M$ (30–40% of maximal contraction). $*p < 0.05$ vs –10 log M; $^{\dagger}p < 0.05$ between groups. Reprinted from ref. *49* with permission.

minimal effects on resting voltage, but nonetheless does function via membrane hyperpolarization involving K^+ channel opening at depolarizing voltages (Fig. 7). Further, TEA, a known inhibitor of high conductance Ca^{2+}-activated K^+ channels, attenuates CNP-mediated changes in whole-cell current. EDHF may cause hyperpolarization and relaxation of VSMC *(51)*. One of the EDHFs may be an activator of high conductance Ca^{2+}-activated K^+ channels. Thus, there appears to be a link between activation of natriuretic peptide–particulate guanylyl cyclase system and stimulation of K^+ channels, and CNP may function via K^+ channels in coronary VSMC. In intact pituitary tumor cells, ANP results in cGMP-stimulated K^+ channel opening through activation of a cGMP-dependent protein kinase *(52)*. Thus, CNP may function via activation of particulate guanylyl cyclase with cGMP accumulation and subsequent vasorelaxation as well as via K^+ channel opening via cGMP-dependent protein kinase activation.

Systemic Cardiovascular Actions

When CNP is infused intravenously in anesthetized dogs, at doses equivalent to those of ANP that produce natriuresis, plasma cGMP rises, and arterial pressure, right atrial pressure, cardiac output, renal blood flow, glomerular filtration rate, and sodium excretion decrease. With a bolus injection, cardiac output declines, renal blood flow and glomerular filtration rate do not change, but sodium excretion still decreases. Thus, CNP lacks the renal effects of ANP, and is therefore a more cardiovascular selective member of the natriuretic peptide family.

In normal humans, infusion of synthetic human CNP-22 (5 pmol/kg/min), achieving supraphysiological levels in plasma, results in no significant hemodynamic action or natriuresis *(53)*. During coinfusion of AII, the expected pressor and aldosterone responses are not altered by CNP *(54)*. Increases in cGMP are much lower than those previously demonstrated with equimolar amounts of ANP or BNP. These results make it improbable that acute increases in circulating CNP are vasoactive or natriuretic in humans. However, like BNP, CNP could affect ANP metabolism and degradation by competing for binding to neutral endopeptidase (EC 24. 11) and/or NPR-C receptors. Clearly, further work is required to assess the effects of more chronic infusions both in experimental animals and in humans.

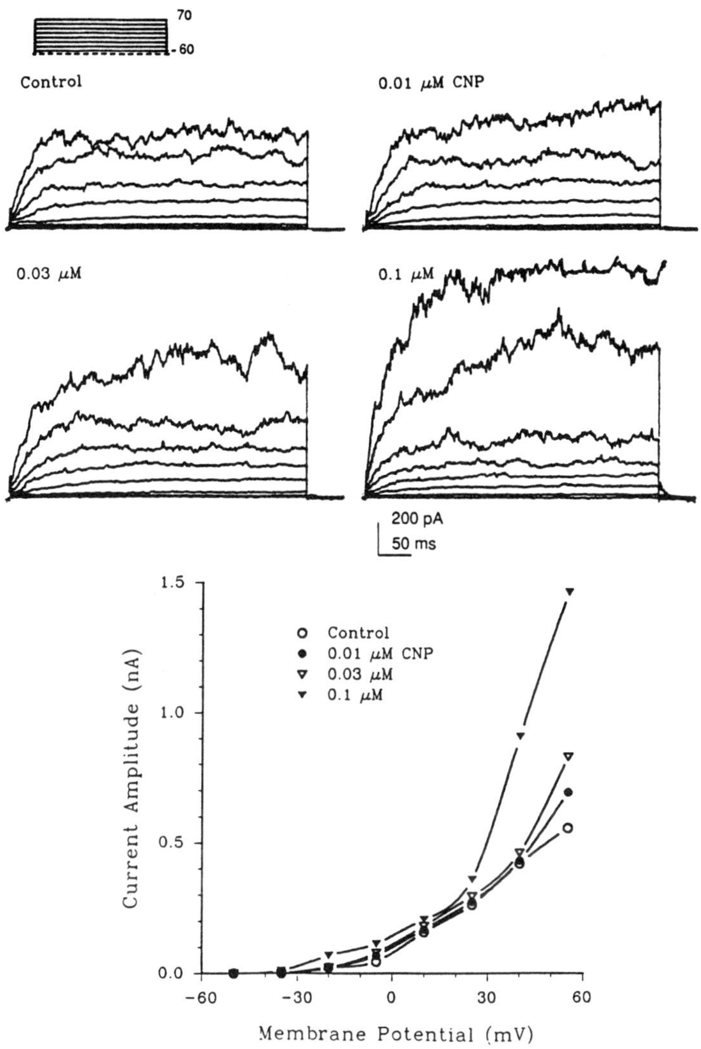

Fig. 7. Augmentation of whole-cell K^+ currents by CNP in smooth muscle cells from porcine coronary arteries. The figure shows the relationship between the amplitude of steady-state K^+ currents and membrane potentials in the absence and presence of CNP at 0.01, 0.03, and 0.1 μ*M*. Reprinted from ref. *50* with permission.

INTERACTIONS OF CNP WITH OTHER VASOACTIVE FACTORS

The vascular NO system involves two pathways for NO generation via activation of the enzyme NO synthase (NOS). These two enzymatic pathways involve a Ca^{2+}-sensitive pathway, termed the constitutive NOS (cNOS); and the Ca^{2+}-independent pathway, termed the inducible NOS (iNOS). Once NOS is activated, NO is produced and cGMP is generated via soluble guanylyl cyclase, in contrast to cGMP generated by CNP via particulate guanylyl cyclase. Although the soluble and particulate guanylyl cyclase systems have been viewed as separate, recent investigations suggest an interaction. In cultured aortic VSMCs, CNP has no effect on basal nitrite, the stable end product of NO. In

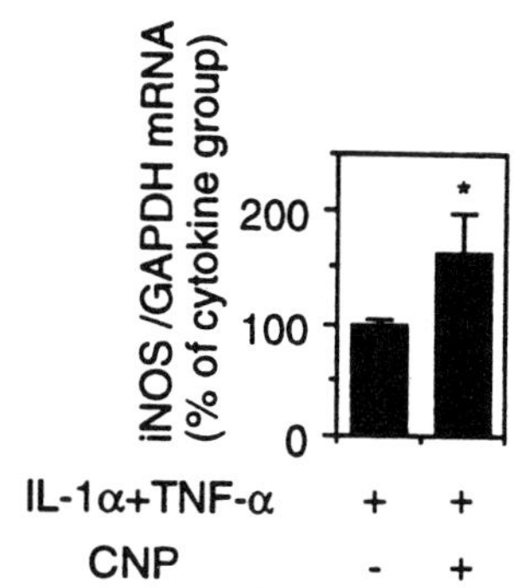

Fig. 8. Northern blot analysis of iNOS mRNA from rat aortic smooth muscle cells treated with combinations of cytokines and CNP. The density of iNOS mRNA relative to GAPDH expression is shown. Modified from ref. *55* with permission.

contrast, when CNP is added with TNF, CNP markedly enhances the ability of TNF to generate cGMP *(55)*. This action is associated with CNP enhancement of iNOS mRNA and mimicked by 8-bromo-cGMP (Fig. 8). These studies thus underscore a unique interaction between the NO and CNP systems in vascular regulation.

Regarding ET-1, several studies provide evidence of interactions. In cultured porcine endothelial cells, CNP inhibits the ET-1 release stimulated by AII and thrombin through a cGMP-dependent process *(56)*. In rat VSMCs, CNP, via a cGMP mechanism, upregulates vascular ET_B receptors. In these studies, ET reduces cGMP formation induced by CNP and sodium nitroprusside by about 50% *(57)*. There appears to be a functional interaction between ET and CNP in the regulation of vascular tone *(58)*, and the two may function as opposing humoral mechanisms in control of an endothelial-VSMC axis.

CNP METABOLISM AND DEGRADATION

The NPR-C receptor functions as a clearance receptor that binds, internalizes, and degrades CNP as well as ANP and BNP. In addition to clearance by the NPR-C receptor, CNP is subject to degradation by the ectoenzyme, neutral endopeptidase (EC 24.11, NEP), which is widely distributed in the kidney, lung, heart, as well as in VSMC and endothelial cells. For natriuretic peptides, kinetic studies show that the rank order of hydrolysis by NEP is CNP < ANP < BNP *(59)*. NEP may limit full biological actions of CNP through rapid degradation. NEP is highly expressed in cultured human coronary endothelial cells from both the epicardial arteries and the microcirculation *(60)*, and there is upregulation of coronary NEP by thrombin. In cardiovascular disease states in which thrombin or its metabolites are increased, the vasorelaxing and growth inhibiting actions of CNP may be limited by enhanced expression of coronary NEP.

CNP IN CARDIOVASCULAR DISEASE

Hypertension

C-type natriuretic peptide has the potential to influence arterial pressure by actions at diverse sites. Via its central nervous system effects it may act to alter autonomic regulation of vascular tone and arterial pressure. Centrally administered CNP lowers blood pressure and adrenocortical secretion in normotensive sheep *(61)*. Infusions of CNP have been shown to lower blood pressure in both anesthetized and conscious dogs *(53)*. By its vasorelaxant and antimitogenic effects on VSMC, CNP may influence vascular remodeling in hypertension. CNP also modulates purinergic and adrenergic transmission in a concentration-dependent manner without altering cGMP or cAMP concentrations *(62)*.

To date, no difference in plasma CNP has been observed between normotensive and hypertensive humans or animals. However, the vasorelaxing action of CNP is markedly attenuated in aortic rings of rats with genetic hypertension *(63)*. This suggests downregulation of NPR-B receptors or alterations in signal transduction mechanisms. The response to ANP in this study was not altered. CNP seems unlikely to participate acutely in sodium or blood pressure homeostasis in humans. However, with its strategic location in the central nervous system and in vascular endothelium adjacent to VSMC, CNP may play a role in the overall regulation of arterial pressure, and in the remodeling associated with hypertension.

Atherosclerosis

Biopsy studies suggest the quiescent nature of many human atherosclerotic plaques *(64)*, implying that, at some stage, factors favoring myoproliferation are balanced by antimitogenic substances, such as heparan sulfate, gamma interferon, and NO. Endothelium-derived CNP has been shown to be potently antimitogenic and may regulate growth of VSMC in a paracrine function, and exert autocrine modulation of endothelial proliferation *(11)*. Increased expression of NPR-B receptors in phenotypically altered VSMC *(65)* suggests that CNP may have an important antimitogenic role in such cells. Indeed, the NPR-B receptor remains present and highly expressed in vascular wall following injury *(66)*. Additionally, CNP production in atherosclerosis could be activated by cytokines that are known to be present in atheromatous lesions. Such cytokines could include IL-1, TNF, and TGF-β. In preliminary studies (unpublished), enhanced CNP immunoreactivity has been identified in atheromatous aortas from rabbits with atherosclerosis induced by cholesterol feeding. This preliminary observation also has been extended to CNP immunoreactivity in atheromata obtained with atherectomy in patients with coronary atherosclerosis. Thus, CNP may play an important role in the pathophysiology of human and experimental atherosclerosis.

Congestive Heart Failure (CHF) and Shock

In CHF, plasma levels of CNP are not elevated, although atrial and ventricular CNP content is increased *(67)*, suggesting a paracrine role of the peptide. In the peripheral vasculature of patients with CHF, vasodilatory effects of ANP are attenuated whereas those of CNP are preserved *(68)*. Since CHF is associated with an elevation of circulating cytokines that are potent stimulators of CNP release, the peptide may have an important paracrine effect on vascular tone in patients with CHF. Additionally, in patients with septic shock, a marked increase in plasma CNP levels has been described *(69)*. This indicates that CNP may be a mediator of the marked vasodilatation that characterizes shock in association with NO activation.

THERAPEUTIC IMPLICATIONS

Atherosclerosis and Restenosis

Vasorelaxing and antimitogenic actions suggest a potential therapeutic role for CNP in cardiovascular disease. However, since CNP is a peptide, oral administration is not feasible, which limits its use to intravenous or transdermal use. To date, no studies have utilized such an approach. An alternative approach is to limit degradation of CNP by orally available inhibitors of neutral endopeptidase (NEP).

Recent preliminary studies have shown, in the hypercholesterolemic rabbit, an upregulation of NEP in the aortic wall *(70)*. Orally administered NEP inhibition in the same model markedly decreases atheromatous plaque formation induced by hypercholesterolemia *(71)*. This effect may be caused by potentiation of the paracrine effects of CNP, which is one of the major substrates of NEP. Vascular injury owing to various agents, including hypercholesterolemia, may thus upregulate NEP activity and thereby diminish the vasorelaxant and antimitogenic effects of CNP. Additionally, in the cholesterol-fed rabbit, NEP inhibition combined with angiotensin-converting enzyme (ACE) inhibition also retards the development of atherosclerosis and reverses the endothelial dysfunction that characterizes atherosclerosis. Specifically, the impaired relaxation to acetylcholine of isolated atheromatous aortas, is reversed by combined inhibition of NEP and ACE *(72)*. Further studies are required to address a therapeutic role of NEP inhibitors in atherosclerosis.

A major problem with angioplasty is restenosis occurring in the area of injury. In the rat carotid artery injury model, CNP, infused at 1 μg/kg/min for 5 d, results in a 60% reduction in neointima formation *(73)* together with enhanced production of cGMP in the injured vessel but not in the intact vessel, indicating increased expression of the NPR-B receptor at the sites of vascular injury. The antimitogenic and vasorelaxing effects of CNP could potentially be used to limit restenosis after balloon injury.

An intriguing approach to vascular disease has been the application of gene transfer of antimitogenic factors. Recent studies have demonstrated the feasibility of viral-mediated gene transfer methodology to overexpress ANP gene in endothelial cells and VSMC *(74)*. The vasodilator and growth inhibitory properties of CNP should make it a candidate for gene therapy of disease states characterized by vasoconstriction and VSMC proliferation, most importantly, atherosclerosis and restenosis.

CONCLUSIONS AND FUTURE AREAS OF RESEARCH

CNP emerges as an additional endothelial-derived vasorelaxing factor with potent actions on vascular tone and VSMC growth. These actions are mediated by activation of particulate guanylyl cyclase as well as by probable hyperpolarization of VSMC membrane potential. The full biological actions of CNP may be limited by the rapid degradation of CNP by NEP, which is highly expressed both on endothelial cells as well as VSMC. Moreover, CNP interacts importantly with other endothelial-derived vasoactive and growth regulating factors such as NO and ET-1.

CNP also may play a compensatory role in vascular wall injury such as in atherosclerosis in which cytokines and/or other factors stimulate production and expression of CNP. CNP may be important in the progression of vascular lesions associated with mechanical or chemical injury of the endothelium. Additionally, the full biological potential of CNP in vascular disease such as in atherosclerosis may be limited by upregulation of NEP, which degrades secreted CNP supporting a role for inhibition of this enzyme in order to potentiate the local actions of CNP. The next few years will certainly provide exciting new insight into this newly discovered endothelial-derived vasoactive factor in vascular biology and disease.

REFERENCES

1. DeBold AJ, Borenstein HB, Veress AT, Sonnenberg H. A rapid and potent natriuretic response to intravenous injection of atrial myocardial extract in rats. Life Sci 1981;28:89–94.
2. Burnett JC Jr, Granger JP, Opgenorth TF. Effects of synthetic atrial natriuretic factor on renal function and renin release. Am J Physiol 1984;247:F863–F866.
3. Koller KJ, Goeddel DV. Molecular biology of the natriuretic peptides and their receptors. Circulation 1992;86:1081–1088.
4. Mukoyama M, Nakao K, Hosoda K, Suga K, Saitu Y, Ogawa Y, Shiralrami G, Jougasaki M, Obata K, Yasue H, Kambayashi Y, Inouye K, Imura H. Brain natriuretic peptide as novel cardiac hormone in humans: evidence for an exquisite dual natriuretic peptide system, atrial natriuretic peptide and brain natriuretic peptide. J Clin Invest 1991;87:1402–1412.
5. Sudoh TN, Minamino N, Kangawa K, Matsuo H. C-type natriuretic peptide (CNP), a new member of natriuretic peptide family identified in porcine brain. Biochem Biophys Res Commun 1990;168:863–870.
6. Heublein DM, Clavell AL, Lerman A, Wold L, Burnett JC Jr. C-type natriuretic peptide immunoreactivity in human breast vascular endothelial cells. Peptides 1992;13:1017–1019.
7. Suga S, Nakao K, Itoh H, Kamatsu Y, Ogawa Y, Hama H, Imura H. Endothelial production of C-type natriuretic peptide and its marked augmentation by transforming growth factor-β. J Clin Invest 1992;90:1145–1149.
8. Stingo AJ, Clavell AL, Heublien DM, Wei CM, Pittelkow MR, Burnett JC, Jr. Presence of C-type natriuretic peptide in cultured human endothelial cells and plasma. Am J Physiol 1992;263(Heart Circ Physiol 32):H1318–H1321.
9. Nakao K, Ogawa Y, Suga S, Imura H. Molecular biology and biochemistry of the natriuretic peptide system I: natriuretic peptides. J Hypertens 1992;10:907–912.
10. Tawaragi Y, Fuchimura K, Tanaka S, Minamino N, Kangawa K, Matsuo H. Gene and precursor structures of human C-type natriuretic peptide. Biochem Biophys Res Commun 1991;175:645–651.
11. Ogawa Y, et al. Human C-type natriuretic peptide: characterization of the gene and peptide. Hypertension 1992;19:809–813.
12. Ogawa Y, Itoh H, Yoshitake Y, Inoue M, Yoshimasa T, Serikawa T, Nakao K. Molecular cloning and chromosomal assignment of the mouse C-type natriuretic peptide (CNP) gene (Nppc): comparison with the human CNP gene (NPPC). Genomics 1994;24:383–387.
13. Minamino N, Kangawa K, Matsuo H. N-terminally extended form of C-type natriuretic peptide (CNP-53) identified in porcine brain. Biochem Biophys Res Commun 1990;170:973–979.
14. Wilkins MR, Needleman P. Effect of pharmacologic manipulation of endogenous atriopeptin activity on renal function. Am J Physiol 1992;262(Renal Fluid Electrolyte Physiol 31):F161–F167.
15. Chinkers M, Garbers DL. The protein kinase domain of the ANP receptor is required for signalling. Science 1989;245:1392.
16. Koller K, deSauvage FJ, Lowe DG, Goeddel DV. Conservation of the kinase like domain is essential for activation of the natriuretic peptide receptor guanylyl cyclases. Mol Cell Biol 1992;12:2581–2590.
17. Koller KJ, Lowe DG, Bennett GL, Minamino N, Goeddel DV, et al. Selective activation of the B-natriuretic peptide receptor by C-type natriuretic peptide (CNP). Science Washington DC 1991; 252:120–123.
18. Suga SK, Nakao K, Mukoyama Y, Ogawa T, Shirakami G, Kambayashi Y, Inouye K, Imura H. Receptor selectivity of natriuretic peptide family, atrial natriuretic peptide, brain natriuretic peptide and C-type natriuretic peptide. Endocrinology 1992;130:229–239.
19. Maack T. Receptors of atrial natriuretic factor. Annu Rev Physiol 1992;54:11–27.
20. Nusseinzveig DR, Lewicki J, Maack T. Cellular mechanisms of the clearance function of type C receptors of atrial natriuretic factor. J Biol Chem 1990;265:20,952.
21. Hirata M, Chang CH, Murad F. Stimulatory effects of atrial natriuretic factor on phosphoinositide hydrolysis in cultured bovine aortic smooth muscle cells. Biochem Biophys Acta 1989;10:346–351.
22. Anandsrivatsva MB, Sairam MR, Cantin M. Ring deleted analogs of atrial natriuretic factor inhibit adenylate cyclase/c AMP system. J Biol Chem 1990;265:8566–8572.
23. Drewett JG, Ziegler RJ, Trachte GJ. Neuromodulatory effects of atrial natriuretic peptides correlate with an inhibition of adenylate cyclase but not an activation of guanylate cyclase. J Pharm Exp Ther 1992;260:689–696.
24. Levin ER. Natriuretic peptide C receptor: more than a clearance receptor. Am J Physiol 1993;264: E483–489.

25. Levin ER, Frank HL. Natriuretic peptides inhibit astroglial cell proliferation: mediation by C-receptor. Am J Physiol 1990;261:R453–R457.
26. Tallerco-Melnyk T, Yip CC, Watt VM. Widespread co-localization of mRNAs encoding the guanylate cyclase coupled natriuretic peptide receptors in rat tissues. Biochem Biophys Res Commun 1992;189:610–616.
27. Nunez DJR, Dickson MC, Brown MJ. Natriuretic peptide receptor mRNAs in the rat and human heart. J Clin Invest 1992;90:1966–1971.
28. Canaankuhl S, Jamison RL, Myers BD, Pratt RE. Identification of "B" receptor for natriuretic peptide in human kidney. Endocrinology 1992;130:550–552.
29. Komatsu Y, Nakao K, Itoh H, Suga S, Ogawa Y, Imura H. Vascular natriuretic peptide system in humans (Letter). Lancet 1992;340:622.
30. Popescu LM, Panoiu C, Hinescu M, Nutu O. The mechanism of cGMP-induced relaxation in VSMC. Eur J Pharmacol 1985;107:393,394.
31. Cornwell TL, Pryzwansky KB, Lincoln TM. Regulation of sarcoplasmic reticulum protein phosphorylation by localized cyclic GMP-dependent protein kinase in VSMCs. Mol Pharmacol 1991;40:923–931.
32. Furukawa KI, Ohshima N, Tawada-Iwata Y, Shigekawa M. Cyclic GMP stimulates Na/Ca exchange in VSMCs in primary culture. J Biol Chem 1991;266:12,337–12,341.
33. O'Donnell ME, Owen NE. Atrial natriuretic factor stimulates Na/K/Cl cotransport in VSMCs. Proc Natl Acad Sci USA 1986;83:6132–6136.
34. Mery PF, Lohmann SM, Fischmeister R. Ca current is regulated by cyclic GMP dependent protein kinase in mammalian cardiac myocytes. Proc Natl Acad Sci USA 1991;88:1197–1201.
35. Meisherei KD, Taylor CJ, Saneii H. Synthetic atrial peptide inhibits intracellular Ca^{2+} release in smooth muscle. Am J Physiol 1986;250:C171–C174.
36. Hirata M, Kohse KP, Chang CH, Ikebe T, Murad F. Mechanism of cyclic GMP inhibition of inositol phosphate formation in rat aorta segments and cultured bovine aortic smooth muscle cells. J Biol Chem 1990;265:1268–1273.
37. Winquist RJ, Faison EP, Waldman SA, Schwartz K, Murad F, Rapoport RM. Atrial natriuretic factor elicits an endothelium-independent relaxation and activates perticulate guanylate cyclase in VSMC. Proc Natl Acad Sci USA 1984;81:7661–7664.
38. Lincoln TM. Cyclic GMP and mechanisms of vasodilation. Pharmacol Ther 1989;41:479–502.
39. Yandle TG. Biochemistry of natriuretic peptides. J Int Med 1994;235:561–576.
40. Edwards BS, Zimmerman RS, Schwab RR, Heublein DM, Burnett JC Jr. Atrial stretch, not pressure is the principal determinant controlling the acute release of atrial natriuretic factor. Circ Res 1988; 62:191–195.
41. Espiner EA. Physiology of natriuretic peptides. J Int Med 1994;235:527–541.
42. Nazario B, Hu RM, Pedram A, Prins B, Levin ER. Atrial and brain natriuretic peptides stimulate the production and secretion of C-type natriuretic peptide from bovine aortic endothelial cells. J Clin Invest 1995;95:1151–1157.
43. Suga S, Itoh H, Komatsu Y, Ogawa Y, Hama N, Yoshimasa T, Nakao K. Cytokine induced C-type natriuretic peptide (CNP) secretion from vascular endothelial cells: evidence for CNP as a novel autocrine/paracrine regulator from endothelial cells. Endocrinology 1993;133:3038–3041.
44. Wennberg PW, Wei CM, Miller VM, Kinoshita MM, Burnett JC Jr. Vascular acions of a natriuretic peptide receptor and particulate guanylate cyclase inhibitor upon isolated canine coronary arteries. Circulation 1994;90:I112.
45. Furuya M, Takehisa M, Minamitake Y, Kitajima Y, Hayashi Y. Novel natriuretic peptide, CNP, potently stimulates cyclic GMP production in rat cultured VSMCs. Biochem Biophys Res Commun 1990; 170:201–208.
46. Furuya M, Yoshida M, Minamino N, Kangawa K, Matsuo H. C-type natriuretic peptide is a growth inhibitor of rat VSMCs. Biochem Biophys Res Commun 1991;177:927–931.
47. Porter JG, Protter AA. C-type natriuretic peptide inhibits growth factor-dependent DNA synthesis in smooth muscle cells. Am J Physiol 1992;263:C1001–1006.
48. Wei C , Hu S, Miller V, Burnett JC Jr. Vascular actions of C-type natriuretic peptide in isolated porcine coronary arteries and coronary VSMCs Biochem Biophys Res Commun 1994;205:765–771.
49. Wie CM, Aarhus LL, Miller VM, Burnett JC Jr. Action of C-type natriuretic peptide in isolated canine arteries and veins. Am J Physiol 1993;264:H71–H73.
50. Wei C, Hu S, Miller V, Burnett JC Jr. Vascular actions of C-type natriuretic peptide in isolated porcine coronary arteries and coronary VSMCs. Biochem Biophys Res Commun 1994;205:765–771.

51. Vanhoulte PM, Cohen RA. Endothelium dependent hyperpolarization: beyond NO and cyclic GMP. Circulation 1996;2:3337–3749.
52. White RE, Lee AB, Scherbatko AD, Lincoln TM, Schonburnn A, Armstrong DL. K^+ channel stimulation by natriuretic peptides through cGMP-dependent dephosphorylation. Nature 1993;361:263–266.
53. Stingo AJ, Clavell A, Aarhus L, Burnett JC Jr. Cardiovascular and renal actions of C-type natriuretic peptide. Am J Physiol 1992;262(Heart Circ Physiol 31):H308–H312.
54. Hunt PJ, Yandle TG. Bioactivity and metabolism of C-type natriuretic peptide in normal man. J Clin Endocrinol Metab 1994;78:1428–1435.
55. Marumo T, Nakaki T, Hishikawa K, Hirahashi J, Suzuki H, Kato R, Saruta T. Natriuretic peptide-augmented induction of NO synthase through cyclic guanosine 3',5'-monophosphate elevation in VSMCs. Endocrinology 1995;136:2135–2142.
56. Kohno M, Horio T, Yokokawa K, Kurihara N, Takeda T. C-type natriuretic peptide inhibits thrombin and AII stimulated ET-1 release via cyclic guanosine 3',5'-monophosphate. Hypertension 1992;19:320–325.
57. Vigne P, Lund L, Frelin C. Cross talk among cyclic AMP, cyclic GMP, and Ca^{+2}-dependent intracellular signalling mechanisms in brain capillary endothelium. J Neurochem 1994;62:2269–2274.
58. Nir A, Clavell AL, Aarhus LL, Burnett JC Jr. The modulating effect of C-type natriuretic peptide on the hemodynamic actions of ET-1. Am J Hypertens 1993;6:74A.
59. Dussaule JC, Stefanski A, Bea ML, Ronco P, Ardailou R. Characterization of neutral endopeptidase in VSMCs of rabbit renal cortex. Am J Physiol 1993;264:F45–F52.
60. Graf K, Koehne P, Grafe M, et al. Regulation and expression of neutral endopeptidase 24.11 in human endothelial cells. Hypertension 1995;26:230–235.
61. Charles CJ, Richards AM, Espiner EA. Central C-type natriuretic peptide but not atrial natriuretic factor lowers blood pressure and adrenocortical secretion in normal conscious sheep. Endocrinology 1992;131:721–726.
62. Trachte GJ, Drewett JG. C-type natriuretic peptide neuromodulates independently of guanylyl cyclase activation. Hypertension 1994;23:38–43.
63. Wei CM, Burnett JC Jr. Atrial natriuretic peptide and CNP in spontaneously hypertensive rats and their vasorelaxing actions in vivo. Hypertension 1994;23(Part 2):903–907.
64. Dartsch PC. In vitro growth characteristics of human atherosclerotic plaque cells: comparison of cells from primary stenosing and restenosing lesions of peripheral and coronary arteries. Res Exp Med 1990;190:77–87.
65. Suga S, Nakao K. Phenotype-related alteration in expression of natriuretic peptide receptors in aortic smooth muscle cells. Circ Res 1992;71:34–39.
66. Brown J, Chen Q. Regional expression of natriuretic peptide receptors during the formation of arterial neointima in the rabbit. Circ Res 1995;77:906–918.
67. Wei CM, Heublein DM, Kao PC, Edwards WD, Burnett JC Jr. Natriuretic peptide system in human heart failure. Circulation 1993;88:1004–1009.
68. Nakamura M, Arakawa N, Yoshida H, Makita S, Hiramori K. Vasodilatory effects of C-type natriuretic peptide in forearm resistance vessels are distinct from those of atrial natriuretic peptide in chronic heart failure. Circulation 1994;90:1210–1214.
69. Hama N, Itoh H, Shirakami G, Suga S, Komatsu Y, Yoshimasa T, Tanaka I, Mori K, Nakas K. Detection of C-type natriuretic peptides in human circulation and marked increase of plasma CNP level on septic shock patients. Biochem Biophys Res Commun 1994;198:1177–1182.
70. Kugiyama K, Sugiyama S, Matsumura T, Yasutaka O. Increased activity of neutral endopeptidase 24.11 inhibits relaxations in response to C-type natriuretic peptide in atherosclerotic arteries. Circulation 1994;90:I–36.
71. Kugiyama K, Sugiyama S, Matsumura T, Yasue H. Suppression of atherosclerotic changes in cholesterol fed rabbits treated with an oral inhibitor of neutral endopeptidase 24.11. Circulation 1993;88:I–521.
72. Kullo IJ, Muller VM, Lawson GM, Burnett JC Jr. Dual inhibition of neutral endopeptidase (NEP) and angiotensin converting enzyme (ACE) suppresses atherogenesis and improves endothelial function in hypercholestemic rabbits. J Am Coll Cardiol 1996;27(2 Suppl. A):164A.
73. Furuya M, Aisaka K, Miyazaki T, Honbou N, Kawashima K, Ohno T, Tanaka S, Minamino H, Kangawa K, Matsuo H. C-type natriuretic peptide inhibits intimal thickening after vascular injury. Biochem Biophys Res Commun 1993;193:248–253.
74. Morishita R, Gibbons GH, Pratt RE, Tomita N, Dzau VJ. Autocrine and paracrine effects of atrial natriuretic peptide gene transfer on VSMCs and endothelial cellular growth. J Clin Invest 1994;94:824–829.

7 Vascular Actions of Insulin in Health and Disease

Role of the Endothelium

Alain D. Baron, MD
and Helmut O. Steinberg, MD

CONTENTS

INTRODUCTION

Insulin has specific and physiologic cardiovascular actions in humans, and causes an increase in skeletal muscle blood flow (SMBF) and a fall in vascular resistance. In this chapter, the physiologic role of insulin-induced skeletal muscle vasodilation and its mechanism including the interaction between insulin and the endothelium to modulate the endothelium-derived nitric oxide (NO) system are reviewed. Finally, the effect of insulin resistance on the vascular actions of insulin is also explored. The latter has important clinical consequences given that insulin resistance is a common feature of obesity, of noninsulin-dependent diabetes mellitus (NIDDM), and hypertension, and is associated with an increased risk of macrovascular disease *(1,2)*.

VASCULAR ACTIONS OF INSULIN IN HEALTH

Global Hemodynamics

That combined infusions of insulin and glucose cause an increase in cardiac output (CO) has long been recognized *(3)*, but it has only recently become clear that insulin has

From: *Contemporary Endocrinology: Endocrinology of the Vasculature*
Edited by: J. R. Sowers Humana Press Inc., Totowa, NJ

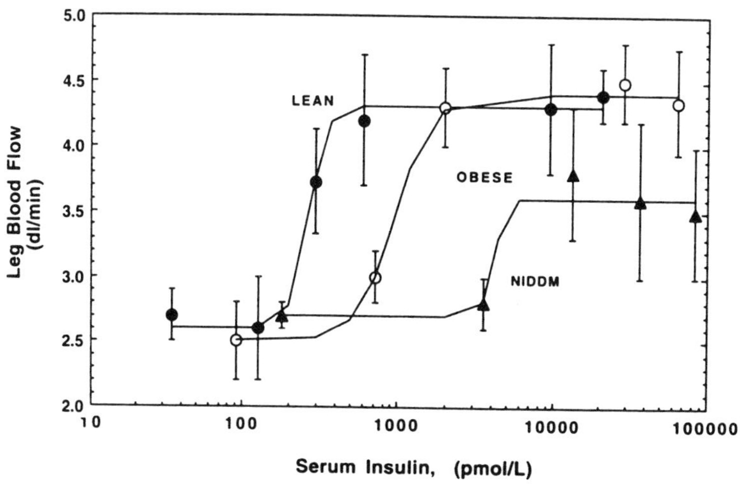

Fig. 1. Rates of LBF determined during euglycemic clamp studies over a wide range of steady state insulin concentrations in lean (●) and obese nondiabetic subjects (○) and patients with NIDDM (▲). Note the log scale on the abscissa. Reprinted from ref. *37* with permission.

effects on the heart independent of the prevailing glucose concentration. In dogs, insulin increases both heart rate and stroke volume resulting in a net increase in cardiac output independent of changes in the prevailing glucose concentration *(4)*. In humans insulin also causes a dose-dependent rise in CO with high physiologic insulin concentrations of ~70 μU/mL causing an ~15% rise in CO via increments in both heart rate and stroke volume *(5)*. This rise in CO is accompanied by a small but significant fall in mean arterial pressure, indicating a reduction in systemic vascular resistance.

Interestingly, when leg (muscle) blood flow (LBF) was simultaneously assessed with CO, doses of insulin, which induce a 15% increase in CO, caused an 80% increase in LBF *(5)*. Thus, physiologic insulin concentrations result in a >40% fall in leg vascular resistance versus a ~20% fall in systemic vascular resistance. Thus, insulin causes both an increase and redistribution of CO to skeletal muscle, with a positive correlation between the increments in CO and SMBF observed during insulin infusion *(5)*.

Regional Hemodynamics

Combining the euglycemic hyperinsulinemic clamp technique with the leg balance technique we have constructed insulin dose-response curves for insulin's effect to increase SMBF. Insulin increases SMBF in a dose-dependent fashion with an apparent ED_{50} (effective dose to produce the half-maximal effect) of ~35–40 μU/mL in lean insulin-sensitive subjects. Maximal vasodilation was observed at insulin concentrations of ~200 μU/mL with some individuals displaying up to 2.5-fold increases in LBF above baseline (Fig. 1) *(6)*. Others, more recently, also have observed similar hemodynamic effects of insulin *(7–10)*. The vasodilating effects of insulin occur relatively slowly compared to its action to stimulate glucose extraction; nevertheless, the hemodynamic action is apparent within the first 30 min of insulin infusion *(6,7,10)*. Insulin infused locally, directly into the brachial *(11)* or femoral artery *(12)*, leads to similar increases in blood flow and perhaps a more rapid time-course, suggesting that insulin's potent vasodilating effects are mediated via local vascular factors.

MECHANISM OF INSULIN-MEDIATED VASODILATION

Role of Endothelium-Derived Relaxing Factors

Endothelium-Derived NO

Since the observation that the presence of an intact endothelium was necessary for vasodilation in response to acetylcholine (ACh) *(13)*, via release of endothelium-derived relaxing factor (EDRF), attention has been directed at the role of the endothelium in the control of vascular tone. More recently this endothelial factor has been identified as NO (14), and endothelial-derived NO (EDNO) is now recognized as the most potent endogenous vasodilator. EDNO is synthesized from the terminal guanidino nitrogen atom(s) of the amino acid L-arginine *(15,16)* in a reaction catalyzed by the endothelium-based, calcium (Ca^{2+})-dependent NO synthase (NOS_3) *(17)*. EDNO is released from the endothelial cell, traverses to the subendothelium to stimulate vascular smooth muscle cell (VSMC) guanylate cyclase *(18)* and possibly Na^+/K^+ adenosine triphosphatase (ATPase) *(19,20)*, which decreases intracellular Ca^{2+} ($[Ca^{2+}]_i$), and results in VSMC relaxation. Substances other than ACh also produce EDNO-dependent vasodilation *(21)*, including a number of peptides *(22)*. EDNO is oxidatively degraded to nitrite (NO_2) and nitrate (NO_3), which can be detected in the urine *(23)*.

Study of endothelium-dependent vasodilation has been expedited by the introduction of a specific inhibitor of NOS, the L-arginine analog, L-*n*-monomethyl-arginine (L-NMMA). L-NMMA impairs ACh-mediated vasodilation *(24)* and this impairment can be overcome by administration of L-arginine. In vivo infusions of L-NMMA have been utilized to gage the contribution of EDNO synthesis/release to the maintenance of vascular tone. In humans, L-NMMA causes vasoconstriction of the forearm *(25,26)* and leg *(12)* arterial circulation, indicating that basal EDNO release contributes to the maintenance of vascular tone in those limbs. L-NMMA has also been shown to cause hypertension in both animals and humans *(27,28)*. Importantly, L-NMMA causes constriction of small resistance arterioles that control microcirculatory flow and capillary recruitment *(29)*.

We recently tested the hypothesis that insulin vasodilates skeletal muscle vasculature via an EDNO-dependent mechanism *(12)*. Intrafemoral artery infusions of the specific inhibitor of EDNO synthesis, L-NMMA, were administered under basal conditions to healthy volunteers and LBF responses were measured by thermodilution. In a separate group, L-NMMA infusions were performed after 3 h of hyperinsulinemia (~270 μU/mL) during a euglycemic clamp designed to increase LBF approximately twofold. At baseline, L-NMMA caused a ~25% fall in LBF. During hyperinsulinemia LBF increased approximately twofold, and in contrast to baseline, L-NMMA caused a ~50% fall in LBF so that LBF returned to basal levels (Fig. 2). These data, confirmed by others *(30)*, indicate that insulin-mediated vasodilation is EDNO dependent.

Insulin potentially causes EDNO-dependent vasodilation by either stimulating the synthesis/release of EDNO or sensitizing the VSMC to EDNO. To test these two possibilities we examined insulin's effect on increments in LBF in response to graded intrafemoral artery infusions of methacholine chloride (MCh), which like ACh increases EDNO production, or sodium nitroprusside (SNP), a NO donor that causes endothelium-independent vasodilation. Low-dose insulin infusion (insulin levels ~25 μU/mL) lead to a significant shift ($p < 0.01$, analysis of variance) to the left in the MCh, but not the SNP dose-response curve (Fig. 3) *(12)*. These observations have been confirmed by others *(31)*. Since MCh causes the synthesis and release of EDNO, these data suggest that insulin

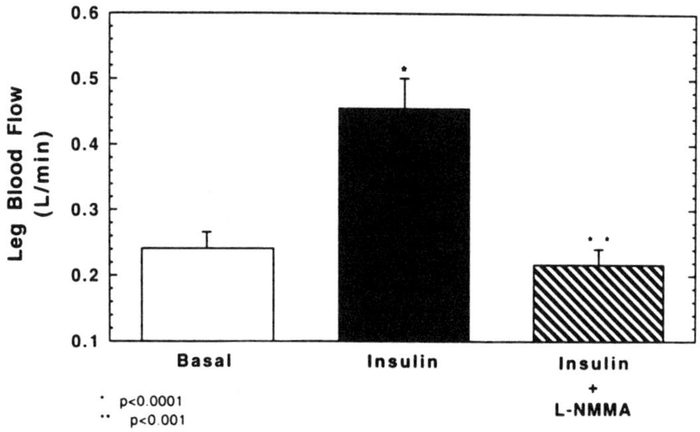

Fig. 2. LBF at baseline during hyperinsulinemia alone and during a superimposed intrafemoral artery infusion of L-NMMA (16 mg/min). Reprinted from ref. *12* with permission.

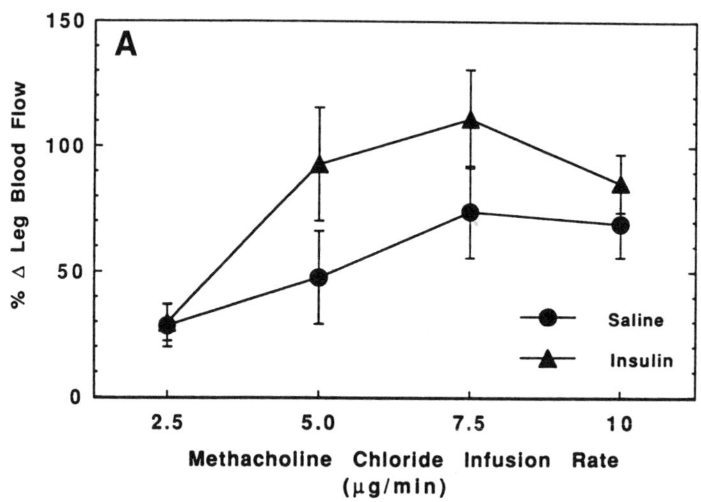

Fig. 3. (A) Percent increment in LBF above baseline in response to graded intrafemoral artery infusions of methacholine chloride (2.5–10.0 μg/min) during saline and during euglycemic hyperinsulinemia (15–40 mU/m²/min).

modulates the endothelial synthesis/release of EDNO, but not EDNO action on VSMC. This physiologic interaction between insulin and the EDNO system is illustrated in the hypothetical schema (Fig. 4).

Endothelium-Derived Hyperpolarizing Factor and Nonendothelial Mechanisms

Since the vasodilatory response to ACh is only partially inhibited by NOS blockade, endothelium-dependent vasodilation in response to acetylcholine is only in part mediated by EDNO. This non-EDNO vasodilatation is suspected to be caused by the release of an endothelium-derived hyperpolarizing factor (EDHF) because it can be partially blocked by ouabain *(32)*. Thus, another potential and theoretical mechanism for insulin-mediated vasodilation is the release of EDHF.

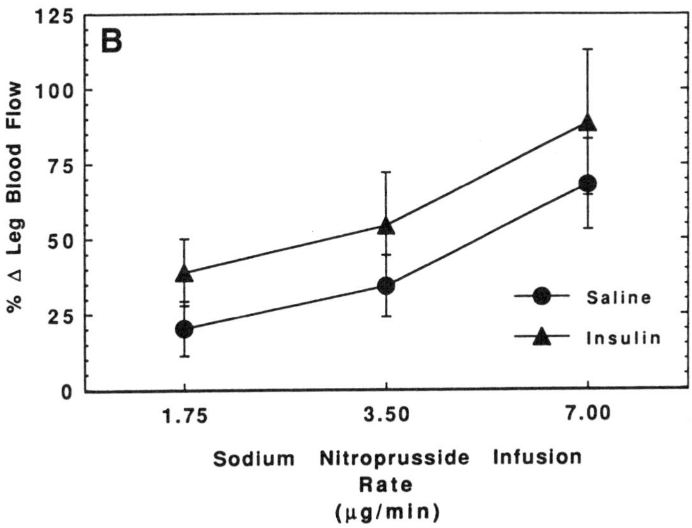

Fig. 3. (B) Percent increment in LBF above baseline in response to graded intrafemoral artery infusions of sodium nitroprusside (1.75–7 μg/min) during saline and during euglycemic hyperinsulinemia (15–20 mU/m²/min). Fig. 3A,B reprinted from ref. *12* with permission.

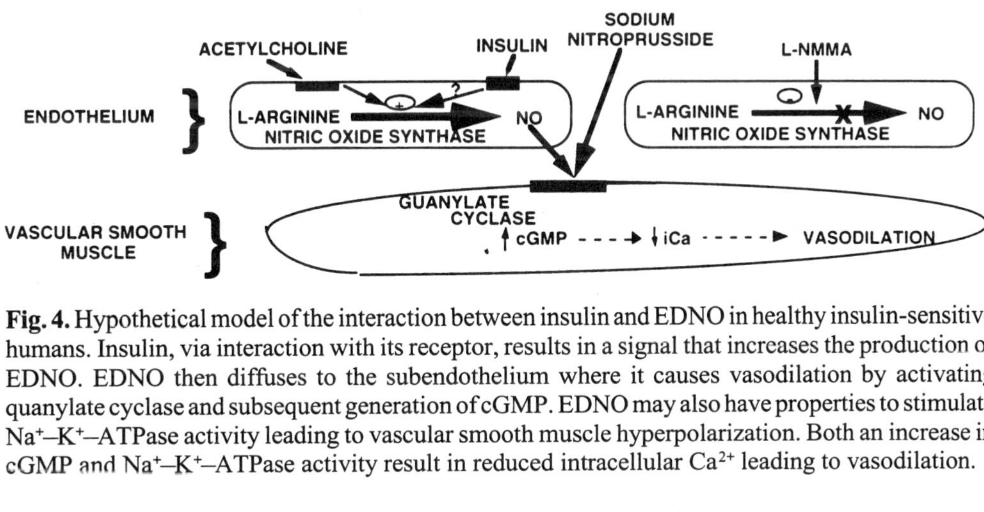

Fig. 4. Hypothetical model of the interaction between insulin and EDNO in healthy insulin-sensitive humans. Insulin, via interaction with its receptor, results in a signal that increases the production of EDNO. EDNO then diffuses to the subendothelium where it causes vasodilation by activating quanylate cyclase and subsequent generation of cGMP. EDNO may also have properties to stimulate Na^+–K^+–ATPase activity leading to vascular smooth muscle hyperpolarization. Both an increase in cGMP and Na^+–K^+–ATPase activity result in reduced intracellular Ca^{2+} leading to vasodilation.

Insulin may also cause vasodilation via direct effects on VSMC. Others have reported that insulin causes hyperpolarization of VSMC leading to reductions in $[Ca^{2+}]_i$ and consequent VSMC relaxation *(33,34)*. Sowers and coworkers *(35,36)* showed that insulin enhances the gene expression and activity of the VSMC Na^+–K^+–ATPase and Ca^+ ATPase, which are the main cellular pumps involved in regulating VSMC $[Ca^{2+}]_i$ metabolism. Although it appears unlikely that these other vasodilating factors have a significant role in the short-term regulation of skeletal muscle vasculature tone, it is possible that they are more important in vasodilation mediated by insulin in other vascular beds or in the long-term regulation of vascular tone. Finally, it is important to consider that insulin may vasodilate by inhibiting the production/release of endothelium-derived constricting factors.

VASCULAR ACTIONS OF INSULIN IN DISEASE

Insulin Resistance

We have measured LBF responses to increasing doses of insulin in insulin-resistant obese and noninsulin-dependent diabetic subjects. Compared to controls, obese and NIDDM exhibit dose-response curves that are markedly right-shifted with an ED_{50} of ~140 and ~720 μU/mL or 3 or 18 times control in obese *(6,37)* and NIDDM subjects, respectively. LBF at maximally effective insulin concentrations was reduced by ~40% in NIDDM. There was a strong correlation between the rate of insulin-mediated glucose uptake (IMGU) and the magnitude of the increase in LBF for all groups, suggesting that muscle perfusion may be an important determinant of IMGU. Thus, these data indicate that insulin augments SMBF in a dose-dependent fashion and this effect is blunted in insulin-resistant groups. There was a modest but consistent (~3–5%) fall in mean arterial pressure (MAP) at all insulin concentrations in controls but only at the higher insulin concentrations in insulin-resistant subjects. Thus, physiological insulin concentrations have specific and coordinated hemodynamic actions to increase blood flow (reduce vascular resistance) to skeletal muscle, and this action is impaired in states of insulin resistance.

Several groups *(37–41)* have reported that 50% of essential hypertensives exhibit reduced rates of IMGU compared to normotensive controls. We explored whether the relationship between blood pressure and insulin sensitivity and insulin-mediated vasodilation is continuous. Since most hypertensives are obese, we studied normotensives exhibiting a wide range of resting blood pressure. Utilizing the euglycemic clamp and leg balance technique, we found a strong inverse relationship between blood pressure and both the rate of IMGU and the ability of insulin to vasodilate (Fig. 5) *(41)*. Thus, those who were most insulin sensitive with respect to IMGU displayed the lowest MAP and also exhibited the greatest SMBF in response to insulin. Others *(4,42)* also found impaired insulin-mediated venodilation in hypertensive subjects.

Thus, obesity, hypertension, and NIDDM are all insulin-resistant states associated with impaired insulin-mediated vasodilation. Given that insulin vasodilates via the release of EDNO, it is reasonable to explore whether these insulin-resistant states are associated with defective endothelium-dependent vasodilation.

ENDOTHELIUM-DEPENDENT VASODILATION AND INSULIN RESISTANCE

Defective ACh-mediated vasodilation has now been reported in essential hypertensives *(43,44)* and their relatives *(45)*. Blunted reductions in forearm blood flow in response to L-NMMA have also been reported in essential hypertensives *(46,47)*, suggesting reduced EDNO production rates in this population. The evidence in human diabetes is not straightforward. Indeed, in insulin-dependent diabetics (IDDM), endothelium-dependent vasodilation has been reported to be either normal *(48,49)* or impaired *(50)*. Endothelium-independent vasodilation to SNP, an exogenous NO donor, has also been found to be normal *(48,50)* or impaired *(49)*. Furthermore, one group *(49)* reported diminished basal EDNO production (reduced L-NMMA-mediated vasoconstriction), but normal vasodilation in response to ACh. In NIDDM, others *(51)* found normal L-NMMA response but impaired vasodilation to ACh and SNP, suggesting impaired vascular smooth muscle responsiveness to EDNO.

These studies do not distinguish between hyperglycemia, insulin deficiency, or insulin resistance as possible causes of any EDNO abnormalities observed. Furthermore, in none

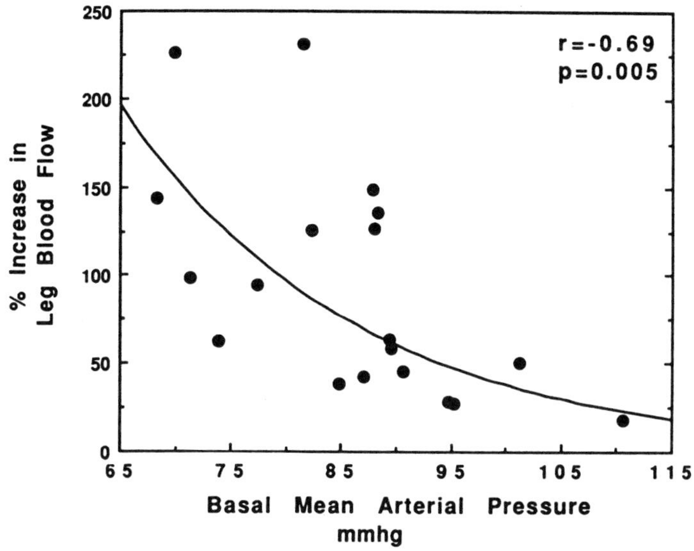

Fig. 5. Scatterplot shows the relation between basal mean arterial pressure and relative increment above baseline in (muscle) LBF during hyperinsulinemic (600 mU/m²/min) euglycemic clamp studies. Reprinted from ref. *41* with permission.

of these reports was EDNO production actually quantitated, leaving the possibility that the functional defects described with ACh may not actually reflect abnormal EDNO production *(52)*. Recently groups have measured urinary excretion of nitrate to quantitate in vivo NO production *(53,54)*. However, given the large overall nitrate pool and the relatively small fraction of total nitrate produced from arginine, measuring urinary excretion of NO oxidative products to quantitate NO production could be misleading.

Hypertension

The mechanism of insulin resistance in essential hypertension *(36)* is not known. We have explored whether insulin resistance in essential hypertension is secondary to impaired insulin-induced vasodilation. We studied normotensive subjects exhibiting a wide range of resting mean arterial pressure at baseline and during a euglycemic hyperinsulinemic clamp. The results indicate that insulin-mediated muscle vasodilation is inversely proportional to the height of the resting mean blood pressure, independent of the obesity status (Fig. 5). Because muscle glucose uptake is determined by the product of the rate of muscle blood flow and glucose extraction, it is important to note that there was no relationship between insulin-stimulated muscle glucose extraction and IMGU. Therefore, if insulin-induced vasodilation is instrumental in amplifying insulin's effect to enhance insulin action, it follows that impaired insulin-mediated vasodilation in patients with essential hypertension could contribute to insulin resistance.

Diabetes

To understand the effect of the diabetic state on insulin-mediated vasodilation, it is important to consider the independent effects of both insulin and hyperglycemia on the vasculature. To examine the effect of glucose concentration independent of changes in insulinemia on LBF, we performed studies *(55)* during somatostatin-induced insulin defi-

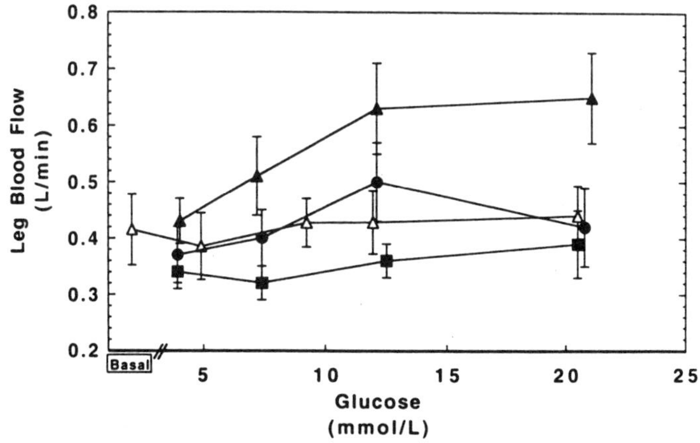

Fig. 6. Rates of LBF during a 120 mU/m²/min insulin infusion as a function of the prevailing serum glucose concentration in obese nondiabetic subjects (●), obese untreated noninsulin-dependent diabetics (■), lean controls (▲), and lean controls during somatostatin induced insulinopenia (△). Reprinted from ref. *55* with permission.

ciency and during fixed hyperinsulinemia. Glucose concentration (during insulinopenia) has no discernible effect to modulate LBF. In contrast, during hyperinsulinemia, glucose concentration had a dose-responsive effect to increase LBF (~2.5-fold) in control but not in obese *(6)*, NIDDM *(35)*, or IDDM (Fig. 6) *(56)*. Insulin-mediated vasodilation is impaired in both insulin-dependent and noninsulin-dependent diabetics, but this response is highly heterogeneous and, the vascular response to insulin is not predictable based on the level of glycemia. Because hyperglycemia has both acute and chronic effects on the vasculature, it is likely that glycemic control does not completely predict vascular response to insulin.

To ascertain whether glucose disposal rate is the determinant for the vasodilation, we combined the aforementioned data to match glucose flux rates between groups (e.g., high insulin/euglycemia vs low insulin/hyperglycemia). At matched glucose flux rates, LBF is similar between lean and obese but remains diminished in NIDDM. Thus, the data suggest that insulin-mediated vasodilation may be related to the rate of glucose metabolism. Since insulin also causes vasodilation in isolated blood vessels *(33)*, skeletal muscle glucose metabolism may be one but not the only or major signal for skeletal muscle vasodilation. This notion is supported by recent work *(10)* demonstrating that when the rate of carbohydrate metabolism is increased with fructose infusion (producing lower insulin levels than an equivalent glucose infusion), vasodilation does not occur. Thus, insulin itself may vasodilate independent of carbohydrate metabolism.

PHYSIOLOGIC ROLE OF INSULIN'S VASCULAR ACTIONS AND PATHOPHYSIOLOGIC IMPLICATIONS

Contribution to Glucose Metabolism

To assess the contribution of insulin-mediated vasodilation to insulin's overall effect to stimulate glucose uptake in skeletal muscle, we utilized an intra-arterial infusion of L-NMMA, a competitive inhibitor of NOS, to reduce LBF to basal levels after 4 h of euglycemic hyperinsulinemia (75–200 μU/mL). Steady-state euglycemic hyperinsulinemia alone caused ~15-fold increase in leg glucose extraction and twofold increase in

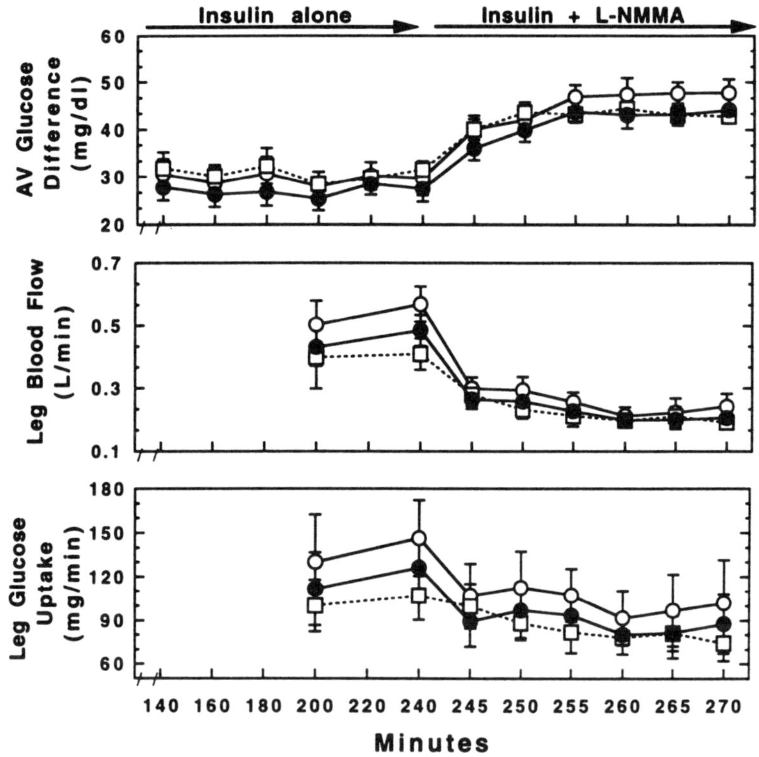

Fig. 7. Femoral arterio-venous glucose differences **(A)**, rates of LBF **(B)**, and rates of leg glucose uptake **(C)** under steady-state conditions after 200 min of euglycemic hyperinsulinemia and at 5-min intervals during a 30-min intrafemoral artery infusion of L-NMMA designed to reduce skeletal muscle LBF in 6 subjects studied at an insulin infusion rate of 40 mU/m²/min (group I, □), 15 subjects studied at an insulin infusion rate of 120 mU/m²/min (group II, ●), and a subgroup of group II (group III, ○) matched for body composition to group I. Reprinted from ref. *57* with permission.

LBF. With the added infusion of L-NMMA, LBF acutely returned back to baseline rates, and the glucose extraction increased by 50% with a net effect to reduce leg glucose uptake by ~25% *(57)*. Therefore, the vasodilation observed with insulin infusion accounts for ~25% of insulin's overall effect to stimulate glucose uptake (Fig. 7). Thus, impairment of insulin-mediated vasodilation in essential hypertension, and other insulin-resistant states, could partially account for the reduced rates of insulin-mediated glucose uptake observed in these patients.

Maintenance of Vascular Tone

Insulin's vasorelaxing properties may be instrumental in the maintenance of vascular tone. To better understand the role of insulin and insulin resistance on vascular tone, we have performed graded systemic infusions of norepinephrine in insulin-sensitive and obese insulin-resistant subjects and assessed the pressor effect of these infusions in the basal state and during euglycemic hyperinsulinemic clamps *(58)*. Insulin caused a shift to the right in the norepinephrine pressor dose-response curve in lean but not in insulin-resistant obese subjects, and similar norepinephrine concentrations resulted in greater elevations in blood pressure in obese than in lean subjects (Fig. 8). Thus, obesity/insulin

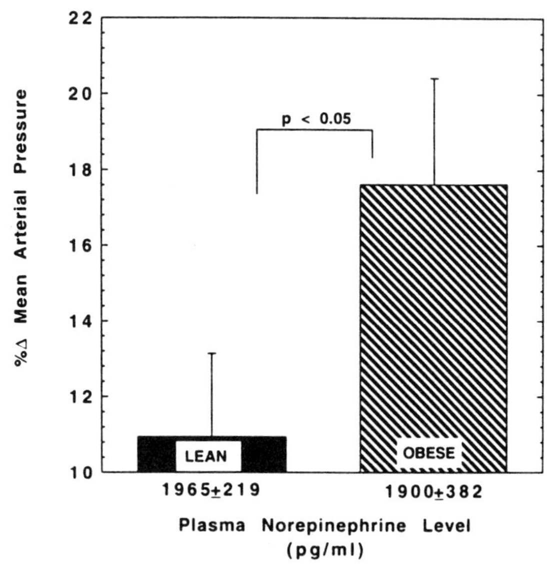

Fig. 8. Relative incremental rise in MAP at equivalent prevailing plasma norepinephrine concentrations in lean and obese subjects during systemic infusions of norepinephrine. Reprinted from ref. *58* with permission.

resistance is associated with increased pressor sensitivity. Moreover, insulin's normal ability to shift the norepinephrine pressor dose-response curve to the right is impaired in obese insulin-resistant subjects, further suggesting that insulin resistance itself is associated with increased sensitivity to norepinephrine's pressor effect.

CONCLUSION

Insulin's vasoactive properties and its ability to release EDNO appear to play a role to amplify insulin's action to stimulate glucose uptake and regulate vascular tone and responsiveness. Dysfunction of the insulin/EDNO interaction is observed in insulin-resistant states, resulting in impaired insulin-mediated vasodilation *(6,37,59)*. This observation suggests that the endothelium itself may exhibit insulin resistance. Given the importance of EDNO as a regulator of vascular tone *(26,28)*, platelet adhesiveness *(60)*, thrombosis *(61)*, and VSMC mitogenesis *(62,63)*, it follows that insulin resistance at the level of the endothelium may have profound implications with respect to the increased risk of hypertension and macrovascular disease seen in insulin-resistant humans. Clearly, more clinical and basic research into the vascular and endothelial action of insulin are needed to better understand its full physiologic and pathophysiologic role. Finally, interactions between the endothelium and other circulating hormones whose traditional roles have not been associated with endothelial function is likely to be a fruitful area of inquiry.

REFERENCES

1. Nosadini R, Manzato E, Solini A, Fioretto P, Brocco E, Zambon S, Morocutti A, Sambataro M, Velussi M, Cipollina MR, Crepaldi G. Peripheral, rather than hepatic, insulin resistance and atherogenic lipoprotein phenotype predict cardiovascular complications in NIDDM. Eur J Clin Invest 1994;24:258–266.
2. Lindahl B, Asplund K, Hallmans G. High serum insulin, insulin resistance and their associations with cardiovascular risk factors. The Northern Sweden Monica population study. J Int Med 1993;234:263–270.

3. Page MM, Smith RBW, Watkins PJ. Cardiovascular effects of insulin. Br J Pharmacol 1976;1:430–432.
4. Liang C-S, Doherty JU, Faillace R, Maekawa K, Arnold S, Gavras H, Hood WB. Insulin infusion in conscious dogs. Effects on systemic and coronary hemodynamics, regional blood flows, and plasma catecholamines. J Clin Invest 1982;69:1321–1336.
5. Baron AD, Brechtel G. Insulin differentially regulates systemic and skeletal muscle vascular resistance. Am J Physiol (Endocrinol Metab 28) 1993;265:E61–E67.
6. Laakso M, Edelman SV, Brechtel G, Baron AD. Decreased effect of insulin to stimulate skeletal muscle blood flow in obese men. J Clin Invest 1990;85:1844–1852.
7. Anderson EA, Hoffman RP, Balon TW, Sinkey CA, Mark AL. Hyperinsulinemia produces both sympathetic neural activation and vasodilation in normal humans. J Clin Invest 1991;87:2246–2252.
8. Bennett WM, Connacher AA, Scrimegeour CM. Euglycemic hyperinsulinemia augments amino acid uptake by human leg tissues during hyperaminoacidemia. Am J Physiol 1990;259:E185–E194.
9. Neahring JM, Stepniakowski K, Greene AS, Egan BM. Insulin does not reduce forearm alpha-vasoreactivity in obese hypertensive or lean normotensive men. Hypertension 1993;22:584–590.
10. Vollenweider P, Tappy L, Randin D, Schneiter P, Jequier E, Nicod P, Scherrer U. Differential effects of hyperinsulinemia and carbohydrate metabolism on sympathetic nerve activity and muscle blood flow in humans. J Clin Invest 1993;92:147–154.
11. Ueda S, Petrie JR, Elliott HL, Connell JM. Insulin mediated vasodilation is dependent on local glucose concentrations. Hypertension 1995;25:561.
12. Steinberg HO, Brechtel G, Johnson A, Fineberg N, Baron AD. Insulin-mediated skeletal muscle vasodilation is nitric oxide dependent. J Clin Invest 1994;94:1172–1179.
13. Furchgott RF, Zawadzki JV. The obligatory role of endothelial cells in the relaxation of arterial smooth muscle by acetylcholine. Nature 1980;288:373–382.
14. Moncada S, Radomski MW, Palmer RMJ. Endothelium derived relaxing factor: identification as nitric oxide and role in the control of vascular tone and platelet function. Biochem Pharmacol 1988;37:2495–2501.
15. Palmer RMJ, Rees DD, Ashton DS, Moncada S. L-arginine is the physiological precursor for the formation of nitric oxide in endothelium-dependent relaxation. Biochem Biophys Res Comm 1988;153:1251–1256.
16. Palmer RMJ, Ashton DS, Moncada S. Vascular endothelial cells synthesize nitric oxide from L-arginine. Nature 1988;333:524–526.
17. Marletta MA. Nitric oxide synthase: aspects concerning structure and catalysis. Cell 1994;78:927–931.
18. Ignarro LJ. Nitric oxide: a novel signal transduction mechanism for transcellular communication. Hypertension 1990;16:477–483.
19. Gupta S, McArthur C, Grady C, Ruderman NB. Stimulation of vascular Na-K-ATPase activity by nitric oxide: a cGMP-independent effect. Am J Physiol 1994;266:H2146–H2151.
20. Gupta S, McArthur C, Grady C, Ruderman NB. Role of endothelium-derived nitric oxide in stimulation of Na(+)-K(+)-ATPase activity by endothelin in rabbit aorta. Am J Physiol 1994;266:H577–H582.
21. Vanhoutte PM, Miller VM. Heterogeneity of endothelium-dependent responses in mammalian blood vessels. J Cardiovasc Pharmacol 1985;7(Suppl. 3):S12–S23.
22. D'Orleans-Juste P, Dion S, Mizrahi J, Regoli D. Effects of peptides and non-peptides on isolated arterial smooth muscles: role of endothelium. Eur J Pharmacol 1985;114:9–21.
23. Suzuki H, Ikenaga H, Hishikawa K, Nakaki T, Kato R, Saruta T. Increases in NO2-/NO3-excretion in the urine as an indicator of the release of endothelium-derived relaxing factor during elevation of blood pressure. Clinical Sci 1992;82:631–634.
24. Rees DD, Palmer RMJ, Hodson HF, Moncada S. A specific inhibitor of nitric oxide formation from L-arginine attenuates endothelium dependent relaxation. Br J Pharmacol 1989;96:418–424.
25. Rees DD, Palmer RMJ, Moncada S. Role of endothelium-derived nitric oxide in the regulation of blood pressure. Proc Natl Acad Sci USA 1989;86:3375–3378.
26. Vallance P, Collier J, Moncada S. Effects of endothelium-derived nitric oxide on peripheral arteriolar tone in man. Lancet 1989;2:997–1000.
27. Baylis C, Mitruka B, Deng A. Chronic blockade of nitric oxide synthesis in the rat produces systemic hypertension and glomerular damage. J Clin Invest 1992;90:278–281.
28. Stammler JS, Loh E, Roddy M-A, Currie KE, Creager MA. Nitric oxide regulates basal systemic and pulmonary vascular resistance in healthy humans. Circulation 1994;89:2035–2040.
29. Nagao T, Illiano S, Vanhoutte PM. Heterogeneous distribution of endothelium-dependent relaxations resistant to Ng-nitro-L-arginine in rats. Am J Physiol 1992;263:H1090–H1094.
30. Scherrer U, Randin D, Vollenweider P, Vollenweider L, Nicod P. Nitric oxide release accounts for insulin's vascular effects in humans. J Clin Invest 1994;94:2511–2515.

31. Taddei S, Virdis A, Mattei P, Natali A, Ferrannini E, Salvetti A. Effect of insulin on acetylcholine-induced vasodilation in the forearm of normotensive subjects. Hypertension 1995;25:552.
32. Brayden JE. Membrane hyperpolarization is a mechanism of endothelium-dependent cerebral vasodilation. Am J Physiol 1990;259:H669–H673.
33. Kahn AM, Allen JC, Seidel CL, Shelat H, Song T. Insulin reduces contraction and intracellular calcium concentration in vascular smooth muscle. Hypertension 1993;22:735–742.
34. Standley PR, Zhang F, Ram JL, Zemel MB, Sowers JR. Insulin attenuates vasopressin-induced calcium transients and a voltage-dependent calcium response in rat vascular smooth muscle cells. J Clin Invest 1991;88:1230–1236.
35. Tirupattur PR, Ram JL, Standley PR, Sowers JR. Regulation on Na^+, K^+-ATPase gene expression by insulin in vascular smooth muscle cells. Am J Hypertens 1993; 6:626–629.
36. Sowers JR, Eptstein M. Diabetes mellitus and associated hypertension, vascular disease, and nephropathy: an update. Hypertension 1995;26:869–879.
37. Laakso M, Edelman SV, Brechtel G, Baron AD. Impaired insulin-mediated skeletal muscle blood flow in patients with NIDDM. Diabetes 1992;41:1076–1083.
38. Ferrannini E, Buzzigoli G, Bonadonna R, Giorico MA, Oleggini M, Graciadei L, Pedrinelli R, Brandi L, Bevilacqua D. Insulin resistance in essential hypertension. N Engl J Med 1987;317:350–357.
39. Pollare T, Lithell H, Berne C. Insulin resistance is a characteristic feature of primary hypertension independent of obesity. Metabolism 1990;39:167–174.
40. Shen D-C, Shieh S-M, Fuh M M-T, Wu C-A, Chen Y-D I, Reaven GM. Resistance to insulin stimulated glucose uptake in patients with hypertension. J Clin Endo Metab 1988;66:580–583.
41. Baron AD, Brechtel-Hook G, Johnson A, Hardin D. Skeletal mule blood flow—a possible link between insulin resistance and blood pressure. Hypertension 1993;21:129–135.
42. Grover A, Padginton C, Wilson MF, Sung BH, Izzo JL Jr, Dandona P. Insulin attenuates norepinephrine-induced venoconstriction. An ultrasonographic study. Hypertension 1995;25(4 Pt 2):779–784.
43. Panza JA, Quyyumy A, Brush JE, Epstein SE. Abnormal endothelium dependent vascular relaxation in patients with essential hypertension. N Engl J Med 1990;323:22–27.
44. Panza JA, Casino PR, Badar DM, Quyyumi AA. Effect of increased availability of endothelium-derived-nitric-oxide precursor on endothelium-dependent vascular relaxation in normal subjects and in patients with essential hypertension. Circulation 1993;87:1475–1481.
45. Taddei S, Virdis A, Mattei P, Arzilli F, Salvetti A. Endothelium-dependent forearm vasodilation is reduced in normotensive subjects with familial history of hypertension. J Cardiovasc Pharmacol 1992;20(Suppl. 12):193–195.
46. Panza JA, Casino PR, Kilcoyne CM, Quyyumi AA. Role of endothelium-derived nitric oxide in the abnormal endothelium-dependent vascular relaxation of patients with essential hypertension. Circulation 1993;87:1468–1474.
47. Calver A, Collier J, Moncada S, Vallance P. Effect of local intra-arterial NG-monomethyl-L-arginine in patients with hypertension: the nitric oxide dilator mechanism appears abnormal. J Hypertens 1992;10:1025–1031.
48. Smits P, Kapma J-A, Jacobs M-C, Lutterman J, Thien T. Endothelium-dependent vascular relaxation in patients with type 1 diabetes. Diabetes 1993;42:148–153.
49. Calver A, Collier J, Vallance P. Inhibition and stimulation of nitric oxide synthesis in the human forearm arterial bed of patients with insulin-dependent diabetes. J Clin Invest 1992;90:2548–2554.
50. Johnstone MT, Craeger SJ, Scales KM, Cusco JA, Lee BK, Craeger MA. Impaired endothelium-dependent vasodilation in patients with insulin-dependent diabetes mellitus. Circulation 1993;88: 2510–2516.
51. McVeigh GE, Brennan GM, Johnston GD, McDermott BJ, McGrath LT, Andrews JW, Hayes JR. Impaired endothelium dependent and independent vasodilation in patients with type 2 (non-insulin-dependent) diabetes mellitus. Diabetologia 1992;35:771–776.
52. Angus JA, Lew M. Interpretation of the acetylcholine test of endothelial dysfunction in hypertension. J Hypertension 1992;10(Suppl. 7):S179–S186.
53. Castillo L, Sanchez M, Vogt J, Chapman TE, DeRojas-Walker TC, Tannenbaum SR, Ajami AM, Young VR. Plasma arginine, citrulline, and ornithine kinetics in adults, with observation on nitric oxide synthesis. Am J Physiol 1995;268:E360–E367.
54. Castillo L, DeRojas TC, Chapman TE, Vogt J, Burke JF, Tannenbaum SR, Young VR. Splanchnic metabolism of dietary arginine in relation to nitric oxide synthesis in normal adult man. Proc Natl Acad Sci USA 1993;90:193–197.

55. Edelman SV, Laakso M, Wallace P, Brechtel G, Olefsky JM, Baron AD. Kinetics of insulin-mediated and non-insulin-mediated glucose uptake in humans. Diabetes 1990;39:955–964.
56. Baron AD, Laakso M, Brechtel G, Edelman SV. Mechanism of insulin resistance in insulin-dependent diabetes mellitus: a major role for reduced skeletal muscle blood flow. J Clin Endo Metab 1991;73:637–643.
57. Baron AD, Steinberg HO, Chaker H, Leaming R, Johnson A, Brechtel G. Insulin-mediated skeletal muscle vasodilation contributes to both insulin sensitivity and responsiveness in lean humans. J Clin Invest 1995;96:786–792.
58. Baron AD, Brechtel G, Johnson A, Fineberg N, Henry DP, Steinberg HO. Interactions between insulin and norepinephrine on blood pressure and insulin sensitivity. J Clin Invest 1994;93:2453–2462.
59. Steinberg H, Brechtel G, Johnson A, Baron AD. Insulin mediated endothelium dependent vasodilation is impaired in obesity. Diabetes 1994;43(Suppl. 1):101A.
60. Radomski MW, Palmer RMJ, Moncada S. The anti-aggregating properties of vascular endothelium: interactions between prostacyclin and nitric oxide. Br J Pharmacol 1987;92:639–646.
61. Mollace V, Salvemini D, Anggard E, Vane J. Nitric oxide from vascular smooth muscle cells: regulation of platelet reactivity and smooth muscle cell guanylate cyclase. Br J Pharmacol 1991;104:633–638.
62. Kopalkov V, Gordon D, Kulik TJ. Nitric oxide-generating compounds inhibit total protein and collagen synthesis in cultured vascular smooth muscle cells. Circ Res 1995;76:305–309.
63. Garg UC, Hassid A. Nitric oxide-generating vasodilators and 8-bromo-cyclic guanosine monophosphate inhibit mitogenesis and proliferation of cultured rat vascular smooth muscle cells. J Clin Invest 1989;83:1774–1777.

8 Angiotensin–Nitric Oxide
Interaction and the Regulation of Renal Vascular Tone

William H. Beierwaltes, PhD
and David H. Sigmon, PhD

CONTENTS

INTRODUCTION

The potent circulating vasoconstrictor angiotensin II (AII) and the ubiquitous endothelium-derived vasodilator, nitric oxide (NO), are endogenous vascular antagonists. The concept that the regulation of blood pressure (and vascular resistance) is the result of a balance between vasoconstriction and vasodilation may be somewhat oversimplified; nevertheless it is a natural place to begin to understand the intricate interaction between these two important modulators of vascular tone.

AII, an octapeptide hormone, is a potent vasoconstrictor. Its substrate, angiotensinogen, is produced in abundance by the liver, circulates, and is converted into angiotensin I (AI) by the enzyme renin, which is predominantly derived from the juxtaglomerular (JG) cells of the renal afferent arteriole *(1)*. Since the substrate is generally in excess, renin is the rate-limiting step in this cascade. Renin is stored in granules in the JG cells. Its release is stimulated through several pathways. These include:

1. The (intra)renal baroreceptor: an undefined mechanism by which diminished renal perfusion pressure and adaptive renal arteriolar dilation stimulates renin, whereas elevated perfusion pressure decreases it;

From: *Contemporary Endocrinology: Endocrinology of the Vasculature*
Edited by: J. R. Sowers Humana Press Inc., Totowa, NJ

2. Renal sympathetic nerves: direct sympathetic innervation of the JG cells can directly affect renin secretion, whereas renal innervation of the afferent arteriole and/or the tubule may also indirectly influence renin release *(2)*;
3. Feedback regulation from the tubular macula densa, which senses distal delivery of sodium chloride, increasing renin in response to diminished delivery, or decreasing it as delivery is increased; and
4. Other endogenous factors (including humoral agents such as prostacyclin *[3]*) that stimulate renin release, or atrial natriuretic peptide *(4)* and even AII *(1,5)*, which depress renin release.

AI is further degraded to the potent biologically active AII by angiotensin-converting enzyme (ACE), which is found in the endothelium and circulation. Although all blood vessels seem to be susceptible to the effects of AII, the resistance vessels of visceral organs are particularly affected *(6)*. The kidney is especially rich in AII, owing to the fact that it is the source of renin and receives a large fraction of the cardiac output and therefore available angiotensinogen. Although it is clear that perturbations that stimulate the renin-angiotensin system may dramatically influence vascular resistance beds and blood pressure, it is not really clear what role AII may play in the quiescent and homeostatic individual, because it seems to function as a buffer rather than contributing to the steady state of vascular tone.

In contrast to the well-established circulating peptide constrictor hormone AII, the endothelium-derived relaxing factor *(7)*, or NO, does not circulate. It is produced within the endothelium by conversion of its amino acid substrate L-arginine by the endothelial isoform of nitric oxide synthase (NOS) into NO and citrulline. This NOS is a constitutive enzyme that is also calcium (Ca^{2+})/calmodulin dependent *(8)*. It is rapidly bound and inactivated by hemoglobin in the circulation, but freely diffuses into the adjacent vascular smooth muscle cells (VSMC), where it reacts with soluble guanylate cyclase to produce cyclic guanosine monophosphate (cGMP), the second messenger in the cascade resulting in vascular relaxation. The primary stimulus for endothelium-derived NO is increased vascular shear stress, though receptor-mediated agonists (acetylcholine, bradykinin) and nonreceptor-mediated stimuli such as Ca^{2+} ionophores stimulate NO synthesis *(7)*. Unlike AII (and most vasoactive hormones), NO is produced continuously and imparts a constant vasodilatory effect. Indeed, competitive antagonists of the L-arginine substrate, which block NO synthesis, induce an immediate 20–30 mmHg increase in blood pressure and total peripheral resistance *(9)*. This phenomenon was first observed when the NO synthesis inhibitor N^G-monomethyl L-arginine (L-NMMA) was given to anesthetized rats and very quickly caused hypertension and a decrease in their heart rate. This observation implies that NO contributes to maintaining resting vascular tone, and to the tonic maintenance of normal blood pressure.

AII AND NO INTERACTIONS IN THE REGULATION OF VASCULAR TONE

The obvious question that arises from these observations is: If removal of NO vasodilation results in significant vasoconstriction in the resistance beds throughout the body, what is the stimulus for this phenomenon? One possibility is the resting tone of VSMC, which is amplified in the absence of the basal dilatory influence of NO. Alternatively (but not exclusively) it could be the result of sympathetic-driven vasoconstriction in the absence of NO. Finally, removing NO-mediated vasodilation could exaggerate the influence of one or more endogenous vasoconstrictor hormones, resulting in a pressor response and increases in some or all vascular resistance beds. An excellent candidate for such a constrictor is AII.

Inhibition of NO synthesis with different agents results in acute hypertension, decreased renal blood flow (RBF), and a disproportionate decrease in glomerular filtration rate (GFR), resulting in an increased filtration fraction *(10)*. These responses are similar to those following direct intrarenal infusion of AII *(11–13)*, in which similar renal vasoconstriction is accompanied by a lesser decrease in GFR such that the filtration fraction increases. Similar renal responses to removing NOS or increasing AII suggest that, in the absence of endogenous NO, the influence of AII on renal hemodynamics is exaggerated. Subsequent studies have been performed to remove or exaggerate the influence of the renin–angiotensin system, and then evaluate the responses to NOS inhibition.

In barbiturate-anesthetized normal rats, the acute pressor response of 20–25 mmHg, seen with NO synthesis inhibition using an L-arginine analog antagonist of NOS, N^{w}-nitro L-arginine methyl ester (L-NAME), is unaltered by treatment with losartan, a selective AII receptor blocker *(14)*. However, the 35% reduction in RBF seen with L-NAME was completely eliminated by blocking AII. Notably, though the decrease in RBF was completely attenuated, there was still a significant (though greatly diminished) increase in renal vascular resistance, suggesting that vasoconstrictors other than AII also influence the renal resistance vessels, though to a much lesser extent. Similar studies showed that an ACE inhibitor does not diminish the systemic pressor response but greatly attenuates renal vasoconstriction *(14)*. Further, a kinin antagonist has no effect on the renal response to L-NAME, suggesting that it is mediated by blocking AII rather than through potentiating endogenous dilator kinins *(14)*. Further, the AII receptor blocker, losartan, attenuates the reductions in RBF, GFR, and sodium excretion observed after NOS inhibition *(15)*.

In renal micropuncture studies, NOS inhibition causes afferent arteriolar vasoconstriction, decreases single nephron GFR, and inhibits glycine-induced renal vasodilation *(16)*. However, prior AII blockade with losartan eliminated all of these changes, suggesting that they were owing to AII in the absence of NO synthesis. If exogenous AII is administered to raise circulating levels artificially, the systemic pressor response to NOS inhibition by L-NAME is only slightly exaggerated, but renal vasoconstriction is greatly exaggerated, leading to a decline in renal function *(17)*. Thus, elevated AII may serve as a stimulus for increased NO production in order to maintain renal vascular tone and renal function. Although renal responses to NOS inhibition can largely be attenuated by AII blockade, the systemic pressor response remains intact *(6,14–18)*. Investigators have tested whether the systemic pressor response to NOS inhibition can be attenuated by prior blockade of various constrictor systems, including the renin–angiotensin system, the sympathetic nervous system, prostanoids, and vasopressin *(19)*. In each case, or when blockers are combined, the systemic response remains intact. In normotensive and hypertensive rats characterized by either low, normal, or high plasma renin activity (PRA), there is little difference in the systemic pressor response to L-NAME, suggesting that AII does not have a major interaction with NO in the maintenance of total peripheral resistance and therefore systemic blood pressure *(20)*. Elevated systemic blood pressure in the absence of endothelium-derived NO is not the result of a general effect of specific constrictor signals. However, renal vasoconstriction in response to NOS inhibition is largely mediated by the unbridled influence of endogenous AII, especially when AII is

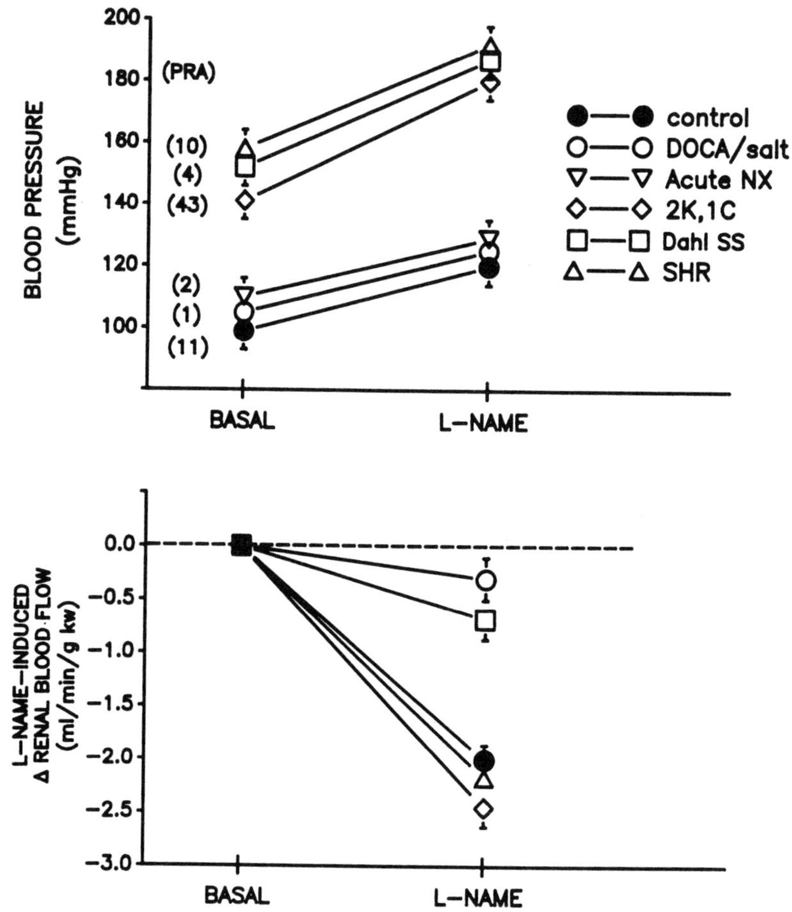

Fig. 1. Relationship between basal PRA (PRA, shown in parentheses in the upper panel) and both the systemic pressor response and decrease in RBF induced by NOS inhibition using L-NAME. Results are from three normotensive and three hypertensive models under inactin anesthesia with different PRAs. These include normal control Sprague Dawley rats (control, PRA = 11 ng A1/mL/h), normotensive rats given deoxycorticosterone acetate and a high sodium diet (DOCA/salt, PRA = 1 ng A1/mL/h) to suppress PRA, and acutely nephrectomized normotensive rats (acute NX, PRA = 2 ng A1/mL/h). The hypertensive rats include two kidney, one clip renovascular hypertensive rats (2K,1C, PRA = 43 ng A1/mL/h; note that RBF is measured in the contralateral nonclipped kidney), Dahl salt-sensitive genetic rats (Dahl SS, PRA = 4 ng A1/mL/h), and SHR (PRA = 10 ng A1/mL/h). Although the different PRAs did not influence the change in blood pressure induced by NOS inhibition in either normotensive or hypertensive rats, the change in RBF was blunted in those rats in which PRA was suppressed below control levels. These data support the particular sensitivity of the renal circulation to the interaction between NO and AII.

increased. It has been noted that the "endothelial modulation of RBF is largely the result of a unique interaction" between the inherent dilation of endothelial NO and the constrictor influence of AII within the kidney *(14)*.

Additional studies have supported the role of AII–NO interaction in controlling renal perfusion by manipulating endogenous levels of AII (Fig. 1) *(18)*. Rats in which AII is suppressed by a chronic high-salt diet and deoxycorticosterone acetate (DOCA) treatment demonstrate a diminished renal response to NOS inhibition, similar to that reported with pharmacological blockade of the renin–angiotensin system. Likewise, with chronic suppression of AII, the systemic pressor response to L-NAME remains intact. With high PRA, and presumably AII, induced by dietary sodium restriction, the systemic response to L-NAME is exaggerated (by 30%) but renal vasoconstriction is not enhanced further. As previously reported in rats on a normal diet, pharmacological blockade of AII receptors diminishes the renal vasoconstriction but not the systemic pressor response in sodium-restricted, high PRA rats *(18)*. Increased AII may stimulate NO production, either directly through elevating $[Ca^{2+}]_i$, which is an essential cofactor for NOS *(8)*, or indirectly by elevating vascular resistance and therefore endothelial shear stress, the most potent endogenous stimulus for NO production *(7)*. Systemic pressor response to NOS inhibition in pithed rats maintained normotensive with exogenous AII infusion is greatly exaggerated *(21)*. Evidence for direct stimulation of NO synthesis by AII or its degradation products has also been reported *(22)*, and indirect evidence in vivo *(17)* and in vitro *(5)* using renal cortical slices (with both endothelium and JG cells intact) suggests that AII may directly stimulate NOS *(5)*.

INTERACTION OF AII AND NO IN REGULATION OF RENAL VASCULAR TONE

There is an interaction between AII and NO in the renal resistance beds. In vivo micropuncture studies *(16)* have shown that renal endothelium-derived NO counteracts the effect of AII in the glomerulus and on sodium handling in the renal tubules. Using microdissected and perfused renal afferent arterioles, investigators have shown that inhibiting NOS results in enhanced vasoconstriction in response to exogenous AII *(23,24)*. These reports suggest that NO buffers the constrictor influence of AII in the renal resistance vessels. Buffering of AII-induced vasoconstriction by endogenous NO is present in the renal afferent but not the efferent arteriole, which may account for the apparent differential sensitivity in these two vascular sites *(25)*. In the blood-perfused JG nephron preparation in afferent and efferent arterioles, NOS inhibition-induced vasoconstriction is attenuated by AII blockade *(26)*. However, if AII is added, the resulting vasoconstriction is not enhanced by NOS inhibition in either arteriolar bed. Thus, in these deep nephron sites, AII and NO interact to maintain tone in both afferent and efferent arterioles. As AII is increased, there is a signal (through one or more possible pathways) to stimulate the counter-regulatory influence of NO.

Contrary to the aforementioned studies, in conscious rats, pharmacological blockade of the renin–angiotensin system does not diminish the renal vasoconstriction induced by blockade of NOS *(27)*. The difference between this report and previous studies *(14,18,28)* is the state of anesthesia. Since barbiturate anesthesia increases PRA two- to threefold *(29)*, the different results involve renal AII:NO interactions, especially in the renal circulation. This notion has been tested by comparing renal and systemic pressor responses to NOS inhibition in normal conscious euvolemic rats, and in conscious rats subjected to chronic sodium restriction to elevate AII *(29)*. In conscious normal rats, renal vasoconstriction and systemic pressor responses to NOS inhibition with L-NAME are unaffected by the AII blocker losartan *(27)*. However, in conscious rats with chronic dietary sodium restriction, the renal vasoconstriction seen with L-NAME (but not the systemic pressor response) is greatly attenuated by pretreatment with losartan. These data help resolve the disparate results and suggest that under quiescent and homeostatic conditions, AII is only a minor regulator of renal vascular resistance. Any influence that elevates AII evokes the dominant interaction between NO and AII in regulating renal hemodynamics *(29)*.

Although the variable influence of AII over renal perfusion is of considerable interest, no experimental manipulation of AII diminishes the systemic pressor response to NOS inhibition. Since NOS inhibition uniformly decreases heart rate and cardiac output, the increase in total peripheral resistance appears to be independent from the influence of AII. Investigations of the influence of NOS inhibition on distribution of blood flow to peripheral blood vessels have focused on the following hypothesis: If NO-mediated vasodilation is a uniform influence in all resistance beds, then alterations in the distribution of blood flow seen under various conditions may reflect the regional influence of different local constricting pathways, including AII. Nonselective inhibition of NOS decreases organ blood flow and increases vascular resistance in the cerebral, mesenteric, and gastric circulations as well as in the kidney *(30–33)*. Hepatic blood flow *(33)* or blood flow to fat *(31)* appears to be the most susceptible to NOS inhibition, visceral circulation is more variable with NOS inhibition than peripheral vasculature *(28)*, and the exaggerated renal response is largely mediated by AII.

Interactions between AII and NO as modulators of the distribution of regional blood flow have been studied in both conscious and anesthetized rats *(6)*. In anesthetized rats, NOS inhibition by L-NAME results in decreased blood flow in visceral organs (kidney, intestine, lung) but not in the brain, heart, or femoral vasculature. Receptor blockade with losartan attenuates the decrease in visceral blood flow. In contrast, in conscious rats, L-NAME increases resistance in visceral and other beds, but there is no further influence of AII blockade *(27,29)*. These studies indicate that NO is important in maintaining regional or organ blood flow, and that the evolution of significant AII–NO interaction in modifying local blood flow is apparent only in visceral vascular beds, and then only when a stimulus (such as anesthesia) elevates AII above normal resting levels.

SYSTEMIC VASCULATURE NO–AII INTERACTIONS

NO buffers the constrictor action of AII, and indirect evidence suggests that AII stimulates NO synthesis *(5,22)*. Whether NO influences the release or secretion of renin (and subsequently AII) is controversial. It was originally reported *(34)* that endothelium-derived NO, through its second messenger cGMP, inhibits renin release in vitro. This suggested that NO might act through a negative feedback loop, in which increases in NO buffer the constrictor influence of AII, and as it increases, exert an inhibitory influence on renin secretion and therefore AII production. Another in vitro study reported that inhibition of NOS resulted in potentiation of renin release *(35)*. These and subsequent studies in vitro were based on earlier observations of renin inhibition by atrial natriuretic peptide via its inhibitory second messenger cGMP, both in vitro *(4)* and in vivo *(36)*. The first in vivo study supported the renin-inhibitory effect of NO only when the renal baroreceptor and sympathetic nervous system were held constant *(37)*, though similar protocols using constant renal perfusion and denervation in vivo arrived at the opposite conclusion *(38)*. In vitro studies have reported a possible stimulation *(39)* or even both inhibition and stimulation *(40)* of renin by NO. In vivo, it has been reported that renin stimulated by the renal baroreceptor pathway, using reduced renal perfusion below the range of autoregulation, is greatly attenuated by NOS inhibition *(6,41,42)*. However, NOS inhibition, even after reducing renal perfusion pressure, results in an increase in renal vascular resistance *(43)*, which should blunt any response of the renal baroreceptor. Thus, the retarded renin release in studies after NOS inhibition may not reflect a direct stimulation of renin by NO at low perfusion, but rather a diminished renin response owing to renal vasoconstriction secondary to NOS inhibition. Clearly, the nature of NO's influence over renin release remains to be elucidated.

ALTERED AII–NO INTERACTIONS AND HYPERTENSION

The observation that inhibition of NO synthesis elicits an acute hypertensive response led to a number of studies on the effects of chronic NOS inhibition. Chronic administration of inhibitors of NOS evolves into dose-dependent and progressive onset of hypertension *(44,45)*. This hypertension, especially with more aggressive inhibition, also may result in such pathologies as vascular hypertrophy *(46)*, focal arteriolar obliteration *(47)*, cardiac hypertrophy *(46,48)*, proteinurea *(48)*, and glomerular sclerosis *(47,49)*. The role of AII in this unique model of hypertension is controversial. Progressive levels of chronic NOS inhibition lead to progressive hypertension without altering GFR or sodium excretion; PRA is decreased only at the highest levels of inhibition *(44)*. Dogs given chronic administration of subpressor levels of NOS inhibitors are hypertensive when fed a high-sodium diet *(45)*. This seems to mitigate against a role for AII in the development of hypertension, because salt-induced hypertension is not usually considered to be AII dependent. However, if hypertensive doses of L-NAME are administered, alterations of salt intake from low to high have no further effect on the increasing blood pressure *(50,51)*, whereas salt loading of rats with chronic NOS inhibition exaggerates the hypertension and results in glomerular damage and proteinurea *(49)*.

Chronic NOS inhibition has a greater influence on stimulating PRA in young rats than in older rats *(46)*, perhaps the result of increased renal damage in the young animals. Concurrent AII receptor blockade *(47,49,51,52)* or an ACE inhibitor *(44,46,48,51)* attenuates or prevents the development of L-NAME-induced hypertension as well as the accompanying renal damage and cardiac hypertrophy. Although the chronic inhibition of the renin–angiotensin system seems to retard or eliminate hypertension induced by chronic NOS inhibition, once the hypertension is established, the role of AII is less clear. Reversal of hypertension by acute blockade of AII is either partial *(47,53)* or slow to evolve *(52)*, sometimes taking weeks for normotensive levels to be attained. Acute reversal of chronic NOS inhibition-induced hypertension requires both AII and ganglionic blockade, since neither perturbation alone results in reversal *(53)*. Thus it appears that AII is involved in the initiating steps of hypertension induced by chronic NOS inhibition, but its role in the maintenance or sustained phase is substantially less. The magnitude of the hypertension and the corresponding renal damage is dose dependent, and these effects may be related to the role of AII in influencing blood pressure under conditions of diminished NO synthesis. These chronic and acute studies, in which the absence of endothelium-derived NO results in hypertension, have led to the hypothesis that various forms of hypertension may be the result of inherent or induced endothelial dysfunction, predisposing the subject to hypertension as in the various NOS inhibition-induced models.

The strongest evidence for endothelial dysfunction in hypertension comes from in vitro studies involving relaxation and contraction of isolated vascular rings or strips *(54)*. There is attenuated endothelium-dependent relaxation in vessels from various models of hypertension; both AII-dependent models such as 2K,1C renovascular hypertension *(55)* and aortic coarctation *(56,57)*, and AII-independent models like the spontaneously hypertensive rat (SHR) *(58–60)*, salt-induced hypertension *(61)*, DOCA-salt hypertension *(56,62)*, and one-kidney, one-clip renovascular hypertension *(63,64)*. There are reports that endothelium-dependent relaxation in the human forearm is blunted in patients with essential hypertension *(65,66)*, and antihypertensive therapy reverses this apparent deficiency *(56)*. However, three further lines of investigation have undermined this (perhaps simplistic) approach to explaining hypertension.

Most reports of impaired endothelium-dependent relaxation in hypertension come from studies using conduit vessels such as the aorta that contribute little to total peripheral resistance. A recent review *(67)* suggests that there are differing degrees of dysfunction, with more in the conduit vessels, and less in the coronary circulation. The diminished response to acetylcholine (ACh) is not always duplicated in response to bradykinin, thus an apparent dysfunctional endothelium-derived vasorelaxation may depend on what agent is used to preconstrict the preparation, or which endothelium-dependent vasodilator is used. Dysfunctional dilation in response to ACh in norepinephrine-preconstricted vessels disappears when the same preparation is preconstricted with vasopressin *(68)*. These types of data suggest that this phenomenon represents something more than just dysfunctional endothelium.

Secondly, the degree of dysfunction may also be related to the role of AII in the model of hypertension. It is now apparent that AII-dependent hypertension *(68,69)* involves normal endothelial NO synthesis, but responses to endothelium-dependent vasodilators such as ACh are blunted by simultaneous release of an endothelium-derived constricting factor (EDCF). This factor has been identified as a cyclooxygenase product acting on the (constrictor) thromboxane receptor. Although there is considerable debate over the precise identity of EDCF, it appears to be the intermediate endoperoxide, prostaglandin H_2 (PGH_2) *(58,68–71)*, or possibly one of its metabolites, thromboxane A_2 (TXA_2;) *(72–75)*. Both of these have been reported to be vasoconstrictors in the systemic as well as the renal circulation *(70,73,76,77)*, both are produced by platelets and blood vessels, and both contract vessels through a common receptor *(76)*. Production of EDCF by vessels has been linked to elevated AII, and AII infusion produces increased vascular tissue levels and renal excretion of TXA_2 *(73,77,78)*. The increase in blood pressure induced by chronic infusion of AII in rats is attenuated by prior treatment with a PGH_2/TXA_2 receptor antagonist *(79)*, and hypertension associated with acute AII infusion is blunted by pretreatment with either a PGH_2/TXA_2 receptor antagonist or an inhibitor of thromboxane synthase *(74,75,80)*. Treatment with a PGH_2/TXA_2 receptor antagonist decreases blood pressure in rats with AII-dependent hypertension *(71,72,77)*. This is different from results using normotensive rats or models of hypertension characterized by normal or low PRA *(75,76,80)*, in which the receptor antagonist has no effect on blood pressure. Thus, if elevations in circulating AII are buffered by a concomitant increase in the synthesis of NO, but also provoke synthesis of an additional constricting factor, PGH_2/TXA_2, the end result would seem to be an apparent decrease in endothelial NO. However, the apparent deficiency is not really a function of diminished NO, but rather a normal or even increased NO synthesis counteracted synergistically by two potent constrictor systems.

Finally, the concept of general endothelial dysfunction is not supported by the in vivo literature (Fig. 1). Acute inhibition of NO synthesis results in an exaggerated pressor response in various models of hypertension, independent of the basal level or role of AII

(20). Exaggerated pressor responses of 50–150% have been reported in acute hypertension by carotid ligation and vagotomy *(20,43)*, in high renin models such as 2K,1C renovascular hypertension *(81–83)*, in low renin models like the Dahl salt sensitive hypertensive rat *(84)*, and in models with apparently normal renin such as the SHR *(85)*.

If under normal conditions, NO buffers the effect of increased circulating AII, will it act similarly when pathological factors result in abnormally elevated AII levels, such as in AII-dependent hypertension in the 2K,1C rat? Induced-renovascular hypertension is characterized by diminished renal perfusion, a rise in systemic pressure, atrophy of the clipped kidney, and an increase in circulating AII and a progressive rise in blood pressure over 3–5 wk *(86)*. Greater stenosis progressively compromises renal function and accelerates the pathogenesis of the disease. Although all the visceral organs, including the contralateral or non-stenotic kidney are exposed to both high perfusion pressure and elevated circulating AII, the clipped (or stenotic) kidney will have high AII but diminished perfusion as a function of the extent of the stenosis. The degree of stenosis correlates with the rise in PRA and the magnitude of the hypertension *(87)*. If data from normotensive rats with elevated AII hold true in this model of hypertension, then NO should act as an antihypertensive factor. The visceral organs, and in particular the nonstenotic kidney, should have elevated NO synthesis owing to increased shear stress associated with the elevated perfusion pressure and vascular resistance. Thus, vasculatures should exhibit a normal or even exaggerated constrictor response to NOS inhibition. If, on the contrary, hypertension leads to some endothelial dysfunction, then we might expect a diminished systemic pressor response to NOS inhibition and a retardation of the increased resistance in the vessels serving that organ.

In 2K,1C hypertensive rats *(83)*, the systemic pressor response to NOS inhibition by L-NAME is exaggerated twofold compared with normotensive rats. In both groups, L-NAME increases vascular resistance in all organ beds investigated and, with the exception of the renal circulation, the increase in vascular resistance is greater in the hypertensive animals than in the controls. The circulation of the brain and heart do not change much after L-NAME in normotensive rats, but the increase in vascular resistance to L-NAME in these beds is exaggerated in 2K, 1C hypertensive rats *(6)*. These observations suggest that in this "induced" model of hypertension, regional vasculatures are not subject to any apparent dysfunctional endothelium, and the influence of the endothelium on local as well as total peripheral resistance may even be exaggerated. Interestingly, an exaggerated systemic pressor response also has been reported in a variety of models of hypertension, both of genetic origin *(84,85)* and induced *(43,81,88)*.

RENAL BLOOD FLOW CHANGES WITH ALTERATIONS OF AII–NO INTERACTIONS

In 2K,1C renovascular hypertension, the kidney's responses to NO synthesis inhibition are confused by reports suggesting that the hemodynamic response to NOS inhibition in a stenotic kidney is either similar to that in a normal kidney *(83,69)* or is completely refractory and without any change after pharmacologic blockade of NOS *(81)*. In contralateral, nonstenotic kidneys, things are clearer. Inhibition of NOS results in profound renal vasoconstriction *(69,81–83)*, and this response is reversed by AII blockade with losartan *(81)*. Thus, NO appears to balance the effect of elevated AII in the nonstenotic kidney. However, the variability of data in the stenotic kidney require further analysis.

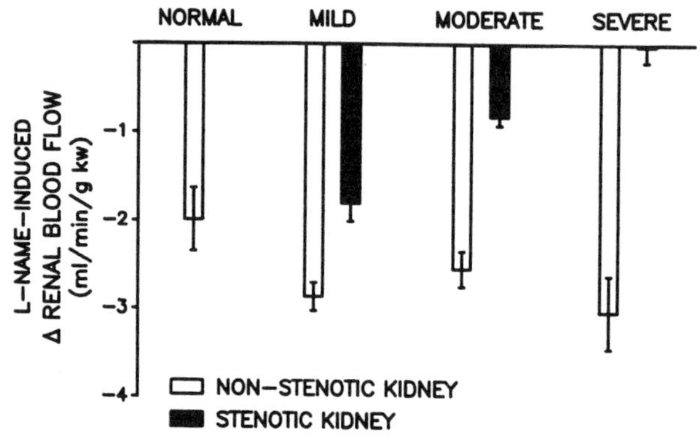

Fig. 2. Decrease in RBF in response to NOS inhibition by L-NAME in kidneys of normotensive control rats (normal), and in the nonstenotic contralateral kidneys and the stenotic or clipped kidneys of 2K,1C renovascular hypertensive rats classified as having either mild, moderate, or severe "functional" renal stenosis. Note that in the nonstenotic kidneys, the decrease in RBF after NOS inhibition is not altered between groups, but in the stenotic kidneys, the decrease in RBF (and by implication, the influence of NO on renal perfusion) is diminished as the degree of stenosis is increased.

If we assume that placing a clip on the renal artery results in a population of different levels of stenosis and renal compromise, then a way is needed to determine whether the magnitude of stenosis alters the influence of NO in the kidney. If increased renal artery stenosis decreases perfusion and subsequently diminishes shear stress, the primary signal for NO synthesis, there should be a progressive decrease in NO production as stenosis becomes greater.

Since renal arteriography in rats is impractical, and neither absolute RBF nor the degree of renal atrophy is a good index of renal stenosis, a separate criterion has been developed, referred to as a "functional index" of stenosis *(82)*. This is based on the degree of renal perfusion and renal adaptation to stenosis after clipping. Renal artery stenosis in this model always results in some degree of renal atrophy. RBF corrected by kidney weight in the clipped kidney has been compared to flow per weight of the nonstenotic kidney and this results in three distinct stenosis populations *(82)*. The first population has essentially normal (corrected) RBF in the stenotic kidney (ratio = 1) was classified as having "mild (functional)" stenosis. A second intermediate group in whom RBF per kidney weight is diminished to only half that in the contralateral kidney is classified as having "moderate" stenosis. Those rats in which the corrected perfusion of the stenotic kidney is only 10–20% of that in the nonstenotic kidney are classified as having "severe" stenosis. Although all three groups are hypertensive, blood pressure is highest in those with severe stenosis, and PRA correlates with the classified degree of stenosis. Additionally, the response of RBF to inhibition of NO synthesis also correlates with the apparent degree of stenosis (Fig. 2) *(82)*. In rats classified with "mild" stenosis, the stenotic kidney behaves much like the contralateral kidney or, for that matter, a normal kidney. Inhibition of NO synthesis produces renal vasoconstriction, which is AII dependent. In contrast, in severely stenotic kidneys, NOS inhibition produces no change in RBF. In the group with moderate stenosis, the renal hemodynamic response is midway between the change seen in "mild" and the absence of change seen in the "severe" groups. These data suggest that the contralateral or nonstenotic kidney has normal or even elevated NO production, which may counteract the high levels of AII, preserving renal function. In the stenotic kidney, the degree of perfusion is the result of the balance between NO and high circulating and intrarenal AII, which can be offset by the restriction of RBF, decreasing shear stress, the primary stimulus for NO formation *(82)*. This results in an imbalance between dilator and constrictor influences in favor of AII, resulting in progressive failure of the stenotic kidney. This, in turn, stimulates AII, further exacerbating the problem.

Does renal artery stenosis lead to a dysfunctional endothelium? To address this problem, removal of the occluding clip (repair of the stenosis) in rats after 4 wk of stenosis has been carried out with and without prior inhibition of NOS. Reversal of hypertension is highly dependent on reperfusion of the underperfused kidney, and this reperfusion is highly NO dependent *(88)*. Clip removal lead to complete restoration of RBF and subsequent normalization of blood pressure within 1 h. However, if NOS is first blocked, RBF does not recover after unclipping, and hypertension remains unabated *(88)*. These observations suggest that even after 4–5 wk of stenosis, the endothelium is intact and remains an important factor in the maintenance of RBF.

It has been suggested that sustained hypertension may damage the endothelium, resulting in dysfunction *(67)*. However, chronic renovascular hypertension (in rats clipped from 12–14 wk) does not eliminate the constrictor response to NOS inhibition. In this chronic model, AII plays a diminished role *(89)*, but inhibitors such as L-NAME still produce a significant though attenuated renal constrictor response. This suggests either that sustained 2K,1C hypertension does not greatly alter endothelial function, or that only those rats able to maintain some degree of endothelial function can survive the insult of prolonged hypertension.

In conclusion, the tonic vasodilator influence of endothelium-derived NO seems to buffer the constrictor effect of AII, particularly in the visceral resistance beds, and most notably in the renal circulation. Under unstressed and quiescent conditions, when circulating AII is low, this interaction is minimal. In this state, NO appears to regulate basal vascular tone. However, any stimulus of AII evokes a corresponding stimulus of NO, and AII itself (or effects secondary to AII's actions) may stimulate NO synthesis. It is also possible (though controversial) that NO, through increases in cGMP, may inhibit renin release. Contrary to early literature, different models of hypertension are not characterized by diminished NO synthesis. In fact, it appears that NOS may be stimulated by hypertension (and in particular AII-dependent hypertension) in an attempt to blunt the developing vasoconstriction and associated elevated blood pressure. In hypertension induced by chronic NOS inhibition, the role of AII is not completely clear, but it appears to be related to renal damage rather than having a direct role in the pathogenesis of this unique form of elevated blood pressure. Finally, the ability to maintain some degree of endothelial function and consequently renal NO synthesis seems to be a key factor in adaptation of the kidney to persistent stenosis or elevated renal perfusion pressure. All of these data suggest that NO is a critical regulator of renal vascular tone, and that in the kidney there is a rather unique interaction between the dilator effect of NO synthesis balancing AII-induced vasoconstriction.

REFERENCES

1. Keeton TK, Campbell WB. The pharmacologic alteration of renin release. Pharm Rev 1980;32:81–227.
2. Barajas L, Powers K. The structure of the juxtaglomerular apparatus (JGA) and the control of renin secretion; an update. J Hypertens 1984;2(Suppl. 1):3–12.

3. Beierwaltes WH, Schryver S, Sanders E, Strand J, Romero JC. Renin release selectively stimulated by prostaglandin I2 in isolated rat glomeruli. Am J Physiol 1982;243:F276–F283.
4. Henrich WL, McAllister EA, Smith PB, Campbell WB. Guanosine 3'5'-cyclic monophosphate as a mediator of inhibition of renin release. Am J Physiol 1988;255:F474–F478.
5. Beierwaltes WH. Nitric oxide participates in Ca^{2+}-mediated regulation of renin release. Hypertension 1994;23(Suppl. I):I40–I44.
6. Sigmon DH, Beierwaltes WH. AII:nitric oxide interaction and the distribution of blood flow. Am J Physiol 1993;265(R34):R1276–R1283.
7. VanHoutte PM. Endothelium and the control of vascular function. Hypertension 1989;13:658–667.
8. Busse R, Mulsch A. Ca^{2+}-dependent nitric oxide synthesis in endothelial cytosol is mediated by calmodulin. FEBS Lett 1990;265:133–136.
9. Rees DD, Palmer RMJ, Moncada S. Role of endothelium-derived nitric oxide in the regulation of blood pressure. Proc Natl Acad Sci USA 1989;86:3375–3378.
10. Baylis C, Harton P, Engles K. Endothelial derived relaxing factor controls renal hemodynamics in the normal rat kidney. J Am Soc Nephrol 1990;1:875–881.
11. Lohmeier TE, Cowley AW. Hypertensive and renal effects of chronic low level intrarenal33. angiotensin infusion in the dog. Circ Res 1979;44:154–160.
12. Porush JG, Kaloyanides GJ, Cacciaguida RJ, Rosen SM. The effects of AII and renal water and electrolyte excretion in normal and caval dogs. J Clin Invest 1967;46:2109–2122.
13. Rosivall L, Naval G. Effects on renal hemodynamics of intraarterial infusion of angiotensin I and II. Am J Physiol 1983;254:F181–F187.
14. Sigmon DH, Carretero OA, Beierwaltes WH. Angiotensin-dependence of endothelium-mediated renal hemodynamics. Hypertension 1992;20:643–650.
15. Takenaka T, Mitchell KD, Navar LG. Contribution of AII to renal hemodynamic and excretory responses to nitric oxide synthesis inhibition in the rat. J Am Soc Neph 1993;4:1046–1053.
16. Di Nicola L, Blantz RC, Gabbai FB. Nitric oxide and AII. Glomerular and tubular interaction in the rat. J Clin Invest 1992;89:1248–1256.
17. Baylis C, Harvey J, Engles K. Acute nitric oxide blockade amplifies the renal vasoconstrictor actions of AII. J Am Soc Neph 1994;5:211–214.
18. Sigmon DH, Carretero OA, Beierwaltes WH. Plasma renin activity and the renal response to nitric oxide synthesis inhibition. J Am Soc Neph 1992;3:1288–1294.
19. Pucci ML, Nasjletti A. Pressor and renal vasoconstrictor effects of NG-nitro-L-arginine as affected by blockade of pressor mechanisms mediated by the sympathetic nervous system, angiotensin prostanoids and vasopressin. J Pharm Exp Ther 1992;261:240–245.
20. Beierwaltes WH, Potter DL, Kiel CS, Pegoraro AA, Sigmon DH, Carretero OA. Pressor response to inhibition of endothelium-derived relaxing factor (EDRF) is amplified in hypertension. Physiologist 1991;34:250.
21. Pegoraro AA, Carretero OA, Sigmon DH, Beierwaltes WH. Sympathetic modulation of endothelium-derived relaxing factor. Hypertension 1992;19:643–647.
22. Haber RL, Decker PJ, Einhaupt KM. Angiotensin degradation products mediate endothelium-dependent dilation of the rabbit brain arterioles. Circ Res 1991;68:1621–1627.
23. Ito S, Johnson CS, Carretero OA. Modulation of AII vasoconstriction by endothelium-derived relaxing factor in the isolated microperfused rabbit afferent arteriole. J Clin Invest 1991;87:1656–1663.
24. Yoshida H, Tamaki T, Aki Y, Kimura S, Takenaka I, Abe Y. Effects of AII on isolated rabbit afferent arterioles. Jpn J Pharmacol 1994;66:457–464.
25. Ito S, Arima S, Ren YL, Juncos LA, Carretero OA. Endothelium-derived relaxing factor/nitric oxide modulates AII action in the isolated microperfused rabbit afferent but not efferent arteriole. J Clin Invest 1993;91:2012–2019.
26. Ohishi K, Carmines P, Inscho EW. Navar LG. EDRF–AII interactions in rat juxtamedullary afferent and efferent arterioles. Am J Physiol 1992;263:F900–F906.
27. Baylis C, Engles K, Samsell L, Harton P. Renal effects of acute endothelium-derived relaxing factor blockade are not mediated by AII. Am J Physiol 1993;26 4:F74–F78.
28. Sigmon DH, Carretero OA, Beierwaltes WH. Renal versus femoral hemodynamic response to endothelium-derived relaxing factor synthesis inhibition. J Vasc Res 1993;30:218–223.
29. Sigmon DH, Beierwaltes WH. AII:endothelium derived nitric oxide interaction in conscious rats. J Am Soc Neph 1994;4:1675–1682.
30. Broten TP, Miyashiro JK, Moncada S, Reigl EO. Role of endothelium-derived relaxing factor in parasympathetic coronary vasodilation. Am J Physiol 1992;262:H1579–H1584.

31. Loeb AL, Longnecher DE. Inhibition of endothelium-derived relaxing factor-dependent circulatory control in intact rats. Am J Physiol 1992;262:H1494–H1500.
32. Pique JM, Whittle BJR, Esplugues JV. The vasodilator role of endogenous nitric oxide in the rat gastric microcirculation. Eur J Pharmacol 1989;174:293–296.
33. Wang YX, Gavras I, Wierzba T, Bernard L, Gavras H. Inhibition of nitric oxide, bradykinin and prostaglandins in normal rats. Hypertension 1991;19(Suppl. II):II225–II261.
34. Vidal MJ, Romero JC, VanHoutte PM. Endothelium-derived relaxing factor inhibits renin release. Eur J Pharm 1988;149:401,402.
35. Beierwaltes WH, Carretero OA. Nonprostanoid endothelium-derived factors inhibit renin release. Hypertension 1992;19(Suppl. II):II68–II73.
36. Villarreal D, Freeman RH, Johnson RA. Renal effects of ANF (95–126), a new atrial peptide analogue, in dogs with experimental heart failure. Am J Hypertens 1991;4:508–515.
37. Sigmon DH, Carretero OA, Beierwaltes WH. Endothelium-derived relaxing factor regulates renin release in vivo. Am J Physiol 1992;263:F256–F261.
38. Johnson RA, Freeman RH. Renin release in rats during blockade of nitric oxide synthesis. Am J Physiol 1994;266:R1723–R1729.
39. Kurtz A, Kaissling B, Busse R, Baier W. Endothelial cells modulate renin secretion from isolated mouse juxtaglomerular cells. J Clin Invest 1991;88:1147–1154.
40. Schricker K, Kurtz A. Liberators of NO exert a dual effect on renin secretion from isolated mouse renal juxtaglomerular cells. Am J Physiol 1993;265:F180–F186.
41. Naess PA, Christensen G, Kirkenboen KA, Kiil F. Effect on renin release of inhibiting renal nitric oxide synthesis in anesthetized dogs. Acta Physiol Scand 1993;148:137–142.
42. Persson PB, Baumann JE, Ehmke H, Hackenthal E, Kirchheim HR, Nafz B. Endothelium-derived NO stimulates pressure dependent renin release in conscious dogs. Am J Physiol 1993;264:F943–F947.
43. Beierwaltes WH, Sigmon DH, Carretero OA. Endothelium modulates renal blood flow but not autoregulation. Am J Physiol 1992;262:F943–F949.
44. Navarro J, Sanchez A, Saiz J, Ruilope LM, Garcia-Estan J, Romero JC, Moncada S, Lahera V. Hormonal, renal and metabolic alterations during hypertension induced by chronic inhibition of NO in rats. Am J Physiol 1994;267:R1516–R1521.
45. Salazar FJ, Alberola A, Pinilla JM, Romero JC, Quesada T. Salt-induced increase in arterial pressure during nitric oxide synthesis inhibition. Hypertension 1993;22:49–55.
46. Morton JJ, Beattie EC, Speirs A, Gulliver F. Persistent hypertension following inhibition of nitric oxide formation in the young Wistar rat: role of renin and vascular hypertrophy. J Hypertens 1993;11:1083–1088.
47. Ribeiro MO, Antunes E, deNucci G, Lovisolo SM, Zatz R. Chronic inhibition of nitric oxide synthesis; a new model of arterial hypertension. Hypertension 1992;20:298–303.
48. Hropo M, Grensch H, Klaus E, Langer KH, Linz W, Wiemer G, Scholkens BA. Ramapril prevents the detrimental sequels of chronic NO synthesis inhibition in rats: hypertension, cardiac hypertrophy and renal insufficiency. Naunyn-Schmiedeberg's Arch Pharm 1994;350:646–652.
49. Okamura M, Konishi Y, Nishimura M, Umetani N, Iwai J, Negoro N, Inoue T, Takeda T, Kanayama Y. Enhancement of hypertension and renal injury by salt loading during chronic nitric oxide inhibition. Effects of TCV-116, a novel AII receptor antagonist. Blood Pressure 1994;5:75–78.
50. Johnson RA, Freeman RH. Sustained hypertension in the rat induced by chronic blockade of nitric oxide production. Am J Hypertension 1992;5:919–922.
51. Jover B, Herizi A, Ventre F, Dupont M, Mimran A. Sodium and angiotensin in hypertension induced by long term nitric oxide blockade. Hypertension 1993;21:944–948.
52. Pollock DM, Polakowski JS, Divish BJ, Opgenorth TJ. Angiotensin blockade reverses hypertension during long-term nitric oxide synthase inhibition. Hypertension 1993;21:660–666.
53. Qui C, Engles K, Baylis C. AII and alpha 1 adrenergic tone in chronic nitric oxide blockade induced hypertension. Am J Physiol 1994;266:R1470–R1476.
54. Furchgott RF, Zawadzki JV. The obligatory role of endothelial cells in the relaxation of arterial smooth muscle by acetylcholine. Nature 1980;288:373–376.
55. Ortenberg JM, Cook AK, Inscho EW, Carmines PK. Attenuated afferent arteriolar response to acetylcholine in Goldblatt hypertension. Hypertension 1992;19:785–789.
56. Lockette W, Otsuka Y, Carretero OA. The loss of endothelium-dependent vascular relaxation in hypertension. Hypertension 1986;8(Suppl. II):II61–II66.
57. Miller MJS, Pinto A, Mullane KM. Impaired endothelium-dependent relaxations in rabbits subjected to aortic coarctation hypertension. Hypertension 1987;10:164–170.

58. Diedrich D, Yang Z, Buhler FR, Luscher TF. Impaired endothelium-dependent relaxation in hypertensive resistance arteries involves cyclooxygenase pathway. Am J Physiol 1988;258:H445–H451.
59. Sim MK, Singh M. Decreased responsiveness of the aortae of hypertensive rats to acetylcholine, histamine and noradrenaline. Br J Pharm 1987;90:147–150.
60. Tesfamariam B, Halpern W. Endothelium-dependent and endothelium-independent vasodilation in resistance arteries from hypertensive rats. Hypertension 1988;11:440–444.
61. Luscher TF, Raij L, Vanhoutte PM. Endothelium-dependent responses in normotensive and hypertensive Dahl rats. Hypertension 1987;9:157–163.
62. Van deVoorde, Leusen I. Endothelium-dependent and independent relaxation of aortic rings from hypertensive rats. Am J Physiol 1986;250:H711–H717.
63. Dohi Y, Criscione L, Luscher TF. Renovascular hypertension impairs formation of endothelium-derived relaxing factor and sensitivity to endothelin-1 in resistance arteries. 1991;104:349–354.
64. Nakamura T, Prewitt RL. Effect of NG-monomethyl-L-arginine on endothelium-dependent relaxation in arterioles of one kidney, one clip hypertensive rats. Hypertension 1991;17:785–789.
65. Lindner L, Kiowski W, Buhler FR, Luscher T. Indirect evidence for release of endothelium-derived relaxing factor in human forearm circulation in vivo. Blunted response in essential hypertension. Circulation 1990;81:1762–1767.
66. Panza JA, Quyyumi AA, Brush JE, Epstein SE. Abnormal endothelium-dependent vascular relaxation in patients with essential hypertension. New Engl J Med 1990;323:22–27.
67. Luscher TF. Heterogeneity of endothelial dysfunction in hypertension. Eur Heart J 1992;13(Suppl. D):50–55.
68. Lin L, Nasjletti A. Prostanoid-mediated vascular contraction in normotensive and hypertensive rats. Eur J Pharm 1992;220:49–53.
69. Sigmon DH, Beierwaltes WH. Interaction between nitric oxide and endothelium-derived constricting factor in renovascular hypertension. Hypertension 1995;25:803–808.
70. Lin L, Balazy M, Pagano PJ, Nasjletti A. Expression of prostaglandin H_2-mediated mechanism of vascular contraction in hypertensive rats; relation to lipoxygenase and prostacyclin synthase activities. Circ Res 1994:74;197–205.
71. Lin L, Mistry M, Stier CT, Nasjletti A. Role of prostanoids in renin-dependent and renin-independent hypertension. Hypertension 1991;17:517–525.
72. Mistry M, Muirhead EE, Yamaguchi Y, Nasjletti A. Renal function in rats with AII-salt-induced hypertension: effect of thromboxane synthesis inhibition and receptor blockade. J Hypertens 1990;8:73–83.
73. Wilcox CS, Welch WJ. AII and thromboxane in the regulation of blood pressure and renal function. Kidney Int 1990:38(Suppl. 30);S81–S83.
74. Wilcox CS, Welch WJ. Thromboxane mediation of the pressor response to infused AII. Am J Hypertens 1990;3:242–249.
75. Wilcox CS, Welch WJ, Snellen H. Thromboxane mediated the renal hemodynamics response to infused AII. Kidney Int 1991;41:1090–1097.
76. Mais DE, Saussy DL, Chaikouni A, Kochel PJ, Knapp DR, Hananaka N, Halushka PV. Pharmacologic characterization of human and canine thromboxane A2/prostaglandin H2 receptors in platelets and blood vessels: evidence for different receptors. J Pharmacol Exp Ther 1985;233:418–424.
77. Mistry M, Nasjletti A. Role of pressor prostanoids in rats with angiotensin-salt induced hypertension. Hypertension 1988;11:758–762.
78. Himmelstein SI, Klotman PE. The role of thromboxane in two-kidney, one-clip Goldblatt hypertension in rats. Am J Physiol 1989;257:F190–F196.
79. Mistry M, Nasjletti A. Contrasting effect of thromboxane synthase inhibitor and a thromboxane receptor antagonist on the development of AII-salt induced hypertension. J Pharmacol Exp Ther 1990;253:90–94.
80. Yamaguchi Y, Fenoy FJ, Roman RJ, Nasjletti A. AII influences the renal hemodynamic responses to blockade of thromboxane A_2 and prostaglandin H_2 response. J Pharmacol Exp Ther 1992;263:905–909.
81. Sigmon DH, Beierwaltes WH. Renal nitric oxide and AII interaction in renovascular hypertension. Hypertension 1993;22:237–242.
82. Sigmon DH, Beierwaltes WH. Degree of renal artery stenosis alters nitric oxide regulation of renal hemodynamics. J Am Soc Nephrol 1994;5:1369–1377.
83. Sigmon DH, Beierwaltes WH. Nitric oxide influences blood flow distribution in renovascular hypertension. Hypertension 1994;23(Suppl. I):I34–I39.
84. Pegoraro AA, Carretero OA, Sigmon DH, Beierwaltes WH. Blood pressure response to nitroarginine is enhanced in young Dahl salt-sensitive rats. FASEB J 1991;5:A380.

85. Ono H, Ono Y, Frohlich ED. Nitric oxide synthase inhibition in spontaneously hypertensive rats: systemic renal and glomerular hemodynamics. Hypertension 1995;26:256–262.
86. Beierwaltes WH. Possible endothelial modulation of prostaglandin-stimulated renin release. Am J Physiol 1990;258:F1363–F1371.
87. Leenen FHH, DeJong W. A solid silver clip for induction of predictable levels of renal hypertension in the rat. J Applied Physiol 1971;31:142–144.
88. Beierwaltes WH, Potter DL, Carretero OA, Sigmon DH. Nitric oxide synthesis inhibition blocks reversal of 2K,1C renovascular hypertension after unclipping. Hypertension 1995;25:174–179.
89. Sigmon DH, Beierwaltes WH. Endothelium-derived nitric oxide (EDNO) in the chronic, angiotensin II (AII) independent phase of 2K,1C renovascular hypertension. J Am Soc Nephrol 1994;5:592.

9 Altered Endothelial Function in Diabetes Mellitus

An Overview

Richard L. Klein, PhD
and John A. Colwell, MD, PhD

Contents

INTRODUCTION

Vascular endothelial cells have received increasing attention as potential contributors to the pathogenesis of vascular disease in diabetes mellitus. Early observations suggested that endothelial injury may be a very early stage in diabetic micro- and macroangiopathy, and subsequent data support this view. A complete review of this rapidly expanding literature is beyond the scope of this chapter; the reader is referred to previous reviews *(1,2)*. Our focus is on recent evidence of endothelial dysfunction in diabetes mellitus.

Vascular endothelial cells participate in a variety of functions that may contribute to vascular disease, and many are altered in the diabetic state (Table 1) *(1,2)*. The focus of this chapter is on the following factors: vasodilators—endothelium-derived relaxing factor (EDRF) or nitric oxide (NO) and prostacyclin (PGI_2); vasoconstrictors—thromboxane (TXA_2) and endothelin; the von Willebrand factor (vWF); cell adhesion molecules—endothelial cell adhesion molecule-1 (ECAM-1) and L-selectin; and the major regulatory proteins of the fibrinolytic system, tissue plasminogen activator (tPA) and plasminogen activator inhibitor (PAI-1) (Fig. 1). Alterations in these factors (Table 1) may promote arteriosclerosis and thrombosis in diabetes.

From: *Contemporary Endocrinology: Endocrinology of the Vasculature*
Edited by: J. R. Sowers Humana Press Inc., Totowa, NJ

Table 1
Alterations in Vascular Endothelium in Diabetes Mellitus

1. Increased plasma levels of vWF.
2. Increased expression, synthesis, and plasma levels of endothelin-1.
3. Diminished prostacyclin production/release.
4. Decreased release of EDRF/NO and reduced responsiveness to NO.
5. Impaired fibrinolytic activity.
6. Increased endothelial cell procoagulant activity.
7. Increased endothelial cell surface thrombomodulin.
8. Impaired plasmin degradation of glycosylated fibrin.
9. Increased levels of advanced glycosylated end products.

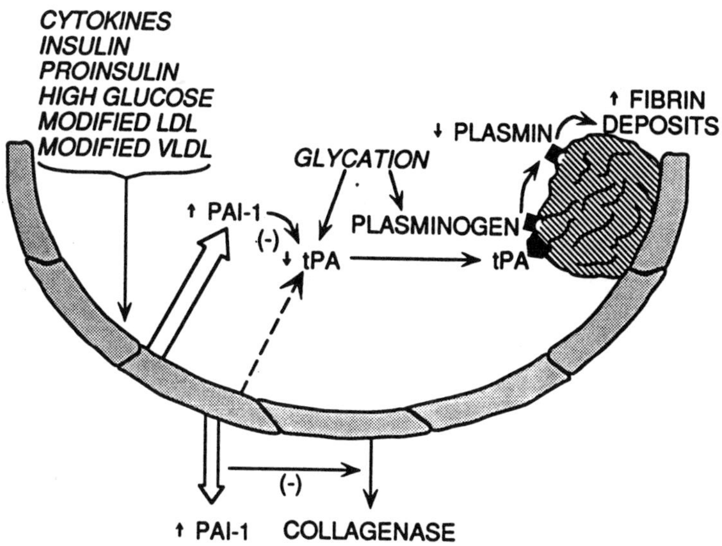

Fig. 1. Effects of diabetes on the fibrinolytic system.

EDRF/NO

There is increasing evidence for depressed release or diminished activity of NO from atherosclerotic arteries, and dietary-induced hypercholesterolemia may inhibit endothelium-dependent relaxation. Defective endothelium-dependent relaxation is a feature of experimental and human diabetes *(3)*. Linkage to advanced glycation products has been shown by inhibition of endothelium-derived relaxation and quenching of NO by these products *(4)*. Lipoprotein oxidation associated with the diabetic state may inactivate EDRF/NO after its release from endothelial cells *(5)*. The role of hyperglycemia in diminishing endothelial cell production and release of NO is extensively discussed in another chapter of this book.

PGI_2

PGI_2 release from endothelial cells is coupled with NO release, and like NO, PGI_2 synthesis and/or release is reduced in both type I and type II diabetes (Table 1) *(1,6,7)*. PGI_2, like NO, is not only a vasodilator, but also an inhibitor of platelet aggregation and vascular growth and remodeling *(2,6,7)*. Thus, decreased endothelial release of PGI_2 in diabetes has been linked to platelet hyperaggregability, increased adhesiveness, and increased thromboxane release in diabetes mellitus *(2,6,7)*. There is also evidence of a deficiency of a plasma-derived stimulatory factor of endothelial PGI_2 release in diabetes *(6)*. Indeed, a deficiency in this factor may contribute to vascular complications in diabetes mellitus by causing a reduction in PGI_2 production by the vascular wall *(6)*. Further, reduced production of NO and PGI_2 in diabetes mellitus may contribute directly to accelerated atherosclerosis, since these factors inhibit the growth and remodeling effects of endothelin, platelet-derived growth factor (PDGF), insulin-like growth factor (IGF-1), and angiotensin II (AII) *(7)*.

TXA_2 AND ENDOTHELIN

The endothelium also synthesizes and releases contracting agents such as TXA_2 and endothelin. TXA_2, a product of cyclo-oxygenase, counteracts the vascular effects of NO *(7)*. Release by the aorta of TXA_2 is increased in hyperglycemic alloxan-diabetic rabbits *(8)*. Generation of this factor appears to be related to hyperglycemia, rather than to elevated lipid levels *(8)*. Diabetes also enhances the contractile response of rat mesenteric veins, which is induced by prostanoids, and is associated with increased vasoconstriction in arteries that are exposed to serotonin and to a thromboxane analog *(2,8)*. TXA_2 and its immediate prostaglandin endoperoxide precursor prostaglandin H_2 (PGH_2) are synthesized from activated platelets as well as vessel wall tissues. Thus, the increased activation of platelets in diabetes mellitus *(7)* may contribute to elevated TXA_2/PGH_2 in this disease state. These eicosanoids (PGH_2 and TXA_2) exert potent vasoconstricting effects on vascular smooth muscle cells (VSMC) that are mediated by a common TXA_2/PGH_2 *(9,10)*. A very recent study *(10)* helped elucidate the intracellular pathways mediating the VSMC growth effects of these eicosanoids. Indeed, the growth-promoting intracellular mechanism of TXA_2/PGH_2 appears to be very similar to those observed for AII, IGF-1, PDGF, endothelin, and thrombin, including increases in VSMC $[Ca^{2+}]_i$, activation of mitogen-activated protein (MAP) kinase, and expression of the immediate growth-response genes (i.e., proto-oncogenes such as c-*jun* and c-*fos*) *(10)*.

There is an accumulating body of evidence that enhanced vascular contraction in both type I and type II diabetes is related to increased production of the potent vasoconstrictor endothelin by both endothelial and VSMC *(11–29)*. Increased circulating levels of endothelin are partly related to the effects of hyperglycemia *(26,27)*, since levels are often elevated in patients with type I diabetes mellitus *(11,12)*. However, insulin is also a potent stimulator of endothelial *(22–24)* and VSMC *(25)* production of endothelin-1, perhaps explaining why levels are often elevated in type II diabetics *(13–18)*. In addition, elevated endothelin levels may contribute to the vascular *(13–17)*, renal *(17–19)*, and neural damage *(21,27)* accompanying diabetes mellitus. Thus, like platelets in diabetes *(7)*, the endothelium is dominated by a balance that favors thromboxane and endothelin release and vasoconstriction, and this is not counterbalanced by an increase in vasodilators EDRF and/or PGI_2 in the diabetic state (Table 1) *(1,2,7)*.

vWF

The vascular endothelium is intimately involved in the regulation of various metabolic processes (e.g., hemostasis, fibrinolysis, vasomotor control, and vascular permeability), all of which may be relevant to the pathogenesis of diabetic complications *(1,2,7,27–30)*.

It is difficult to measure these endothelial functions in vivo; however, it has been suggested that the plasma level of vWF, a glycoprotein synthesized mainly by endothelial cells, may serve as a nonspecific marker of endothelial dysfunction *(15,28,30)*. Diabetic nephropathy and retinopathy are serious complications of diabetes mellitus. Indeed, dysfunction of the vascular endothelium may play a significant role in development of these diabetic complications.

Recent studies have investigated the relationship between urinary and plasma levels of vWF and diabetic nephropathy and retinopathy. A prospective, 3-yr study of 52 type I diabetic patients with and without nephropathy has been conducted *(28)* to investigate the relationship between plasma vWF concentration and nephropathy. Patients were divided into three groups: no nephropathy (urinary albumin excretion [UAE] rate < 15 μg/min), incipient nephropathy (UAE rate 15–200 μg/min), and clinical nephropathy (UAE rate > 200 μg/min). Incipient nephropathy developed or worsened in 17 patients, and clinical nephropathy worsened in 1 patient during the study period. Plasma vWF concentrations increased significantly in all patients in this group. A decrease in UAE was observed in 3 patients with incipient UAE at baseline; this was accompanied by a decrease in plasma vWF concentration. There was a slight but significant increase in plasma vWF concentration in the remaining 38 patients without nephropathy. In a subsequent study *(30)*, endothelial dysfunction, as estimated by plasma vWF concentration, preceded and appeared to predict development of microalbuminuria in type I diabetic patients. Similar studies were conducted in patients with type I diabetes with similar conclusions and further demonstrated that vWF was strongly related to the occurrence of cardiovascular events in these patients *(29)*.

Diabetic retinopathy appears linked to diabetic nephropathy *(27)*. Although the nature of this linkage is uncertain, it has been suggested that endothelial dysfunction may represent the pathophysiological basis for these epidemiological observations *(28–31)*. The relationship between retinal status and plasma vWF concentration was investigated in a cohort of 17 type I diabetic patients who were followed prospectively for 42 mo *(31)*. UAE rates remained normal in all patients throughout the study. Plasma vWF concentrations were similar in patients with or without retinopathy (if less than three microaneurysms were observed by an ophthalmologist after dilation of the pupils on two occasions and after fluorescein angiography on a third occasion). Patients in whom plasma vWF concentration increased had higher systolic blood pressure when compared to those in whom the concentration did not increase. This observation suggests that pulse pressure and related shear stress may be determinants of endothelial cell production and secretion of vWF *(7)*.

One recent study compared the plasma vWF concentration in type II diabetic patients before and after consuming a diet high in monounsaturated fatty acids for 3 wk compared to levels attained while consuming an isocaloric high-carbohydrate diet *(32)*. Plasma vWF concentration significantly decreased while consuming the monounsaturated fat diet. In contrast, there were no significant changes observed in plasma vWF concentration when the patients consumed the high carbohydrate diet *(32,33)*. The diet high in monounsaturated fatty acids also reduced blood pressure, further supporting a relationship between vWF, blood pressure, and vascular injury in patients with diabetes mellitus.

CELL ADHESION MOLECULES

Endothelial cells elaborate leukocyte-specific adhesion molecules both constitutively and in response to cytokines and other mediators *(34–46)*. Circulating monocytes display receptors for these cell adhesion molecules. Adhesion of leukocytes to the endothelium is an important step for migration into inflamed tissue. Intercellular adhesion molecule-1 (ICAM-1) is found on vascular endothelial cells and a variety of other cell types, and a form of circulating ICAM-1 has been described in plasma during ongoing inflammation or tissue damage *(34)*. L-selectin is a recently identified cell adhesion molecule found on lymphocytes *(35)*. ICAM-1 and L-selectin levels in plasma are increased in patients with recent-onset type I diabetes and in subjects at risk for type I diabetes *(35)*. In contrast, the expression of ICAM-1 is decreased on monocytes isolated from patients with recent onset type I diabetes *(36)*. These studies suggest that an ongoing immune process in type I diabetes may cause increased levels of soluble adhesion molecules to be released from monocytes. Recent studies indicate that one endothelial cell adhesion molecule, E-selectin (ELAM-1), and a vascular cell adhesion molecule (VCAM) are increased in type II diabetic patients; however, ICAM-1 is not *(37)*.

Type I diabetes mellitus is caused by a T-cell-mediated destruction of the β-cells in the islets of Langerhans. The interaction between T-cells and their antigens or targets is assisted by adhesion molecules on the surfaces of lymphocytes and counter-receptors on antigen-presenting or other cells. As indicated, soluble forms of these adhesion molecules are increased in diabetic patients *(35,37,38)*. ICAM-1 immunoglobulin fusion proteins have been demonstrated to stop proliferation of T-cells in vitro *(38)*. Similarly, monoclonal antibodies to ICAM-1 reduce the development of hyperglycemia in streptozotocin-induced diabetic rats *(39)*. Administrations of antileukocyte-associated antigen-1 (anti-LFA-1) and anti-ICAM-1 inhibit development of diabetes in nonobese, diabetic mice *(40)*. Monoclonal antibodies to the α-4-lymphocyte adhesion molecule administered to nonobese mice also suppress development of diabetes in these animals *(41,42)*, suggesting that prevention of lymphocyte homing to the pancreatic islets may provide a selective target for prevention/treatment of type I diabetes mellitus. For autoreactive T-cells to cause disease, the cells must be able to leave the blood and enter into the target tissue. Interaction between VCAM-1 and α4-integrin is critical to T-cell entry into the islets of Langerhans and in the pathogenesis of diabetes in a mouse model *(43)*. Thus, elaboration of adhesion molecules is important in the pathogenesis of insulin-deficient diabetes as well as the vascular disease accompanying this condition.

FIBRINOLYSIS AND DIABETES

Cardiovascular disease caused by accelerated atherosclerosis is the leading cause of death in patients with diabetes mellitus *(7,44,45)*. Lipoprotein abnormalities including increased glyco-oxidation of low-density lipoprotein (LDL) cholesterol contribute to this acceleration of atherosclerosis (Table 2) *(7)*. Impaired endogenous fibrinolytic activity may accelerate atherosclerosis by exposing vascular luminal wall surfaces to persistent and recurrent thrombi and clot-associated mitogens (Table 2). PAI-1 and tPA are the major regulators of fibrinolysis. Fibrinolytic activity is reduced in patients with type II diabetes mellitus (Table 2) *(7,46–48)*, but may be unaffected in patients with type I diabetes *(1,2,7,45–49)*.

Recent studies have investigated factors responsible for altered levels of tPA and PAI-1 in diabetic patients. Diabetes treatment may affect the levels of PAI-1 and tPA in diabetic patients *(50–52)*. PAI-1 activity in type II diabetic patients treated with metformin is reduced toward normal; however, platelet aggregation does not change *(51)*. Glycemic control and insulin resistance are both improved when the drug is administered *(51)*.

Table 2
Lipid, Fibrinolytic, and Coagulation Abnormalities Seen in Patients with Diabetes Mellitus

1. Increased glycooxidation.
2. Elevated small dense LDL.
3. Elevated plasma insulin/proinsulin levels.
4. Decreased lipoprotein lipase activity.
5. Increased fibrinogen and PAI-1.
6. Decreased fibrinolytic activity.
7. Decreased ATIII, protein C and S levels.
8. Elevated plasma levels of VLDL and Lp(a).
9. Decreased plasma HDL cholesterol.

Insulin therapy in type II diabetic patients, however, reduced PAI activity independently of glycemic control *(52)*. Further, PAI-1 concentration is correlated with the level of peripheral insulin resistance *(53,54)* and insulin concentration *(55)*. Proinsulin and proinsulin split products, both known to be present in relatively high concentration in plasma in type II patients (Table 2), directly stimulate PAI-1 synthesis *(56,57)*. The presence of diabetic complications may influence fibrinolysis since type II patients without retinopathy have higher levels of tPA than patients with retinopathy *(58)*, but tPA and PAI-1 concentrations are reduced in type I patients with retinopathy *(59)*. PAI-1 levels are significantly higher in type I patients with microalbuminuria compared to normoalbuminuric patients *(60)* and in type II patients with nephropathy compared to nondiabetic subjects with nephropathy *(61)*.

The gene coding for PAI-1 is localized to specific locus of chromosome 7 and the gene is polymorphic; genetic variation at the PAI-1 locus is associated with altered levels of PAI-1 activity in nondiabetic subjects *(62)*. Whether genotype contributes to the difference in PAI-1 levels in diabetic patients is currently under investigation. In a study of 192 type I and 327 type II diabetic patients and 123 nondiabetic subjects, there was no difference in the frequency of the restriction alleles between diabetic patients and control subjects and between the type of diabetes or the presence of retinopathy *(63)*. In contrast, when the promoter region of the PAI-1 gene was investigated in type II diabetic patients, there was a difference in PAI-1 activity among the three different genotypic groups described *(64)*. This study further demonstrated that the interactions of PAI-1 genotype with plasma triglyceride level and with insulin sensitivity were the major determinants of PAI-1 activity in these patients. Therefore, it may be possible to target individuals with unfavorable genotypes for early intervention with lipid-lowering drugs to reduce their overall risk of atherogenesis and thrombosis.

PAI is present in human platelets *(65)*, and platelets account for more than 90% of the PAI-1 in blood *(66)*. The concentration of PAI-1 is higher in platelets isolated from type II diabetic patients compared to nondiabetic subjects *(67)*. We have investigated the release of PAI-1 from platelets isolated from type II diabetic patients compared to healthy, nondiabetic subjects. Platelets from patients with type II diabetes release significantly more PAI-1 than platelets from normal subjects at the same level of platelet aggregation *(68)*. Thus, in type II diabetes, increased platelet aggregation and release of PAI-1 may delay endogenous thrombolysis and contribute to increased thrombogenesis and atherogenesis in diabetic patients.

In summary, endothelial dysfunction is clearly a component of diabetic vascular disease. One can easily visualize a scenario of endothelial damage, possibly by glycemia (and/or glycation products), hyperlipemia, hypertension, increased shear force, and other alterations that characterize the diabetic state. Evidence of endothelial damage in animal models and in acutely insulin-deficient people supports the view that this process occurs early in the course of diabetes and may be related to acute as well as chronic metabolic decompensation. Effects of endothelial damage appear to be supportive of the initiation and progression of both diabetic microangiopathy (clinically, of the retinal and renal microcirculation) and diabetic macroangiopathy (clinically, of the coronary, leg, and cerebral artery). The process may be driven by hyperglycemia and potentiated by hyperlipidemia. The net effect can be vascular damage which initiates and propagates clinical events that are characterized by vasoconstriction, adherence of platelets and monocytes, atherosclerosis and/or micro-occlusive vascular disease and, ultimately, vascular thrombosis, and tissue or organ death.

CONCLUSION

It is recognized that this formulation is a major extension of existing knowledge. Many questions remain to be answered. In particular, if such a sequence of events is correct, intervention at various steps in the process could slow down or even prevent the progression of diabetic vascular disease. This is the challenge for the future.

REFERENCES

1. Colwell JA, Lyons TJ, Klein RL, Lopes-Virella M. New concepts about the pathogenesis of atherosclerosis and thrombosis in diabetes mellitus. In: Levin MJ, ed. The Diabetic Foot. Mosby, St. Louis, MO, 1992, pp. 79–114.
2. Colwell JA, Jokl R. Vascular thrombosis in diabetes. In: Porte D, Sherwin R, Rifkin H, ed. Diabetes Mellitus: Theory and Practice, 5th ed. Appleton and Lange, Norwalk, CT, 1996, in press.
3. Abiru T, Watanabe Y, Kamata K, Miyata N, Kasuya Y. Decrease in endothelium-dependent relaxation and levels of cyclic nucleotides in aorta from rabbits with alloxan-induced diabetes. Res Commun Chem Pathol Pharmacol 1990;68:13–25.
4. Bucala R, Tracey KJ, Cerami A. Advanced glycosylation products quench nitric oxide and medicate defective endothelium-dependent vasodilation in experimental diabetes. J Clin Invest 1991;87:432–438.
5. Simon BC, Cunningham LD, Cohen RA. Oxidized low density lipoproteins cause contraction and inhibit endothelium-dependent relaxation in the pig coronary artery. J Clin Invest 1990;86:75–79.
6. Umeda F, Inoguchi T, Nawata H. Reduced stimulatory activity on prostacyclin production by cultured endothelial cells in serum from aged and diabetic patients. Atherosclerosis 1989;75:61–66.
7. Epstein M, Sowers JR. Diabetes mellitus and hypertension. Hypertension 1992;19:403–418.
8. Tesfamariam B, Jakubowski JA, Cohen RA. Contraction of diabetic rabbit aorta due to endothelium-derived PGH_2/TXA_2. Am J Physiol 1989;257:H1327–H1333.
9. Morinelli TA, Oatis JE, Okwu AK, Mais DE, Halushka P. Characterization of an ^{125}I-labelled thromboxane A_2/prostaglandin H_2 receptor agonist. J Pharmacol Exp Ther 1989;251:557–562.
10. Sachinidis A, Flesch M, Ko Y, Schrör K, Böhm M, Düsing R, Vetter H. Thromboxane A_2 and vascular smooth muscle cell proliferation. Hypertension 1995;26:771–780.
11. Takahashi K, Ghatei MA, Lam H-C, O'Halloran DJ, Bloom SR. Elevated plasma endothelin in patients with diabetes mellitus. Diabetologia 1990;33:306–310.
12. Collier A, Leach JP, McLellan A, Jardine A, Morton J, Small M. Plasma endothelin like immunoreactivity levels in IDDM patients with microalbuminuria. Diabetes Care 1992;15:1038–1040.
13. Kawamura M, Ohgawara H, Naruse M, Suzuki N, Iwasaki N, Naruse K, Hori S, Demura H, Omori Y. Increased plasma endothelin in NIDDM patient with retinopathy. Diabetes Care 1992;15:1396,1397.
14. Bertello P, Veglio F, Pinna G, Gurioli L, Molino P, Alban S, Chiandussi L. Plasma endothelin in NIDDM patients with and without complications. Diabetes Care 1994;17:574–577.

15. Morise T, Takeuchi Y, Kawano M, Koni I, Yakeda R. Increased plasma levels of immunoreactive endothelin and von Willebrand factor in NIDDM patients. Diabetes Care 1995;18:87–89.
16. Properzi G, Terenghi G, Gu XH, Poccia G, Pasqua R, Francavilla S, Polak JM. Early increase precedes a depletion of endothelin-1 but not of von Willebrand factor in cutaneous microvessels of diabetic patients. A quantitative immunohistochemical study. J Pathol 1995;175:243–252.
17. Abassi ZA, Klein H, Golomb E, Keiser HR. Urinary endothelin: a possible marker of renal damage. Am J Hypertens 1993;6:1046–1054.
18. Lee Y-J, Shin S-J, Tsai J-H. Increased urinary endothelin-1-like immunoreactivity excretion in NIDDM patients with albuminuria. Diabetes Care 1994;17:263–266.
19. Fukui M, Nakamura T, Ebihara I, Osada S, Tomino Y, Masaki T, Goto K, Furuichi Y, Koide H. Gene expression for endothelins and their receptors in glomeruli of diabetic rats. J Lab Clin Med 1993;122: 149–156.
20. Takeda Y, Miyamori I, Yoneda T, Takeda R. Production of endothelin-1 from the mesenteric arteries of streptozotocin-induced diabetic rats. Life Sci 1991;48:2553–2556.
21. Cameron NE, Dines KC, Cotter MA. The potential contribution of endothelin-1 to neurovascular abnormalities in streptozotocin-diabetic rats. Diabetologia 1994;37:1209–1215.
22. Ferri C, Carlomagno A, Coassin S, Baldoncini R, Cassone Faldetta MR, Laurenti O, Properzi G, Santucci A, De Mattia G. Circulating endothelin-1 levels increase during euglycemic hyperinsulinemic clamp in lean NIDDM men. Diabetes Care 1995;18:226–233.
23. Wolpert HA, Steen SN, Istfan NW, Simonson DC. Insulin modulates circulating endothelin-1 levels in humans. Metabolism 1993;42:1027–1030.
24. Hu R, Levin ER, Pedram A, Frank HJ. Insulin stimulates production and secretion of endothelin from bovine endothelial cells. Diabetes 1993;42:351–358.
25. Anfossi G, Cavalot F, Massucco P, Mattiello L, Mularoni E, Hahn A, Trovati M. Insulin influences immunoreactive endothelin release by human vascular smooth muscle cells. Metabolism 1993;42:1081–1083.
26. Hattori Y, Kasai K, Nakamura T, Emoto T, Shimoda S-I. Effects of glucose and insulin on immunoreactive endothelin-1 release from cultured porcine aortic endothelial cells. Metabolism 1991;40:165–169.
27. Parving HH, Hommel E, Mathiesen E, Skøtt P, Edsberg B, Bahnsen M, Lauritzen M, Hougaard P, Lauritzen E. Prevalence of microalbuminuria, arterial hypertension retinopathy and neuropathy in patients with insulin-dependent diabetes mellitus. Br Med J 1988;296:156–160.
28. Stehouwer CDA, Stroes ESG, Hackeng WHL, Mulder PGH, Den Ottolander GJH. von Willebrand factor and development of diabetic nephropathy in IDDM. Diabetes 1991;40:971–976.
29. Stehouwer CDA, Nauta JJP, Zeldenrust GC, Hackeng WHL, Donker AJM, Den Ottolander GJH. Urinary albumin excretion, cardiovascular disease, and endothelial dysfunction in non-insulin dependent diabetes mellitus. Lancet 1992;340:319–323.
30. Stehouwer CDA, Fischer HRA, van Kuijk AWR, Polak BCP, Donker AJM. Endothelial dysfunction precedes development of microalbuminuria in IDDM. Diabetes 1995;44:561–564.
31. Stehouwer CDA, Zellenrath P, Polak BCP, Baarsma GS, Nauta JJP, Donker AJM, den Ottolander GJH. von Willebrand factor and early diabetic retinopathy: no evidence for a relationship in patients with Type 1 (insulin-dependent) diabetes mellitus and normal albumin excretion. Diabetologia 1992;35:555–559.
32. Rasmussen O, Thomsen C, Ingerslev J, Hermansen K. Decrease in von Willebrand factor levels after a high-monounsaturated-fat diet in non-insulin-dependent diabetic subjects. Metabolism 1994;43:1406–1409.
33. Thomsen C, Rasmussen OW, Ingerslev J, Hermansen K. Plasma levels of von Willebrand factor in non-insulin-dependent diabetes mellitus are influenced by dietary monounsaturated fatty acids. Thromb Res 1995;77:347–356.
34. Rothlein R, Mainolfi EA, Czajkowski M, Marlin SD. A form of circulating ICAM-1 in human serum. J Immunol 1991;147:3788–3793.
35. Lampeter ER, Kishimoto TK, Rothlein R, Mainolfi EA, Bertrams J, Kolb H, Martin S. Elevated levels of circulating adhesion molecules in IDDM patients and in subjects at risk for IDDM. Diabetes 1992;41:1668–1671.
36. Martin S, Rothe H, Tschoepe D, Schwippert B, Kolb H. Decreased expression of adhesion molecules on monocytes in recent onset IDDM. Immunology 1991;73:123–125.
37. Steiner M, Reinhardt KM, Krammer B, Ernst B, Blann AD. Increased levels of soluble adhesion molecules in type 2 (non-insulin-dependent) diabetes mellitus are independent of glycemic control. Thromb Haemostas 1994;72:979–984.
38. Roep BO, Heidenthal E, de Vries RR, Kolb H, Martin S. Soluble forms of intercellular adhesion molecule-1 in insulin-dependent diabetes mellitus. Lancet 1994;343:1590–1593.

39. Herold KC, Vezys V, Gage A, Montag AG. Prevention of autoimmune diabetes by treatment with anti-LFA-1 and anti-ICAM-1 monoclonal antibodies. Cell Immunol 1994;157:489–500.
40. Hasegawa Y, Yokono K, Taki T, Amano K, Tominaga Y, Yoneda R, Yagi M, Maeda S, Yagita H, Okumura K, Kasuga M. Prevention of autoimmune insulin-dependent diabetes in non-obese diabetic mice by anti-LFA-1 and anti-ICAM-1 mAb. Int Immunol 1994;6:831–838.
41. Yang XD, Michie SA, Tisch R, Karin N, Steinman L, McDevitt HO. A predominant role of integrin alpha 4 in the spontaneous development of autoimmune diabetes in nonobese diabetic mice. Proc Natl Acad Sci USA 1994;91:12,604–12,608.
42. Yang XD, Michie SA, Tisch R, Karin N, Steinman L, McDevitt HO. Cell adhesion molecules: a selective therapeutic target for alleviation of IDDM. J Autoimmun 1994;7:859–864.
43. Baron JL, Reich E-P, Visintin I, Janeway CA Jr. The pathogenesis of adoptive murine autoimmune diabetes requires an interaction between α4-integrins and vascular cell adhesion molecule-1. J Clin Invest 1994;93:1700–1708.
44. Sowers JR, Sowers PS, Peuler JD. Role of insulin resistance and hyperinsulinemia in development of hypertension and atherosclerosis. J Lab Clin Med 1994;123:647–652.
45. Colwell JA, Lopes-Virella MF, Winocour PD, Halushka PV. New concepts about the pathogenesis of atherosclerosis in diabetes mellitus. In: Levin ME, O'Neal LW, eds. The Diabetic Foot. Mosby, St. Louis, 1988, pp. 51–70.
46. Schneider DJ, Nordt TK, Sobel BE. Attenuated fibrinolysis and accelerated atherogenesis in type II diabetic patients. Diabetes 1993;42:1–7.
47. Carmassi F, Morale M, Puccetti R, De Negri F, Monzani F, Navalesi R, Mariani G. Coagulation and fibrinolytic system impairment in insulin dependent diabetes mellitus. Thromb Res 1992;67:643–654.
48. Gray RP, Patterson DLH, Yudkin JS. Plasminogen activator inhibitor activity in diabetic and nondiabetic survivors of myocardial infarction. Arterioscler Thromb 1993;13:415–420.
49. Vicari AM, Vigano D'Angelo S, Testa S, Comi G, Galardi G, Orsi E, D'Angelo A. Normal tissue plasminogen activator and plasminogen activator inhibitor activity in plasma from patients with type 1 diabetes mellitus. Horm Metab Res 1992;24:516–519.
50. Vukovich T, Proidl S, Knobl P, Teufelsbauer H, Schnack C, Schernthaner G. The effect of insulin treatment on the balance between tissue plasminogen activator and plasminogen activator inhibitor-1 in type 2 diabetic patients. Thromb Haemostas 1992;68:253–256.
51. Nagi DK, Yudkin JS. Effects of metformin on insulin resistance, risk factors for cardiovascular disease, and plasminogen activator inhibitor in NIDDM subjects. A study of two ethnic groups. Diabetes Care 1993;16:621–629.
52. Jain SK, Nagi DK, Slavin BM, Lumb PJ, Yudkin JS. Insulin therapy in type 2 diabetic subjects suppresses plasminogen activator inhibitor (PAI-1) activity and proinsulin-like molecules independently of glycemic control. Diabetic Med 1993;10:27–32.
53. Potter van Loon BJ, Kluft C, Radder JK, Blankenstein MA, Meinders AE. The cardiovascular risk factor plasminogen activator inhibitor type 1 is related to insulin resistance. Metabolism 1993;42:945–949.
54. Gough SC, Rice PJ, McCormack L, Chapman C, Grant PJ. The relationship between plasminogen activator inhibitor-1 and insulin resistance in newly diagnosed type 2 diabetes mellitus. Diabetic Med 1993;10:638–642.
55. McGill JB, Schneider DJ, Arfken CL, Lucore CL, Sobel BE. Factors responsible for impaired fibrinolysis in obese subjects and NIDDM patients. Diabetes 1994;43:104–109.
56. Nordt TK, Schneider DJ, Sobel BE. Augmentation of the synthesis of plasminogen activator inhibitor type-1 by precursors of insulin. A potential risk factor for vascular disease. Circulation 1994;89:321–330.
57. Nordt TK, Sawa H, Fujii S, Sobel BE. Induction of plasminogen activator inhibitor type-1 (PAI-1) by proinsulin and insulin in vivo. Circulation 1995;91:764–770.
58. Takeda Y, Urano T, Watanabe I, Taminato A, Yoshimi T, Takada A. Changes in fibrinolytic parameters in male patients with type 2 (non-insulin-dependent) diabetes mellitus. Thromb Res 1993;71:405–415.
59. Cho YW, Yang DH, Oh DY, Baick SH, Kim SK, Kim SJ, Hong SY. Plasma t-PA and PAI-1 antigen concentrations in non-insulin dependent diabetic patients: implication for diabetic retinopathy. Diabetes Res Clin Pract 1994;22:123–128.
60. Gruden G, Cavallo-Perin P, Bazzan M, Stella S, Vuolo A, Pagano G. PAI-1 and factor VII activity are higher in IDDM patients with microalbuminuria. Diabetes 1994;43:426–429.
61. Schleiffer T, Hellstern P, Freitag M, Brass H. Plasminogen activator inhibitor 1 activity in lipoprotein(a) in nephropathic patients with non-insulin-dependent diabetes mellitus versus patients with nondiabetic nephropathy. Haemostasis 1994;24:49–54.

62. Dawson S, Hamsten A, Wiman B, Henney A, Humphries S. Genetic variation at the plasminogen activator inhibitor-1 locus is associated with altered levels of plasminogen activator inhibitor-1 activity. Arterioscler Thromb 1991;11:183–190.
63. Mansfield MW, Stickland MH, Carter AM, Grant PJ. Polymorphisms of the plasminogen activator inhibitor-1 gene in type 1 and type 2 diabetes, and in patients with diabetic retinopathy. Thromb Haemostas 1994;71:731–736.
64. Panahloo A, Mohamed-Ali V, Lane A, Green F, Humphries SE, Yudkin JS. Determinants of plasminogen activator inhibitor 1 activity in treated NIDDM and its relation to a polymorphism in the plasminogen activator inhibitor 1 gene. Diabetes 1995;44:37–42.
65. Erickson LA, Ginsberg MH, Loskutoff DJ. Detection and partial characterization of an inhibitor of plasminogen activator in human platelets. J Clin Invest 1984;74:1465–1472.
66. Booth NA, Anderson JA, Bennett B. Platelet release protein which inhibits plasminogen activators. J Clin Pathol 1985;38:825–830.
67. Jokl R, Laimins M, Klein RL, Lyons TJ, Lopes-Virella MF, Colwell JA. Platelet plasminogen activator inhibitor 1 in patients with type II diabetes. Diabetes Care 1994;17:818–823.
68. Jokl R, Klein RL, Lopes-Virella MF, Colwell JA. Release of platelet plasminogen activator inhibitor 1 in whole blood is increased in patients with Type 2 diabetes. Diabetes Care 1995;18:1150–1155.

10 Vascular Abnormalities in Diabetes Mellitus

Katherine D. Hein, MD *and George L. King,* MD

CONTENTS

INTRODUCTION

Diabetes mellitus causes a variety of changes in the vascular system, affecting both the micro- and macrovasculature. Classical pathologies in the microvasculature are manifested as diabetic retinopathy and nephropathy. Macrovascular diseases are observed in the coronary arteries, large peripheral vasculature involving mostly the lower limbs, and cerebral vessels. In addition, diabetes and insulin resistance are strongly associated with essential hypertension, and appear to accelerate the development of atherosclerosis *(1,2)*. Vascular abnormalities of diabetes include nutrient delivery, defense against foreign agents, hemostasis/fibrinolysis, and repair of injury. Recent clinical and epidemiologic studies have shown that intensive insulin treatment with partial normalization of glycemic control delays the appearance and possibly slows the progression of diabetic microvascular complications and neuropathy in type I diabetic patients. However, the evidence that good glycemic control can prevent or slow the progression of macrovascular diseases is not clear *(3)*. In this chapter, we discuss the cellular and molecular mechanisms that may explain the underlying pathological and clinical abnormalities observed in the vascular complications of diabetes.

In discussing possible mechanisms causing vascular dysfunction we first describe some of the physiological and pathological changes reported in diabetic macro- and microvascular tissues. Vascular abnormalities are usually classified as extracellular or cellular. For the extracellular changes, the most common and classical finding in diabetes is the thickening of capillary basement membrane (BM) *(4)*, found commonly in all tissues as well as in retinal and renal glomeruli *(5)*. Increased thickening of BM involves both protein and carbohydrate components. Most of the increase in the protein content is probably owing to type IV collagen secreted by the capillary endothelial cells *(6)*. In the renal mesangium, which is thickened or expanded to give the nodular appearance

From: *Contemporary Endocrinology: Endocrinology of the Vasculature*
Edited by: J. R. Sowers Humana Press Inc., Totowa, NJ

Table 1
Changes in Cell Number in Vascular Tissues from the Diabetic State

Retina	*Macrovessels*	*Renal glomeruli*
Endothelial cells ↑	Endothelial cells ↓	Endothelial cells ↔ then ↓
Pericytes ↓	Smooth muscle cells ↑	Mesangial cells ↔ then might ↑
		Epithelial cells ↔ then ↓

known as nodular sclerosing disease, type VI collagen is also increased *(7,8)*. Other components of extracellular matrix such as fibronectin and laminin do not show a generalized increase in the renal glomeruli of diabetic patients. In contrast, proteoglycans, which have been shown to be mainly of the heparan sulfate variety, are decreased both in the sulfate component as well as in the protein core *(9)*.

The carbohydrate contribution to vascular disease involves both enzymatic glycosylation as well as nonenzymatic glycation. The main component is probably the result of enzymatic glycosylation rather than glycation, since most of the carbohydrates in vascular proteins and in vascular cells result from enzymatic glycosylation *(10)*. However, the percent of increase is probably greater in the nonenzymatic glycation carbohydrate pool since that component is quite low in the basal state, comprising probably <5% of the carbohydrate in most cells. The role of the BM in causing vascular dysfunction could potentially be caused by several mechanisms. First, a decrease in negative charges could change the filtration properties in the renal glomeruli. Second, changes in the BM composition can affect vascular cell metabolism and contribute to alterations in migration, cell adhesion, and growth. Third, nonenzymatic glycation of extracellular protein and its byproducts may affect vascular endothelial and smooth muscle cell (VSMC) metabolism and function directly by binding to specific receptors. In addition, degraded products of the BM can alter VSMC growth indirectly by initially activating macrophages, which then release vasoactive cytokines *(11,12)*. However, it is not clear whether a quantitative relationship exists between capillary BM thickening and glomerular BM dysfunction. Furthermore, it is not clear whether the BM thickening in tissues other than the kidney plays a major part in the development of diabetic vascular complications.

Similarly, the vascular cellular changes are quite diverse depending on the vasculature involved (Table 1). Cells involved include endothelial cells and the vascular supporting cells, which are VSMC in large vessels and pericytes in capillaries. In the renal glomeruli, there are also mesangial cells and epithelial cells that are different both biochemically and functionally from other vascular tissues. Some general statements can be made, however. In microvessels, endothelial cells exhibit an activated or proliferative histology when exposed to hyperglycemia *(12)*. This is manifested by the appearance of microaneurysms, a group or cluster of endothelial cells not only in the retina but also in other vascular beds such as the brain, heart, and adipose tissue *(13,14)*. In large vessels however, endothelial cells may have a reduced ability to proliferate or migrate possibly owing to hyperglycemia and other metabolic factors such as oxidized lipids *(15)*.

Table 2
Possible Mechanisms of Glucose's Adverse Effects

Nonenzymatic glycation
Sorbitol-myoinositol changes
Redox potential alterations
DAG-PKC pathway activation

For vascular supporting cells, a diverse picture is also observed. In the microvessels, the classical finding is that there is a loss of pericytes not only in the retina, but also in peripheral tissues *(16)*. However, the clearest example of pericyte loss is observed in the retinal capillaries, which normally have a ratio of 1:1 with respect to pericytes and endothelial cells. This ratio is reduced to 1:10 after several years of diabetes with poor glycemic control. Loss of pericytes is unique to diabetes and is not observed in other chronic diseases or in aging *(17,18)*.

Mesangial cells are modified vascular contractile cells located in the renal glomeruli. In contrast to retinal pericytes, the growth of mesangial cells is not inhibited by hyperglycemia. In fact, a small increase in cell number has been reported in the early stages of diabetic nephropathy *(4,19)*. However, in the renal glomeruli, the hallmark of diabetic nephrology is the expansion of the mesangium and BM thickening, which have been consistently observed in diabetic animals or patients *(4,19)*. In large vessels, proliferation of VSMC may be increased when exposed to the diabetic milieu resulting in the acceleration of atherosclerosis. Diabetic macrovascular disease is pathologically very similar to atherosclerosis, which is accelerated by diabetes, especially in the lower extremities *(20,21)*. Manifestation of a variety of pathologies in different vascular beds when exposed to the same set of altered systemic metabolic parameters suggests that local tissue factors have an important modulating effect on the vascular cellular responses. Therefore, studies to identify the mechanism by which diabetes causes vascular disease need to be characterized in specific vasculature. For example, data derived from the arterial vascular cells cannot be generalized to explain disease processes in the microvessels. Furthermore, findings derived from vascular cells of the retina may not be applicable to disease processes occurring in the renal glomeruli.

Multiple risk factors have been identified in diabetic patients for the development of vascular complications. One factor, hyperglycemia, has been shown to be responsible for the development and progression of microvascular complications involving the retina, glomeruli, and neuronal tissues. Hyperglycemia was established as the major risk factor by the recently completed Diabetes Complications and Control Trial, which provided clinical data to show that better glycemic control can delay and reduce microvascular complications in type I diabetic patients *(3)*. Mechanisms for the development of vascular dysfunction caused by hyperglycemia are not clearly understood, but it is likely hyperglycemia can affect many vascular metabolic pathways. Studies using cultured vascular cells support the fact that elevated glucose levels can affect the metabolism and regulation of many metabolites and proteins in the vascular cells.

Although multiple mechanisms have been proposed to explain the adverse effects of hyperglycemia, we discuss only four major ones that have generated a large amount of data as well as several therapeutic trials (Table 2). One of the oldest theories involves the aldose reductase (AR) pathway and postulates that elevations of glucose levels intracellularly channel some free glucose through the AR pathway, which is activated only at high glucose concentrations since the Km for glucose is in the millimolar range. Glucose is subsequently metabolized by AR into sorbitol, which can be slowly processed into fructose and channeled back into the glycolysis pathway. The increase in sorbitol level has been postulated to effect osmotic changes intracellularly or to alter the myoinositol uptake, which is postulated to alter vascular cell response to various cytokines and hormones *(22,23)*. Animal studies using inhibitors of AR (ARI) have suggested that ARI can normalize functions and possible pathologies in the retina, neurons, and kidney in diabetic rats. However, results from studies using ARI to treat diabetic dogs as well as clinical studies for the prevention of various vascular or neuropathic complications have been equivocal *(24)*. To determine whether AR has a role in diabetic complications, some investigators have used a hypergalactosemic model in dogs and rats to test the polyol model. The hypergalactosemic model is based on the finding that galactose can be metabolized by AR, but cannot be broken down further by polyol dehydrogenase, thereby exaggerating the increase in the polyol level to a much greater extent than glucose. These animals will develop a similar retinopathy and neuropathy to diabetic animals. However, in the hypergalactosemic dog, no obvious nephropathy developed *(24)*. This suggests that AR may possibly have a role in neuropathy and retinopathy, but does not have a major role in nephropathy. In addition, we and others have found that galactose can be metabolized through pathways other than aldose reductase, thereby inducing increases in diacyglycerol (DAG) and protein kinase C (PKC) activation *(25)*. Therefore, it cannot be assumed that the hypergalactosemic model is testing only the polyol theory. At this point it is not clear whether polyol pathways play a major role in diabetic vascular complications.

A second possible mechanism involves altering the ratio between NADH/NAD or the oxidative reductive stress experienced by vascular cells. This theory is different from the oxidative stress theory of hyperglycemia since it postulates that an increase in NADH causes the problem rather than a primary increase in oxidative metabolites *(23)*. The increase in the reductive metabolites is postulated to come from the metabolism of glucose either through AR pathway or through glycolysis. Abnormalities such as vascular permeability and flow could possibly be related to an increase in NADH/NAD ratio since the use of pyruvate, which will decrease NADH, appears to normalize some vascular abnormalities in diabetic rats *(23)*. One possible problem with the NADH/NAD hypothesis resides in the fact that the oxidative reductive potential induced by AR pathway may not be substantial enough to alter the total cellular NADH/NAD ratio in relation to that produced overall by the cell. Further studies using larger populations are needed to determine the role of reductive stress in the development of diabetic vascular complications. Concomitant measurements of NADH/NAD levels also will be needed to test the hypothesis.

Third, elevated glucose levels increase the level of intracellular VSMC DAG levels. Elevated DAG levels can activate the PKC pathway, an important signal transduction system. Hyperglycemia increases PKC activity levels in the membrane fraction of cultured VSMC and in vascular tissue involving the retina, aorta, heart, and renal glomeruli of diabetic animals (Table 3) *(25,26)*. Once PKC has been activated, it may affect vascular permeability, contractility, BM turnover, adhesion molecule expression, cell growth, and regulation of coagulation and fibrinolysis. Studies of cultured vascular cells with activation of DAG and PKC pathway by hyperglycemia show altered expression of

Table 3
List of Vascular Cells and Tissues in which DAG and PKC Levels Have Been Reported in Diabetic or Hyperglycemic State

Cells	*DAG*	*PKC*
Endothelial cells (bovine retina, bovine aorta, rat capillary)	↑	↑
Aortic smooth muscle cells (rat, bovine, human)	↑	↑
Pericyte (bovine)	↑	↔
Mesangial cells (rat and human)	↑	↑
Tissue		
Retina	↑	↑
Heart	↑	↑
Aorta	↑	↑
Renal glomeruli	↑	↑
Platelets	?	↑

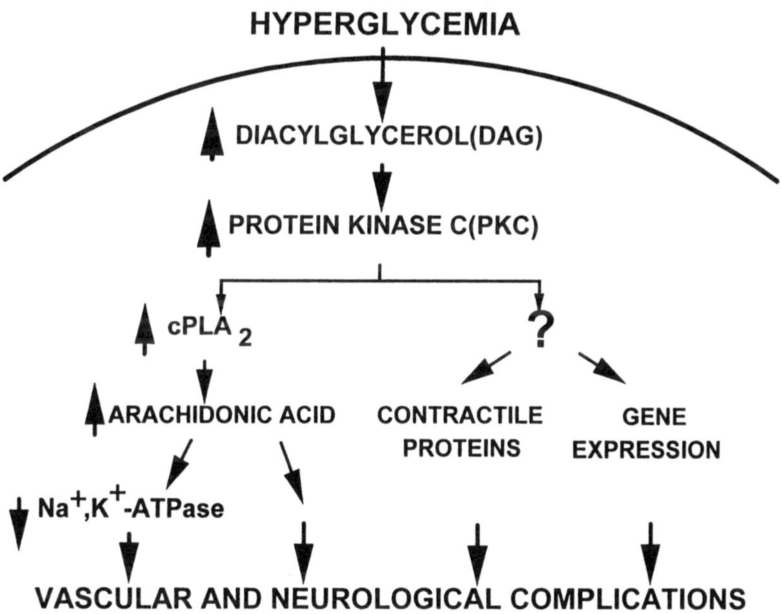

Fig. 1. Scheme for DAG/PKC activation and cellular dysfunction and hyperglycemia.

various genes such as caldesmon and fibronectin. We have shown that hyperglycemia can increase the levels of DAG and PKC in aortic VSMC, which, in turn, can activate other kinases such as cytosolic phospholipase A_2 ($cPLA_2$) *(26)*. $cPLA_2$ is an important regulatory enzyme since one of its products is arachidonate, and it can regulate many cellular functions directly. In addition, arachidonate is a precursor for the cyclo-oxygenase pathway in the production of prostaglandins (PGs). Since PGs can affect many cellular functions, the activation of $cPLA_2$ clearly shows that activation of PKC can have important cellular consequences. Furthermore, the activation of $cPLA_2$ with the release of arachidonate and PGs such as PGE2, has been shown to inhibit another important cellular enzyme called Na^+, K^+-ATPase (Fig. 1). These studies may explain the previous finding that hyperglycemia can inhibit Na^+, K^+-ATPase through the activation of PKC. Normalization of Na^+, K^+-ATPase in the presence of hyperglycemia can be prevented with inhibitors of PKC and $cPLA_2$ *(26)*. Besides cellular and biochemical changes inhibitors of PKC have been reported to normalize hemodynamic changes in the retina and kidney, indicating that PKC activation has a major role in the establishment of diabetic vascular complications *(26)*.

In addition to the previously described mechanisms that affect mainly intracellular metabolism, the last theory focuses on the effect of hyperglycemia on extracellular pathways specifically involving the formation of nonenzymatic glycation products between glucose and primary amines on proteins, and possibly on DNA as well, by nucleophilic addition *(11,12)*. The rate of glycation is in proportion to the plasma glucose level and the duration of hyperglycemia. Early glycation products, which are reversible, are best known as Amadori products and can be used to quantitate the level of glycemic control, as hemoglobin A_{1c}. After a duration of several days, the early reversible products will undergo a transformation to form irreversible products such as advanced glycosylation products (AGE). AGE products are a family of complex chemicals that can be formed by crosslinking of glucose to matrix proteins such as collagen and other BM matrix components and to plasma proteins such as low-density lipoprotein (LDL) and albumin *(11,12)*. Therefore, the advanced glycation reaction could affect the function of the extracellular proteins in their interaction with glycated proteins. For example, a glycated LDL may not bind to its receptor with the same affinity as the native LDL. In addition, glycated BM matrix may bind to receptors such as the integrins differently on the vascular cell. Alternatively, products of glycated protein such as AGE as well as their degradation products can interact with specific proteins or receptors on macrophages, which in turn release cytokines such as tumor necrosis factor to cause vascular changes *(27)*.

An inhibitor of glycation product, aminoguanadine, has been used to test this hypothesis. Aminoguanadine can prevent the increase in vascular permeability, reduce BM thickening, and decrease albuminuria, thereby reducing risk for diabetic macrovascular disease as well as nephropathy in diabetic animals *(11,12)*. Aminoguanadine can also inhibit the adverse effects of infused AGE products *(28)*. Further studies are needed to explain this finding, since aminoguanadine reportedly prevents formation of AGE rather than inhibits the adverse effects of AGE directly. In addition, the formation of AGE cannot explain all the findings in the vascular complications since the AGE hypothesis suggests that the basic disease process of diabetes and that of aging are similar except the rate is accelerated in diabetics. However, many of the vascular pathologies found in the diabetic patient are clearly not observed in aging. For example, the loss of pericytes in diabetic retinopathy is not observed in aging, with loss of endothelial cells occurring in aging.

Besides these hypotheses, a large amount of data has been accumulated to support a potential role for oxidative stress as a causal factor in the development of diabetic complications *(29)*. Clinical studies to support the definitive use of antioxidants as therapeutic agents in diabetic patients are still lacking. However, a wealth of data are available in cultured vascular cells as well as in vivo studies in diabetic animals and patients to support that hyperglycemia can induce oxidative stress in vascular tissues. Oxidative stress byproducts can be derived from multiple sources, such as byproducts of nonenzymatic glycation. In addition, the increase in NADH level has been postulated to activate oxidative enzymes. Similarly, the activation of PKC is known to regulate and activate various NADP oxidases. Therefore, hyperglycemia can induce oxidation stress by a variety of mechanisms. Further studies are necessary to identify clearly the various cellular mechanisms by which hyperglycemia can induce oxidants and whether they are responsible for vascular dysfunction.

Besides hyperglycemia, the role of growth factors in the vascular complications of diabetes has received considerable attention. For diabetic proliferative retinopathy, vascular endothelial growth factor (VEGF) is elevated in the vitreous of patients with active proliferative disease *(30)*. The level of VEGF was decreased after photocoagulation or when the disease progressed into an inactive phase, indicating that VEGF is the main growth factor causing neoproliferative retinopathy. Further, the major stimulator of VEGF expression is hypoxia, which has been suggested as the major underlying impetus for the development of diabetic proliferative retinopathy *(31)*. In addition, inhibitors of VEGF action or binding have been reported to prevent angiogenesis in the retina. Definitive studies are needed to show that inhibitor of VEGF action can prevent diabetic proliferative disease in patients. Transforming growth factor-β (TGF-β) is increased in early diabetic nephropathy and can stimulate mesangial cells in culture to produce type IV collagen and fibronectin *(32)*. In addition, hyperglycemia can also induce the expression of collagen and fibronectin, which can be inhibited by antibodies to TGF-β, suggesting that TGF-β may play a role in the increase in BM thickness observed in diabetic nephropathy.

Insulin and insulin-like growth factors (IGF) have been studied intensively *(33)*; however, discussion in this chapter is limited to effects of insulin, IGF, and growth hormone (GH) on the vascular cells only. Early clinical studies have suggested that, in patients with severe progressive diabetic retinopathy, pituitary ablation treatment appears to diminish the aggressive neovascularization process in the retina *(31)*. These studies led to the notion that GH and possibly IGF-1 may be involved in the development of proliferative diabetic retinopathy. Multiple studies have found IGF receptors in cultured cells from the retinal vasculature suggesting that IGF has both metabolic and growth effects *(33)*. However, studies from diabetic patients measuring either GH or IGF-1 from the retina and the plasma have not shown a consistent correlation with the activity of the neovascularizing process in the retina. Thus, it is not clear what the exact role of IGF-1 or GH is in the development of proliferative diabetic retinopathy. It is possible that IGF-1, a relatively weak mitogen in the retinal vasculature, may enhance the growth promoting effect of other angiogenic factors such as VEGF in the development of diabetic proliferative retinopathy.

For diabetic nephropathy, both IGF-1 and GH infusion have been shown to increase glomerular filtration rate as well as renal plasma flow. Again, in cultured vascular cells from the renal glomeruli, IGF receptors and action have been demonstrated, suggesting that GH and IGF-1 may be involved in the development of early diabetic nephropathic changes such as increased glomerular filtration rate and nephromegaly. However, patients with acromegaly who have elevated levels of GH and IGF-1 do not develop diabetic nephropathy. In addition, in transgenic mice overexpressing either GH or IGF-1, the pathology of the renal glomeruli that leads to the nephropathy in these mice does not parallel exactly what is observed in diabetic patients *(33)*. Therefore, it is still unclear what role GH and IGF-1 play in the development of diabetic nephropathy, but they can not explain the totality of the morphology in the renal glomeruli of diabetics.

Table 4
Some of Insulin's Actions on Vascular Cells in Tissues

Metabolic	*Chronic*
Glucose incorporation	Endothelin expression
Amino acid transport	PAI-1 expression
Insulin receptor tyrosine phosphorylation	Protein synthesis
MAP kinase activation	DNA synthesis
Blood flow	c-*fos*
	c-*myc* activators

Studies of insulin in diabetic vascular complications have focused mainly on its role as a risk factor for the development of hypertension and macrovascular disease *(34)*. Insulin resistance and possibly hyperinsulinemia appear to be risk factors for the development of hypertension and atherosclerosis *(34)*. Vascular cells as well as capillary vessels have insulin receptors and are responsive to insulin (Table 4) *(35)*. These actions include both metabolic actions, such as glycogen incorporation and amino acid transport, and regulation of gene expression. Insulin can regulate a variety of genes in the vasculature which has not been considered a classical insulin target. Insulin may not regulate vasculature glucose transport since the predominate glucose transporter in the vascular cells is GLUT-1 *(36)*. It has been suggested that the existence of insulin resistance causes hyperinsulinemia, which can stimulate vascular VSMC to proliferate, leading to acceleration of atherosclerosis. However, the mitogenic effect of insulin on the vascular VSMC is quite weak and requires insulin concentration 100–1000 times greater than that encountered in physiological or pathophysiological conditions *(35)*, and epidemiology studies have not uniformly demonstrated that hyperinsulinemia is a risk factor for macrovascular disease. Vascular tissues normally are responsive to insulin for a whole variety of actions, ranging from regulation of various enzymes such as glycogen phosphorylase, to gene regulation, such as the expression of endothelin *(37)*. However, the actions of insulin may not be the same as those from the classical insulin-sensitive tissues such as liver, muscle, and brain. In the insulin-resistant state, the vasculature may also become resistant to insulin action, and with the modulating action of insulin on the vasculature diminished, other cytokines such as angiotensin or tumor necrosis factor may mediate their growth effects unimpeded. For example, if insulin can modulate the action of vasoactive hormones such as endothelin, angiotensin, or the production of nitric oxide, then, in insulin-resistant states, these modulating actions of insulin will be decreased, allowing the vasoactive hormones to mediate their activities without mitigation.

In summary, the varied metabolic changes induced by diabetes can cause multiple changes in the cells of micro- and macrovessels. The actions of the metabolic changes are then either exacerbated or modulated by genetic factors, which then leads to a wide range of severity observed in the diabetic vascular complications in the retina, kidney, and macrovascular disease. In this chapter we have described several of the better known biochemical pathways by which hyperglycemia can cause these vascular dysfunctions. In addition, a brief discussion regarding the role of growth factors was presented. Therapeutic agents that reduce the adverse reactions of hyperglycemia and improve insulin resistance are in clinical trials and will provide interesting results in the near future.

ACKNOWLEDGMENTS

The authors wish to thank Joan C. Taylor for her secretarial assistance. The studies in this publication have been supported by National Institute of Health (NIH) grants EY05110, EY09178, DK23811, and ST32-HL07734-03, and NIH Diabetes Endocrinology Research Center grant DK-36836.

REFERENCES

1. Kannel WB, McGee DL. Diabetes and glucose tolerance as risk factors for cardiovascular disease: The Framingham Study. Diabetes Care 1979;2:120–126.
2. Krolewski AS, Warram JH, Rand LI, Kahn CR. Epidemiologic approach to etiology of type I diabetes mellitus and its complications. N Engl J Med 1987;317:1390–1398.
3. The Diabetes Control and Complications Trial Research Group. The effect of intensive treatment of diabetes on the development and progression of long-term complications in insulin-dependent diabetes mellitus. N Engl J Med 1993;329:977–986.
4. Morgensen CE, Osterby R, Gundersen HJG. Early functional and morphologic vascular renal consequences of the diabetic state. Diabetologia 1979;17:71–76.
5. Williamson JR, Kilo C. Extracellular matrix changes in diabetes mellitus. In: Scarpelli DG, Migaki G, eds. Comparative Pathobiology of Major Age-Related Diseases. Liss, New York, 1984, pp. 269–278.
6. Danne T, Spiro MJ, Spiro RG. Effect of high glucose on type IV collagen production by cultured glomerular epithelial endothelial and mesangial cells. Diabetes 1993;42:170–177.
7. Mohan PS, Carter WG, Spiro RG. Occurrence of type VI collagen in extracellular matrix of renal glomeruli and its increase in diabetes. Diabetes 1990;39:31–37.
8. Wakisaka M, Spiro MJ, Spiro RG. Synthesis of type VI collagen by cultured glomerular cells and comparison of its regulation by glucose and other factors with that of type IV collagen. Diabetes 1994;43:95–103.
9. Shimomura H, Spiro RG. Studies on macromolecular components of human glomerular BM and alterations in diabetes. Diabetes 1987;36:374–381.
10. Garlick RL, Bunn HF, Spiro RG. Nonenzymatic glycation of basement membranes from human glomeruli and bovine sources. Effect of diabetes and age. Diabetes 1988;37:1144–1150.
11. Brownlee M, Lecture L. Glycation and diabetic complications. Diabetes 1994;43:836–841.
12. Brownlee M. Advanced protein glycosylation in diabetes and aging. Annu Rev Med 1995;46:223–234.
13. King GL, Shiba T, Oliver J, Inoguchi T, Bursell S-E. Cellular and molecular abnormalities in the vascular endothelium of diabetes mellitus. Annu Rev Med 1994;45:179–188.
14. King GL, Banskota NK. Mechanisms of diabetic microvascular complications. In: Kahn CR, Weir GC, eds. Joslin's Diabetes Mellitus, 13th ed. Lea & Febiger, Philadelphia, PA, 1994, pp. 633–647.
15. Lorenzi M. Glucose toxicity in the vascular complications of diabetes: the cellular perspective. Diab Metab Rev 1992;8:85–103.
16. Merimee TJ. Diabetic retinopathy: a synthesis of perspectives. N Engl J Med 1990;322:978–983.
17. Cogan DG, Toussaint D, Kuwabara T. Retinal vascular patterns IV: diabetic retinopathy. Arch Ophthalmol 1961;60:100–112.
18. Kuwabara T, Cogan DG. Retinal vascular patterns VI: mural cells of the retinal capillaries. Arch Ophthalmol 1963;69:492a–502a.
19. Spiro RG. Biochemistry of the renal glomerular BM and its alterations in diabetes mellitus. N Engl J Med 1973:388:1337–1342.
20. Colwell JA, Lopes-Virella M, Halushka PV. Pathogenesis of atherosclerosis in diabetes mellitus. Diabetes Care 1981;4:121–133.
21. LoGerfo FW, Coffman JD. Current concepts: vascular and microvascular disease of the foot in diabetes. Implications for foot care. N Engl J Med 1984;311:1615–1619.
22. Greene D, Lattimer SA, Sima AAF. Sorbitol, phosphoinositides and sodium-potassium-ATPase in the pathogenesis of diabetic complications. N Engl J Med 1987;316:599–606.
23. Williamson JR, Chang K, Frangos M, Hasan KS, Ido Y, Kawamura T, Nyengaard JR, Van den Enden M, Kilo C, Tilton RG. Hyperglycemic pseudohypoxia and diabetic complications. Diabetes 1993;42:801–813.
24. Engerman RL, Kern TS. Aldose reductase inhibition fails to prevent retinopathy in diabetic and galactosemic dogs. Diabetes 1993;42:820–825.

25. Xia P, Inoguchi T, Kern TS, Engerman RL, Oates PJ, King GL. Characterization of the mechanism for the chronic activation of diacylglycerol-protein kinase C pathway in diabetes and hypergalactosemia. Diabetes 1994;43:1122–1129.
26. Xia P, Kramer RM, King GL. Identification of the mechanism for the inhibition of Na,K-adenosine triphosphatase by hyperglycemia involving activation of protein kinase C and cytosolic phospholipase A_2. J Clin Invest 1995;96:733–740.
27. Vlassara H, Brownlee M, Manogue KR, Dinarello CA, Pasagian A. Role in normal tissue remodeling. Science 1988;240:1546–1548.
28. Hammes HP, Martin S, Federlin K, Geisen K, Brounlee M. Aminoguanidine treatment inhibits the development of experimental diabetic retinopathy. Proc Natl Acad Sci USA 1991;88:11,555–11,558.
29. Baynes JW. Perspectives in diabetes. Role of oxidative stress in development of complications in diabetes. Diabetes 1991;40:405–412.
30. Ferrara N, King GL. Vascular endothelial growth factor in ocular fluid of patients with diabetic retinopathy and other retinal disorders. N Engl J Med 1994;331:1480–1487.
31. Merimee TJ. Diabetic retinopathy: a synthesis of perspectives. N Engl J Med 1990;322:978–983.
32. Sharma K, Ziyadeh FN. The emerging role of transforming growth factor-beta in kidney diseases. Am J Physiol 1994;266(6 Pt 2):F829–F842.
33. Grant M, King GL. IGF-1 and blood vessels: implications for microvascular and macrovascular disease. Diabetes Rev 1995;3:113–128.
34. Ferrannini E. Hypertension as an insulin resistant disorder: role of obesity. In: Smith U, Bruun NE, Hedner T, Hokfelt B, eds. Novo Nordisk Foundation Symposium No. 5. Excerpta Medica, Amsterdam, 1991,123–135.
35. King GL, Davidheiser S, Banskota N, Oliver J, Inoguchi T. Insulin receptors and actions on vascular cells. In: Smith U, Bruun NE, Hedner T, Hokfelt B, eds. Novo Nordisk Foundation Symposium No. 5, Excerpta Medica, Amsterdam, 1991,183–187.
36. Kaiser N, Sasson S, Feener EP, Moller DE, King GL. Differential regulation of glucose transport and transporters by glucose in vascular endothelial and smooth muscle cells. Diabetes 1992;42:80–89.
37. Oliver FJ, de la Rubia G, Feener EP, Lee M-E, Loeken MR, Shiba T, Quertermous T, King GL. Stimulation of endothelin-1 gene expression by insulin in endothelial cells. J Biol Chem 1991;266: 23,251–23,256.

11 Effects of Hyperglycemia on Vascular Endothelium Nitric Oxide Metabolism

Steven B. Magill, MD, PhD
and Jamie Dananberg, MD

Contents

INTRODUCTION

Vascular complications remain the leading cause of increased mortality in the diabetic population. There are many theories as to the etiology of these effects, but vascular endothelial dysfunction appears to play an extremely important role. Accumulating data suggests that exposure to increased concentrations of glucose leads to endothelial dysfunction. Studies in diabetes have demonstrated elevations in plasma von Willebrand's factor *(1)*, diminished release of prostacyclin (PGI) *(2)*, a vasodilatory prostaglandin (PG), enhanced secretion of endothelin *(3)*, and lowered lipoprotein lipase activity *(4)* as evidence of abnormal endothelial function.

The endothelium participates in vascular regulation by modulating release of various vasorelaxing factors such as nitric oxide (NO), endothelium-derived hyperpolarization factor, and PGI; and vasoconstricting factors such as thromboxane and endothelin. Recent studies have shown that NO-mediated endothelium-dependent vasorelaxation is impaired in both animal and human forms of diabetes mellitus. Investigators utilizing isolated vessels have demonstrated that agonist-stimulated relaxation is decreased in diabetes *(5–9)*.

From: *Contemporary Endocrinology: Endocrinology of the Vasculature*
Edited by: J. R. Sowers Humana Press Inc., Totowa, NJ

In humans, impairment of endothelium-dependent vascular relaxation has been shown in forearm blood flow in both insulin-dependent *(10,11)* as well as in noninsulin-dependent diabetic subjects *(12)*.

Cellular mechanisms leading to altered endothelial cell function have been examined. In streptozotocin-treated diabetic rats, the impairment in aortic relaxation is caused by a diminished production of NO *(13)*. Similar findings were found utilizing mesenteric artery preparations in the same diabetic model *(14)*. However, abnormal relaxation of rabbit aortic rings exposed to high levels of glucose is caused by increased endothelial production of vasoconstrictive PGs (thromboxane and prostaglandin $F_{2\alpha}$ [$PGF_{2\alpha}$]), as a function of protein kinase C (PKC) activation *(15,16)*. Increases in oxygen-derived free radicals *(17,18)*, diminished activation of Na^+, K^+-ATPase *(19,20)*, or the excess production of advanced glycosylation endproducts (AGE; *21*), may play important roles leading to endothelial dysfunction secondary to chronic hyperglycemia. This chapter concentrates on the cellular mechanisms that lead to impairment of endothelial cell NO production in hyperglycemic environments.

VASCULAR ENDOTHELIAL DYSFUNCTION IN DIABETES MELLITUS

Diabetes is associated with micro- and macrovascular complications, an important early component of which is endothelium dysfunction. The endothelium is a key component in regulation of vascular tone through release of both contracting and relaxing factors. Endothelium-dependent vasodilation induced by infusion of acetylcholine (ACh) has been demonstrated to be mediated by NO *(22)*. NO causes vasodilation by stimulating guanylyl cyclase activity and elevating cyclic GMP (cGMP) in vascular smooth muscle cells (VSMC). Reductions in NO may lead to vascular injury by enhanced platelet aggregability *(23)*, adhesion of monocytes to the endothelium *(24)*, and/or to enhanced mitogenesis of VSMC *(25)*.

Impaired endothelium-dependent vascular relaxation has been found in several models of diabetes *(5,7,26)*. Similarly, impaired relaxation to ACh has been demonstrated in aortic rings obtained from diabetic rabbits *(27)*, as well as in rings obtained from normal rabbits exposed to high concentrations of glucose for 6 h *(15)*. Impaired endothelium-dependent relaxation has been observed in corpora cavernosa tissue obtained from impotent diabetic men *(28)*. There is abnormal endothelium-dependent vasodilation in the forearms of diabetic patients *(10,29)*. These effects appear to be mediated by impaired basal release of NO. However, reduced vasodilatory response to both ACh and nitroglycerin has been observed in type II diabetic subjects, implicating both the endothelium and vascular smooth muscle as sites of dysregulation *(12)*.

MECHANISMS OF ENDOTHELIAL CELL DYSFUNCTION IN DIABETES MELLITUS: ROLE OF NO

NO, a short-lived free radical, is synthesized from L-arginine by NO synthase utilizing the reduced form of nicotinamide adenine dinucleotide phosphate (NADPH), O_2, tetrahydrobiopterin, flavin adenine dinucleotide (FAD), and flavin mononucleotide (FMN) as cofactors *(30)*. There are multiple isoforms of NO synthase (NOS) that fall into two distinct categories. Constitutively expressed forms (cNOS) are present in endothelial cells (138 kDa, type II NOS) and in brain (150 kDa, type II NOS) and are regulated by the availability and binding of calcium (Ca^{2+})/calmodulin. An additional isoform expressed only after activation by cytokines is found principally in macrophages (iNOS). Although this form binds calcium/calmodulin, such binding is not required for NO generation. Following stimulation with γ-interferon or tumor necrosis factor-α (TNF-α), the inducible isoform is also expressed in VSMC, heart, chondrocytes, liver, and endothelium *(31)*. That both cNOS and iNOS appear to be expressed in both VSMC and endothelial cells *(32)* is potentially important because NO is an inhibitor of platelet aggregation and vascular growth *(31,33)*. In animal models, NO-mediated vasodilation is impaired in diabetes *(8,26,34)*. Both basal and agonist-stimulated levels of cGMP are also reduced in animal models of diabetes *(26,35)*. Thus, impairment in NO production or release could lead to the development of vascular injury and accelerated atherosclerosis associated with diabetes. There is abnormal endothelium-dependent vasodilation but preserved endothelium-independent (i.e., smooth muscle dependent) vasodilation in forearm blood flow studies from diabetic patients *(10,29)*. However, moderately controlled diabetic subjects have no impairment in endothelium-dependent vasodilation *(36)*. The latter observation has been confirmed in animal studies *(15,16)*, and indicates that moderate hyperglycemia (5.5–10 m*M* glucose) may not impair endothelial dysfunction. Others have reported a correlation between the length of diabetes and the degree on impairment of endothelium-dependent relaxation *(37)*.

Although endothelial NO synthesis or release is impaired, VSMC responses appear to be intact in diabetes, based on studies that have relied on measurement of relaxation in isolated precontracted arterial strips or on measurement of forearm blood flow. These are reflective of integrated events involving the endothelium, VSMC, and other tissues. We have studied events related to glucose-mediated alteration in NO production. Utilizing rat aortic endothelial cells, we used the accumulation of intracellular cGMP as a measure of the effects of high glucose concentration on NO. We found that ACh-induced elevations in cGMP were completely abolished in endothelial cells that had been exposed to 22 m*M* glucose for 24 h. In contrast, under normoglycemic conditions (5.5 m*M* glucose), plus either 15.5 m*M* mannitol (equiosmolar concentrations compared to 22 m*M* glucose) or 3-*o*-methylglucose (15.5 m*M*; a nonmetabolizable substrate), NO-dependent cGMP production was not impaired (Fig. 1). Furthermore, the inhibition was at the level of NO production and not guanylyl cyclase responsivity, in that sodium nitroprusside (NTP; a direct generator of NO) caused a substantial increase in cGMP that was unaffected by elevated glucose concentrations. These data have been corroborated by some *(5,8,26)*, but not others *(38)*. Others found that guanylyl cyclase activity in glomeruli from diabetic rats was attenuated, but only after exposure of cells to high glucose for 7–14 d *(39)*. However, these latter effects have been attributed to hyperglycemia-induced quenching of NO by advanced glycosylation end products rather than direct interaction with guanylyl cyclase *(21,40)*. We have concluded that AGE cannot account for the metabolic effects we observed given the short incubatory conditions utilized in our experiments.

The reduced endothelium-dependent vasodilation that occurs in experimental or clinical diabetes may be the result of a combination of effects on NO-induced vasodilation. There may be decreased synthesis or release of NO via inhibition of NOS. Alternatively, there may be a reduced responsiveness of VSMC soluble guanylyl cyclase to NO. Free radicals produced under hyperglycemic conditions may limit availability of NO; similarly, vasoconstrictive prostanoids may interact directly or indirectly to limit the effects of NO. These latter issues are discussed more fully in the next section.

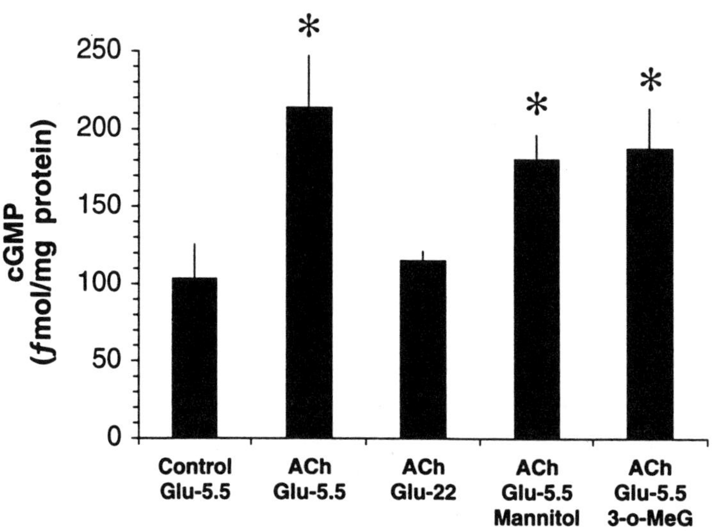

Fig. 1. Effect of 22 m*M* glucose (Glu-22), 16.5 m*M* mannitol, or 16.5 m*M* 3-*o*-methylglucose (3-*o*-MeG) vs 5.5 m*M* glucose on ACh-induced stimulation of endothelial cGMP. Control cells were exposed to 5.5 m*M* glucose (Glu-5.5). Treated cells were incubated with 22 or 5.5 m*M* glucose plus either mannitol or 3-o-methylglucose for 24 h then stimulated with $10^{-6}M$ ACh for 10 min. $*p < 0.05$ compared to untreated, control cells.

HYPERGLYCEMIA-RELATED ALTERATIONS IN OTHER FACTORS

Several groups have demonstrated elevation in vasoconstrictive prostanoids under hyperglycemic conditions *(15,41)*. The precursor prostanoid, prostaglandin H_2 (PGH_2), appears to be the major contributor because exogenous PGH_2 impairs ACh-induced relaxation in an equivalent manner to that seen in experimental diabetes *(42)*. Following exposure of cultured endothelial cells to high glucose concentrations for 6 h or more, there is an abnormal release of prostanoids. These effects have been attributed to abnormal release of arachidonic acid *(43)*. It has been suggested that altered metabolism of arachidonic acid leads to increased production of free radicals, such as superoxide. Both increased production of free radicals and decreased activity of free radical scavengers occur in experimental diabetes *(44)*. Similarly, superoxide dismutase (superoxide scavenger) partially corrects abnormal endothelium-dependent relaxation in diabetic rat aorta *(45)*. A decrease in endothelial cell superoxide dismutase activity leads to reduced NO release *(46,47)*. The decreased endothelium-dependent relaxation seen in diabetes may be linked to increased production of free radicals through cyclo-oxygenase activation and catalysis in the endothelium. Cyclo-oxygenase produces superoxide by conversion of NADPH to a nicotinamide adenine dinucleotide phosphate (NADP) radical during conversion of prostaglandin G_2 (PGG_2) to PGH_2; NADP subsequently interacts with oxygen to produce superoxide *(18)*. Finally, superoxide causes endothelium-dependent vasoconstriction by dampening basal release of NO in diabetic rat aorta *(48)*.

Taken together, these data support the conclusion that vasoconstrictive prostanoids and free radicals play a substantive role in endothelial dysfunction associated with diabetes. An interaction between arachidonic acid metabolism, free radical generation, and NO production in endothelial cells *(16)* is illustrated in Fig. 2. The exact mechanism by which these systems may alter NO production is still, however, under intense investigation.

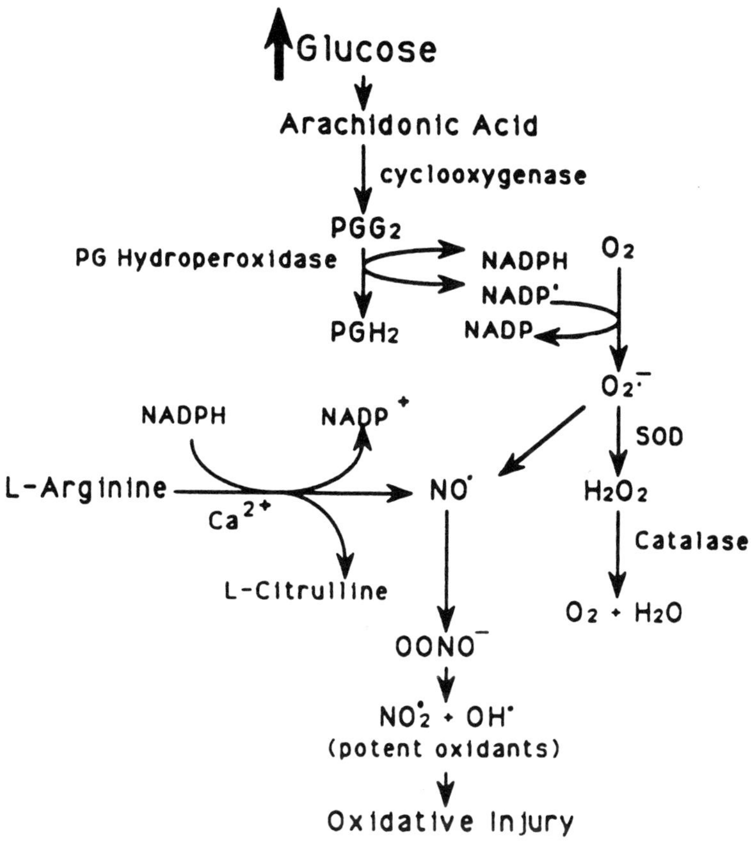

Fig. 2. A hyperglycemic environment is proposed to lead to abnormal arachadonic acid metabolism in the endothelium, which enhances free radical formation and limits NO availability. The cyclo-oxygenase pathway produces PGH_2 from PGG_2 and, reciprocally, NADP formation from NADPH. NADP in turn reacts with O_2 to yield superoxide (O_2^-). Superoxide can be scavenged by superoxide dismutase to hydrogen peroxide (H_2O_2) and by further action of catalase, to oxygen and water. NO is formed by conversion of L-arginine to citrulline utilizing the cofactors NADPH, O_2, and calcium/calmodulin. Superoxide may also interact with NO to form peroxynitrite ($OONO^-$), which can form potent oxidants such as hydroxyl radical (NO_2) or nitrogen dioxide (NO_2), leading to oxidative damage. Modified from ref. *18* with permission.

AGE

AGE involve nonenzymatic glycosylation and crosslinking of proteins following exposure of tissues to high concentrations of glucose *(49)*, and these products inactivate NO in experimental diabetes *(21)*. Aminoguanidine, which inhibits formation of AGE, can reverse, in part, abnormal endothelium-dependent relaxation in aortic strips taken from diabetic rats *(21)*. Aminoguanidine is a structural analog of L-arginine and may inhibit NOS *(50)*. Aminoguanidine is also proposed to limit the hyperemia associated with diabetic vascular dysfunction. AGE form over a period of time and cannot play an important role in many of the acute in vitro studies discussed. However, these results suggest that activation of iNOS in conjunction with AGE may paradoxically contribute to diabetic vascular injury.

POLYOL PATHWAY METABOLISM AND NO IN DIABETES MELLITUS

Heightened polyol pathway metabolism is seen in experimental diabetes *(51–53)*. Metabolism of glucose to sorbitol by the polyol pathway under conditions of hyperglycemia serves to shunt excess glucose. The first and rate-limiting reaction consists of reduction of glucose to sorbitol (polyol) by aldose reductase (AR) utilizing NADPH as the hydrogen donor. Of note, AR has been found to be abundant in endothelial cells *(54)*. Oxidation of sorbitol to fructose by sorbitol dehydrogenase (SDH), the second step of the polyol pathway, is coupled to reduction of NAD^+ to NADH. Since AR and sorbitol dehydrogenase are coupled to NADPH/$NADP^+$ and NAD^+/NADH, respectively, hyperglycemic conditions may deplete NADPH, a critical cofactor for NOS. Additionally, endogenous antioxidants such as glutathione reductase require NADPH, and depletion of NADPH has been shown to augment production of oxidants under the stress of hyperglycemia *(55)*.

Metabolism of glucose via the polyol pathway leads to depletion of myoinositol and other intracellular osmolytes, as well as reduced Na^+, K^+-ATPase activity and altered phosphoinositide metabolism *(56)*. In nerve tissue, sorbitol itself acts as an osmolyte and competitively inhibits uptake of myoinositol resulting in disruption in the inositol signaling pathway *(57)*. The polyol pathway has been previously linked to microvascular complications of diabetes in that AR inhibitors reverse impaired endothelium function both in aortic relaxation in diabetic animals *(51)* and in cultured endothelial cells *(38)*. Finally, inhibition of NOS reproduces the effect hyperglycemia has on diminishing Na^+, K^+-ATPase activity in nerves from diabetic rats *(20)*.

We explored the cellular basis for glucose-mediated inhibition of NOS. We hypothesized that a decrease in NO production might be linked to increased metabolism of glucose through the polyol pathway during prolonged hyperglycemic states. Endothelial cells were treated with sorbinil ($10^{-3}M$; an inhibitor of AR) in the presence of 22 m*M* glucose. Following the addition of sorbinil, the ability of these cells to produce NO following ACh stimulation was restored to normal (Fig. 3). To examine the interaction between polyol metabolism and NOS inhibition, we also investigated the altered redox potential-coupled ratios. As noted, AR may compete for NADPH under hyperglycemic conditions and may limit the availability of the cofactor for NOS *(58,59)*. We tested whether changes in the NADPH/NADP ratio were associated with dampened NO production following incubation of cells in 22 m*M* glucose. We found no difference in NADPH, NADP, or the ratio of NADPH/NADP in cells incubated in control (5.5 m*M* glucose) vs high glucose conditions. Thus, altered redox potential is not an important factor in limiting NO production under hyperglycemic environments in endothelial cells.

DIACYLGLYCEROL AND PKC ACTIVATION IN DIABETES

Increased de novo synthesis of diacylglycerol (DAG) or enhanced concentrations of DAG have been found in a variety of tissues under hyperglycemic environments *(60–62)*. Others, however, have found that DAG levels were unchanged in thoracic aorta of diabetic rats *(63)*. Enhanced DAG production leads to activation of PKC, which participates in regulation of receptor turnover and function, ion flux, and contraction of vascular smooth muscle. PKC activation has been found in cultured aortic VSMC incubated under hyperglycemic conditions *(64)*. Augmented PKC activity has been linked to a variety of metabolic changes in diabetes and theorized to lead to microvascular complications *(60)*.

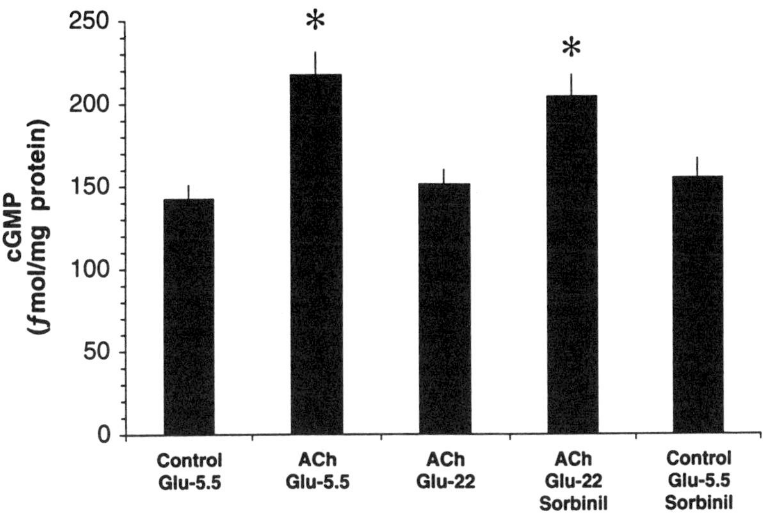

Fig. 3. Effect of 22 m*M* glucose (Glu-22) and $10^{-3}M$ sorbinil on ACh-induced stimulation of endothelial cGMP. Control cells were exposed to 5.5 m*M* glucose (Glu-5.5) and treated cells to 22 m*M* glucose and/or $10^{-3}M$ sorbinil for 24 h, then stimulated with $10^{-6}M$ ACh for 10 min. $*p < 0.05$ compared to untreated cells.

PKC activation has also been implicated in generation of vasoconstrictive prostanoids *(65,66)*, and production and release of superoxide *(67)*. Activation of PKC has also been demonstrated in endothelial cells exposed to high concentration of glucose *(68)*. Others have suggested that polyol metabolism reduces PKC activation owing to cellular accumulation of sorbitol, leading to a decrease in myoinositol, reduced phosphoinositide turnover, and subsequent decrease in activity of PKC *(69)*. It has been proposed that this differential response between tissues may relate to the degree of AR expression. In endothelial cells exposed to high glucose, de novo DAG synthesis predominates and may lead to enhanced microvascular dysfunction. On the other hand, in nerves under hyperglycemic conditions, glucose-induced AR-mediated sorbitol accumulation has been shown to induce a reciprocal decrease in myoinositol rather than de novo production of DAG, leading to diminished Na^+, K^+-ATPase activity *(70)*.

In endothelial cells we found that PKC activity translocated from the cytosolic to the membranous compartment following exposure of cells to 22 m*M* glucose, or after brief exposure (10 min) to phorbol ester, findings consistent with in vivo activation of PKC *(71)*. Finally, we demonstrated that activation of PKC was linked to polyol metabolism in that sorbinil completely blocked the hyperglycemic-induced activation of PKC (Fig. 4).

These data support the hypothesis that high-glucose conditions enhance polyol metabolism and lead to activation of PKC, which, directly or indirectly, reduces activation of NOS through putative phosphorylation effects. Cerebellar NOS can be phosphorylated by several kinases including PKC, and NOS activity is reduced by these effects *(72)*. Purified cerebellar NOS can be phosphorylated by protein kinase A and two calmodulin-dependent kinases but not by PKC *(73)*. Since there is only approx 50% homology between the neural and endothelial NOS, it is difficult to equate phosphorylation effects by separate kinases in these two isoforms. In endothelial cells, stimulation of phosphorylation of NOS leads to translocation of the enzyme from the cytosolic to the

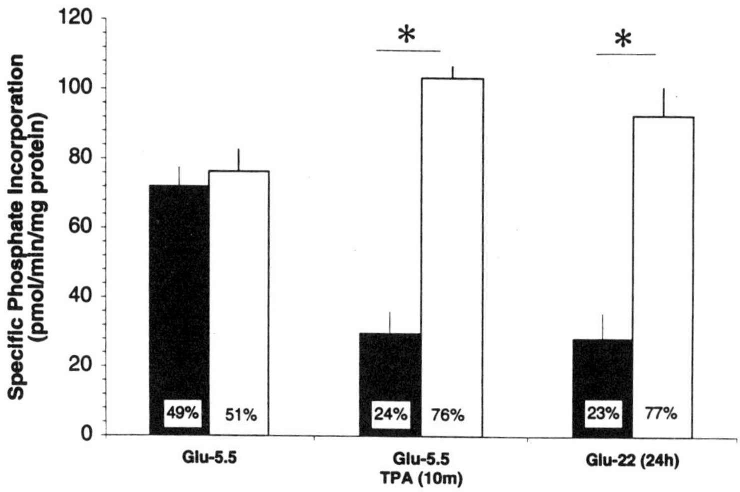

Fig. 4. Effect of 22 m*M* glucose (Glu-22) or the phorbol ester TPA on DEAE-cellulose-purified PKC activity extracted from endothelial cells. PKC activity was measured as specific ^{32}P incorporation into a kinase specific substrate in both membranous *(o)* and cytosolic *(n)* fractions. The cells were treated with either 5.5 m*M* glucose (Glu-5.5) or 22 m*M* glucose for 24 h. One group of cells was treated with TPA for 10 min. The percentage figures indicate the relative proportion of total activity in each compartment. $^*p < 0.05$ compared to 5.5 m*M* glucose-treated cells.

membranous fraction *(74)*. Additionally, phorbol esters have been demonstrated to reduce NO-dependent cGMP levels in cells transfected with the cDNA for NOS *(72)*. Finally, endothelium-dependent NO production is inhibited by brief treatment of cells with phorbol ester, thus implicating PKC activation as a link to reduction of NOS activity *(75)*.

We tested the notion that activation of PKC can link the decreased activity of NOS with metabolic changes in cells exposed to high-glucose concentrations. Endothelial cells were incubated in the presence of either 12-*o*-tetradecanoylphorbol-13-acetate (TPA) or calphostin C (a highly specific inhibitor of PKC) for 24 h to prevent PKC activation. Both treatments fully prevented glucose-mediated inhibition of cGMP accumulation (Fig. 5). These data strongly implicate activation of PKC as a key event in the inhibition of endothelial NOS. In preliminary experiments we have shown that NOS protein expression is unchanged following exposure of cells to high glucose as measured by Western blotting techniques. We have further shown in immunoprecipitation experiments that PKC is able to phosphorylate type III NOS in intact endothelial cells.

Thus, acute elevations in glucose concentration activates PKC, which secondarily phosphorylates NOS. We speculate that this phosphorylation event inhibits the Ca^{2+}/calmodulin-induced stimulation of NOS. Indeed, a PKC-phosphorylation site consensus sequence (rkKTFK) lies within the putative Ca^{2+}/calmodulin binding domain of type III NOS. Of note, this threonine site is not present in other NOS isoforms despite an otherwise highly conserved Ca^{2+}/calmodulin binding domain.

Other kinase systems may or may not be activated by high-glucose concentrations and could directly or indirectly affect NOS as well. However, these remain to be elucidated. We theorize that uncontrolled hyperglycemia in the clinical setting causes similar changes in the endothelium and could be an early marker for impaired endothelial function. Such dysfunction can play an important role in the vascular complications seen in diabetes

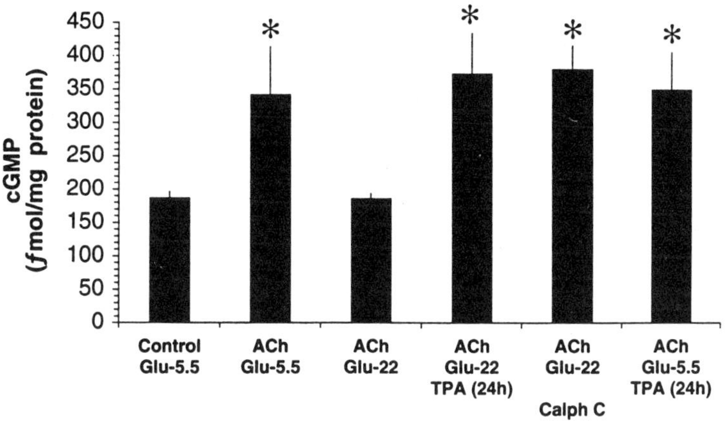

Fig. 5. Effect of 22 m*M* glucose (Glu-22) and/or TPA on ACh-induced stimulation of endothelial cGMP. Control cells were exposed to 5.5 m*M* glucose for 24 h. Samples were exposed to 22 m*M* glucose with or without TPA for 24 h, then stimulated with 10^{-6} *M* ACh for 10 min. Another group of cells was exposed to 22 m*M* glucose in addition to pretreatment with calphostin C (Calph C) prior to stimulation with ACh. $*p < 0.05$ compared to untreated cells.

mellitus. Identification of the molecular mechanisms of endothelial dysfunction presents targets to which future therapeutic interventions can be aimed at prevention of diabetic vascular disease.

ACKNOWLEDGMENTS

This work was supported in part by a Research Advisory Group Grant 142A7C from the Veterans Administration. Additional support came from the American Heart Association and its Michigan affiliate and from the Michigan Diabetes and Research Training Center. J. Dananberg performed this work during the tenure of a Clinician-Scientist Award from the American Heart Association. S. B. Magill was supported by the Michigan Diabetes Research and Training Center Grant DK 07245-19. Part of this work was presented at the 75th Annual Scientific Meeting of the Endocrine Society, Las Vegas, NV, June 1993. A portion of this work is under review for publication in the *Journal of Clinical Investigation*.

REFERENCES

1. Bensousan D, Levy-Toledano S, Passa P, Caen J, Canivet J. Platelet hyperaggregation and increased plasma level of von Willebrand factor in diabetic patients with retinopathy. Diabetologia 1975;11:307–312.
2. Harrison HE, Reece AH, Johnson M. Decreased vascular PGI in experimental diabetes. Life Sci 1978;23:351–356.
3. Yamauchi T, Ohnaka K, Takayanagi R, Umeda F, Nawata H. Enhanced secretion of endothelin-1 by elevated glucose levels from cultured bovine aortic endothelial cells. FEBS Lett 1990;267:16–18.
4. Steiner G. Diabetes and atherosclerosis. Diabetes 1981;30(Suppl. 2):1–7.
5. Oyama Y, Kawasaki H, Hattori Y, Kanno M. Attenuation of endothelium-dependent relaxation in aorta from diabetic rats. Eur J Pharmacol 1986;131:75–78.
6. Ignarro LJ, Lippton H, Edwards JC, Baricos WH, Hyman AL, Kadowitz PJ, Gruetter CA. Mechanism of VSMC relaxation by organic nitrates, nitrites, nitroprusside and NO: evidence for the involvement of S-nitrosothiols as active intermediates. J Pharmacol Exp Ther 1981;218:739–749.

7. Meraji S, Jayakody L, Senaratne MPJ, Thompson ABR, Kappagoda T. Endothelium-dependent relaxation in aorta of BB rat. Diabetes 1987;36:978–981.
8. Durante W, Sen AK, Sunahara FA. Impairment of endothelium-dependent relaxation in aortae from spontaneously diabetic rats. Br J Pharmacol 1988;94:463–468.
9. Abiru T, Watanabe Y, Kamata K, Kasuya Y. Changes in endothelium-dependent relaxation and levels of cyclic nucleotides in the perfused mesenteric arterial bed from streptozotocin-induced diabetic rats. Life Sci 1993;53:PL7–PL12.
10. Calver A, Collier J, Vallance P. Inhibition and stimulation of NO synthesis in the human forearm arterial bed of patients with insulin-dependent diabetes. J Clin Invest 1992;90:2548–2554.
11. Elliot TG, Cockcroft JR, Groop P, Viberti GC, Ritter M. Inhibition of NO synthesis in forearm vasculature of insulin-dependent diabetic patients: blunted vasoconstriction in patients with microalbuminuria. Clin Sci 1993;85:687–693.
12. McVeigh GE, Brennan GM, Johnston GD, McDermott BJ, McGrath LT, Henry WR, Andrews JW, Hayes JR. Impaired endothelium-dependent and independent vasodilation in patients with type 2 (non-insulin-dependent) diabetes mellitus. Diabetologia 1992;35:771–776.
13. Chang KSK, Stevens WC. Endothelium-dependent increase in vascular sensitivity to phenylephrine in long-term streptozotocin diabetic rat aorta. Br J Pharmacol 1992;107:983–990.
14. Taylor PD, McCarthy AL, Thomas CR, Poston L. Endothelium-dependent relaxation and noradrenaline sensitivity in mesenteric resistance arteries of streptozotocin-induced diabetic rats. Br J Pharmacol 1992;107:393–399.
15. Tesfamariam B, Brown ML, Deykin D, Cohen RA. Elevated glucose promotes generation of endothelium-derived vasoconstrictor prostanoids in rabbit aorta. J Clin Invest 1990;85:929–932.
16. Tesfamariam B, Brown ML, Cohen RA. Elevated glucose impairs endothelium-dependent relaxation by activating protein kinase C. J Clin Invest 1991;87:1643–1648.
17. Tesfamariam B, Cohen RA. Free radicals mediate endothelial cell dysfunction caused by elevated glucose. Am J Phys 1992;263:H321–H326.
18. Tesfamariam B. Free radicals in diabetic endothelial cell dysfunction. Free Radic Biol Med 1994;16:383–391.
19. Gupta S, Sussman I, McCarthur CS, Tornheim K, Cohen RA, Ruderman NB. Endothelium-dependent inhibition of Na/K-ATPase activity in rabbit aorta by hyperglycemia. J Clin Invest 1992;90:727–732.
20. Stevens MJ, Dananberg J, Feldman EL, Lattimer SA, Kamijo M, Thomas TP, Shindo H, Sima AF, Greene DA. The linked roles of NO, aldose reductase and, (Na^+, K^+)-ATPase in the slowing of nerve conduction in the streptozotocin diabetic rat. J Clin Invest 1994;94:853–859.
21. Hogan M, Cerami A, Bucala R. Advanced glycosylation endproducts block the antiproliferative effect of NO. Role in the vascular and renal complications of diabetes mellitus. J Clin Invest 1992;90:1110–1115.
22. Vallance P, Collier J, Moncada S. Effects of endothelium-dependent NO on peripheral arteriolar tone in man. Lancet 1989;ii:997–1000.
23. Radomski MW, Palmer RMJ, Moncada S. An L-arginine/nitric oxide pathway present in human platelets regulates aggregation. Proc Natl Acad Sci USA 1990;87:5193–5197.
24. Kubes P, Suzuki M, Granger DN. NO: an endogenous modulator of leukocyte adhesion. Proc Natl Acad Sci USA 1991;88:4651–4656.
25. Garg UC, Hassid A. NO generating vasodilation and 8-bromo-cyclic guanosine monophosphate inhibit mitogenesis and proliferation of cultured rat VSMC cells. J Clin Invest 1989;83:1774–1777.
26. Kamata K, Miyata N, Kasuya Y. Impairment of endothelium-dependent relaxation and changes in levels of cyclic GMP in aorta from streptozotocin-induced diabetic rats. Br J Pharmacol 1989;97:614–618.
27. Tesfamariam B, Jakabowsky JA, Cohen RA. Contraction of diabetic rabbit aorta caused by endothelium-derived PGH_2-TXA_2. Am J Physiol 1989;257:H1327–H1333.
28. Saenz de Tejada IS, Goldstein J, Azadzoik K, Krane K, Cohen RA. Impaired neurogenic and endothelium-mediated relaxation of penile smooth muscle from diabetic men with impotence. N Engl J Med 1989;320:1025–1030.
29. Johnstone MT, Creager SJ, Scales KM, Casco JA, Lee BK, Creager MA. Impaired endothelium-dependent vasodilation in patients with insulin-dependent diabetes mellitus. Circ 1993;88:2510–2516.
30. Moncada S, Palmer RMJ, Higgs EA. NO, physiology, pathophysiology, and pharmacology. Pharmacol Rev 1991;43:109–142.
31. Marletta MA. NOS structure and mechanism. J Biol Chem 1993;268:12,231–12,234.
32. Forstermann U, Closs EI, Pollock JS, Nakane M, Schwarz P, Gath I, Kleinert H. Nitric oxide synthase isozymes: characterization, purification, molecular cloning, and functions. Hypertension 1994;23(part 2): 1121–1131.

33. Radomski MW, Palmer RMJ, Moncada S. Endogenous NO inhibits platelet adhesion to vascular endothelium. Lancet 1987;ii:1057,1058.
34. Mayhan WG. Impairment of endothelium-dependent dilatation of cerebral arterioles during diabetes mellitus. Am J Physiol 1989;256:H621–H625.
35. Abiru T, Watanabe Y, Kamata K, Miyata N, Kasuya Y. Decrease in endothelium-dependent relaxation and levels of cyclic nucleotide in aorta from rabbits with alloxan-induced diabetes. Res Comm Chem Pathol Pharmacol 1990;68:13–25.
36. Smits P, Kapma JA, Jacobs MC, Lutterman J, Thien T. Endothelium-dependent vascular relaxation in patients with type I diabetes. Diabetes 1993;42:148–153.
37. Orie N, Aloamaka C, Iyawe VI. Duration-dependent attenuation of acetylcholine but not histamine-induced relaxation of the aorta in diabetes mellitus. Gen Pharmacol 1993;24:329–332.
38. Tesfamariam B, Palacino JJ, Weisbrod RM, Cohen RA. Aldose reductase inhibition restores endothelial cell function in diabetic rabbit aorta. J Cardiovasc Pharmacol 1993;21:205–211.
39. Craven PA, Studer RK, DeRubertis FR. Impaired NO-dependent cyclic guanosine monophosphate generation in glomeruli from diabetic rats. Evidence for protein kinase C-mediated suppression of the cholinergic response. J Clin Invest 1994;93:311–320.
40. Bucala R, Tracey KJ, Cerami A. Advanced glycosylation products quench NO and mediate defective endothelium-dependent vasodilatation in experimental diabetes. J Clin Invest 1991;87:432–438.
41. Rosen P, Schror K. Increased PGI release from perfused hearts of acutely diabetic rats. Diabetologia 1980;18:391–394.
42. Tesfamariam B, Cohen RA. Role of superoxide anion and endothelium in vasoconstrictor action of PG endoperoxide. Am J Physiol 1992;262:H1915–H1919.
43. Weisbrod RM, Brown ML, Cohen RA. Elevated glucose alters endothelial cell NO and prostanoid circulation. Circ 1991;84(Suppl. II):II43.
44. Wolff SP, Dean RT. Glucose autooxidation and protein modification: the role of oxidative glycosylation in diabetes. Biochem J 1987;245:234–250.
45. Hattori Y, Kawasaki H, Abe K, Kanno M. Superoxide dismutase recovers altered endothelium-dependent relaxation in diabetic rat aorta. Am J Physiol 1991;261:H1086–H1094.
46. Mugge A, Elwell JH, Peterson TE, Harrison OG. Release of intact endothelium dependent derived relaxing factor depends on endothelial superoxide dismutase. Am J Physiol. 1991;260: C219–C225.
47. Omar HA, Cherry PD, Mortelliti MP, Burke-Wolin T, Wolin MS. Inhibition of coronary artery superoxide dismutase attenuates endothelium-dependent and -independent nitrovasodilator relaxation. Circ Res 1991;69:601–608.
48. Pieper GM, Gross GJ. Oxygen free radicals abolish endothelium-dependent relaxation in diabetic rat aorta. Am J Physiol 1988;255:H825–H833.
49. Brownlee MA, Cerami A, Vlassara H. Advanced glycosylation endproducts in tissue and the biochemical basis of diabetic complications. N Engl J Med 1988;318:1315–1321.
50. Corbett JA, Tilton RG, Chang K, Hasan KS, Ido Y, Wang JL, Sweetland MA, Lancaster JR, Williamson JR, McDaniel ML. Aminoguanidine, a novel inhibitor of NO formation, prevents diabetic vascular dysfunction. Diabetes 1992;41:552–556.
51. Cameron NE, Cotter MA. Impaired contraction and relaxation in aorta from streptozotocin-diabetic rats: role of polyol pathway. Diabetologia 1992;35:1011–1019.
52. Hodgson WC, King RG. Effects of glucose, insulin or aldose reductase inhibition on responses to endothelin-1 of aortic rings from streptozotocin-induced diabetic rats. Br J Pharmacol 1992;106:644–649.
53. Yamashita T, Umeda F, Hashimoto T, Inoguchi T, Yamauchi T, Mimura K, Watanabe J, Nawata H. Effect of glucose on Na, K-ATPase activity in cultured bovine aortic endothelial cells. Endocrinol Jpn 1992;39:1–7.
54. Kern TS, Engerman RL. Immunohistochemical distribution of aldose reductase. Histochem J 1982;14:507–515.
55. Gonzalez RG, Barnett P, Aguayo J, Cheng HM, Chylack LT. Direct measurement of polyol pathway activity in the ocular lens. Diabetes 1984;33:196–199.
56. Stevens MJ, Lattimer SA, Kamijo M, Van Huysen C, Sima AAF, Greene DA. Osmotically induced nerve taurine depletion and the compatible osmolyte hypothesis in experimental diabetic neuropathy. Diabetologia 1993;36:608–614.
57. Greene DA, Lattimer SA, Sima AAF. Sorbitol, phosphoinositides and sodium-potassium-ATPase in the pathogenesis of diabetic complications. N Engl J Med 1987;316:599–606.

58. Tilton RG, Chang K, Hasan KS, Smith SR, Petrash JM, Misko TP, Moore WM, Currie MG, Corbett JA, McDaniel ML, Williamson JR. Prevention of diabetic vascular dysfunction by guanidines: inhibition of NOS versus advanced glycation end-product formation. Diabetes 1993;42:221–232.
59. Greene DA, Sima AAF, Stevens MJ, Feldman EL, Killen PD, Henry DN, Thomas T, Dananberg J, Lattimer SA. Aldose reductase inhibitors: an approach to the treatment of diabetic nerve damage. Diab Metab Rev 1993;9:189–217.
60. Wolf BA, Williamson JR, Easom RA, Chang K, Sherman WR, Turk J. Diacylglycerol accumulation and microvascular abnormalities induced by elevated glucose levels. J Clin Invest 1991;87:31–38.
61. Craven PA, Davidson CM, DeRubertis FR. Increase in diacylglycerol mass in isolated glomeruli by glucose from de novo synthesis of glycerolipids. Diabetes 1990;39:667–674.
62. Pugliese G, Tilton RG, Williamson JR. Glucose-induced metabolic imbalances in the pathogenesis of diabetic vascular disease. Diab Metab Rev 1991;7:35–39.
63. Okumura K, Nishiura T, Awaji Y, Kondo J, Hashimoto H, Ito T. 1, 2 diacylglycerol content and its fatty acid composition in thoracic aorta of diabetic rats. Diabetes 1991;40:820–824.
64. Williams B, Schrier RW. Characterization of glucose-induced in situ protein kinase C activity in cultured vascular smooth cells. Diabetes 1992;41:464–472.
65. Pfeilschifter J, Bauer C. Role of phospholipase C and protein kinase C in vasoconstrictor-induced PG synthesis in cultured rat mesangial cells. Biochem J 1986;236:289–294.
66. Wu KK, Hatzakis H, Lo SS, Seong DC, Sanduja SK, Tai HH. Stimulation of de novo synthesis of PG G/H synthase in human endothelial cells by phorbol ester. J Biol Chem 1988;263:19,043–19,047.
67. Robinson JM, Badwey JA, Karnovsky ML, Karnovsky MJ. Superoxide release by neutrophils: synergistic effects of a phorbol ester and a calcium ionophore. Biochem Biophys Res Comm 1984;122:734–739.
68. Craven PA, DeRubertis FR. Protein kinase C is activated in glomeruli from streptozotocin diabetic rats. Possible mechanisms by glucose. J Clin Invest 1989;83:1667–1675.
69. Greene DA, Lattimer-Greene S, Sima AAF. Pathogenesis of diabetic neuropathy: role of altered phosphoinositide metabolism. Clin Rev Neurobiol 1989;5:143–219.
70. Thomas TP, Porcellati F, Kato K, Stevens MJ, Sherman WR, Greene DA. Effects of glucose on sorbitol pathway activation, cellular redox, and metabolism of myo-inositol, phosphoinositide, and diacylglycerol in cultured human retinal pigment epithelial cells. J Clin Invest 1994;93:2718–2724.
71. Shiba T, Inoguchi T, Sportsman JR, Heath WF, Bursell S, King GI. Correlation of diacylglycerol level and protein kinase C activation in rat retina to retinal circulation. Am J Physiol 1993;265:E783–E793.
72. Bredt DS, Ferris CD, Snyder SH. NOS regulatory sites. Phosphorylation by cyclic AMP-dependent protein kinase, protein kinase C, and calcium/calmodulin protein kinase; identification of flavin and calmodulin binding sites . J Biol Chem 1992;267:10,976–10,981.
73. Brune B, Lapetina EG. Phosphorylation of NOS by protein kinase A. Biochem Biophys Res Comm 1991;181:921–926.
74. Michel T, Li GK, Busconi L. Phosphorylation and subcellular translocation of endothelial NOS. Proc Natl Acad Sci, USA 1993;90:6252–6256.
75. Tsukahara H, Gordienko DV, Goligorsky MS. Continuous monitoring of NO release from human umbilical vein endothelial cells. Biochem Biophys Res Comm 1993;193:722–729.

12 Evidence Linking Fatty Acids, the Risk Factor Cluster, and Vascular Pathophysiology

Implications for the Diabetic Hypertensive Patient

Brent M. Egan, MD
and Konrad T. Stepniakowski, MD, PHD

CONTENTS

INTRODUCTION

This chapter focuses on nonesterified fatty acids (NEFAs), the risk factor cluster, and vascular pathophysiology. The discussion begins with an overview of the cluster and the possible pathogenetic link to the defect of insulin-mediated glucose disposal. Selected controversies in the insulin resistance–hypertension theory are addressed and another defect of insulin action, namely suppression of lipolysis and plasma NEFAs, is offered

From: *Contemporary Endocrinology: Endocrinology of the Vasculature*
Edited by: J. R. Sowers Humana Press Inc., Totowa, NJ

Table 1
Established and Putative Components of the Cardiovascular Risk Factor Cluster

Cardiovascular neurohumoral	*Dyslipidemia*	*Glucose metabolism*	*Neurohumoral*
Hypertension[a]	↑ VLDL/triglyceride[a]	Insulin resistance[a]	↑ renin[b]
Vascular remodeling[b]	↓ HDL cholesterol[a]	Hyperinsulinemia[a]	↑ aldosterone[b]
Cardiac hypertrophy[b]	Dense LDL (↑ Apo B)[b]	Elevated fatty acids[b]	↑ Sympatetic drive[b]
Diastolic dysfunction[b]		IGT and NIDDM[a,c]	↓ Parasymp[b]

[a]Well-established.
[b]Possible or probable.
[c]IGT, impaired glucose tolerance; NIDDM, noninsulin-dependent diabetes mellitus.

as an alternative explanation linking insulin resistance to hypertension. The emphasis moves to mechanisms by which NEFAs may modulate vascular function and structure with a focus on neurovascular tone and endothelium-dependent vasodilation. The chapter closes with thoughts on the implications of increased plasma NEFAs and their effects on neurovascular tone and endothelium-dependent vasodilation to the pathophysiology in the diabetic hypertensive.

RISK FACTOR CLUSTERING

Obesity, particularly abdominal obesity, is associated with noninsulin-dependent diabetes mellitus, hypertension, dyslipidemia, and other components of a syndrome known as the cardiovascular risk factor cluster (Table 1). Clustering of risk factors exceeds that expected by chance implying a common pathogenetic denominator underlying their association. Elucidation of common pathogenetic denominator(s) have centered principally on resistance to insulin-mediated glucose disposal.

ABDOMINAL OBESITY, DIABETES, AND HYPERTENSION

The Insulin-Resistance Hyperinsulinemia Connection

Abdominal obesity, diabetes, and hypertension are associated with resistance to insulin-mediated glucose disposal *(1)*. Hyperinsulinemia is also a characteristic feature of insulin resistance until frank hyperglycemia occurs in the diabetic subset *(2)*. These individuals also may be more resistant than normal controls to insulin's depressor actions including vasodilation *(3–6)*. Thus, hyperinsulinemia and insulin resistance associated with high-risk obesity may comprise the pathogenetic link between weight *(7)* and salt-sensitive *(8)* elevations of systemic blood pressure *(9)*.

Vascular Insulin Resistance: Potential Role in Blood Pressure and Glucose Homeostasis

Insulin is a vasodilator *(9–11)*, and insulin's vasodilator action may be inversely related to both insulin-mediated glucose disposal and blood pressure *(6)*. In fact, this attenuated vasodilator response may contribute to the defect in glucose disposal by impairing the delivery of glucose and insulin to skeletal muscle, the major site of glucose utilization *(12,13)*. Thus, resistance to insulin's vasodilator action could contribute both to increased vascular resistance *(14)* and impaired glucose metabolism *(15)*, which characterize human essential hypertension.

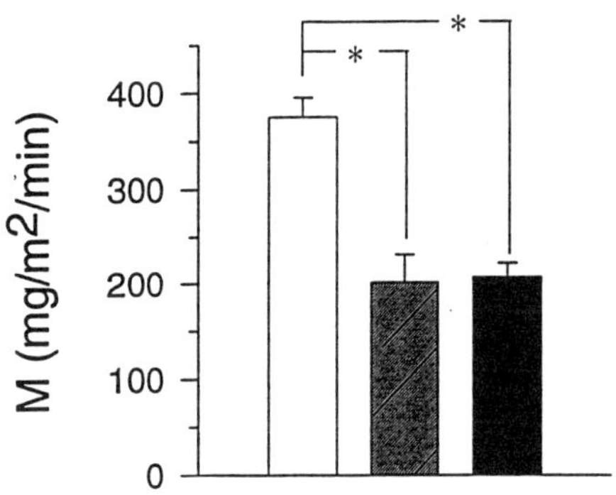

Fig. 1. Glucose disposal (M, mg/m^2/min) is shown during the final 30 min of a 2-h euglycemic clamp period with insulin infused at 40 mU/m^2/min for lean normotensives (□), obese normotensives (▨), and obese hypertensives (■). As depicted, glucose disposal was similarly reduced in both abdominally obese hypertensives and normotensives compared to lean normotensive subjects.

Hyperinsulinemia and Sympathetic Drive

Obese hypertensives have increased plasma norepinephrine concentrations that decline with weight loss *(16)*. Hyperinsulinemia may contribute to the greater sympathetic drive in obesity, since insulin's capacity to activate the sympathetic nervous system is retained in these individuals, despite their defective glucose disposal *(17)*. Insulin antagonizes vascular α-adrenoceptor responses *(18)*, and this action is impaired in patients with hypertension *(19)*. Consequently, in obese hypertensives, preservation of insulin's capacity to activate the sympathetic nervous system combined with a defect of insulin's capacity to antagonize vascular α-adrenergic tone could play an important role in the heightened neurovascular tone and impaired glucose utilization. The clinical relevance of vascular α-adrenergic tone to the glucose metabolism in obese hypertensives is strengthened by evidence that treating these patients with prazosin, an α_1-adrenoceptor agonist, markedly improved their defect of insulin-mediated glucose disposal *(20)*.

EVIDENCE AGAINST THE HYPERINSULINEMIA–INSULIN RESISTANCE–HYPERTENSION CONNECTION

Evidence is not uniformly corroborative of a clear link among hyperinsulinemia, resistance to insulin-mediated glucose disposal, and hypertension. For example, prolonged euglycemic hyperinsulinemia in dogs does not induce hypertension or exacerbate the salt sensitivity during angiotensin infusion *(21,22)*. Euglycemic hyperinsulinemia does not raise blood pressure in normotensive or hypertensive humans *(23,24)*. And, some epidemiologic studies are unable to link insulin to hypertension *(25)*. Age, body mass index, and body fat distribution, which are determinants of insulin action, may confound efforts to discern the pathogenetic relationship of hyperinsulinemia and insulin resistance to hypertension, since hypertensive patients tend to be older, heavier, and have a more centralized body fat distribution than normotensive controls *(1,26)*. To address these concerns, glucose disposal during euglycemic hyperinsulinemia has been assessed in abdominally obese hypertensives, abdominally obese normotensives, and in lean normotensives *(27)*. Glucose disposal is equally and markedly reduced in both abdominally obese groups compared to lean normotensive controls (Fig. 1). Thus, the presence of

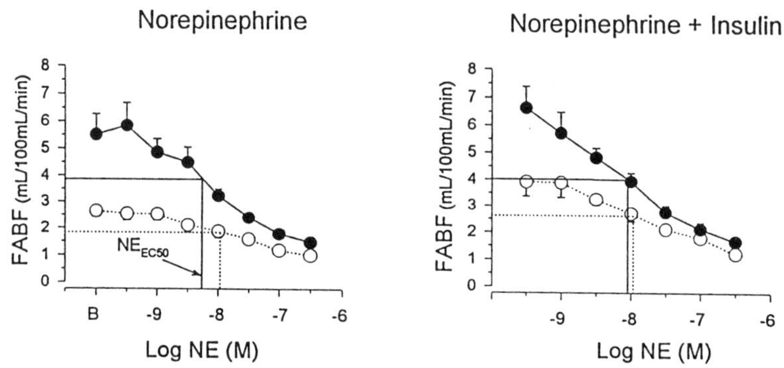

Fig. 2. The effects of a local (brachial artery) insulin infusion on forearm vascular resistance responses to regional norepinephrine are shown in both obese hypertensive patients (●) and lean normotensive controls (○). Raising local insulin concentrations from fasting values to ~100 μU/mL did not significantly change the EC_{50} for norepinephrine in either group.

hypertension does not appear to exacerbate the severe insulin resistance associated with abdominal obesity. Thus, marked resistance to insulin-mediated glucose disposal is not necessarily associated with hypertension, although the blood pressures of insulin-resistant normotensives might be even lower if it were not for their defects of insulin action.

Insulin and α-Adrenergic Vasoconstriction

The effects of insulin on vascular α-adrenergic reactivity have been variable with increases *(28–31)*, decreases *(10,18,19,32)*, and no changes *(32,33)*. Insulin did not antagonize forearm responses to α-adrenoceptor agonists in obese, insulin-resistant hypertensives, or lean normotensives (Fig. 2) *(33)*. Others report insulin does not antagonize regional vasoconstrictor responses to an α_1-adrenoceptor agonist *(32)*, even though reflex vasoconstrictor responses are reduced by insulin *(34)*. These data may be explained *(35)* by insulin-mediated enhancement of endothelium-dependent vasodilation *(36)*, which interferes with neurally mediated vasoconstriction but not vasoconstriction elicited by an exogenously administered α_1-adrenoceptor agonist *(32,33)*.

Insulin and Salt Sensitivity

Although some reports demonstrate that hyperinsulinemia and insulin resistance are associated with salt sensitivity of the blood pressure *(7,8)*, these findings have not been universally confirmed *(21,22,37,38)*. In obese humans, we have not observed differences in indices of hyperinsulinemia and insulin resistance between the salt-sensitive and salt-resistant subsets *(37)*. Those with higher plasma insulin concentrations are more likely to manifest a pressor response to salt restriction *(38)*. The pressor response to salt restriction in the insulin-resistant subset coincide with evidence for greater activation of the renin–angiotensin–aldosterone system with volume depletion *(39)*.

NEFAS AND RISK FACTOR CLUSTERING: AN ALTERNATIVE HYPOTHESIS

Abdominal obesity is associated with increased NEFA concentrations and turnover *(40)*. NEFAs may contribute to the risk factor cluster by reducing hepatic insulin uptake; increasing hepatic glucose output, apoprotein B, and very low density lipoprotein synthesis; and decreasing skeletal muscle glucose utilization *(40,41)*. An important role for fatty acids in the defective glucose homeostasis of diabetes was proposed by Randle and colleagues more than 30 yr ago *(41)* and confirmed by subsequent reports (i.e., *42*). Thus, an extensive literature implicates NEFAs in the metabolic defects of the risk factor cluster which include impaired glucose tolerance and noninsulin-dependent diabetes.

NEFAS AND BLOOD PRESSURE REGULATION

Evidence for NEFAs as a player in blood pressure homeostasis includes observations on the hemodynamic effects of increasing the molar ratio of NEFAs to albumin in minipigs *(43)*. Raising NEFAs systemically to ~2 m*M* increased resistance in most vascular beds and elevated blood pressure *(43)*, and NEFAs in the 1.5–2 m*M* range are seen after a high-fat meal in patients with familial combined hyperlipidemia *(44)*. High NEFAs in these patients probably play an important role in their dyslipidemia, hypertension, and excess risk for cardiovascular disease *(44,45)*. Thus, defective NEFA metabolism may contribute to both dyslipidemia and hypertension in patients with familial combined hyperlipidemia.

EVIDENCE OF A ROLE FOR NEFAS IN THE PATHOPHYSIOLOGY OF OBESITY HYPERTENSION

Abdominal obesity is more common among hypertensive patients than the general population. Abnormalities of fatty acid (FA) metabolism in abdominally obese subjects may serve as one common denominator underlying this to the cluster. For example, abdominal obesity is associated with greater FA turnover, which is more resistant to suppression by insulin and stimulation by exercise and epinephrine than in lean or lower body obese subjects *(40,46)*. Similarly, plasma FA concentrations in noninsulin-dependent diabetics are more resistant to suppression by insulin compared to nondiabetic controls. And, patients with hypertension have higher plasma NEFAs than normotensive subjects, although the differences are not always statistically significant *(15)*. Collectively, these findings raise the possibility that defective NEFA metabolism in abdominally obese subjects may underlie the risk factors of hypertension, diabetes, and dyslipidemia. NEFAs may contribute by direct and indirect mechanisms to increased neurovascular tone in high-risk obesity (Fig. 3) *(10,17)*.

Evidence that Neurovascular Tone is Elevated in High-Risk Obesity

Plasma norepinephrine, an index of sympathetic drive, is elevated in obese hypertensives and declines with blood pressure during weight loss *(16)*. Similarly, obesity-induced hypertension in dogs appears to have a strong neurogenic component *(50,51)*. Our previous studies were conducted on overweight younger men, since this group is disproportionately affected by the cardiovascular risk factor cluster *(52)*. Consequently, studies on this high-risk group may be helpful in unraveling pathophysiological mechanisms underlying the cluster. As shown in Fig. 4, an overweight group of comparatively young men with mild hypertension had greater α-adrenergic tone, assessed by the forearm vasodilator response to a regional phentolamine infusion, than overweight normotensive men of similar age. The data also suggest that the heightened α-adrenergic tone plays an important role in their elevated vascular resistance, since regional vascular resistances in the overweight hypertensives and overweight normotensives were nearly identical after blocking endogenous α-adrenergic tone *(53)*.

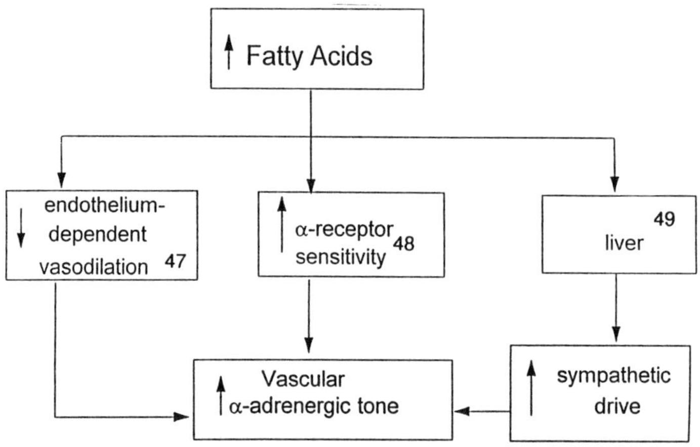

Fig. 3. Potential mechanisms by which FA may augment vascular α-adrenergic tone are provided. As indicated, FA may increase neurovascular tone by inhibiting endothelium-dependent vasodilation, enhancing α_1-adrenoceptor sensitivity, and raising sympathetic drive.

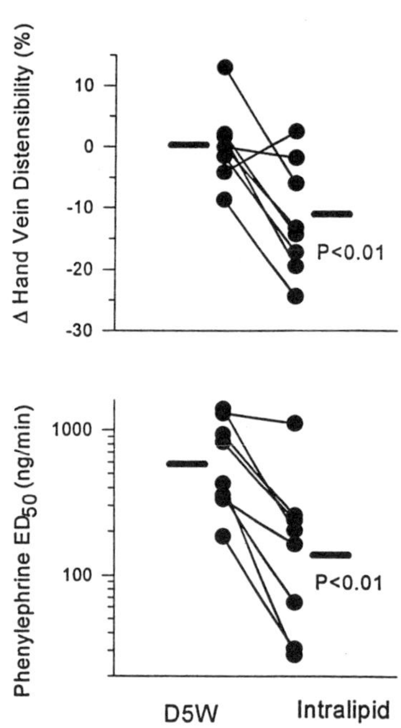

Fig. 4. Effects of raising FA locally with an infusion of intralipid/heparin as compared to a control infusion of D5W/heparin on dorsal hand vein responses are provided. Raising FA locally decreased baseline hand vein distensibility and reduced the phenylephrine dose required to cause 50% of the maximally obtained response (ED_{50}).

NEFA Concentrations and Turnover in Obese Hypertensive Patients

We have observed that fasting plasma NEFAs are greater in nine obese hypertensives than in lean normotensives, and the NEFA present in highest concentrations are oleic followed by palmitic then linoleic acids (Table 2). Plasma NEFAs are also more resistant

Table 2
Fasting Plasma NEFAs in Lean Normotensives and Obese Hypertensives

	NEFA, μM	
Nonesterified FA	*Lean normotensive* (8)	*Obese hypertensive* (9)
Palmitic (16:0)	79 ± 15	135 ± 6[a]
Stearic (18:0)	30 ± 5	47 ± 3[a]
Oleic (18:1[cis])	113 ± 20	195 ± 15[a]
Linoleic (18:2[cis])	57 ± 10	80 ± 8
Total	313 ± 54	626 ± 40[a]

[a] $p < 0.05$.

to insulin suppression in persons with lower high-density lipoproteins (HDL)-cholesterol values, and evidence for risk factor clustering *(39)*. NEFA concentration and turnover are higher during euglycemic hyperinsulinemia in obese hypertensives than in obese normotensives *(54)*. The FA turnover during euglycemic hyperinsulinemia is strongly and directly related to blood pressure across these three groups. Moreover, correlations of FA concentrations and turnover to blood pressure are independent of insulin and insulin-mediated glucose disposal which indirectly supports a pathogenetic role for NEFAs in obesity hypertension.

EFFECTS OF FA ON NEUROVASCULAR TONE

FA may augment vascular α-adrenergic tone by various pathways (Fig. 3), which include increasing sympathetic drive *(49)* and α-adrenoceptor responsiveness *(48)*, as well as indirect effects such as impaired endothelium-dependent vasodilation *(47)*, and structural vascular remodeling *(53)*.

NEFAs and Sympathetic Drive

The adipose depot most consistently and strongly related to blood pressure is abdominal visceral fat *(55)*. Turnover of fat (i.e., lipolysis and reesterification) appears to be especially high in those with high-risk abdominal obesity *(40)*. In rats, infusing oleic acid, the most abundant plasma FA (Table 2), into the portal vein elicits a neurogenic reflex and raises blood pressure *(49)*. This pressor effect of portal vein oleate is sustained and can be prevented by prazosin, a selective α_1-adrenoceptor antagonist. These data support the notion that visceral obesity elicits a rise in blood pressure by increasing the delivery of FA, especially oleic acid, to the liver thus enhancing α_1-adrenergic tone *(49)*. Two weeks on a high-fat diet in normal volunteers raise heart rate and ambulatory blood pressure *(56)*. Pyrazinoylguanidine, a novel compound which inhibits hormone-sensitive lipase and lower NEFAs, reduces blood pressure and other components of the cluster in patients with diabetes, renal disease, and hypertension *(57,58)*. These provocative data serve as a basis for further research to better elucidate the relationship of FA metabolism to short- and long-term blood pressure regulation in humans.

NEFAS AND VASCULAR α-ADRENOCEPTOR RESPONSES

Overweight hypertensives have increased vascular α-adrenergic tone *(17)* and higher plasma NEFA concentrations and turnover rates that are resistant to suppression by insulin *(53)*. Studies have been conducted to determine if FA enhance vascular tone and α-adrenergic reactivity *(43,48)*. Raising local FA concentrations within the physiological range reduced basal hand vein distensibility and the dose of phenylephrine required to induce 50% of the maximum venoconstrictor response (Fig. 4). These results indicate that NEFAs, and quite likely, linoleic and oleic acids, the main NEFAs infused, can increase vascular tone and α-adrenergic reactivity in vivo *(48,59)*. Furthermore, these FA effects appear to be mediated by local and direct vascular action(s) *(60)*. Raising dorsal hand vein NEFAs enhances α_1-adrenoceptor sensitivity to phenylephrine but may not reflect effects on more physiologically relevant responses to endogenously released norepinephrine, a nonselective α-adrenoceptor agonist. However, evidence has been obtained that raising NEFAs locally increases the magnitude and duration of the venoconstrictor response to thigh cuff inflation *(60)*. These data suggest that NEFAs augment reflex neurovascular responses and strengthen the probability that fatty acid abnormalities augment endogenous neurovascular tone.

NEFAS AND ENDOTHELIUM-DEPENDENT VASODILATION

Effects on Endothelial Cells

Phorbol esters, which activate protein kinase C (PKC), inhibit endothelium-dependent vasodilation in vitro *(61)* and nitric oxide synthase (NOS) activity in cultured endothelial cells *(62)*. Endothelial dysfunction, in turn, enhances vascular α-adrenergic reactivity. Thus, the notion that cis-unsaturated NEFAs, such as oleic and linoleic acids, which activate PKC, might reduce nitric oxide (NO) production by the endothelium was examined. Oleic and linoleic acids, within the physiological range of 10–100 μ*M*, induce a concentration-dependent inhibition of NOS activity in cultured endothelial cells. Inhibition of NO production is observed under basal conditions and during adenosine triphosphate and ionomycin stimulation. Unlike oleic and linoleic acids, neither stearic nor elaidic acids, at 100 μ*M* concentrations, have effects on ionomycin-stimulated NO generation (Fig. 5) *(47)*. Our findings with linoleic acid are consistent with an earlier report that this NEFA impairs endothelium-dependent vasodilation by a PKC-independent mechanism—namely by effects on Ca^{2+}-activated K^+ channels.

Effects of Oleic Acid on Endothelium-Dependent Vasodilation In Vitro

Aortic and femoral artery ring studies were performed to determine if the inhibitory effects of oleic acid observed in cell culture extended to endothelium-dependent responses in vascular tissue. Oleic acid, 100 μ*M*, inhibits the relaxation to acetylcholine by ~50% in rabbit femoral artery rings preconstricted with phenylephrine (Fig. 6) *(47)*. These data suggest that oleic acid inhibits endothelium-dependent vasodilation by reducing the generation of NO and not by inhibiting guanylate cyclase or the cellular effects of cyclic guanosine monophosphate.

Fig. 5. *(opposite page)* The effects of four different 18-carbon FA on NOS activity (conversion of arginine to citrulline) are compared to control (vehicle-treated) cells. Both oleic and linoleic acids, at concentrations of 100 μ*M*, impaired NO generation, whereas identical concentrations of stearic and elaidic acids did not. □, Lonomycin (2 μ*M*); ■, lonomycin + 18-carbon FA.

Fig. 6. *(opposite page)* Oleic acid reduces the relaxation response to the endothelium-independent vasodilator acetylcholine in rabbit femoral artery rings preconstricted with phenylephrine. Equivalent (100 μ*M*) concentrations of oleic acid had no effect on the endothelium-independent responses to nitroprusside.

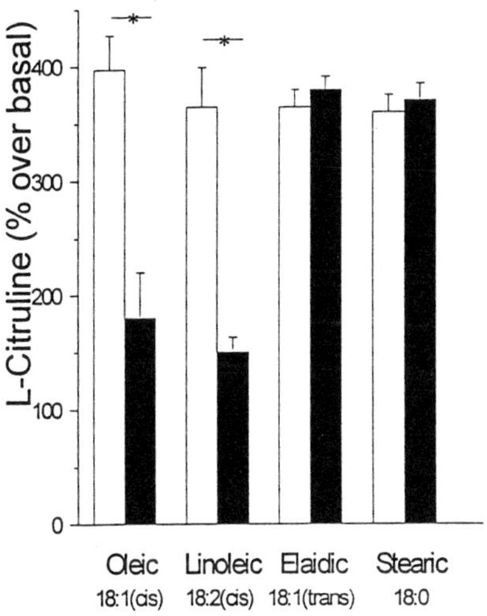
L-Citruline (% over basal)
400
300
200
100
0
*
*
Oleic 18:1(cis)
Linoleic 18:2(cis)
Elaidic 18:1(trans)
Stearic 18:0

Fig. 5.

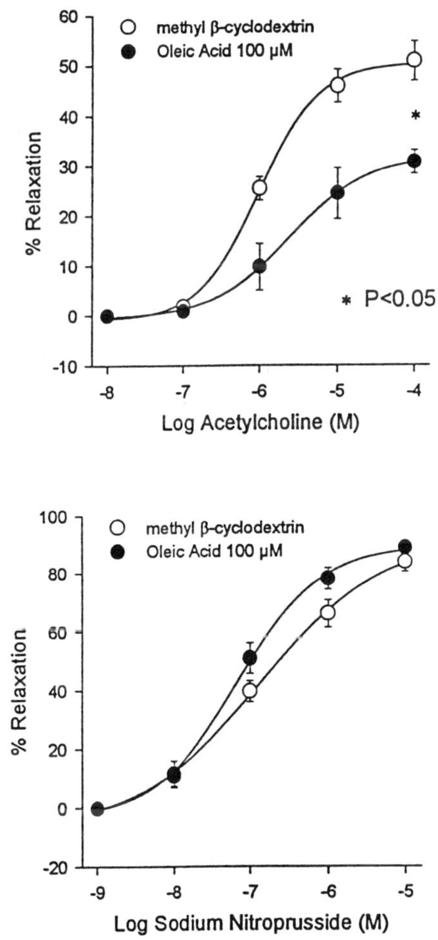
methyl β-cyclodextrin
Oleic Acid 100 μM
% Relaxation
60
50
40
30
20
10
0
-10
*
* P<0.05
-8
-7
-6
-5
-4
Log Acetylcholine (M)
methyl β-cyclodextrin
Oleic Acid 100 μM
% Relaxation
100
80
60
40
20
0
-20
-9
-8
-7
-6
-5
Log Sodium Nitroprusside (M)

Fig. 6.

NEFAS AND VASCULAR STRUCTURE

Several vasoconstrictors which activate PKC also function as mitogens in vascular smooth muscle cells (VSMC). Since FA, especially cis-unsaturated NEFAs activate PKC *(63)*, it was intriguing that linoleic acid increases expression of several proto-oncogenes and enhanced thymidine uptake in rat VSMC *(64)*. And, the mitogenic effect of linoleic acid are linked to stimulation of mitogen-activated protein kinase *(64,65)*. We have preliminary evidence indicating that the mitogenic effect of oleic acid on human aortic smooth muscle cells is mediated by activation of PKC *(66)*. Changes in vascular structure may predispose to vascular complications of hypertension and serve to nonspecifically alter vascular reactivity and support the elevated blood pressure *(53)*. Indeed, FA may contribute to VSMC proliferation and lesion formation in atherosclerotic plaques.

POSSIBLE SIGNAL TRANSDUCTION MECHANISMS BY WHICH NEFAS MEDIATE THEIR ACTIONS ON VSMC AND ENDOTHELIAL CELLS

Activation of PKC is a potentially important mechanism by which FA may contribute to vascular disease. FA, especially cis-unsaturated NEFAs such as oleic, linoleic, linolenic, and arachidonic acids, activate PKC *(63,67)*. Putative mechanisms involved in the NEFA PKC signaling pathway are depicted in Fig. 7. Movement of NEFAs from the extracellular fluid to the cytosol is facilitated by high-capacity, low-affinity ($K_d \sim 1\ \mu M$) FA binding proteins in the cell membrane *(68)*. The estimated intracellular concentration of NEFAs is ~3–5 μM. This is in the same range as the EC_{50} of 5 μM for activation of the Ca^{2+}-independent isoforms of PKC by cis-unsaturated NEFAs *(68)*. The EC_{50} for these FA to activate Ca^{2+}-dependent isoforms of PKC is much higher at 50 μM *(69)*. Moreover, FA fully activate Ca^{2+}-independent isoforms of PKC but only partially activate (~50%) Ca^{2+}-dependent PKC isoforms *(69)*. NEFAs activate PKC by binding to the regulatory domain at a site distinct from that for diacylglycerol *(67,70)*. These observations suggest that intersubject differences of intracellular FA may contribute to differences in PKC activity, and the associated vascular disease risk.

Evidence Suggesting a Role for PKC in Cardiovascular Risk Factor Clustering

Activation of PKC may induce insulin resistance, alter lipid metabolism *(71)*, decrease integrity of the endothelial barrier *(72,73)*, and impair endothelium-dependent dilation which could reduce glucose disposal and accelerate atherogenesis *(74)* and increase neurovascular tone *(75–77)*. Activation of PKC can stimulate VSMC growth while inhibiting endothelial cell growth and microvessel formation *(78)*. These events may contribute to vascular remodeling *(54)*; augment vascular reactivity; and exacerbate the defects in delivery of oxygen *(79)*, glucose, and insulin *(12,80)* to their metabolic targets.

Diabetic individuals often have abnormalities in FA metabolism as well as elevations in blood sugar. Hyperglycemia enhances the production of diacylglycerol, a major regulator of PKC. The implications of PKC activation by glucose in the diabetic patient were recently the subject of a comprehensive review *(81)*. Theoretically, the combined effects of defective FA and glucose homeostasis may produce an even greater activation of PKC and worsening of cardiovascular risk and injury than either defect alone.

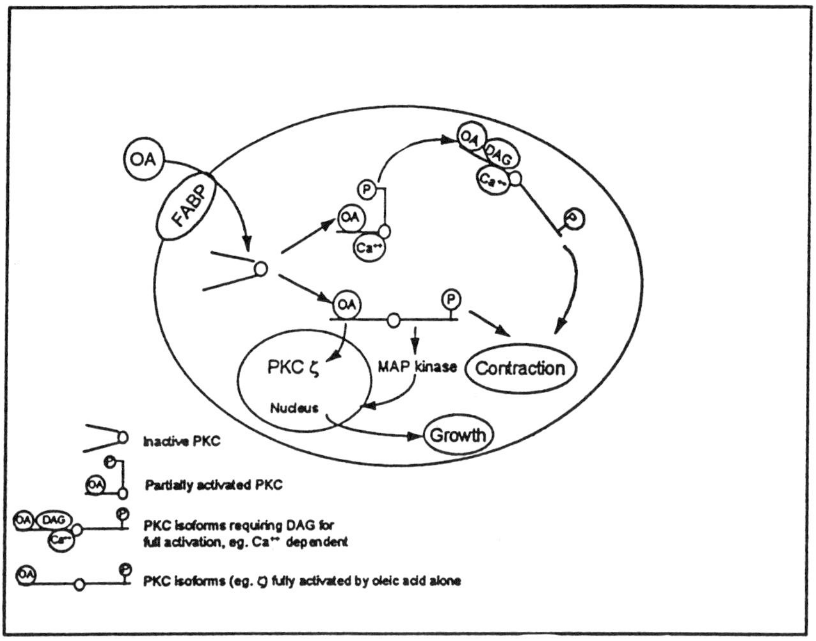

Fig. 7. FA and PKC in VSMC. FA may mediate some significant effects by activating both the Ca^{2+}-dependent isoforms of PKC in concert with diacylglycerol and the Ca^{2+}-independent isoforms of PKC which may have a diacylglycerol binding site. The cellular effects of activating PKC with FA could enhance both VSMC tone and growth.

NEFAs have other actions which could also affect cellular events important in blood pressure regulation. These actions include alterations of membrane fluidity and the activity of several cation transporters including Na^+/K^+ ATPase, Na^+ and K^+ channels, and Ca^{2+} currents *(82,83)*. FA can also influence signal transduction pathways important in regulating vascular tone and growth through effects on the composition of membrane phospholipids *(83)*. In fact, diabetic and hypertensive patients have abnormalities in membrane FA content that appear pathogenetically linked to disturbances in glucose and blood pressure homeostasis *(84,85)*. Some of these changes in membrane lipids very likely affect products of the cycloxygenase, lipoxygenase, and epoxygenase (P450) pathways which are important modulators of cardiovascular and renal function *(86,87)*.

VASCULAR EFFECTS OF NEFAS: IMPLICATIONS FOR THE DIABETIC HYPERTENSIVE PATIENT

Glucose and blood pressure homeostasis are complex processes reflecting the integration of multiple physiologic controllers. Control of glucose and blood pressure appear more closely intertwined as our understanding on the links between metabolism and blood flow grows. As noted, FA may enhance vascular α-adrenergic tone and impair endothelium-dependent vasodilation. In turn, vascular α-adrenergic tone and endothelium-dependent vasodilation may affect not only blood pressure regulation by altering pressure natriuresis *(88)* and peripheral vascular resistance *(53)*, but also play an important part in determining the sensitivity to insulin-mediated glucose disposal. Indeed, increased neurovascular tone and impaired endothelium-dependent vasodilation contribute to hyper-

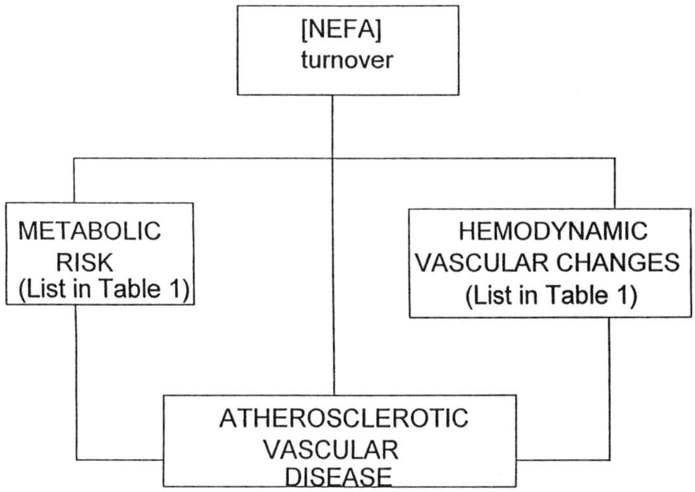

Fig. 8. A hypothetical relationship is shown among FA, metabolic (lipids, lipoproteins, glucose), and hemodynamic risk factors (endothelium-dependent dilation, vascular α-adrenergic tone, blood pressure), and cardiovascular disease. As depicted, FA may be a common pathogenetic denominator that contributes both to the more readily recognized metabolic and hemodynamic risk factors as well as to vascular disease.

tension, resistance to insulin-mediated glucose disposal, vascular remodeling, and atherosclerosis *(6,12,74)*. Thus, abnormalities of FA in patients with noninsulin-dependent diabetes mellitus may contribute to the constellation of adverse metabolic, hemodynamic, and vascular changes *(47)*. In patients with noninsulin-dependent diabetes, the resistance to insulin action combined with the relative insulin deficiency would be expected to further exacerbate the defect in NEFA metabolism and associated vascular disease.

From a therapeutic perspective, interventions that decrease the defects in FA turnover, such as pyrazinoylguanidine *(57)*, and oxidation, such as metformin *(89)*, may work closer to the primary cause of the cluster and may be more effective in reducing cardiovascular disease in diabetic patients than a multimodal regimen directed at each clinical manifestation of the cluster. One mechanism by which intensive insulin therapy decreases cardiovascular complications, in addition to tighter glucose control, may be the lowering of FA concentrations and turnover and thus minimizing the adverse cardiovascular effects of these lipids on a number of other more visible risk factors (Fig. 8).

This chapter summarizes evidence suggesting that FA may be one common pathogenetic denominator underlying the risk factor cluster and the excess of vascular disease in affected individuals (Fig. 8). Correction of the defective NEFA metabolism may serve to more efficiently and effectively manage the risk factor cluster and reduce cardiovascular complications than conventional approaches directed at multiple facets of the cluster.

REFERENCES

1. Stern M, Haffner S. Body fat distribution and hyperinsulinemia as risk factors for diabetes and cardiovascular disease. Arteriosclerosis 1986;6:123–129.
2. Reaven GM, Hollenbeck CD, Y-DI Chen. Relationship between glucose tolerance, insulin secretion, and insulin action in non-obese individuals with varying degrees of glucose tolerance. Diabetologia 1989;32:52–55.

3. Sowers JR. Relationship between hypertension and subtle and overt abnormalities of carbohydrate metabolism. J Am Soc Nephrol 1990;1:S39–S47.
4. Sowers JR, Sowers PS, Peuler JD. Role of insulin resistance and hyperinsulinemia in development of hypertension and atherosclerosis. J Lab Clin Med 1994;123:647–652.
5. Sowers JR, Epstein M. Diabetes mellitus and hypertension: an update. Hypertension 1995;26(Part 1): 869–879.
6. Baron AD, Brechtel-Hook G, Johnson A, Hardin D. Skeletal muscle blood flow: a possible link between insulin resistance and blood pressure. Hypertension 1993;21:129–135.
7. Rocchini AP, Key J, Bondie D, Chico R, Morehead C, Ketch V, Mertiu M. The effect of weight loss on the sensitivity of blood pressure to sodium in obese adolescents. N Engl J Med 1989;321:580–585.
8. Sharma AM, Ruland K, Spies K-P, Distler A. Salt sensitivity in young normotensive subjects is associated with a hyperinsulinemic response to oral glucose. J Hypertens 1991;9:329–335.
9. Sowers JR, Standley PR, Ram JL, Jacober S. Hyperinsulinemia, insulin resistance, and hyperglycemia: contributing factors in the pathogenesis of hypertension and atherosclerosis. Am J Hypertens 1993;6:260S–270S.
10. Alexander WD, Oake RJ. The effect of insulin on vascular reactivity to norepinephrine. Diabetes 1977;26:611–614.
11. Andres R, Baltzan MA, Cader G, Kierler KL. Effect of insulin on carbohydrate metabolism and on potassium in the forearm of man. J Clin Invest 1962;41:108–115.
12. Laakso M, Edelman SV, Brechtel G, Baron AD. Decreased effect of insulin to stimulate skeletal muscle blood flow in obese man: a novel mechanism of insulin resistance. J Clin Invest 1990;85:1844–1852.
13. Hall JE, Summers FL, Brands MW, Keen H, Alonso-Galicia M. Resistance to metabolic actions of insulin and its role in hypertension. Am J Hypertens 1994;7:772–788.
14. Fries ED. Hemodynamics of hypertension. Physiol Rev 1960;40:27–54.
15. Ferrannini E, Buzzigoli G, Bonadonna R, Giorico MA, Oleggini M, Gradziadei L, Pedrinelli R, Brandi L, Bevilacqua S. Insulin resistance and hypertension. N Engl J Med 1987;317:350–357.
16. Sowers JR, Nyby M, Stern N, Beck F, Baron S, Catania R, Vlachis N. Blood pressure and hormone changes associated with weight reduction in the obese. Hypertension 1982;4:686–691.
17. O'Hare JA, Minaker KL, Rowe JW, Pallotta JA, Young JB. Effect of insulin on plasma norepinephrine and 3,4-dihydroxyphenylalanine in obese men. Metabolism 1989;38:322–329.
18. Zemel MB, Reddy S, Sowers JR. Insulin attenuation of vasoconstrictor responses to phenylephrine in Zuker lean and obese rats. Am J Hypertens 1991;4:537–539.
19. Feldman RD, Bierbrier GS. Insulin-mediated vasodilation: impairment with increased blood pressure and body mass. Lancet 1993;342:707–709.
20. Pollare T, Lithell H, Selinus I, Berne C. Application of prazosin is associated with an increase of insulin sensitivity in obese patients with hypertension. Diabetologia 1988;31:415–420.
21. Hall JE, Brands MW, Hildebrandt DA, Mizelle HL. Obesity-associated hypertension: hyperinsulinemia and renal mechanisms. Hypertension 1992;19(Suppl. I):I45–I55.
22. Hall JE, Coleman TG, Mizelle HL, Smith MJ. Chronic hyperinsulinemia and blood pressure regulation. Am J Physiol 1990;258:F722–F731.
23. Anderson EA, Hoffman RP, Balon TW, Sinkey CA, Mark AL. Hyperinsulinemia produces both sympathetic neural activation and vasodilation in normal humans. J Clin Invest 1991;87:2246–2252.
24. Anderson EA, Balon TW, Hoffman RP, Sinkey CA, Mark AL. Insulin increases sympathetic activity but not blood pressure in borderline hypertensive humans. Hypertension 1992;19:621–627.
25. Muller DC, Elahi D, Pratley RE, Tobin JD, Andres R. An epidemiological test of the hyperinsulinemia-hypertension hypothesis. J Clin Endocrinol Metab 1991;76:544–548.
26. Gillum RF. The association of body fat distribution with hypertension, hypertensive heart disease, coronary heart disease, diabetes and cardiovascular risk factors in men and women aged 18–79 years. J Chron Dis 1987;40:421–428.
27. O'Shaughnessy IM, Myers TJ, Stepniakowski K, Nazzaro P, Kelly TM, Hoffmann RG, Egan BM, Kissebah AH. Glucose metabolism in abdominally obese hypertensive and normotensive subjects. Hypertension 1995;26:186–192.
28. Gans ROB, Bilo JJG, Maarschalkerweerd WWA, Heini RJ, Nauta JJP, Donker AJM. Exogenous insulin augments in healthy volunteers the cardiovascular reactivity to noradrenaline but not to angiotensin II. J Clin Invest 1991;88:512–518.
29. Townsend RR, Yamamoto R, Nickols M, DiPette DJ, Nickols GA. Insulin enhances pressor responses to norepinephrine in rat mesenteric vasculature. Hypertension 1992;19(Suppl. II):II105–II110.

30. Henrion D. Insulin potentiates norepinephrine-induced vascular tone by activation of PKC and tyrosine kinase. Can J Physiol Pharmacol 1993;72:849–854.
31. Peuler JD, Johnson BAB, Phare SM, Sowers JR. Sex-specific effects of an insulin secretagogue in stroke-prone hypertensive rats. Hypertension 1993;22:214–220.
32. Lembo G, Rendina V, Iaccarino G, Lamenza F, Volpe M, Trimarco B. Local hyperinsulinemia selectively attenuates α_2-adrenoceptor mediated forearm vasoconstriction in healthy humans. Hypertension 1993;22:451A.
33. Neahring JM, Stepniakowski K, Greene AS, Egan BM. Insulin does not reduce forearm α-vasoreactivity in obese hypertensive or lean normotensive men. Hypertension 1993;22:584–590.
34. Lembo G, Rendina V, Iaccarino G, Lamenza F, Volpe M, Trimarco B. Insulin reduces reflex forearm sympathetic vasoconstriction in healthy humans. Hypertension 1993;21:1015–1019.
35. Egan BM, Stepniakowski KT. Vascular alpha-adrenergic tone in obesity and salt-sensitive hypertension. In: Laragh JH, Brenner BM, eds. Hypertension: Pathophysiology, Diagnosis and Management, 2nd ed. Raven, New York, 1995, pp. 160:2693–2702.
36. Steinberg HO, Brechtel G, Johnson A, Fineberg N, Baron AD. Insulin-mediated skeletal muscle vasodilation is NO dependent: a novel action of insulin to increase NO release. J Clin Invest 1994;94: 1172–1179.
37. Egan BM, Stepniakowski K, Nazzaro P. Insulin levels are similar in obese salt-sensitive and salt-resistant hypertensive subjects. Hypertension 1994;23(Suppl. I):I1–I7.
38. Egan BM, Stepniakowski K, Goodfriend TL. Renin and aldosterone are higher and the hyperinsulinemic effect of salt restriction greater in subjects with risk factor clustering. Am J Hypertens 1994;7:886–893.
39. Goodfriend TL, Egan B, Stepniakowski K, Ball DL. Relationships among plasma aldosterone, high-density lipcprotein cholesterol, and insulin in humans. Hypertension 1995;25:30–36.
40. Jensen MD, Roust LR. Postprandial free fatty acid kinetics are abnormal in upper body obesity. Diabetes 1993;42:1567–1573.
41. Randle PJ, Garland PB, Hales CN, Newsholme EA. The glucose fatty-acid cycle: Its role in insulin sensitivity and the metabolic disturbances of diabetes mellitus. Lancet 1963;1:785–789.
42. Fanelli C, Calderone S, Epifano L, De Vincenzo A, Modarelli F, Pampanelli S, Perriello G, De Feo P, Brunetti P, Gerich JE, Bolli GB. Demonstration of a critical role for free fatty acids in mediating counter regulatory stimulation of gluconeogenesis and suppression of glucose utilization in humans. J Clin Invest 1993;92:1617–1622.
43. Bülow J, Madsen J, Hojgaard L. Reversibility of the effects on local circulation of high lipid concentrations in blood. Scand J Clin Lab Invest 1990;50:291–296.
44. Cabezas MC, deBruin TWA, deValk HW, Shoulders CC, Jansen H, Erkelens DW. Impaired fatty acid metabolism in familial combined hyperlipidemia. J Clin Invest 1993;92:160–168.
45. Lewis GF, Uffelman KD, Szeto LW, Weller B, Steiner G. Interaction between free fatty acids and insulin in the acute control of very low density lipoprotein production in humans. J Clin Invest 1994;95:158–166.
46. Kanaley JA, Cryer PE, Jensen MD. Fatty acid kinetic responses to exercise: effects of obesity, body fat distribution, and energy-restricted diet. J Clin Invest 1993;92:255–261.
47. Davda RK, Stepniakowski KT, Lu G, Ullian ME, Goodfriend TL, Egan BM. Oleic acid inhibits endothelial cell NOS by a PKC-independent mechanism. Hypertension 1995;764–770.
48. Stepniakowski KT, Goodfriend TL, Egan BM. Fatty acids enhance vascular α-adrenergic sensitivity. Hypertension 1995;25(Part 2):774–778.
49. Grekin RJ, Vollmer AP, Sider RS. Pressor effects of portal venous oleate infusion: a proposed mechanism for obesity hypertension. Hypertension 1995;26:193–198.
50. Rocchini AP, Moorehead CP, DeRemer S, Blondi D. Pathogenesis of weight related changes of blood pressure in dogs. Hypertension 1989;13:922–928.
51. Dominguez LJ, Davidoff AJ Srinivas PR, Standley PR, Walsh MF, Sowers JR. Effects of metformin on tyrosine kinase activity, glucose transport, and intracellular calcium in vascular smooth muscle. Endocrinology 1996;137(1):113–121.
52. Egan BM, Bassett DR, Block WD. Comparative effects of overweight on cardiovascular risk in younger vs older men. Am J Cardiol 1991;67:248–252.
53. Egan BM, Schork N, Panis R, Hinderliter A. Vascular structure enhances regional resistance responses in mild hypertension. J Hypertens 1988;6:41–48.
54. Egan BM, Hennes MMI, O'Shaughnessy IM, Stepniakowski KT, Kissebah AH, Goodfriend TL. Obesity hypertension is more closely related to impairment of insulin's fatty acid than glucose lowering action. Hypertension 1996;27(Part 2):723–728.

55. Kanai H, Matsuzawa U, Kotani K, Keno Y, Kobatake T, Nagai R, Fujioka S, Todunaga K, Tarui S. Close correlation of intra-abdominal fat accumulation to hypertension in obese women. Hypertension 1990;16:484–490.
56. Straznicky NE, Louis WJ, McGrade P, Howes LG. The effect of dietary lipid modification on blood pressure, cardiovascular reactivity and sympathetic activity in man. J Hypertens 1993;11: 427–437.
57. Vesell ES, Chambers CE, Passananti T, Demers LM, Beyer KH. Effects of pyrazinoylguanidine on the glucose-fatty cycle in normal subjects and patients with non-insulin dependent diabetes mellitus. J Clin Pharmacol 1993;33:823–831.
58. Chambers CE, Vesell ES, Helm C, Passananti GT, Beyer KH. Pyrazinoylguanidine: antihypertensive, hypocholesterolemic, and renin effects. J Clin Pharmacol 1992;32:1128–1134.
59. Stspniakowski KT, Egan BM. Additive effects of hypertension and obesity to limit venous distensibility: hemodynamic correlates and metabolic mechanisms. Am J Physiol 1995;268:R562–R568.
60. Stepniakowski KT, Sallee FR, Goodfriend TL, Egan BM. Fatty acids enhance neurovascular reflex responses by effects on α_1-adrenoceptors. Am J Physiol 1996; accepted for publication.
61. Morrison KJ, Pollock D. Impairment of relaxation to acetylcholine and NO by a phorbol ester in rat isolated aorta. Br J Pharmacol 1990;101:432–436.
62. Davda RK, Chandlet LJ, Guzman NJ. PKC modulates receptor-independent activation of endothelial NOS. Eur J Pharmacol 1994;266:237–244.
63. Murakami K, Chan SY, Routtenberg A. PKC activation by cis-fatty acid in the absence of Ca^{2+} and phospholipids. J Biol Chem 1986;261:15,424–15,429.
64. Rao GN, Alexander RW, Runge MS. Linoleic acid and its metabolites, hydroperoxyoctadeadienoic acids, stimulate c-fos, c-jun, and c-myc mRNA expression, mitogen-activated protein kinase activation, and growth in rat aortic smooth muscle cells. J Clin Inves 1994;96:842–847.
65. Khalil RA, Morgan KG. PKC-mediated redistribution of mitogen-activated protein kinase during smooth muscle cell activation. Am J Physiol 1993;265:C406–C411.
66. Lu G, Morinelli TA, Meir KE, Rosenzweig SA, Egan BM. Oleic acid-induced mitogenic signalling in human aortic smooth muscle cells: role for PKC. J Inves Med 1995;43:208 (abstract).
67. Nakanishi H, Exton JH. Purification and characterization of the ζ isoform of PKC from bovine kidney. J Biol Chem 1992;267:1347–1354.
68. Glatz JFC. Involvement of fatty acid translocase and fatty-acid binding protein in signal transduction. Fatty Acids and Cell Signalling: Second International Round Table, Madison WI, June 1994.
69. Khan WA, Blobe G, Halpern A, Taylor W, Wetsel WC, Burns D, Loomis C, Hannun YA. Selective regulation of PKC isoenzymes by oleic acid in human platelets. J Biol Chem 1993;268:5063–5068.
70. Hug H, Sarre TF. PKC isoenzymes: divergence in signal transduction? Review article. Biochem J 1993;291:329–343.
71. Heydrick SJ, Ruderman NB, Kurowski TG, Adams HB, Chen KS. Enhanced stimulation of diacylglycerol and lipid synthesis by insulin in denervated muscle: altered PKC activity and possible link to insulin resistance. Diabetes 1991;40:1707–1711.
72. Oliver JA. Adenylate cyclase and PKC mediate opposite actions on endothelial junctions. J Cell Physiol 1990;145:536–542.
73. Lynch JJ, Ferro TJ, Blumenstock FA, Brockenauer AM, Malik AB. Increased endothelial albumin permeability mediated by PKC activation. J Clin Invest 1990;85:1991–1998.
74. Osterud B, Hansen JB. Fatty acids, platelets, and monocytes: something to do with atherogenesis. Ann Med 1989;21:47–51.
75. Osol G, Laher I, Cipolla M. PKC modulates basal myogenic tone in resistance arteries from the cerebral circulation. Circ Res 1991;68:359–367.
76. O'Donnell ME. Endothelial cell sodium-potassium-chloride cotransport evidence of regulation by Ca^{2+} and PKC. J Biol Chem 1991;266:11,559–11,566.
77. Schuhmann K, Groschner K. Protein kinase-C mediates dual modulation of L-type Ca^{2+} channels in human vascular smooth muscle. FEBS J 1994;341:208–212.
78. Doctrow SR, Folkman J. PKC activators suppress stimulation of capillary endothelial cell growth by angiogenic endothelial mitogens. J Cell Biol 1987;104:679–687.
79. Greene AS, Tonellato PJ, Lui J, Lombard JH, Cowley AW. Microvascular rarefaction and tissue vascular resistance in hypertension. Am J Physiol 1989;256:H126–H131.
80. Egan BM. Neurohumoral, hemodynamic and microvascular changes as mechanisms of insulin resistance: a provocative but partial picture. Int J Obesity 1991;15:133–139.

81. Williams B. Glucose-induced vascular smooth muscle dysfunction: the role of PKC. Review. J Hypertens 1995;13:477–486.
82. Swarts HBP, Stekhoven FMAHS, DePont JJHHM. Binding of unsaturated fatty acids to Na^+, K^+-ATPase leading to inhibition and activation. Biochim Biophys Acta 1990;1024:32–40.
83. Ordway RW, Singer JJ, Walsh JV. Direct regulation of ion channels by fatty acids. TINS 1991;14: 96–100.
84. Borkman M, Storlien LH, Pan DA, Jenkins AB, Chisholm DJ, Campbell LV. The relation between insulin sensitivity and the fatty-acid composition of skeletal-muscle phospholipids. N Engl J Med 1993;328:238–244.
85. Ruiz-Gutierrez V, Stiefel P, Villar J, Garcia-Donas MA, Acosta D, Carneado J. Cell membrane fatty acid composition in type I (insulin-dependent) diabetic patienb: relationship with sodium transport abnormalities and metabolic control. Diabetologia 1993;36:850–856.
86. Ajayi AAL, Mathur R, Halushka PV. Testosterone increases human platelet thromboxane A_2 receptor density and aggregation responses. Circulation 1995;91:2742–2747.
87. Harder DR, Campbell WB, Roman RJ. Role of cytochrome P-450 enzymes and metabolites of arachidonic acid in the control of vascular tone. Review. J Vasc Res 1995;32:79–92.
88. Salom MG, Lahera V, Miranda-Guardiola F, Romero JC. Blockage of pressure natriuresis induced by inhibition of renal synthesis of NO in dogs. Am J Physiol 1992;262(5 Part 2):F718–F722.
89. Landin K, Tengborn L, Smith U. Treating insulin resistance in hypertension with metformin reduces both blood pressure and metabolic risk factors. J Int Med 1991;229(2):181–187.

13 Effects of Low Density Lipoproteins on Endothelial Cell Signaling and Adhesion Molecule Expression

Hermann Haller, MD
and Friedrich C. Luft, MD

CONTENTS

INTRODUCTION

Endothelial cell activation plays an important role in the physiological regulation of healthy and diseased blood vessels *(1)*. Endothelial cell intracellular free calcium concentration $[Ca^{2+}]_i$ is an important mediator of this activation *(2)*. Hypercholesterolemia, particularly the low-density lipoprotein (LDL) fraction, is an important risk factor for the development of atherosclerosis, a disease process intimately involving endothelial cells *(3)*. LDL stimulates endothelial cell $[Ca^{2+}]_i$ (receptor mediated), promotes the release of prostacyclin (PGI), and facilitates inactivation of endothelial-derived relaxing factor (EDRF) or nitric oxide (NO) *(4,5)*. LDL also stimulates $[Ca^{2+}]_i$ in vascular smooth muscle cells (VSMC) *(6,7)*, and in cardiac myocytes *(8)*.

LDL not only activates endothelial cell signals but also results in endothelial cell responses that eventually lead to vascular injury. For instance, LDL fosters monocyte recruitment within the vascular wall and promotes adhesion to intimal surfaces *(9,10)*. Monocyte adhesion may involve interaction with adhesion molecules on endothelial cells *(11)*. The vascular cell adhesion molecule-1 (VCAM) is an inducible receptor that mediates endothelial adhesion of monocytes and lymphocytes *(12–14)*. VCAM is expressed on the surface of endothelial cells overlying early "fatty streak" lesions *(12)*. In rabbits fed cholesterol, the expression of VCAM precedes the subendothelial accumulation of monocytes *(13)*, which suggests a role for VCAM in the early stages of vascular damage *(15)*. The effect of a high cholesterol diet on VCAM expression in vivo suggests

From: *Contemporary Endocrinology: Endocrinology of the Vasculature*
Edited by: J. R. Sowers Humana Press Inc., Totowa, NJ

that LDL modified by oxidation (oLDL) may be responsible for the induction of VCAM *(15)*. Cultured endothelial cells incubated with LDL *(16)* or oLDL *(17,18)* show an increased stickiness of monocytes. VCAM expression is enhanced by lysophosphatidylcholine, a component of LDL *(19)*. In these studies, no effect of native LDL or oLDL on VCAM expression in cultured endothelial cells was observed, suggesting that the biological properties of modified LDL may be different in living organisms than in in vitro.

Endothelial cells clearly possess G-protein-coupled LDL receptors *(4,5)*. Activation of these receptors leads to a $[Ca^{2+}]_i$ instead of a signal that is active in the cytoplasm and the cell nucleus *(4,20–22)*. This signal is augmented by the simultaneous stimulation of other endothelial cell receptors such as thrombin *(20)*. Incubation of endothelial cells with LDL leads to VCAM expression and the adhesion of monocytes via protein kinase C (PKC)-dependent mechanisms *(21)*. Ca^{2+} channel blockers diminish both the LDL induced $[Ca^{2+}]_i$ signals and the LDL-induced VCAM expression, suggesting an intimate relationship *(21)*.

LDL AND $[Ca^{2+}]_i$ SIGNALS

Effects of LDL and thrombin on $[Ca^{2+}]_i$ in endothelial cells *(20)* are shown in Fig. 1, corroborating prior observations. The abscissa shows the time-course of the $[Ca^{2+}]_i$ response. Both stimuli result in prompt increases in $[Ca^{2+}]_i$, with a sustained plateau phase. In the upper panels, the cells were maintained in a solution containing 1 m*M* extracellular Ca^{2+}. The experiments (middle panels) were repeated under the condition of absent extracellular Ca^{2+} with 2.5 m*M* EGTA. The initial increase in $[Ca^{2+}]_i$ was again observed; however, the sustained nature of the effect was abolished with both agonists. Preincubation with thapsigargin reduces the initial $[Ca^{2+}]_i$ peak, but does not affect the sustained effects of the two agonists. Confocal photomicrographs showing $[Ca^{2+}]_i$ in endothelial cells in response to LDL with normal extracellular Ca^{2+} (A), in the presence of EGTA (C), as the response to thrombin with normal extracellular Ca^{2+} (B) and with EGTA (D) are shown in Fig. 2. $[Ca^{2+}]_i$ signal provoked by both LDL and thrombin showed a rapid increase in $[Ca^{2+}]_i$ followed by an increase in the nuclear Ca^{2+} concentration. The endothelial cell $[Ca^{2+}]_i$ signal after thrombin was prolonged, compared to LDL (representative experiment from 8–11 experiments). LDL shows a $[Ca^{2+}]_i$ dose–response relationship up to 100 μg/mL, whereas that for thrombin increased progressively up to 0.1 U/mL. The sustained portion of the LDL response is flat for all doses, ranging from 10–500 μg/mL, whereas that for thrombin increases up to 0.05 U/mL and decreased thereafter. There are downregulating effects of LDL on its receptor, as 24 h with LDL abolished the calcium response to LDL. Prior exposure to LDL does not influence the effects of thrombin on $[Ca^{2+}]_i$ indicating that downregulation of LDL receptors does not significantly influence the $[Ca^{2+}]_i$ to other agonists. To investigate the specificity of the LDL-induced $[Ca^{2+}]_i$ signal, we incubated the endothelial cells with modified, acetylated LDL (acLDL) for 24 h. Preincubation with acLDL does not influence the LDL-induced $[Ca^{2+}]_i$ signal. Pertussis toxin arrests the effects of LDL of endothelial cell $[Ca^{2+}]_i$ (Fig. 3), but had no inhibitory effect on the response to thrombin (sustained effect of thrombin was enhanced). Finally, LDL enhances the effect induced by thrombin. In summary, experiments performed in the absence of extracellular Ca^{2+} and with thapsigargin corroborated a contribution of both an influx of extracellular Ca^{2+} and a contribution from $[Ca^{2+}]_i$ stores to the initial peak in $[Ca^{2+}]_i$. Furthermore, the effect of LDL is receptor

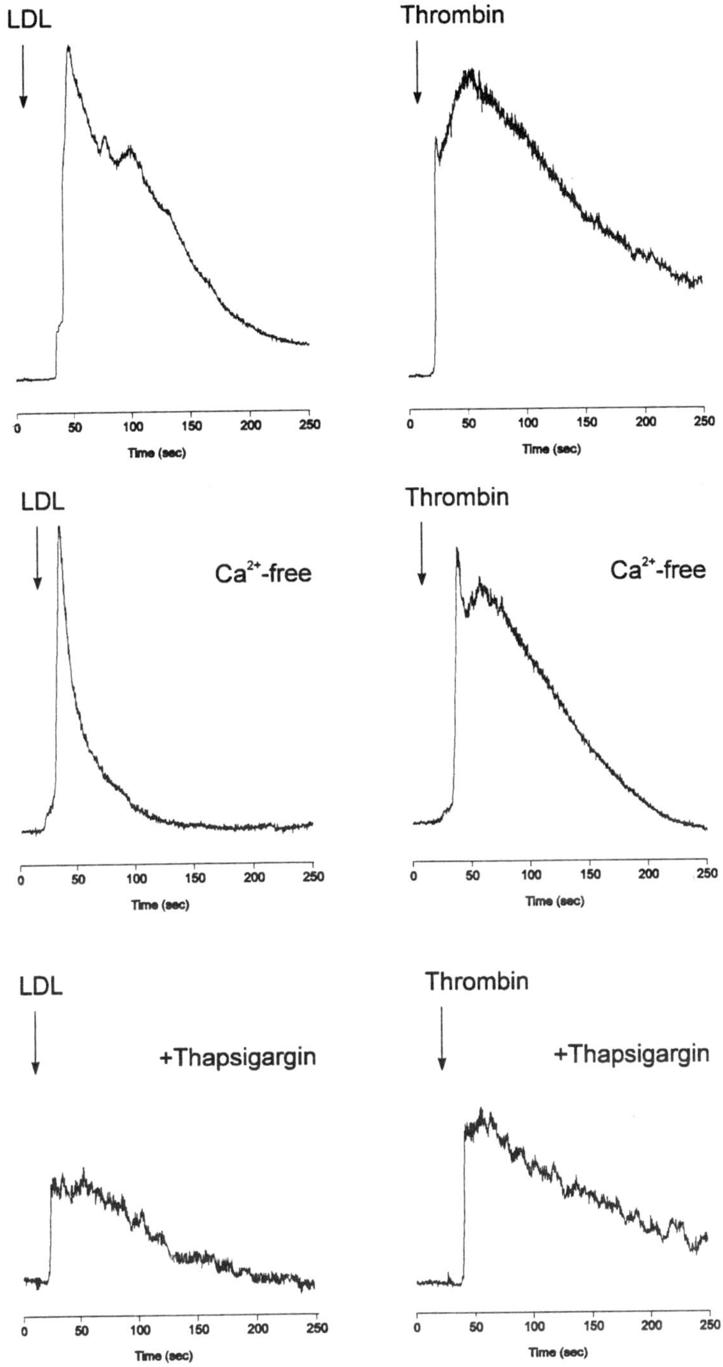

Fig. 1. Effects of LDL (left panel) and thrombin (right panel) on $[Ca^{2+}]_i$ in endothelial cells. Each panel represents the time-course of $[Ca^{2+}]_i$ in response to LDL (100 mg/mL) and thrombin (0.1 U/mL). Addition of agonists is indicated by arrows. The upper panels show the response in the presence of 1 m*M* extracellular Ca^{2+} concentration. The middle panels show the Ca^{2+} response in the absence of extracellular Ca^{2+} (2.5 m*M* EGTA). In lower panels the stimulation of the endothelial cells with LDL (left panel) and thrombin (right panel) after the preincubation with thapsigargin (10^{-5}*M*, 15 min) are shown. Reprinted from ref. *20* with permission.

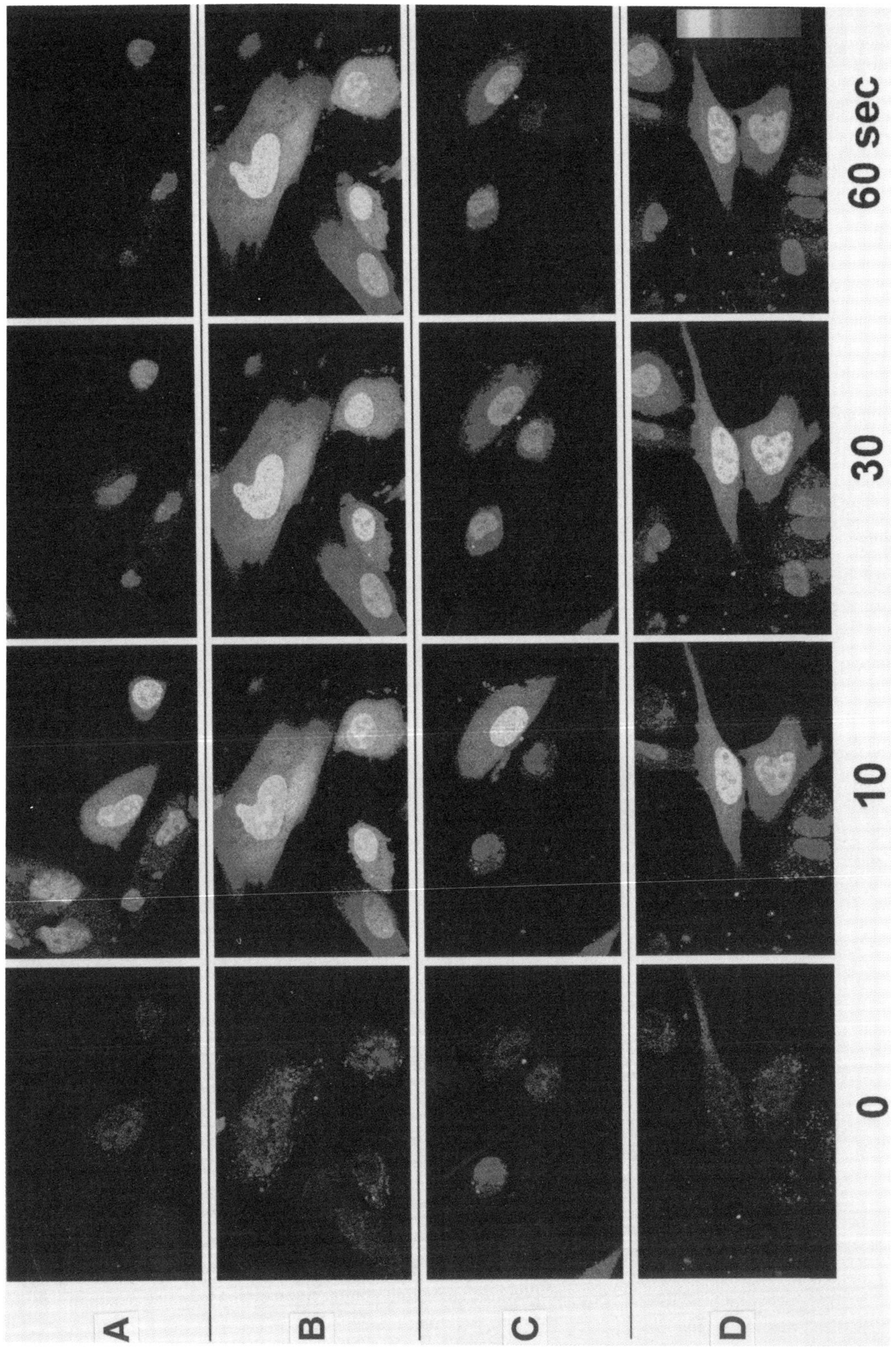

Fig. 2.

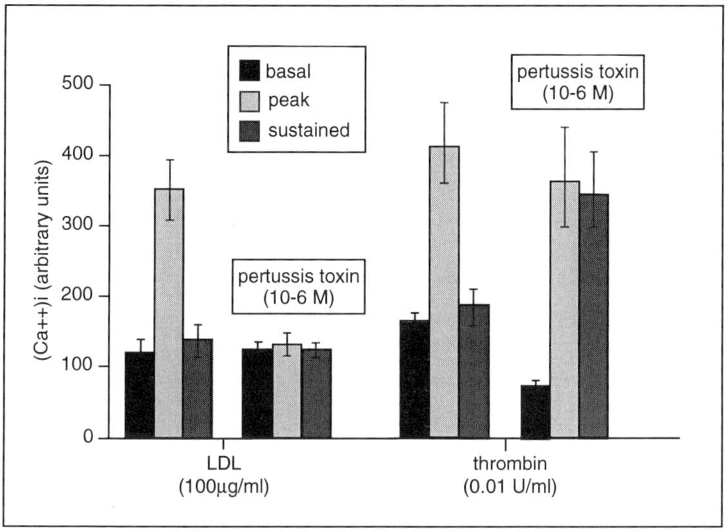

Fig. 3. Effects of pertussis-toxin ($10^{-6}M$) on LDL- (left panel) and thrombin-induced (right panel) Ca^{2+} response in endothelial cells. Endothelial cells were incubated with pertussis toxin ($10^{-6}M$) for 24 h. Cells were then incubated with fura-2, washed three to four times and exposed to LDL or thrombin. Reprinted from ref. *20* with permission.

mediated and the receptor is G-protein coupled, whereas the response to thrombin is not. Finally, LDL and thrombin have additive effects on $[Ca^{2+}]_i$ endothelial responses.

$[Ca^{2+}]_i$ increases in response to LDL, even in the presence of antibodies directed against the LDL receptor *(4)*, but it has been suggested that $[Ca^{2+}]_i$ responses may still be related to receptor activation, rather than a nonspecific interference with cell membrane integrity or ionophore-like properties *(4)*. In VSMC, LDL stimulated Ca^{2+} uptake, an effect not blocked by Ca^{2+} antagonists *(6)*. These data are also consistent with a receptor-operated, rather than a potential-operated Ca^{2+} channel being responsible for the increase in $[Ca^{2+}]_i$. Further, our observation that the $[Ca^{2+}]_i$ response to LDL is inhibited by preincubation with LDL, suggests downregulation of the LDL receptor. Experiments with pertussis toxin suggest that a G-protein coupled receptor is involved *(4)* with activation of phosphatidylinositol-specific phospholipase C and generation of inositol triphosphate (IP_3). Inositol phosphate isomers increase after stimulation with LDL, angiotension II (AII), and platelet-derived growth factor (PDGF), consistent with a G-protein coupled receptor mechanism. The possibility that activation of pertussis toxin-sensitive G-proteins is owing to other ligands delivered by the apo B/E–LDL receptor complex is not ruled out. Such a mechanism would require the internalization of the LDL receptor

---

Fig. 2. *(previous page)* Confocal microscopy of $[Ca^{2+}]_i$ in endothelial cells in response to LDL with **(A)** and without **(C)** extracellular Ca^{2+} as well as in response to thrombin with **(B)** and without **(D)** extracellular Ca^{2+} allowed the visualization of the $[Ca^{2+}]_i$ signal. Each panel represents the time-course of $[Ca^{2+}]_i$ in response to LDL (100 mg/mL) and thrombin (0.1 U/mL). Addition of the agonists caused a rapid increase in $[Ca^{2+}]_i$ followed by an increase in nuclear Ca^{2+} at 10 s. This response is sustained with thrombin compared to LDL, even in the absence of extracellular calcium Ca^{2+}. Reprinted from ref. *20* with permission.

(8). However, a comparison of the time-course of the LDL-induced $[Ca^{2+}]_i$ transients in our experiments and the effects observed in cardiac myocytes *(8)* does not support a role for LDL receptor internalization in $[Ca^{2+}]_i$ signaling.

These findings may have relevance to the behavior of arteries affected with atheromatous lesions and perhaps the pathogenesis of the lesions themselves. In this regard, endothelial cells stimulated with LDL acutely release PGI *(4)*. Chronic effects of LDL on endothelial cells or the release of other phospholipase A_2-dependent products are less well defined. Both native and oLDL inactivate EDRF/NO after release from endothelial cells *(5)*, which could explain the reduced response to nitrates by atherosclerotic vessels. LDL is able to induce expression of surface adhesion molecules on endothelial cells, which, activated in this manner, attract inflammatory cells that participate in the atherosclerotic process *(21)*. Finally, $[Ca^{2+}]_i$ is an important second messenger system involved in many atherogenic processes such as hypertrophy, cell migration, and cell damage. The effect of LDL could initiate any or all of these in endothelial cells. Moreover, a similar activation of VSMC has been described *(22)*, and oLDL evokes a greater response in the $[Ca^{2+}]_i$ signal than does native LDL. Finally, morphological changes in endothelial cells occur after a 5-h exposure to LDL. The cells develop blebbing and exhibit loss of viability, which may also contribute to the atherosclerotic process.

Generation of thrombin is pivotal to coagulation, and perhaps the atherosclerotic process. In longitudinal studies in atherosclerotic patients, an increased risk of major cardiovascular events has been related to baseline abnormalities in plasma fibrinogen *(23,24)*, factor VII *(25)*, antithrombin III *(26)*, and plasminogen activator inhibitor *(27)*. Active thrombin is directly or indirectly related to the actions of all these coagulation factors. The $[Ca^{2+}]_i$ signal in response to thrombin in endothelial cells is more persistent than with LDL. A rapid increase in $[Ca^{2+}]_i$ is followed by an increase in the nuclear $[Ca^{2+}]_i$ concentration. In VSMC, an increase in nuclear Ca^{2+} is observed following various agonists, including thrombin *(28)*. Thus, it is possible that Ca^{2+} plays a role in nuclear signaling. The response to LDL was blocked completely by pertussis toxin, whereas that to thrombin is not, suggesting that the LDL receptor and the thrombin receptor couple to phospholipase C by means of different transduction mechanisms. It is very likely that the thrombin receptor also relies on G proteins *(29)*. However, not all G proteins are pertussis toxin sensitive. The receptor coupling to phospholipase C may involve both pertussis toxin sensitive and insensitive G proteins *(30)*.

Thrombin is known to stimulate phospholipase C in endothelial cells, a process that is sensitive to PKC activation *(31)*. Further, thrombin is known to trigger a cascade of events, such as IP_3 generation, F-actin reorganization, and an increase in endothelial cell permeability *(32)*. We hypothesize that especially the latter attribute may predispose endothelial cells exposed to long-term elevated LDL concentrations to overly express adhesion molecules, develop superficial damage, and lead to decreased cell viability.

LDL AND VASCULAR ADHESION MOLECULE EXPRESSION

VCAM surface expression on endothelial cells exposed to LDL as assessed by flow cytometry is presented in Fig. 4 *(21)*. Tumor necrosis factor-α (TNF-α) (positive control) causes a dramatic shift of the fluorescence curve to the right, indicating increased surface expression of VCAM compared to controls. LDL also shifts the fluorescence curve to the right, albeit to a lesser degree. VCAM expression on endothelial cells following LDL exposure was measured by a modified enzyme-linked immunosorbent assay (ELISA)

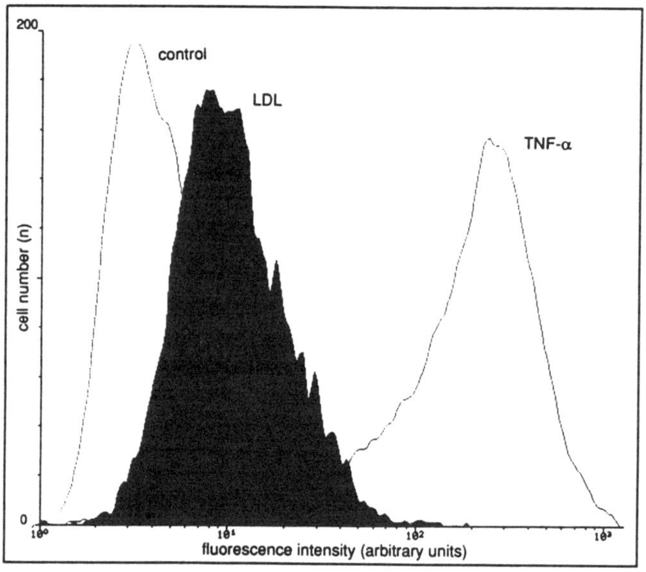

Fig. 4. VCAM surface expression on endothelial cells was assessed by flow cytometry. Cells were treated for 6 h with LDL or TNF-α. TNF-α (positive control) caused a shift of the fluorescence curve to the right indicating increased surface expression of VCAM compared to controls. LDL shifted the fluorescence curve to the right, albeit to a lesser degree. Reprinted from ref. *21* with permission.

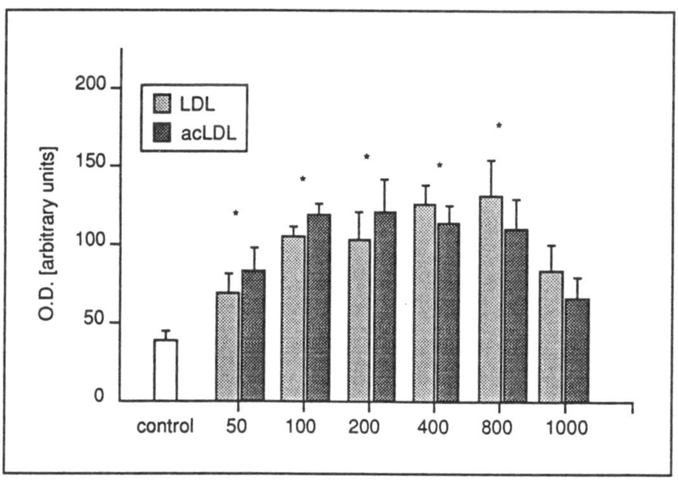

Fig. 5. VCAM surface expression on endothelial cells as induced by LDL, acetylated LDL (acLDL), or TNF-α. Surface expression was determined by ELISA and measured by optical density, and is given on the ordinate in arbitrary units. Shown is a dose–response relationship for increasing doses of LDL and acLDL on the abscissa. The values increased up to 100 mg/mL and stabilized thereafter. With the highest dose of LDL, a decrease was observed, probably because of cell damage. Reprinted from ref. *21* with permission.

(Fig. 5). Incubation of cultured human umbilical vein endothelial cells with LDL resulted in a dose-dependent increase in VCAM expression. Concentrations of LDL at 50 mg/mL induced a significant increase in VCAM expression above baseline. The elevated values

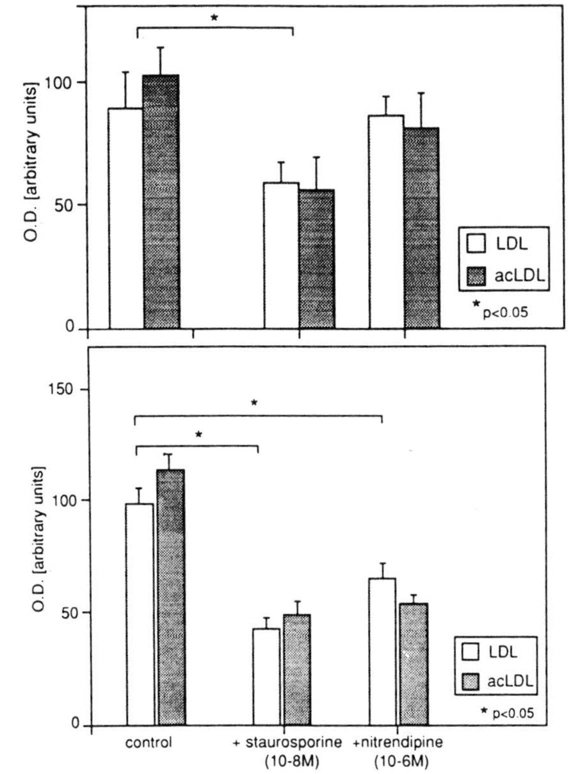

Fig. 6. Effect of the PKC-inhibitor staurosporine ($10^{-8}M$) and the Ca^{2+} antagonist nitrendipine ($10^{-7}M$) on VCAM surface expression induced by LDL and acLDL after 5 (upper panel) and 24 h (lower panel). Controls were effects of LDL and acLDL alone. Staurosporine inhibited the response completely to basal OD values. Nitrendipine had no effect at 5 h, but reduced VCAM surface expression by 24 h ($p < 0.05$). Reprinted from ref. *21* with permission.

stabilized after 100 mg/mL. LDL concentrations at 1000 mg/mL and those above (data not shown) actually decreased VCAM expression, probably because of damage to the cells.

Possible mechanisms of LDL-induced VCAM expression were subsequently investigated (Fig. 6). When endothelial cells were incubated with LDL (100 mg/mL) and the PKC inhibitor staurosporine ($10^{-8}M$) for 5 h, the stimulatory effect of LDL on VCAM expression was abolished completely. Staurosporine at the dose used in these studies had no toxic effects on endothelial cells, and no effects on VCAM expression. However, higher concentrations of staurosporine ($>10^{-7}M$) induced an increase in VCAM expression. Although staurosporine completely blocked the LDL effect on VCAM expression, the effect of TNF-α on VCAM surface expression is only partially inhibited (data not shown). Incubation of the cells with LDL and a Ca^{2+} antagonist also reduce VCAM surface expression significantly, but only after 24 h.

To determine whether or not the effect of LDL on VCAM expression is specific for this surface adhesion molecule, the effect of LDL on the intercellular adhesion molecule-1 (ICAM-1) and on the endothelial leukocyte adhesion molecule (ELAM) was examined. LDL (100 mg/mL) induces a slight, but significant increase in endothelial surface expression of ICAM after 2 and 6 h, while the surface expression of ELAM is not affected by

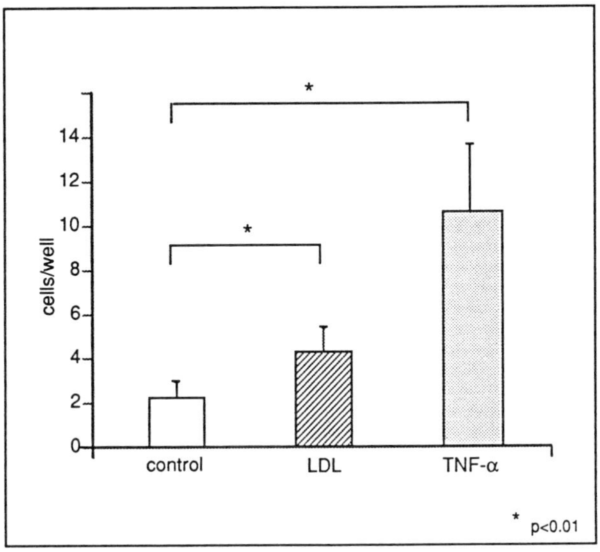

Fig. 7. Effect of LDL (100 mg/mL) and TNF-α on monocyte (U 937) adhesion on endothelial cells. Endothelial cells were exposed to LDL (100 mg/mL) for 24 h, incubated with monocytes for 30 min, and the adherent cells counted under the microscope. LDL induced a significant increase in monocyte adhesion to endothelial cells. This effect is about 20% of the TNF-α induced monocyte binding. Reprinted from ref. *21* with permission.

exposure of endothelial cells to LDL. The functional significance of the LDL-induced upregulation of endothelial cell adhesion molecules was studied by exposing to LDL (100 mg/mL) for 6 and 24 h, incubated with monocytes for 30 min, and the adherent cells counted under the microscope. LDL after 24 h induces a significant increase in monocyte adhesion to endothelial cells (Fig. 7). A stimulatory effect of LDL on monocyte adhesion was also observed after 6 h. Approximately 20% of positive control TNF-α induced monocyte binding; attempts to specifically block the VCAM-dependent adhesion using specific antibodies have been unsuccessful. Instead, the antibodies augment the LDL-induced effect on monocytes by 30%, indicating that the antibodies do not block the specific binding site.

The link between hyperlipidemia and monocyte attachment to endothelium is well established *(33)*, and native LDL, when added to endothelial cells, increased monocyte binding to the cell surface *(34)*. VCAM surface expression is very important in the monocyte recruitment process *(12–15)*, and LDL leads to a small but significant increase in VCAM surface expression on human endothelial cells. It was recently shown that the surface expression of VCAM and ICAM is induced by lysophosphatidylcholine, as well *(19)*. The effect of LDL is small compared to the TNF-α mediated response. A similar response of ICAM to stimulation with LDL was also observed; however, no effect on ELAM could be demonstrated. These data suggest that LDL exerts a specific, stimulatory effect on adhesion molecules of the integrin family, but not on the selectins.

Although acetylated LDL is not abundant in humans, acetylation alters the biological properties of the lipoprotein similar to oxidation *(35)*. oLDL and acLDL both bind to a so-called "scavenger" receptor, which differs from the native LDL receptor *(36–38)*. Numerous studies demonstrated that oLDL leads to a more pronounced cellular stimulation, compared to native LDL *(39)*. However, there seems to be no difference between the two forms of LDL with respect to the effects of LDL on surface expression of VCAM and ICAM. Further, we did not observe a difference in the response of VCAM surface expression between native and acLDL. It is possible that the observed effects of LDL in our study are not the result of receptor–ligand interactions, but instead reflect a nonspecific interaction of LDL with plasma membranes. Other investigators also have observed no difference between the effect of LDL and acLDL on the synthesis of plasminogen activator inhibitor-1 in cultured human endothelial cells *(40)*.

The inhibitory effect of the PKC inhibitor staurosporine suggests that the induction of VCAM by LDL is mediated by PKC. This enzyme complex is also involved in the induction of adhesion molecules by other stimuli such as TNF-α and lipopolysaccharides *(41,42)*. Although staurosporine inhibits other protein kinases as well, at the concentrations the inhibition of PKC is predominant *(43)*. There is activation of PKC by LDL, which is in agreement with several studies showing that LDL leads to an intracellular mobilization of $[Ca^{2+}]_i$ via generation of inositol trisphosphate *(44,45)*.

The Ca^{2+} antagonist does not influence the LDL-induced surface expression of VCAM after 5 h, but does reduce VCAM surface expression after 24 h. This suggests that the early and late induction of VCAM by LDL is controlled by two different mechanisms. Since endothelial cells have no voltage-sensitive (L-type) Ca^{2+} channels *(46)*, Ca^{2+} antagonists likely exert effects on endothelial cells that are not dependent on their inhibitory effect on L-type Ca^{2+} channels. A decrease in leukocyte adhesion in the coronary microcirculation also has been observed after exposure to a Ca^{2+} antagonist *(47)*. In experiments where LDL resulted in a $[Ca^{2+}]_i$ signal within endothelial cells (diminished by thapsigargin and completely blocked by the G-protein inhibitor pertussis toxin), thrombin was used as the positive control for the $[Ca^{2+}]_i$ signal *(20)*. Thrombin is also known to stimulate monocyte adhesion to endothelial cells *(48)*. Although $[Ca^{2+}]_i$ signals were not measured in the VCAM study, the effects of Ca antagonists on VCAM expression are consistent, with an important role for $[Ca^{2+}]_i$ in mediating endothelial cell surface expression of adhesion molecules.

CONCLUSIONS

Recent investigations suggest that LDL leads to both a release of $[Ca^{2+}]_i$ from intracellular stores and a transmembranous $[Ca^{2+}]_i$ influx. The effect of LDL is dependent on binding to a specific G-protein-coupled receptor. LDL enhances the activation induced by other agonists such as thrombin. Thrombin induces PKC-sensitive endothelial cell activation and F-actin reorganization, and increases endothelial cell permeability *(23)*. The notion that LDL exposure results in adhesion molecule expression is substantiated by the observation of stimulant effects of LDL and acLDL on the surface expression of VCAM in endothelial cells. The effect is blocked completely by the concomitant incubation with staurosporine, which suggests that the LDL response is mediated by PKC. The Ca^{2+} antagonist also reduces VCAM expression. Perhaps hypercholesterolemia increases the recruitment of leukocytes via a PKC-mediated increase in adhesion molecule surface expression. Although the effect is small compared to agonists such as TNF-α, atherogenesis is an interactive process that takes years to develop. It is hypothesized that, under in vivo circumstances, which may include the influence of hypertension *(49)*, cigarette smoking *(50)*, and other concomitant noxious influences, small effects may be clinically significant.

REFERENCES

1. Bassenge E, Busse R. Endothelial modulation of coronary tone. Prog Cardiovasc Dis 1988;30:349–380.
2. Weintraub WH, Negulescu PA, Machen TE. Ca^{2+} signalling in endothelia: cellular heterogeneity and receptor internalization. Am J Physiol 1992;263:C1029–C1039.
3. Steinberg D, Parthasarathy S, Carew TE, Khoo JC, Witztum JL. Beyond cholesterol: modifications of low-density lipoprotein that increase its atherogenicity. N Engl J Med 1989;320:915–924.
4. Galle J, Lückhoff A, Busse R, Bassenge E. Low-density lipoproteins stimulate internal free Ca^{2+} and PGI release in endothelial cells. Eicosanoids 1990;3:81–86.
5. Galle J, Mülsch A, Busse R, Bassenge E. Effects of native and oxidized low density lipoproteins on formation and inactivation of endothelium-derived relaxing factor. Arterioscler Thromb 1991;11:198–203.
6. Orlov S, Resink TJ, Bernhardt J, Ferracin F, Bühler FR. Vascular smooth muscle cell Ca^{2+} fluxes: regulation by angiotensin II and lipoproteins. Hypertension 1993;21:195–203.
7. Bochkov V, Tkachuk V, Bühler FR, Resink TJ. Phosphoinositide and Ca^{2+} signalling responses in smooth muscle cells: comparison between lipoproteins, ANG II and PDGF. Biochem Biophys Res Comm 1992;188:1295–1304.
8. Liu K, Pierce GN. The effects of low density lipoprotein on Ca^{2+} transients in isolated rabbit cardiomyocytes. J Biol Chem 1993;268:3767–3775.
9. Faggiotto A, Ross R, Harker L. Studies of hypercholesterolemia in the non-human primate. Changes that lead to fatty streak formation. Arteriosclerosis 1986;4:323–340.
10. Gerrity RG. The role of monocyte in atherogenesis. 1. Transition of blood-borne monocytes into foam cells in fatty lesions. Am J Pathol 1981;103:181–190.
11. Schwartz CJ, Valente AJ, Sprague EA. A modern view of atherogenesis. Am J Cardiol 1993;71:21–29.
12. Cybulsky MI, Gimbrone MJ. Endothelial expression of a mononuclear leukocyte adhesion molecule during atherogenesis. Science 1991;251:788–791.
13. Li H, Cybulsky MI, Gimbrone MJ, Libby P. An atherogenic diet rapidly induces VCAM-1, a cytokine-regulatable mononuclear leukocyte adhesion molecule, in rabbit aortic endothelium. Arterioscler Thromb 1993;13:197–204.
14. Oppenheimer MN, Davis LS, Bogue DT, Ramberg J, Lipsky PE. Differential utilization of ICAM-1 and VCAM-1 during the adhesion and transendothelial migration of human T lymphocytes. J Immunol 1991;147:2913–2921.
15. Libby P, Hansson GK. Involvement of the immune system in human atherogenesis: current knowledge and unanswered questions. Lab Invest 1991;64:5–15.
16. Alderson LM, Endemann G, Lindsey S, Pronczuk A, Hoover RI, Hayes KC. LDL enhances monocyte adhesion to endothelial cells in vitro. Am J Pathol 1986;123:334–341.
17. Berliner JA, Territo MC, Sevanian A, et al. Minimally modified LDL stimulates monocyte endothelial interactions. J Clin Invest 1990;85:1260–1267.
18. Frostegard J, Haegerstrand A, Gidlund M, Nilsson J. Biologically modified LDL increases the adhesive properties of endothelial cells. Atherosclerosis 1991;90:119–126.
19. Kume N, Cybulsky MI, Gimbrone MJ. Lysophosphatidylcholine, a component of atherogenic lipoproteins, induces mononuclear leukocyte adhesion molecules in cultured human and rabbit arterial endothelial cells. J Clin Invest 1992;90:1138–1144.
20. Haller H, Rieger M, Kuhlmann M, Philipp S, Distler A, Luft FC. LDL increases $[Ca^{2+}]_i$ in human endothelial cells and augments thrombin-induced cell signalling. J Lab Clin Med 1994;124:708–714.
21. Haller H, Schaper D, Ziegler W, Kuhlmann M, Distler A, Luft FC. LDL induces surface expression of vascular adhesion molecule (VCAM) on endothelial cells via activation of protein kinase C. Hypertension 1995;25:511–516.
22. Negre-Salvayre A, Fitoussi G, Reaud V, Pieraggi MT, Thiers JC, Salvayre R. A delayed and sustained rise of cytosolic Ca^{2+} is elicited by oxidized LDL in cultured bovine aortic endothelial cells. FEBS Lett 1992;299:60–65.
23. Wilhelmsen L, Svardsudd K, Korsan-Bentsen K, et al. Fibrinogen as a risk factor for stroke and myocardial infarction. N Engl J Med 1984;311:501–505.
24. Meade TW, Mellows S, Brozovic M, et al. Haemostatic function and ischaemic heart disease: principal results of the Northwick Park Heart Study. Lancet 1986;ii:533–537.
25. Yarnell JWG, Baker IA, Sweetnam PM, et al. Fibrinogen, viscosity and white blood cell count are major risk factors for ischemic heart disease: the Caerphilly and Speedwell Collaborative Heart Disease Studies. Circulation 1991;83:836–844.

26. Meade TW, Cooper J, Miller GJ, et al. Antithrombin III and arterial disease. Lancet 1991;337:850,851.
27. Hamsten A, de Faire U, Walldius G, et al. Plasminogen activator inhibitor in plasma: risk factor for recurrent myocardial infarction. Lancet 1987;ii:3–8.
28. Himpens G, De Smedt H, Casteels R. Kinetics of nucleocytoplasmic transients in DDT1MF-2 smooth muscle cells. Am J Physiol 1992;263(Cell Physiol 32):C978–C985.
29. Coughlin SR, Vu TKH, Hung DT, Wheaton VI. Characterization of a functional thrombin receptor: issues and opportunities. J Clin Invest 1991;89:351–355.
30. Johnson RM, Connelly PA, Sisk RB, Pobiner BF, Hewlett EL, Garrison JC. Pertussis toxin or phorbol 12-myristate 13-acetate can distinguish between epidermal growth factor- and angiotensin-stimulated signals in hepatocytes. Proc Natl Acad Sci USA 1986;83:2032–2036.
31. Brock TA, Capasso EA. Thrombin and histamine activate phospholipase C in human endothelial cells via a phorbol ester sensitive pathway. J Cell Physiol 1988;136:54–62.
32. Lum H, Aschner JL, Phillips PG, Fletcher PW, Malik AD. Time course of thrombin-induced increase in endothelial permeability: relationship to Ca^{2+} and inositol polyphosphates. Am J Physiol 1992;263:L219–L225.
33. Li H, Cybulsky MI, Gimbrone MA Jr, et al. An atherogenic diet rapidly induces VCAM-1, a cytokine regulatable mononuclear leukocyte adhesion molecule in rabbit aortic endothelium. Arteriosclerosis 1993;13:197–204.
34. Pritchard KA Jr, Tota RR, Lin JH-C, et al. Native low density lipoprotein. Endothelial cell recruitment of mononuclear cells. Arterioscler Thromb 1991;11:1175–1181.
35. Steinberg D, Parthasarathy S, Carew TE, Khoo JC, Witztum JL. Beyond cholesterol. Modifications of low-density lipoprotein that increase its atherogeneity. N Engl J Med 1989;320:915–919.
36. Matsumoto A, Naito M, Itakura H, et al. Human macrophage scavenger receptors: primary structure, expression and localization in atherosclerotic lesions. Proc Natl Acad Sci USA 1990;87:9133–9137.
37. Kodama T, Freeman M, Rohrer L, Zabrecky J, Matsudaira P, Krieger M. Type I macrophage scavenger receptor contains a-helical and collagen-like coils. Nature 1990;343:531–534.
38. Nagelkerke JF, Barto KP, Berkel TJ. In vivo and in vitro uptake and degradation of acetylated low density lipoprotein by rat liver endothelial, Kupffer and parenchymal cells. J Biol Chem 1983;258:12,221–12,227.
39. Witztum JL, Steinberg D. Role of oxidized low density lipoprotein in atherogenesis. J Clin Invest 1991;88:1785–1792.
40. Tremoli E, Camera M, Maderna P, et al. Increased synthesis of plasminogen activator inhibitor-1 by cultured human endothelial cells exposed to native and modified LDLs. An LDL receptor-independent phenomenon. Arterioscler Thromb 1993;13:338–346.
41. Mattila P, Majuri ML, Mattila PS, Renkonen R. TNF alpha-induced expression of endothelial adhesion molecules, ICAM-1 and VCAM-1, is linked to protein kinase C activation. Scand J Immunol 1992;36:159–165.
42. Herbert J-M. Protein kinase C: a key factor in the regulation of tumor cell adhesion to the endothelium. Biochem Pharmacol 1993;45:527–537.
43. Palkama T, Majuri ML, Mattila P, Hurme M, Renkonen R. Regulation of endothelial adhesion molecules by ligands binding to the scavenger receptor. Clin Exp Immunol 1993;92:353–360.
44. Bochkow V, Tschachuk V, Buhler F, Resink T. Phosphoinositide and Ca^{2+} signalling responses in smooth muscle cells: comparison between lipoproteins, Ang II, and PDGF. Biochem Biophys Res Commun 1992;188:1295–1304.
45. Myers DE, Fidge NH, Stanton H, Larkins RG. The effects of low density lipoprotein and high density lipoprotein on phosphoinositide hydrolysis in bovine aortic endothelial. Atherosclerosis 1992;92:9–16.
46. Himmel HM, Whorton AR, Strauss HC. Intracellular Ca^{2+}, currents, and stimulus-response coupling in endothelial cells. Hypertension 1993;21:112–127.
47. McDonagh PF, Rauzzino MJ. Stimulated leukocyte adhesion in coronary microcirculation is reduced by a Ca^{2+} antagonist. Am J Physiol 1993;265:H476–H483.
48. DiCorleto PE, de la Motte CA. Thrombin causes increased monocytic cell adhesion to endothelial cells through a protein kinase C-dependent pathway. Biochem J 1989;264:71–77.
49. Mai M, Geiger H, Hilgers KF, Veelken R, Mann JFE, Luft FC. Early interstitial changes in hypertension-induced renal injury. Hypertension 1993;22:754–765.
50. Schaberg T, Rau M, Kaiser D, Fassbender M, Lode H, Haller H. Increased number of alveolar macrophages expressing adhesion molecules of the leukocyte adhesion molecule family in smoking subjects: association with cell-binding ability and superoxide anion production. Am Rev Respir Dis 1992;146:1287–1293.

II Vascular Smooth Muscle Cells

14 Angiotensin II Signal Transduction in Vascular Smooth Muscle

Bradford C. Berk, MD, PHD,
Jennifer L. Duff, PHD,
Mario B. Marrero, PHD,
and Kenneth E. Bernstein, MD

CONTENTS

INTRODUCTION

The octapeptide hormone of the renin–angiotensin system, angiotensin II (AII), regulates a wide variety of physiological responses including salt and water balance, blood pressure, and vascular tone. AII is produced both systemically and locally in the vessel wall by the actions of renin, which converts angiotensinogen into AI, and angiotensin-converting enzyme (ACE), which cleaves AI to form AII. In addition to its vasoconstrictor activity, AII has recently been shown to stimulate vascular smooth muscle cell (VSMC) growth, increase the expression of inflammatory mediators such as phospholipase A_2 and NADH oxidase, and activate gene transcription of proto-oncogenes such as c-*fos,* as well as genes activated by the signal transducers and activators of transcription (STAT) pathway. These data suggest that AII plays an important role in various cardiovascular diseases associated with VSMC growth and vessel wall inflammation such as hypertension, restenosis following balloon angioplasty, and atherosclerosis.

From: *Contemporary Endocrinology: Endocrinology of the Vasculature*
Edited by: J. R. Sowers Humana Press Inc., Totowa, NJ

THE AT_1 RECEPTOR

AII binds to at least two high affinity receptors, AT_1 and AT_2 *(1)*. The signal transduction pathways activated by the AT_2 receptor remain unknown, so this chapter focuses on AT_1 signaling. The signal transduction events stimulated by AII binding to the AT_1 receptor are similar to those stimulated by growth factors and cytokines, and include activation of phospholipase C (PLC) *(2)*, calcium mobilization *(3)*, activation of protein kinase C (PKC) *(4)*, induction of proto-oncogenes *(5)*, protein tyrosine phosphorylation *(6)*, and activation of mitogen-activated protein (MAP) kinase *(7,8)*.

The first molecular insight into the AT_1 receptor was the cloning of the receptor by two laboratories in 1991 *(9,10)*. The structure of the AT_1 receptor shows that it is a member of the seven transmembrane-spanning G-protein-coupled receptor family. Other receptors in this family include the α- and β-adrenergic receptors, the muscarinic receptor, the various serotonin receptors, and important vascular receptors such as the thrombin, bradykinin, and endothelin receptors. These receptors share the property of binding to heterotrimeric G-proteins and lacking intrinsic tyrosine kinase activity in contrast to growth factor receptors such as platelet-derived growth factor (PDGF), fibroblast growth factor (FGF), and epidermal growth factor (EGF).

Based on cDNA sequence, the AT_1 receptor is composed of 359 amino acids. The AT_1 receptor is a glycoprotein and contains extracellular glycosylation sites at the amino terminus (Asn^4) and the second extracellular loop (Asn^{176} and Asn^{188}) *(11)*. Based on the location of these glycosylation sites, hydropathy plots, and comparisons with other G-protein-coupled receptors, it is proposed that, following insertion into the membrane, the AT_1 receptor should have seven transmembrane domains arranged as shown in Fig. 1. Interactions among these domains and the corresponding intracellular loops are responsible for determining the nature of AII binding and receptor activation following binding.

For example, the AII binding site appears to be the result of interactions among several of these domains (Fig. 1 and Table 1) *(12–15)*. Several transmembrane domains are responsible for G-protein interactions with the receptor. These domains are present at the amino terminal extension, and in first and third extracellular loops *(16)*. Recent modeling analysis suggests that an interaction between Asp^{74} and Tyr^{292} is critical for AII binding and AT_1 receptor activation *(17)*. Site-directed mutagenesis has established that Asp^{74}, a conserved residue within the second transmembrane domain, is important in G-protein binding and activation *(14,18)*, as well as the conserved residues Tyr^{292} *(17)* and Tyr^{215} *(19)*. In addition, the motif Asp^{125}-Arg^{126}-Tyr^{127} in the amino terminal region of the second cytoplasmic loop is important in G-protein activation *(18)*. These same residues may also be important in AII-stimulated growth *(14)*.

Many G-protein-coupled receptors have been shown to undergo palmitoylation or farnesylation in the carboxyl tail, which may be important for receptor activation *(20,21)*. Palmitoylation usually occurs within the terminal 12 amino acids of the seventh transmembrane domain. In the AT_1 receptor, the only potential palmitoylation or farnesylation site is Cys^{355}, which is 59 amino acids removed from the seventh transmembrane domain. Thus, modification at this site, if demonstrated, would be very atypical.

Receptor phosphorylation is a critical event in the internalization of G-protein-coupled receptors. G-protein coupled receptors do not contain intrinsic kinase activities but are nonetheless phosphorylated on serine and threonine residues by members of the G-protein

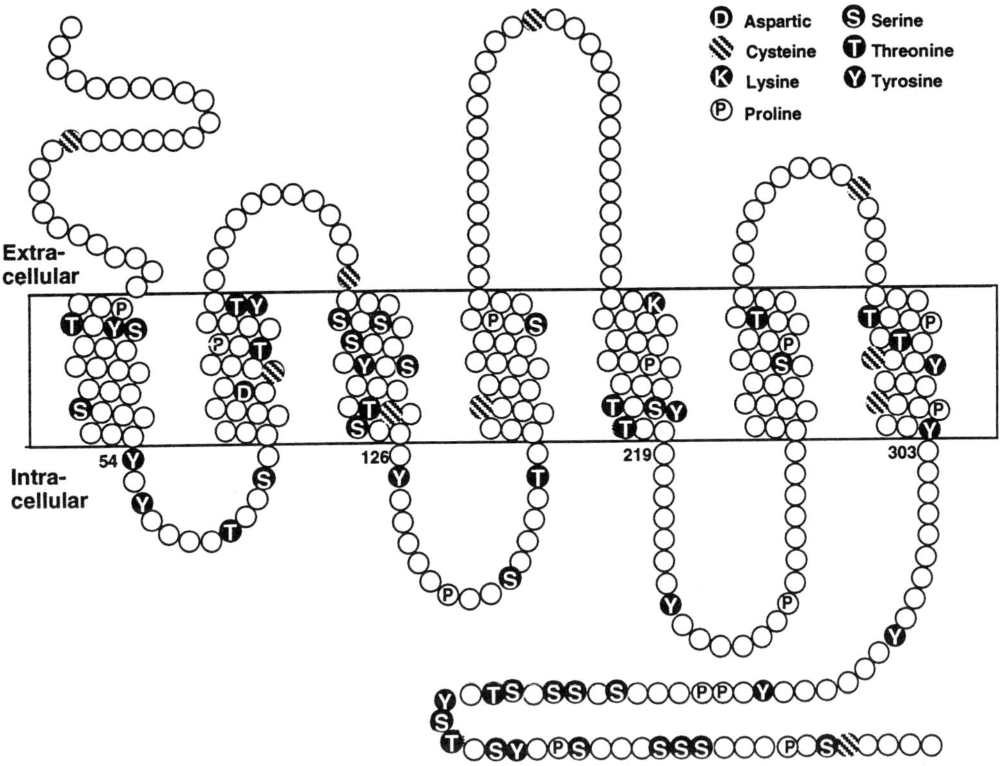

Fig. 1. Representation of amino acids in the rat AT_{1a} receptor. The helices were positioned based on modeling of G-protein-coupled receptors. Depicted in white letters on black circles are the amino acids discussed as critical to ligand binding and signal transduction.

Table 1
Molecular Analysis of AT_1 Receptor Signal Transduction

Function	*Amino acids or domains identified as regulatory*[a]
AII binding	N terminal extension (Ile14, His24, Tyr26, Ile27); Extracellular loop 1 (Tyr92)
	Extracellular loop 3 (Asp278, Asp281) *(16)*
	Lys199 *(16a)*
	Tyr292 *(17)*
	Tyr215 *(19)*
G-protein and/or PLC activation	Asp74 *(14,26)*
	Tyr292 *(17)*
	Tyr215 *(19)*
	Intracellular loop 2, COOH-portion of loop 3, and COOH-tail *(18)*
Internalization	Thr332…Ser335-Thr336-Leu337-Ser338 *(28)*
	Tyr215 *(19)*
	Ala221-Leu222-Lys223-Lys224-Ala225-Tyr226 *(26)*
DNA synthesis	Asp74 *(14)*

[a]The assignment of these amino acids to the indicated actions of the AT_1 receptor are based on the deletion and mutagenesis studies referenced. When mutagenesis of a single amino acid has multiple effects (e.g., Tyr215), this may reflect inhibition of a very proximal step in signal transduction. It should be noted that most of these experiments have been carried out in Chinese hamster ovary (CHO) cells and the signal events may be coupled differently in other tissues such as vascular smooth muscle, heart, and adrenal.

receptor kinase (GRK) family of which the β-adrenergic receptor kinase (βARK) is the prototypic member *(22)*. Recently our group *(23)* and others *(24)* have shown that the AT_1 receptor is phosphorylated basally and in response to AII. The majority of phosphorylation in vivo was found on serine and there was a small increase in total phosphoserine content following agonist exposure. In the β-adrenergic receptor, phosphorylation by βARK is required for receptor internalization and downregulation *(22)*. Phosphorylation occurs at a motif in the third intracellular loop involving Ser^{296}-Ser^{299}, which appears to be shared with the α_{2A} adrenergic receptor *(25)*. G-protein receptor internalization is usually associated with phosphorylation of the large third cytoplasmic loop (e.g., 53 amino acids in the β-adrenergic receptor). In the AT_1 receptor, however, the third loop is only 24 amino acids in length, but it has been suggested that Tyr^{215} and the residues from Ala^{221} to Tyr^{226} in this loop may serve a role in internalization *(19,26)*. The implication that phosphorylation on these tyrosines is important in internalization is probably incorrect in that phosphorylation on serines is important in other G-protein-coupled receptors. Instead it appears likely that these residues in the third loop are required for G-protein activation, which leads to generation of βγ dimers. It has been demonstrated that βγ dimers are required for membrane location of the GRKs, which associate with the βγ subunits via a pleckstrin homology domain present in the GRK (e.g., βARK) *(27)*. However, it has been shown recently that AT_1 receptor internalization is regulated by a motif in the cytoplasmic tail involving Thr^{332}...Ser^{335}-Thr^{336}-Leu^{337}-Ser^{338}, which is similar to the phosphorylation motif present in the third loop of the adrenergic receptors *(25)*. Based on this finding, it appears that the AT_1 carboxyl tail may serve as the mediator of functions normally mediated by the third loop in other G-protein-coupled receptors. In fact, the cytoplasmic tail of the AT_1 receptor is very large compared to most G-protein-coupled receptors, and contains 63 amino acids. The carboxyl tail contains 11 serine, 2 threonine, and 4 tyrosine resides. Thus it appears that, in the AT_1 receptor, a series of threonine and serine residues between Thr^{332} and Ser^{338} is required for receptor internalization *(28)*.

Surprisingly, tyrosine phosphorylation of the AT_1 receptor also occurs *(23,24)*. There is controversy regarding the extent to which tyrosine phosphorylation is regulated by agonist exposure. By immunoprecipitation of the AT_1 receptor and Western blot analysis using antiphosphotyrosine antibody we found no agonist-dependent increase in tyrosine phosphorylation up to 6 min after AII treatment *(29)*. In contrast, when VSMC were metabolically labeled with ^{32}P orthophosphate and the AT_1 receptor immunoprecipitated, phosphotyrosine could be demonstrated by amino acid analysis and there was a slow increase in the phosphotyrosine content following AII exposure *(24)*. It should be noted that both of these techniques measure total phosphotyrosine content; increases and decreases in phosphorylation of individual tyrosine residues could be overlooked. There are several potential tyrosine phosphorylation sites within the AT_1 receptor (Fig. 1), including amino acids 302, 312, 319, and 339 within the carboxyl tail. The tyrosine at position 319 is of special interest because it is part of the motif Tyr-Ile-Pro-Pro, which is analogous to an src-homology 2 (SH2) binding motif found within the PDGF receptor (Tyr-Ile-Ile-Pro), and within the EGF receptor (Tyr-Leu-Pro-Pro) *(30,31)*. In the PDGF and EGF receptors these motifs have been shown to be target sequences when the tyrosine is phosphorylated. SH2 binding domains contain a critical tyrosine residue that, when phosphorylated, bind to signaling proteins that contain the SH2 domain and act as important mechanisms for protein–protein interactions. For example, PLC-γ

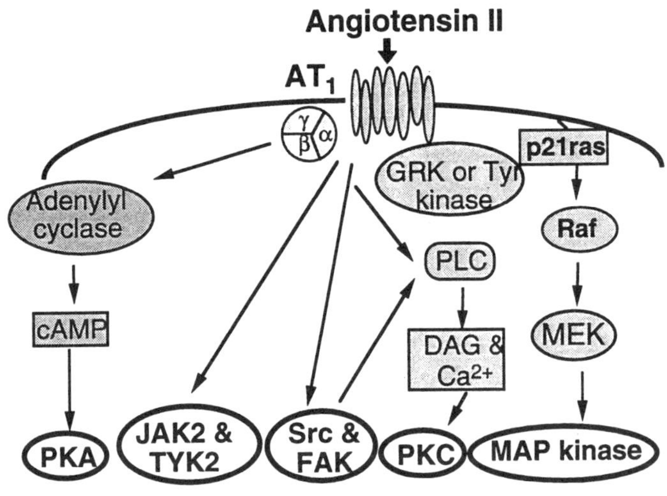

Fig. 2. Summary of kinase-mediated signal transduction pathways stimulated by AII in VSMC. Depicted are five protein kinases potentially activated by AII in VSMC. Protein kinase A (PKA) is likely activated indirectly via formation of prostaglandins. JAK2 and TYK2 are directly activated at the receptor. Src and FAK are not directly activated by the receptor, but as yet to be identified intermediate adapter/activator is probably required. Src is shown as stimulating PLC, which, in this case, is PLC-γ. In addition, PLC-β may be activated by AII in cells where PLC-β is present. PKC is activated by diacylglycerol (DAG) and increases in intracellular Ca^{2+}. Novel and atypical PKC isozymes may be activated independently of these second messengers and are not depicted. MAP kinase is activated by the ras-Raf-MEK pathway. In addition there may be additional upstream regulators of MAP kinase including PKC and Src, not shown here.

contains an SH2 domain that interacts with the Tyr-Ile-Ile-Pro and Tyr-Leu-Pro-Pro sequences present in the PDGF and EGF receptors *(31)*. The tyrosine kinases potentially responsible for tyrosine phosphorylation of the AT_1 receptor are discussed in the following section.

OVERVIEW OF SIGNAL TRANSDUCTION BY THE AT_1 RECEPTOR

Recent findings demonstrate that the AT_1 receptor couples to a wide variety of intracellular signal transduction events. These are summarized in Fig. 2. Four major pathways are discussed in this chapter based on activation of specific kinases: PLC and PKC, STAT proteins and Janus kinases (JAK), $pp60^{c\text{-}src}$ kinase (Src) and focal adhesion kinase (FAK), and Raf kinase and MAP kinase. The purpose of these multiple receptor-activated kinases is to provide an integrated series of regulated cellular events. These events may be delineated based on their temporal features into rapid (<1 min), early (<30 min), late (30 min to 24 h), and very late (>24 h) events as shown in Fig. 3. Alternatively they may be classified according to presumptive physiological relevance into responses related to growth, vasoconstriction, inflammation, migration, and miscellaneous as shown in Table 2. It is clear from this overview that AII has a multiplicity of effects; yet it is unlikely that all these effects occur simultaneously in vivo. Thus, an important area of future research is to determine the physiologic variables that determine the relative extent to which these signal transduction pathways are activated in the vessel itself.

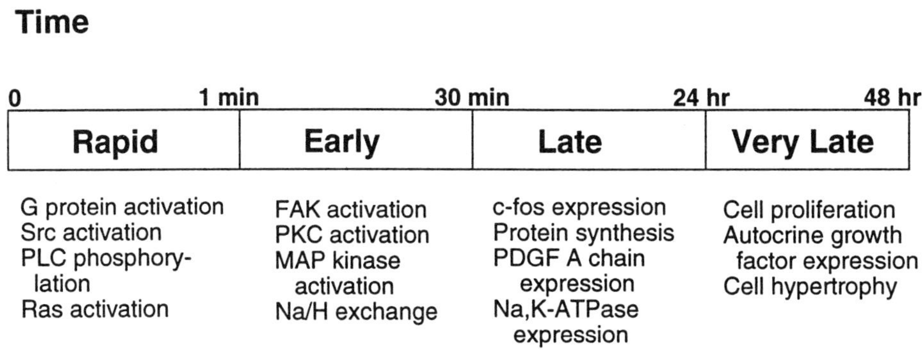

Fig. 3. Time-course for activation of signal transduction stimulated by AII in VSMC. Shown are several of the important events that may be involved in growth, vasoconstriction, migration, and inflammation stimulated by AII.

Table 2
Relationship Between the Physiologic Effects of AII and Specific Protein Kinases[a]

Physiologic effect	*Growth*	*Vasoconstriction*	*Inflammation*	*Migration*
Kinases	Src MAP kinase JAK2	PKC MAP kinase Src	JAK2 TYK2	FAK

[a]The correlation of physiologic effect with specific kinases is a speculative concept that has not been clearly proven for any of these kinases to date. In fact, these "assignments" are only relative. It is likely that under various circumstances (e.g., following balloon injury or in hypertension), different kinases may assume different physiologic roles. The kinases in smaller text have potential but uncertain roles in the indicated effects.

ACTIVATION OF PLC AND PKC

AII binding to the G-protein-coupled AT_1 receptor stimulates the phosphoinositide-specific PLC to hydrolyze phosphatidylinositol 4,5-bisphosphate (PIP_2), thereby generating the second messengers inositol *(1,4,5)*-trisphosphate (IP_3) and diacylglycerol (DAG) (Fig. 4). The IP_3 released into the cytoplasm stimulates the mobilization of calcium from intracellular stores and DAG activates PKC. In contrast to PLC activity, which is transient, the production of DAG in response to AII is biphasic and sustained *(2)*. The sustained production of DAG may be the result of the activity of phospholipase D (PLD), which also has been shown to be stimulated by AII in VSMC *(32)*. PLD hydrolyzes phosphatidylcholine causing a sustained release of choline and phosphatidic acid, which is converted to DAG by phosphatidate phosphohydrolase (Fig. 4).

Our group has made several observations regarding activation of PLC by AII in VSMC. PLC is a family of at least three related genes: PLC-β, PLC-γ, and PLC-δ *(33)*. Isoforms of PLC-β are differentially regulated by α and βγ subunits of G proteins *(34,35)*. In contrast, the PLC-γ isoforms are regulated by tyrosine phosphorylation *(36)*. Regulation of PLC-δ isoforms is unclear but may involve changes in intracellular calcium. For most G-protein-coupled receptors it appears that PLC-β is critical for production of IP_3. However, in VSMC, the PLC-β isoforms are undetectable *(37–39)*, suggesting that another

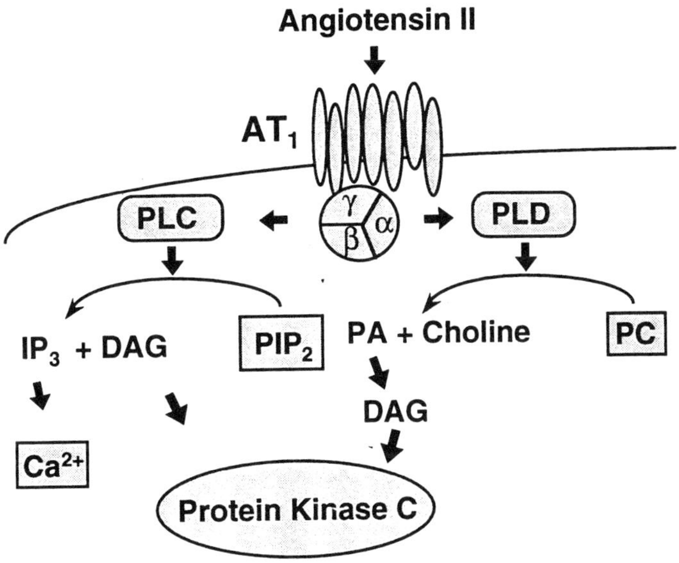

Fig. 4. Classical signal transduction pathways stimulated by AII in VSMC. AII binding to the G-protein-coupled AT_1 receptor stimulates the activity of PLC to hydrolyze PIP_2 to form IP_3 and DAG. IP_3 stimulates the release of Ca^{2+} from intracellular stores and DAG stimulates the activity of protein kinase C. AII also stimulates the activity of PLD to hydrolyze phosphatidylcholine (PC) to form phosphatidic acid (PA) and choline. Through the action of phosphatidate phosphohydrolase, PA can form DAG, which again may stimulate PKC. From ref. *29* with permission.

PLC isoform is responsible for signal transduction in these cells. Our laboratory has shown that among the various isoforms of PLC, the PLC-γ isoform is activated by tyrosine phosphorylation in response to AII. Within 1 min of AII stimulation there is an increase in the tyrosine phosphorylation of PLC-γ *(39)*. The phosphorylation is transient and returns to control levels within 6 min. The time-course for tyrosine phosphorylation of PLC-γ is very similar to the time-course for IP_3 formation, suggesting that PLC-γ activation by tyrosine phosphorylation is responsible for IP_3 generation. This concept is strengthened by several additional findings. Pretreating VSMC with 0.1 m*M* Na_2VO_4, a potent inhibitor of tyrosine phosphatases, for 30 min, then exposing the cells to AII for 3 min, increased AII-induced IP_3 formation (unpublished observations). In addition, as discussed in the Src Family Kinases section, Src, the kinase presumed responsible for tyrosine phosphorylation of PLC-γ is present in VSMC and activated by AII. When Src activity is inhibited by electroporation of anti-Src antibodies, there is a corresponding inhibition of PLC-γ phosphorylation and IP_3 formation, suggesting that PLC-γ is the predominant pathway for IP_3 formation in response to AII in cultured VSMC *(40)*. Finally, the role of PLC-δ was investigated by measuring the effect of calcium chelation on IP_3 formation. When VSMC were incubated with BAPTA-AM, a calcium chelator, AII-stimulated calcium mobilization was completely blocked (for up to 6 min), but no effect on AII-stimulated IP_3 formation occurred. All these responses were completely inhibited by losartan, indicating that the AT_1 receptor is the receptor by which AII stimulates PLC-γ.

Activation of PKC by increases in DAG and calcium is likely to play a role in AII-mediated effects on VSMC. PKC is a serine/threonine kinase that is a member of a multigene family consisting of at least 11 isozymes *(41)*. PKC serves as the receptor for phorbol esters, which are known tumor promoters, and PKC substrates include proteins involved in the regulation of cell proliferation, such as lamins and histone *(41,42)*. AII stimulates the activity of PKC as measured by the phosphorylation of the exogenous substrate histone III-S *(43)*, translocation of PKC from the cytosol to the membrane *(44)*, and phosphorylation of the myristolylated alanine-rich C kinase substrate (MARCKS) protein *(45)*. The role of PKC in AII-signaling processes has been studied by downregulating PKC by prolonged treatment with phorbol esters. Downregulation of PKC significantly reduced the AII-mediated induction of c-*fos* mRNA in VSMC *(5)*. On the other hand, AII stimulation of protein synthesis in VSMC was not dependent on PKC *(46)*, and stimulation of Na^+/H^+ exchange in VSMC was only partially dependent on PKC *(47)*. Crosstalk between signal pathways may be mediated in part by PKC as suggested by the findings that activities of both PLC and PLD are regulated by PKC *(32)*. The data indicate that both PKC-dependent and -independent mechanisms are involved in the regulation of VSMC growth stimulated by AII and that other pathways must also exist to transduce AII signals.

ACTIVATION OF TYROSINE KINASES BY AII

JAK and TYK

A substantial body of evidence indicates that G-protein-coupled receptors such as the AT_1 receptor mediate signal events by activation of tyrosine kinases. AII stimulates the phosphorylation of a variety of VSMC proteins on tyrosine, including the AT_1 receptor itself and PLC-γ1 *(39)*. In the case of the cytokine receptors, such as the interferons and interleukins, tyrosine phosphorylation is mediated by several protein tyrosine kinases that associate with the receptor, including the Src-related kinases Lck and Fyn *(48)*. A variety of recent studies indicate that the AT_1 receptor is likely to share properties with cytokine receptors. In parallel with classical cytokine receptors, such as the interleukin-2, interferon-γ, and interferon-α receptors, the AT_1 receptor stimulates tyrosine phosphorylation, activates the MAP kinase pathway, and induces c-*fos* mRNA expression *(5–8,49,50)*. Perhaps most revealing is the recent demonstration that, in cultured neonatal cardiac fibroblasts, AII activates Stat91 *(51)*, a member of the STAT family of transcription factors characteristically activated by cytokines such as interferon-α and interferon-γ *(52,53)*. Activation of Stat91 and related STAT proteins by cytokines is caused by phosphorylation by tyrosine kinases of the JAK and TYK families *(54)*. We recently found that AII stimulates the tyrosine phosphorylation of JAK2 and Stat113 in VSMC *(55)*. Specifically as shown in Table 3, we observed that JAK2 and TYK2 were stimulated within 5 min of AII treatment. Comparison with the cytokine receptors suggests that AII is most similar to the interferon-γ receptor. These observations and the recent demonstration that thrombin activates JAK2 *(56)* suggest that seven transmembrane receptors may signal using some of the same mechanisms employed by cytokine and growth factor receptors.

Src Family Kinases

An increasing body of evidence suggests that Src plays an important role in AII signal transduction. Two studies demonstrated that Src activity was stimulated by G-protein coupled receptors. Dhar and Shukla *(57)* showed that inhibiting Src activity

Table 3
Comparison of JAK and TYK2 Activation by AII, Cytokines, and Growth Eactors[a]

Agonist	*JAK1*	*JAK2*	*TYK2*	*Stat1*	*Stat2*
AII	–	+ Transient	+ Persistent	+	+
IFN-γ	+	+ Persistent	–	+	–
EGF	+	–	–	+	–
IFN-α	+	–	+	+	+

[a]Results are a summary of data presented in two recent publications *(51,55)*.

blocked platelet-activating factor-mediated PLC-γ phosphorylation and IP_3 formation. It has also been shown that Src, as well as Fyn, is rapidly activated by thrombin in fibroblasts *(58)*. To investigate the role of Src activity in VSMC, our group has performed two types of experiments. First, we electroporated a monoclonal anti-Src antibody into cultured VSMC and measured PLC-γ phosphorylation and IP_3 formation. In comparison to electroporation with purified IgG there was significantly greater inhibition of both signal events by the anti-Src antibody *(40)*. Second, we stimulated VSMC with AII and then immunoprecipitated Src. The activity of Src was then measured by both autophosphorylation and kinase activity toward enolase. Both assays demonstrated a two- to threefold increase in Src activity that peaked within 2 min of AII stimulation *(59)*. These findings demonstrate that Src activation is one of the earliest signal events stimulated by AII and strongly suggest that Src is the kinase responsible for tyrosine phosphorylation of PLC-γ. However, we could not demonstrate that Src was physically associated with the AT_1 receptor by immunoprecipitation. It is possible, therefore, that other signal molecules are required for the interaction of Src with the AT_1 receptor.

FAK

The AT_1 receptor also exhibits similarities to integrin receptors based on several recent studies *(60–62)*. Integrin-mediated signal transduction requires activation of the integrin receptor (e.g., $\alpha_2\beta_1$) by interactions with extracellular matrix ligands (e.g., fibronectin) and recruitment of intracellular kinases. Integrin activation leads to phosphorylation of a 125 kDa tyrosine kinase, shown to be localized to focal adhesions *(63)*, and termed FAK. Tyrosine phosphorylation of FAK appears to be the result of autophosphorylation, and activation occurs by unclear mechanisms. Autophosphorylation of FAK on tyrosine generates a site for binding of SH2-domain containing proteins and leads to recruitment and activation of Src-like protein kinases including Src itself, Fyn, and Csk *(64,65)*. The signal transduction particle consisting of FAK and a Src-like kinase then phosphorylates another focal adhesion protein, paxillin *(66)*. It has become clear that phosphorylation of FAK and paxillin in response to AII is one of the earliest and most prominent tyrosine phosphorylation events in VSMC *(60–62)*. The functional significance of this activation and the alterations in integrin signal remain unknown. However, the finding that Src may be recruited to integrins following FAK activation indicates that Src activation by the AT_1 receptor is indirect, and may involve an integrin-mediated mechanism.

RAF KINASE AND MAP KINASE PATHWAYS

One of the first molecules to be identified as being phosphorylated on tyrosine in response to AII was MAP kinase *(7,8)*. MAP kinases, encoded by the extracellular signal regulated kinase (ERK) genes, are serine/threonine protein kinases activated in response to a variety of extracellular stimuli involved in cell growth, transformation, and differentiation *(67)*. Activation of the p42 and p44 isoforms (ERK2 and ERK1, respectively) requires dual phosphorylation on a threonine and tyrosine residue found within the motif Thr-Glu-Tyr *(68)*. The in vivo substrates for MAP kinases are unknown; however, MAP kinases can phosphorylate a wide variety of proteins in vitro including the kinase that phosphorylates ribosomal S6 protein, $pp90^{rsk}$ *(69)*, cytosolic phospholipase A_2 *(70)*, the transcription factors c-*jun* and $p62^{TCF}$ (also called elk-1) *(71,72)*, and myelin basic protein *(73)*. AII rapidly and transiently stimulates the activity of the p42 and p44 isoforms of MAP kinase in VSMC as determined by phosphorylation of myelin basic protein *(7,8,74)*. The activation of MAP kinase by AII is partially dependent on PKC, as determined by prolonged exposure to phorbol ester *(8)*; however, a significant amount of MAP kinase activation by AII is PKC-independent (unpublished observation). These data suggest that, although separate pathways for MAP kinase and PKC may exist in VSMC, there is considerable crosstalk between the two pathways allowing for greater regulation of downstream events.

AII has also been shown to rapidly activate the kinase responsible for phosphorylation of MAP kinase, MAP kinase kinase, or MEK (MAP or ERK kinase) *(74,75)*. MEK is a unique protein kinase because it can phosphorylate both tyrosine and threonine residues on MAP kinase and is thus considered to be a dual specificity kinase *(76)*. Overexpression of a constitutively active MEK protein in NIH 3T3 cells stimulates mitogenesis and transformation *(77)*, indicating the importance of MAP kinase in the transduction of growth stimulatory signals. MEK is in turn regulated by serine phosphorylation by the Raf-1 kinase and/or the MEK kinase. Recently, Minden et al. *(78)* found that MEK kinase functions upstream of the Jun kinase (JNK, or stress-activated protein kinase [SAPK]) cascade involved in c-Jun phosphorylation rather than the MEK/MAP kinase cascade, suggesting that Raf-1 is the probable upstream regulator of MAP kinase.

AII stimulates the serine/threonine hyperphosphorylation of Raf-1 kinase in VSMC *(6)*. The serine/threonine kinase Raf is regulated by phosphorylation *(79)*, as well as by recruitment to the plasma membrane by the small molecular weight guanine-nucleotide-binding protein, p21ras *(80,81)*. The regulation of p21ras activity is complex, involving several adapter proteins and guanine-nucleotide exchange factors as demonstrated by analysis of the response to growth factors that utilize tyrosine kinase receptors (Fig. 5). In brief, growth factor binding stimulates autophosphorylation of the receptor, which then binds the SH2 domain of the adapter protein, Grb2 *(82)*. Grb2 is complexed to the guanine nucleotide exchange factor, mammalian son-of-sevenless (Sos), which then stimulates the exchange of GDP for GTP on p21ras *(83)*. Tyrosine kinase receptors, therefore, utilize tyrosine phosphorylation to connect receptor activation to the p21ras pathway. On the other hand, G-protein-coupled receptors, such as thrombin, lysophosphatidic acid (LPA), and m2 muscarinic agonists, lack intrinsic tyrosine kinase activity, yet have also been shown to activate p21ras *(84,85)*.

The mechanisms by which these G-protein-coupled receptors activate p21ras are unclear. Two nonexclusive mechanisms that appear likely are activation by G-protein

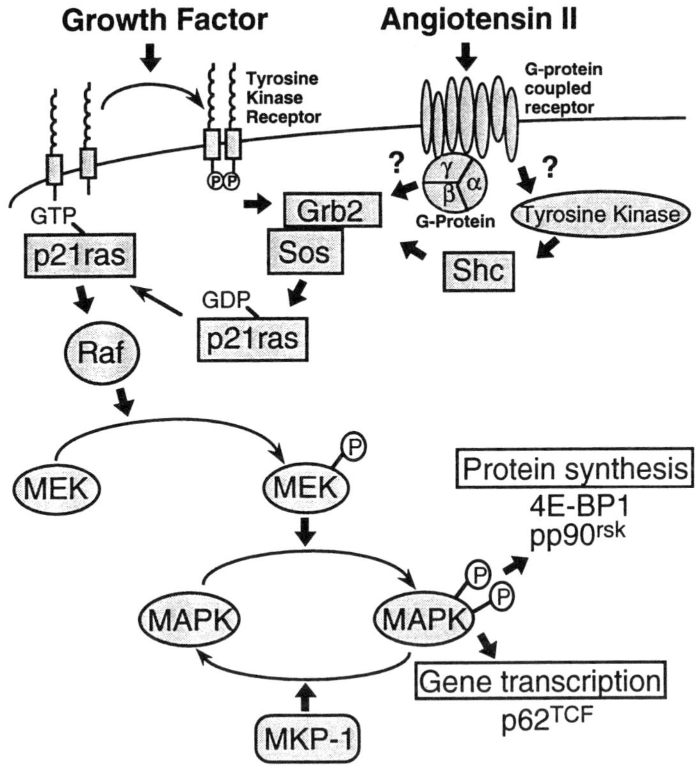

Fig. 5. Stimulation of the MAP kinase pathway by growth factors and AII in VSMC. Growth factor binding stimulates receptor dimerization and tyrosine phosphorylation via intrinsic tyrosine kinase activity. The linker protein Grb2 binds to the phosphorylated receptor via an SH2 domain and also binds to the guanine-nucleotide exchange factor Sos via SH3 domains. Sos stimulates the release of GDP for GTP on p21ras, which then recruits Raf kinase to the plasma membrane where it is then activated. Active Raf kinase phosphorylates and activates MEK, which can then phosphorylate and activate MAP kinase. Activated MAP kinase substrates include proteins involved in protein synthesis such as 4E-BP1 and $pp90^{rsk}$, as well as transcription factors such as $p62^{TCF}$. Dephosphorylation of MAP kinase occurs via the activity of MKP-1, whose expression is induced on growth factor activation. It is not known how AII, which binds to a G-protein-coupled receptor that lacks tyrosine kinase activity, feeds into the MAP kinase pathway. However, two possible mechanisms include binding of the G-protein βγ subunits via PH domains to the Grb2/Sos complex, or via the activity of a receptor-associated tyrosine kinase, which phosphorylates the linker protein Shc, which then interacts with the Grb2/Sos complex. From ref. *29* with permission.

βγ subunits, or by a receptor-associated tyrosine kinase (Fig. 5). Crespo et al. *(86)* found that overexpression of a βγ subunits in COS-7 cells stimulated the activity of MAP kinase that could be blocked by a dominant negative mutant of p21ras. Based on studies done with βARK, they hypothesized that the βγ dimer may bind to a pleckstrin-homology (PH) domain found on a p21ras regulatory protein linking heterotrimeric G-proteins to the p21ras pathway. A candidate p21ras regulatory protein, which contains a PH domain is Sos, which binds Grb2 via SH3 domains and p21ras via SH2 domains *(87)*. Alternatively, tyrosine phosphorylation of a linker protein called Shc may be the predominant mechanism utilized by AII *(88)*. For example, Shc is tyrosine phosphorylated in response to IL-2 receptor stimulation enabling it to act as the phosphorylated receptor and bind to

Grb2, thus linking the receptor to Grb2-Sos *(89,90)*. AII was recently shown to stimulate the tyrosine phosphorylation of Shc in cardiac fibroblasts *(91)*, and Shc was shown to serve as the docking protein for Grb2 in response to PDGF in VSMC *(92)*. We also have found that the tyrosine kinase inhibitor genistein inhibits MAP kinase activation and PLC-γ1 phosphorylation in response to AII, suggesting that a receptor-associated tyrosine kinase may link AII signaling through the AT_1 receptor to the p21ras/MAP kinase pathway (Fig. 5).

S6 KINASE AND STIMULATION OF PROTEIN SYNTHESIS

One of the most important actions of AII on VSMC is the stimulation of cell growth *(46,93)*. Substrates for MAP kinase include both nuclear proteins and cytosolic proteins involved in the initiation of DNA and protein synthesis. The serine/threonine protein kinase $pp90^{rsk}$ *(94)*, which phosphorylates the S6 ribosomal protein and stimulates protein synthesis, has been demonstrated to be a substrate for MAP kinase. AII has been shown to stimulate the phosphorylation of ribosomal S6 protein in VSMC within 30 min *(95)*. This early event may explain the rapid increase in protein synthesis stimulated by AII that precedes VSMC hypertrophy *(46,93)*. Another potential MAP kinase substrate involved in the initiation of the rate-limiting step in protein synthesis is the mRNA cap-binding protein eIF-4E *(96)*. This protein forms a complex with eIF-4A and p220 and binds mRNA to facilitate attachment of the ribosome *(97)*. The eIF-4E protein is phosphorylated in response to mitogenic stimuli *(98)*, resulting in partial enhancement of eIF-4E activity and initiation of translation. eIF-4E is also regulated by association with an inhibitory binding protein, 4E-BP1 (also known as PHAS-1) *(99)*. MAP kinase was recently shown to phosphorylate 4E-BP1 and stimulate the release of eIF-4E allowing it to interact with mRNA *(99)*. This phosphorylation event provides a direct link between growth factor receptor binding and protein synthesis (independent of new gene expression) via the MAP kinase pathway. The role of this pathway in AII stimulation of VSMC hypertrophy is not known; however, Rao et al. *(100)* recently showed that AII stimulates the serine phosphorylation of eIF-4E in VSMC.

SUMMARY

AII was initially identified by its physiologic ability to regulate salt and water metabolism, blood pressure, and vascular tone. However, as demonstrated in this chapter, AII may participate in a diversity of VSMC functions via its effects mediated by the AT_1 receptor. We propose that these functions, shown schematically in Table 2, may be mediated by activation of specific kinases. Although there is overlap and integration between the kinases and these cellular actions, we believe that this concept will be useful to guide future investigations into pathophysiological roles of the renin angiotensin system. Thus, functions related to growth and vasoconstriction (mediated by Src, PKC, Raf, and MAP kinases) would be important to investigate in hypertension, whereas functions related to inflammation and migration (mediated by JAK, TYK, Src, and FAK) might be more relevant to study in atherosclerosis. It is clear that future work will be required to determine the nature of the interactions among these different kinase pathways.

The concept that the AT_1 receptor acts as a multifunctional receptor is well illustrated by the complex nature of the regulation of c-*fos* expression by AII (Fig. 6). As discussed, AII induces c-*fos* mRNA expression rapidly in a PKC- and calcium-dependent fashion *(5)*. Regulation of c-*fos* gene expression may be controlled by at least four AII-stimulated

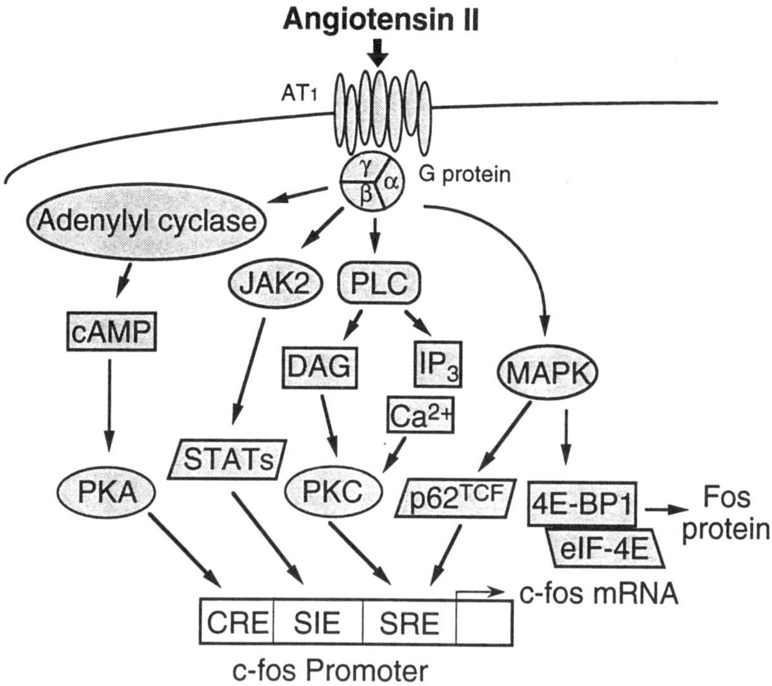

Fig. 6. Regulation of c-*fos* expression by AII. AII stimulates several pathways involved in the expression of the proto-oncogene c-*fos*. The c-*fos* promoter contains a CRE that is sensitive to PKA and cAMP. AII stimulates cAMP production in some cell types via the activity of adenylyl cyclase. The c-*fos* promoter also contains SIE that interacts with members of the STAT family of transcription factors. AII stimulates the phosphorylation and activity of Stat91 and Stat113 through the action of JAK2, thus providing a direct link between the AT_1 receptor and the nucleus. The SRE found on the c-*fos* promoter is also sensitive to PKC, which activated in the presence of DAG and Ca^{2+}. AII stimulates the activity of PLC, which releases DAG and IP_3, which releases Ca^{2+} from intracellular stores. AII also stimulates the activity of MAP kinase, whose substrates include the transcription factor $p62^{TCF}$, which forms a complex at the SRE also found on the c-*fos* promoter, and 4E-BP1, which releases the mRNA cap-binding protein eIF-4E to stimulate translation of c-*fos* mRNA. From ref. *29* with permission.

pathways based on our present knowledge of regulatory elements present in the c-*fos* promoter and the control of protein synthesis.

1. The c-*fos* promoter contains a cAMP/calcium response element (CRE), which has been shown to be regulated by protein kinase A *(101)*. It is likely that, in intact vessels, AII increases cAMP via its effects on prostaglandins *(102)*.
2. The c-*fos* promoter also contains the serum response element (SRE). Induction of the SRE occurs on formation of a ternary complex with serum response factor (SRF), ternary complex factor ($p62^{TCF}$), and the SRE *(103)*. Interestingly, MAP kinase was shown to phosphorylate $p62^{TCF}$ (also known as elk-1 or SAP-1) resulting in enhanced ternary complex formation *(72)*. Thus the SRE present in the c-*fos* promoter may be regulated by MAP kinase phosphorylation of $p62^{TCF}$ *(103)*.
3. A *sis*-inducing factor element (SIE) is present in the c-*fos* promoter and interacts with members of the STAT family of transcription factors (including Stat91 and Stat113) in a tissue- and hormone-specific manner *(51,101)*.

4. Initiation of c-*fos* protein expression may be controlled by AII-mediated regulation of the mRNA cap-binding protein, eIF-4E *(100)*.

Other early growth response genes, such as c-*jun* and collagenase, also contain a TPA-response element (TRE), which is sensitive to activators of PKC such as AII *(104)*. The diversity of signal transduction pathways stimulated by AII which lead to the expression of c-*fos* and other early growth response genes, demonstrate the ability of AII to act as a cytokine and regulate more general cellular functions.

It should be noted that this chapter has focused exclusively on kinases activated in VSMC in response to AII. There are also likely to be kinases inhibited by AII and phosphatases both stimulated and inhibited by AII. In particular, activation of phosphatases that "turn off" AII-mediated signal transduction is an important area for future study. We have shown that the MAP kinase phosphatase (MKP-1) is the dominant regulator of MAP kinase inactivation in response to AII in VSMC *(74)*. The nature of the phosphatases that regulate other components of the AII signaling pathways discussed remain unknown. In summary, there has been a dramatic increase in our understanding of AII signal transduction in VSMC since the cloning of the AT_1 receptor in 1991. Our challenge for the future is to develop new strategies for therapeutic intervention based on the expanding knowledge.

REFERENCES

1. Nakajima M, Mukoyama M, Pratt RE, Horiuchi M, Dzau VJ. Cloning of cDNA and analysis of the gene for mouse angiotensin II type 2 receptor. Biochem Biophys Res Commun 1993;197:393–399.
2. Griendling KK, Rittenhouse SE, Brock TA, Ekstein LS, Gimbrone MA Jr, Alexander RW. Sustained diacylglycerol formation from inositol phospholipids in angiotensin II-stimulated vascular smooth muscle cells. J Biol Chem 1986;261:5901–5906.
3. Brock TA, Alexander RW, Ekstein LS, Atkinson WJ, Gimbrone MA Jr. Angiotensin increases cytosolic free calcium in cultured vascular smooth muscle cells. Hypertension 1985;7:I105–I109.
4. Griendling KK, Tsuda T, Berk BC, Alexander RW. Angiotensin II stimulation of vascular smooth muscle. J Cardio Pharm 1989;14:S27–S33.
5. Taubman MB, Berk BC, Izumo S, Tsuda T, Alexander RW, Nadal-Ginard B. Angiotensin II induces c-fos mRNA in aortic smooth muscle. J Biol Chem 1989;264:526–530.
6. Molloy CJ, Taylor DS, Weber H. Angiotensin II stimulation of rapid protein tyrosine phosphorylation and protein kinase activation in rat aortic smooth muscle cells. J Biol Chem 1993;268:7338–7345.
7. Duff JL, Berk BC, Corson MA. Angiotensin II stimulates the pp44 and pp42 mitogen-activated protein kinases in cultured rat aortic smooth muscle cells. Biochem Biophys Res Commun 1992;188:257–264.
8. Tsuda T, Kawahara Y, Ishida Y, Koide M, Shii K, Yokoyama M. Angiotensin II stimulates two myelin basic protein/microtubule-associated protein 2 kinases in cultured vascular smooth muscle cells. Circ Res 1992;71:620–630.
9. Murphy TJ, Alexander RW, Griendling KK, Runge MS, Bernstein KE. Isolation of a cDNA encoding the vascular type-1 angiotensin II receptor. Nature 1991;351:233–236.
10. Sasaki K, Yamamo Y, Bardham S, Iwai N, Murray JJ, Hasegawa M, Matsuda Y, Inagami T. Cloning and expression of a complementary DNA encoding a bovine adrenal angiotensin type-1 receptor. Nature 1991;351:230–232.
11. Desarnaud F, Marie J, Lombard C, Larguier R, Seyer R, Lorca T, Jard S, Bonnafous JC. Deglycosylation and fragmentation of purified rat liver angiotensin II receptor: application to the mapping of hormone-binding domains. Biochem J 1993;289:289–297.
12. Ji H, Leung M, Zhang Y, Catt KJ, Sandberg K. Differential structural requirements for specific binding of nonpeptide and peptide antagonists to the AT1 angiotensin receptor. Identification of amino acid residues that determine binding of the antihypertensive drug losartan. J Biol Chem 1994;269:16,533–16,536.
13. Noda K, Saad Y, Kinoshita A, Boyle TP, Graham RM, Husain A, Karnik SS. Tetrazole and carboxylate groups of angiotensin receptor antagonists bind to the same subsite by different mechanisms. J Biol Chem 1995;270:2284–2289.

14. Bihoreau C, Monnot C, Davies E, Teutsch B, Bernstein KE, Corvol P, Clauser E. Mutation of Asp74 of the rat angiotensin II receptor confers changes in antagonist affinities and abolishes G-protein coupling. Proc Natl Acad Sci USA 1993;90:5133–5137.
15. Yamano Y, Ohyama K, Kikyo M, Sano T, Nakagomi Y, Inoue Y, Nakamura N, Morishima I, Guo DF, Hamakubo T, Inagami T. Mutagenesis and the molecular modeling of the rat angiotensin II receptor (AT1). J Biol Chem 1995;270:14,024–14,030.
16. Hjorth SA, Schambye HT, Greenlee WJ, Schwartz TW. Identification of peptide binding residues in the extracellular domains of the AT1 receptor. J Biol Chem 1994;269:30,953–30,959.
16a. Yamano Y, Ohyama K, Chaki S, Guo DF, Inagami T. Identification of amino acid residues of rat angiotensin II receptor for ligand binding by site directed mutagenesis. Biochem Biophys Res Commun 1992;187:1426–1431.
17. Marie J, Maigret B, Joseph MP, Larguier R, Nouet S, Lombard C, Bonnafous JC. Tyr292 in the seventh transmembrane domain of the AT1A angiotensin II receptor is essential for its coupling to phospholipase C. J Biol Chem 1994;269:20,815–20,818.
18. Ohyama K, Yamano Y, Chaki S, Kondo T, Inagami T. Domains for G-protein coupling in angiotensin II receptor type I: studies by site-directed mutagenesis. Biochem Biophys Res Commun 1992;189: 677–683.
19. Hunyady L, Bor M, Balla T, Catt KJ. Critical role of a conserved intramembrane tyrosine residue in angiotensin II receptor activation. J Biol Chem 1995;270:9702–9705.
20. Moffett S, Mouillac B, Bonin H, Bouvier M. Altered phosphorylation and desensitization patterns of a human beta 2-adrenergic receptor lacking the palmitoylated Cys341. EMBO J 1993;12:349–356.
21. Kennedy MF, Limbird LE. Mutations of the alpha 2A-adrenergic receptor that eliminate detectable palmitoylation do not perturb receptor-G-protein coupling. J Biol Chem 1993;268:8003–8011.
22. Lefkowitz RJ, Inglese J, Koch WJ, Pitcher J, Attramadal H, Caron MG. G-protein coupled receptors: regulatory role of receptor kinases and arrestin proteins. Cold Spring Harb Symp Quant Biol 1992;57:127–133.
23. Paxton WG, Marrero MB, Klein JD, Delafontaine P, Berk BC, Bernstein KE. The angiotensin II AT_1 receptor is tyrosine and serine phosphorylated and can serve as a substrate for the src family of tyrosine kinases. Biochem. Biophys Res Commun 1994;200:260–267.
24. Kai H, Griendling KK, Lassegue B, Ollerenshaw JD, Runge MS, Alexander RW. Agonist-induced phosphorylation of the vascular type 1 angiotensin II receptor. Hypertension 1994;24:523–527.
25. Eason MG, Moreira SP, Liggett SB. Four consecutive serines in the third intracellular loop are the sites for beta-adrenergic receptor kinase-mediated phosphorylation and desensitization of the alpha 2A-adrenergic receptor. J Biol Chem 1995;270:4681–4688.
26. Hunyady L, Baukal AJ, Balla T, Catt KJ. Independence of type I angiotensin II receptor endocytosis from G protein coupling and signal transduction. J Biol Chem 1994;269:24,798–24,804.
27. Pitcher J, Touhara K, Payne E, Lefkowitz R. Pleckstrin homology domain-mediated membrane association and activation of the β-adrenergic receptor kinase requires cocoordinate interaction with $G_{\beta\gamma}$ subunits and lipid. J Biol Chem 1995;270:11,707–11,710.
28. Hunyady L, Bor M, Balla T, Catt KJ. Identification of a cytoplasmic Ser-Thr-Leu motif that determines agonist-induced internalization of the AT1 angiotensin receptor. J Biol Chem 1994; 269:31,378–31,382.
29. Marrero MB, Schieffer B, Paxton WG, Duff JL, Berk BC, Bernstein KB. The role of tyrosine phosphorylation in angiotensin II mediated intracellular signalling. Cardiovasc Res 1995;30:530–536.
30. Pascal SM, Singer AU, Gish G, Yamazaki T, Shoelson SE, Pawson T, Kay LE, Forman KJD. Nuclear magnetic resonance structure of an SH2 domain of phospholipase C-gamma 1 complexed with a high affinity binding peptide. Cell 1994;77:461–472.
31. Fantl WJ, Johnson DE, Williams LT. Signalling by receptor tyrosine kinases. Annu Rev Biochem 1993;62:453–481.
32. Lassegue B, Alexander RW, Clark M, Akers M, Griendling KK. Phosphatidylcholine is a major source of phosphatidic acid and diacylglycerol in angiotensin II-stimulated vascular smooth muscle cells. Biochem J 1993;292:509–517.
33. Rhee SG, Choi KD. Regulation of inositol phospholipid-specific phospholipase C isozymes. J Biol Chem 1992;267:12,393–12,396.
34. Smrcka AV, Hepler JR, Brown KO, Sternweis PC. Regulation of polyphosphoinositide-specific phospholipase C activity by purified Gq. Science 1991;251:804–807.
35. Taylor SJ, Chae HZ, Rhee SG, Exton JH. Activation of the beta 1 isozyme of phospholipase C by alpha subunits of the Gq class of G proteins. Nature 1991;350:516–578.

36. Kim HK, Kim JW, Zilberstein A, Margolis B, Kim JG, Schlessinger J, Rhee SG. PDGF stimulation of inositol phospholipid hydrolysis requires PLC-gamma 1 phosphorylation on tyrosine residues 783 and 1254. Cell 1991;65:435–441.
37. Homma Y, Sakamoto H, Tsunoda M, Aoki M, Takenawa T, Ooyama T. Evidence for involvement of phospholipase C-gamma 2 in signal transduction of platelet-derived growth factor in vascular smooth-muscle cells. Biochem J 1993;290:649–653.
38. Kato H, Fukami K, Shibasaki F, Homma Y, Takenawa T. Enhancement of phospholipase C delta 1 activity in the aortas of spontaneously hypertensive rats. J Biol Chem 1992; 267:6483–6487.
39. Marrero MB, Paxton WB, Duff JL, Berk BC, Bernstein KE. Angiotensin II stimulates tyrosine phosphorylation of phospholipase C-γ1 in vascular smooth muscle cells. J Biol Chem 1994;269:10,935–10,939.
40. Marrero MB, Schieffer B, Bernstein KE. Electroporation of pp60$^{c\text{-}src}$ antibodies inhibits the angiotensin II activation of phospholipase C-γ1 in rat aortic smooth muscle cells. J Biol Chem 1995;270: 15,734–15,738.
41. Hug H, Sarre TF. Protein kinase C isoenzymes: divergence in signal transduction? Biochem J 1993;291:329–343.
42. Tsuda T, Alexander RW. Angiotensin II stimulates phosphorylation of nuclear lamins via a protein kinase C-dependent mechanism in cultured vascular smooth muscle cells. J Biol Chem 1990;265:1165–1170.
43. Lang U, Vallotton MB. Effects of angiotensin II and of phorbol ester on protein kinase C activity and on prostacyclin production in cultured rat aortic smooth-muscle cells. Biochem J 1989;259: 477–484.
44. Haller H, Quass P, Lindschau C, Luft FC, Distler A. Platelet-derived growth factor and angiotensin II induce different spatial distribution of protein kinase C-α and -β in vascular smooth muscle cells. Hypertension 1994;23:848–852.
45. Tsuda T, Griendling KK, Ollerenshaw JD, Lassegue B, Alexander RW. Angiotensin II- and endothelin-induced protein phosphorylation in cultured vascular smooth muscle cells. J Vasc Res 1993;30:241–249.
46. Berk BC, Vekshtein V, Gordon HM, Tsuda T. Angiotensin II-stimulated protein synthesis in cultured vascular smooth muscle cells. Hypertension 1989;13:305–314.
47. Berk BC, Aranow MS, Brock TA, Cragoe EJ, Gimbrone MAJ. Angiotensin II-stimulated Na^+/H^+ exchange in cultured vascular smooth muscle cells. J Biol Chem 1987;262:5057–5064.
48. Bernstein KE. Molecular analysis of the renin-angiotensin system. Semin Nephrol 1992; 12:524–530.
49. Huckle WR, Prokop CA, Dy RC, Herman B, Earp S. Angiotensin II stimulates protein-tyrosine phosphorylation in a calcium-dependent manner. Mol Cell Biol 1990;10:6290–6298.
50. Huckle WR, Dy RC, Earp HS. Calcium-dependent increase in tyrosine kinase activity stimulated by angiotensin II. Proc Natl Acad Sci USA 1992;89:8837–8841.
51. Bhat GJ, Thekkumkara TJ, Thomas WG, Conrad KM, Baker KM. Angiotensin II stimulates sis-inducing factor-like DNA binding activity. J Biol Chem 1994; 269:31,443–31,449.
52. Darnell JEJ, Kerr IM, Stark GR. Jak-STAT pathways and transcriptional activation in response to IFNs and other extracellular signaling proteins. Science 1994;264:1415–1421.
53. Ruff-Jamison S, Chen K, Cohen S. Induction by EGF and interferon-gamma of tyrosine phosphorylated DNA binding proteins in mouse liver nuclei. Science 1993;261:1733–1736.
54. Ihle JN, Witthuhn BA, Quelle FW, Yamamoto K, Thierfelder WE, Kreider B, Silvennoinen O. Signaling by the cytokine receptor superfamily: JAKs and STATs. Trends Biochem Sci 1994;19:222–227.
55. Marrero MB, Schieffer B, Paxton WG, Heerdt L, Berk BC, Delafontaine P, Bernstein KE. Direct stimulation of Jak/STAT pathway by the angiotensin II AT1 receptor. Nature 1995;375:247–250.
56. Rodriguez-Linares B, Watson SP. Phosphorylation of JAK2 in thrombin-stimulated human platelets. FEBS Lett 1994;352:335–338.
57. Dhar A, Shukla SD. Electrotransjection of pp60v-src monoclonal antibody inhibits activation of phospholipase C in platelets. A new mechanism for platelet-activating factor responses. J Biol Chem 1994;269:9123–9127.
58. Chen YH, Pouysségur J, Courtneidge SA, Van Obberghen-Schilling E. Activation of Src family kinase activity by the G protein-coupled thrombin receptor in growth-responsive fibroblasts. J Biol Chem 1994;269:27,372–27,377.
59. Ishida M, Marrero MB, Schieffer B, Ishida T, Bernstein KE, Berk BC. Angiotensin II activates pp60$^{c\text{-}src}$ in vascular smooth muscle cells. Circ Res 1995;77:1053–1059.
60. Polte TR, Naftilan AJ, Hanks SK. Focal adhesion kinase is abundant in developing blood vessels and elevation of its phosphotyrosine content in vascular smooth muscle cells is a rapid response to angiotensin II. J Cell Biochem 1994;55:106–119.

61. Leduc I, Meloche S. Angiotensin II stimulates tyrosine phosphorylation of the focal adhesion-associated protein paxillin in aortic smooth muscle cells. J Biol Chem 1995;270:4401–4404.
62. Turner CE, Pietras KM, Taylor DS, Molloy CJ. Angiotensin II stimulation of rapid paxillin tyrosine phosphorylation correlates with the formation of focal adhesions in rat aortic smooth muscle cells. J Cell Sci 1995;108:333–342.
63. Schaller MD, Hildebrand JD, Shannon JD, Fox JW, Vines RR, Parsons JT. Autophosphorylation of the focal adhesion kinase, pp125FAK, directs SH2-dependent binding of pp60src. Mol Cell Biol 1994;14:1680–1688.
64. Sabe H, Hata A, Okada M, Nakagawa H, Hanafusa H. Analysis of the binding of the Src homology 2 domain of Csk to tyrosine-phosphorylated proteins in the suppression and mitotic activation of c-Src. Proc Natl Acad Sci USA 1994;91:3984–3988.
65. Yamaguchi R, Maki M, Hatanaka M, Sabe H. Unphosphorylated and tyrosine-phosphorylated forms of a focal adhesion protein, paxillin, are substrates for calpain II in vitro: implications for the possible involvement of calpain II in mitosis-specific degradation of paxillin. FEBS Lett 1994; 356:114–116.
66. Burridge K, Turner CE, Romer LH. Tyrosine phosphorylation of paxillin and $pp125^{FAK}$ accompanies cell adhesion to extracellular matrix: a role in cytoskeletal assembly. J Cell Biol 1992;119:893–903.
67. Boulton TG, Nye SH, Robbins DJ, Ip NY, Radziejewska E, Morgenbesser SD, DePinho RA, Panayotatos N, Cobb MH, Yancopoulos GD. ERKs: a family of protein-serine/threonine kinases that are activated and tyrosine phosphorylated in response to insulin and NGF. Cell 1991;65:663–675.
68. Payne DM, Rossomando AJ, Martino P, Erikson AK, Her J-H, Shadanowitz J, Hunt DF, Weber MJ, Sturgill TW. Identification of the regulatory phosphorylation sites in pp42/mitogen-activated protein kinase (MAP kinase). EMBO J 1991;10:885–892.
69. Sturgill TW, Ray BL, Erikson E, Maller JL. Insulin-stimulated MAP-2 kinase phosphorylates protein S6 kinase II. Nature 1988;334:715–718.
70. Lin LL, Wartman M, Lin AY, Knopr JL, Seth A, Davis RJ. $cPLA_2$ is phosphorylated and activated by MAP kinase. Cell 1993;72:269–278.
71. Paxton WG, Runge M, Horaist C, Cohen C, Alexander RW, Bernstein KE. Immunohistochemical localization of rat angiotensin II AT1 receptor. Am J Physiol 1993;264:F989–F995.
72. Gille H, Sharrocks AD, Shaw PE. Phosphorylation of transcription factor $p62^{TCF}$ by MAP kinase stimulates ternary complex formation at c-*fos* promoter. Nature 1992;358:414–417.
73. Ahn NG, Seger R, Bratlien RL, Diltz CD, Tonks NK, Krebs EG. Multiple components in an epidermal growth factor-stimulated protein kinase cascade. J Biol Chem 1991;266:4220–4227.
74. Duff JL, Monia BP, Berk BC. Mitogen-activated protein (MAP) kinase is regulated by the MAP kinase phosphatase (MKP-1) in vascular smooth muscle cells. J Biol Chem 1995;270:7161–7166.
75. Ishida Y, Kawahara Y, Tsuda T, Yokoyama M. Involvement: of MAP kinase activators in angiotensin II-induced activation of MAP kinases in cultured vascular smooth muscle cells. FEBS Lett 1992;310:41–45.
76. Crews CM, Alessandrini A, Erickson RL. The primary structure of MEK, a protein kinase that phosphorylates the ERK gene product. Science 1992;258:478–480.
77. Cowley S, Paterson H, Kemp P, Marshall CJ. Activation of MAP kinase kinase is necessary and sufficient for PC12 differentiation and for transformation of NIH 3T3 cells. Cell 1994;77:841–852.
78. Minden A, Lin A, McMahon M, Lange-Carter C, Dérijard B, Davis RJ, Johnson GL, Karin M. Differential activation of ERK and JNK mitogen-activated protein kinases by Raf-1 and MEKK. Science 1994;266:1719–1723.
79. Daum G, Eisenmann-Tappe I, Fries H-W, Troppmair J, Rapp UR. The ins and outs of Raf kinases. Trends Biochem Sci 1994;19:474–480.
80. Leevers SJ, Paterson HF, Marshall CJ. Requirement for Ras in Raf activation is overcome by targeting Raf to the plasma membrane. Nature 1994;369:411–414.
81. Stokoe D, MacDonald SG, Cadwallader K, Symons M, Hancock JF. Activation of Raf as a result of recruitment to the plasma membrane. Science 1994;264:1463–1467.
82. Lowenstein EJ, Daly RJ, Betzer AG, Li W, Margolis B, Lammers R, Ullrich A, Skolnik EY, Bar-Sagi D, Schlessinger J. The SH2 and SH3 domain-containing protein GRB2 links receptor tyrosine kinases to ras signalling. Nature 1992;70:431–442.
83. McCormick F. Activators and effectors of ras p21 proteins. Curr Opin Genet Dev 1994;4:71–76.
84. van-Corven EJ, Hordijk PL, Medema RH, Bos JL, Moolenaar WH. Pertussis toxin-sensitive activation of p21ras by G protein-coupled receptor agonists in fibroblasts. Proc Natl Acad Sci USA 1993;90: 1257–1261.

85. Winitz S, Russell M, Qian N-X, Gardner A, Dwyer L, Johnson GL. Involvement of ras and raf in the G_i-coupled acetylcholine muscarininc m2 receptor activation of mitogen-activated protein (MAP) kinase kinase and MAP kinase. J Biol Chem 1993;268:19,196–19,199.
86. Crespo P, Xu N, Simonds WF, Gutkind JS. Ras-dependent activation of MAP kinase pathway mediated by G-protein beta gamma subunits. Nature 1994:369(6479):418–420.
87. Buday L, Downward J. Epidermal growth factor regulates p21ras through the formation of a complex of receptor, Grb2 adapter protein, and Sos nucleotide exchange factor. Cell 1993;73:611–620.
88. Bernstein KE, Shai SY, Howard T, Balogh R, Frenzel K, Langford K. Structure and regulated expression of angiotensin-converting enzyme and the receptor for angiotensin II. Am J Kidney Dis 1993;21:53–57.
89. Ravichandran KS, Lee KK, Songyang Z, Cantley LC, Burn P, Burakoff SJ. Interaction of Shc with the Z-chain of the T cell receptor upon T cell activation. Science 1993; 262:902–904.
90. Rozakis-Adcock M, McGlade J, Mbamalu G, Pelicci G, Daly R, Li W, Batzer A, Thomas S, Brugge J, Pelicci PG, Schlessinger J, Pawson T. Association of the Shc and Grb2/Sem5 SH2-containing proteins is implicated in activation of the Ras pathway by tyrosine kinases. Nature 1992;360:689–692.
91. Schorb W, Peeler TC, Madigan NN, Conrad KM, Baker KM. Angiotensin II-induced protein tyrosine phosphorylation in neonatal rat cardiac fibroblasts. J Biol Chem 1994;269:19,626–19,632.
92. Howard T, Balogh R, Overbeek P, Bernstein KE. Sperm-specific expression of angiotensin-converting enzyme (ACE) is mediated by a 91-base-pair promoter containing a CRE-like element. Mol Cell Biol 1993;13:18–27.
93. Geisterfer AAT, Peach MJ, Owens GK. Angiotensin II induces hypertrophy, not hyperplasia, of cultured rat aortic smooth muscle cells. Circ Res 1988;62:749–756.
94. Sturgill TW, Wu J. Recent progress in characterization of protein kinase cascades for phosphorylation of ribosomal protein S6. Biochem Biophys Acta 1991;1092:350–357.
95. Scott-Burden T, Resink TJ, Baur U, Burgin M, Buhler FR. Activation of S6 kinase in cultured vascular smooth muscle cells by submitogenic levels of thrombospondin. Biochem Biophys Res Commun 1988;150:278–286.
96. Rhoads RE. Protein synthesis, cell growth and oncogenesis. Curr Opin Cell Biol 1991;3:1019–1024.
97. Hershey JW. Translational control in mammalian cells. Annu Rev Biochem 1991;60:717–755.
98. Joshi-Barve S, Rychlik W, Rhoads RE. Alteration of the major phosphorylation site of eukaryotic protein synthesis initiation factor 4E prevents its association with the 48 S initiation complex. J Biol Chem 1990;265:2979–2983.
99. Lin T-A, Kong X, Haystead TAJ, Pause A, Belsham G, Sonenberg N, Lawrence JCJ. PHAS-1 as a link between mitogen-activated protein kinase and translation initiation. Science 1994;266:653–656.
100. Rao GN, Greindling K, Fredrickson RM, Sonenberg N, Alexander RW. Angiotensin II induces phosphorylation of eukaryotic protein synthesis initiation factor 4E in vascular smooth muscle cells. J Biol Chem 1994;269(10):7180–7184.
101. Wagner BJ, Hayes TE, Hoban CJ, Cochran BH. The SIF binding element confers sis/PDGF inducibility onto the c-fos promoter. EMBO J 1990;9:4477–4484.
102. Alexander RW, Gimbrone MAJ. Stimulation of prostaglandin E synthesis in cultured human umbilical vein smooth muscle cells. Proc Natl Acad Sci USA 1976;73:1617–1620.
103. Herrera RE, Shaw PE, Nordheim A. Occupation of the c-fos serum response element in vivo by a multiprotein complex is unaltered by growth factor induction. Nature 1989;340:68–70.
104. Delafontaine P, Lou H, Harrison DG, Bernstein KE. Sequence of a cDNA encoding dog insulin-like growth factor I. Gene 1993;130:305,306.

15 The Vascular Renin System

Peter Eggena, PHD *and Jack D. Barrett,* PHD

CONTENTS

INTRODUCTION

In the classical endocrine renin–angiotensin system (RAS), renin secreted from the kidney cleaves hepatic angiotensinogen in the circulation to launch a cascade of angiotensin peptides including angiotensin (A) I, II, and III. AII, the most prominent of these peptide hormones, initiates through specific plasma membrane receptors, a host of physiological actions ranging from vasoconstriction to volume and growth regulation *(1–4)*. Circulating plasma levels of renin and/or AII do not always correlate with their purported functions *(5,6)*, because of inaccuracies of renin and/or AII measurements, or not considering the sodium status *(7)*. Studies with angiotensin-converting enzyme (ACE) inhibitors, and more recently with specific AII receptor antagonists, have demonstrated that even when the circulating levels are low, AII remains a major regulator of many biological responses, including blood pressure *(8)*.

A recent hypothesis suggests that the circulating picomolar levels of AII are augmented by tissue-generated AII to attain the nanomolar concentrations required by the plasma membrane receptor *(9)* to initiate physiological responses (Fig. 1). Certain tissues are able to release AII *(10,11)*, but the source of the components responsible for local AII generation remains controversial. Regarding renin system precursors, three broad and often opposing opinions have evolved:

1. Local or tissue AII generation is mediated exclusively by plasma-derived renin and angiotensinogen, with participation of locally synthesized ACE;
2. All components required for AII production are of local origin; and
3. Local generation of AII comprises a combination of locally synthesized and plasma-derived components.

Mechanisms that regulate local AII remain to be resolved. Another unresolved topic is whether renin system components are compartmentalized, either within the cell *(12)*

From: *Contemporary Endocrinology: Endocrinology of the Vasculature*
Edited by: J. R. Sowers Humana Press Inc., Totowa, NJ

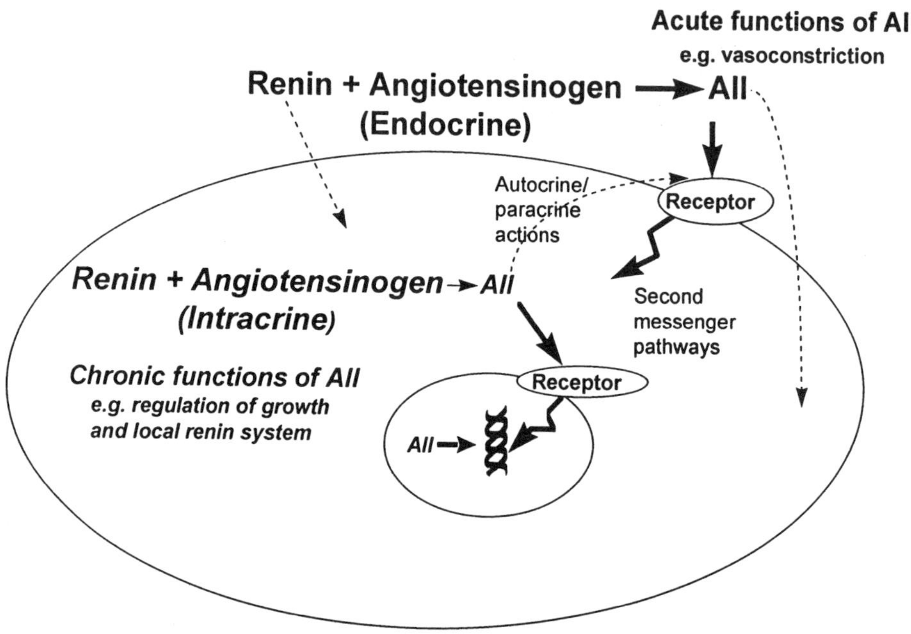

Fig. 1. A proposed model for the interrelationship of the endocrine and intracrine renin systems in the vasculature. The diagram depicts a vascular smooth muscle cell exposed to both the intracrine (italics) and endocrine (normal) renin systems. Solid arrows indicate documented pathways of AII actions, dotted arrows, postulated pathways; broken arrows indicate AII actions via second messenger pathways.

or within particular types of cells, such that component transport is required to initiate AII generation. That blockade of AII generation results in reversal of AII-related pathophysiological manifestations suggests that local renin systems have the ability to generate AII.

A wide variety of disciplines including biochemistry, pharmacology, molecular biology, physiology, and immunology have been employed to address the questions of source and regulation of local renin system components. Potential tissue renin systems have been identified in such diverse tissues as the adrenal *(13)*, heart *(14–17)*, brain *(18–20)*, kidney *(21–23)*, and vascular wall *(24–26)*. This chapter focuses on AII generation in vascular tissue. Initially, studies concerning local synthesis of components of the renin system are addressed, followed by a discussion of potential functions for AII generated within the vascular wall.

RENIN ANGIOTENSIN SYSTEM COMPONENTS IN VASCULAR TISSUE

Renin

In the classical endocrine RAS, renin is considered to originate primarily from juxtaglomerular cells of the kidney *(27,28)*. However, as early as 1964, physical chemical and immunological studies provided evidence for extrarenal sources of renin in such tissues as brain *(20)* and the vasculature *(29–31)*. Application of techniques for quantitation of renin mRNA in vascular tissue provided evidence for renin synthesis within the vascular wall *(32)*. Although some investigators have readily measured vascular renin mRNA by solution or slot blot hybridization *(21)*, others have required amplification techniques to detect its presence *(33)*.

In renal juxtaglomerular cells, posttranslational processing of the enzyme renin proceeds through a constitutive pathway by which the renin precursor prorenin is released *(34)* and a regulated pathway through which active renin is stored and then secreted *(35,36)*. Similar renin processing pathways or renin storage have not been observed in vascular tissue. Although certain isolated tissue enzymes are known to cleave prorenin to generate the active enzyme, their physiological relevance in the vascular wall has yet to be determined *(37–39)*. Active renin has been detected in cultured vascular smooth muscle cells (VSMC) *(40)*, though it has yet to be established whether the enzyme is locally synthesized or sequestered from culture media. Several studies have suggested that vascular renin may be of renal origin. For example, vascular renin activity correlates well with the plasma level of the enzyme *(41–43)* and diminishes following bilateral nephrectomy *(32)*. Infused renin has also been reported to increase vascular renin activity and have a longer half-life in vascular tissue than in the circulation *(32)*. A recent report of intracellular renin transport proteins confirms the notion that vascular renin can be sequestered from the plasma *(44)*; similar conclusions have been presented by others *(45)*. These data suggest that binding of plasma renin to vascular tissue accounts for a portion of vascular renin activity, and the binding mechanism is more complex than simple equilibration. In summary, renin is present in the vascular wall, but further studies are required to delineate the local versus peripheral origin of the enzyme and to determine their relative contribution to local AI formation.

Angiotensinogen

Early studies using physical, chemical, and immunological techniques reported the presence of angiotensinogen in vascular tissues. There are differences in the isoelectric focusing patterns of vascular and plasma angiotensinogen *(31)*, reflecting mainly altered glycosylation. This observation and failure of tissue angiotensinogen to crossreact with antibodies generated against plasma counterpart suggest an origin other than the circulation. The angiotensinogen content of rat aorta can be elevated by central infusion of glucocorticoids such as dexamethasone without changes in the plasma level of the protein *(19)*. Subsequent studies documented that cultured VSMC release angiotensinogen into culture medium *(46)*; however, little protein was detected within VSMC. This in vitro release is modulated by addition of angiotensinogen stimulating and suppressing factors, providing further support for local synthesis and local control of angiotensinogen production within the vascular wall *(46)*. Further support for local synthesis has been derived from reports demonstrating the presence of angiotensinogen mRNA in endothelial, VSMC, and fat cells *(47–49)*. In addition, vascular angiotensinogen mRNA can be modulated by chronic in vivo administration of either recombinant human erythropoietin (rhEPO) *(21)*, or varying dietary salt intake *(50)*.

Thus, angiotensinogen, as well as renin, is present and synthesized locally within the vascular wall. Whether, under physiological conditions, plasma angiotensinogen of hepatic origin also contributes to VSMC angiotensinogen concentration, and hence participates in the regulation of local AI or AII generation, remains to be fully explored. Intracellular levels of angiotensinogen, however, may not be influenced by the plasma level of the protein. Although no specific study with vascular cells has been reported, isolated pituitary cells cultured in the presence of radiolabeled angiotensinogen failed to demonstrate uptake of this protein *(51)*.

ACE

Presence of ACE and its mRNA in the vessel wall have been demonstrated by both in vitro and in vivo studies *(52)*. Vascular ACE has also been reported to be stimulated by dexamethasone *(53)*. Although ACE is present within VSMC *(54)*, the vast majority appears to be located on the luminal surface of the endothelium *(52)*. This observation suggests that local formation of AII from AI is primarily extracellular. Experiments with isolated perfused rat hindquarter have revealed AII release from tissue and alternately AI release when perfusion is conducted in the presence of ACE inhibitors *(10)*. These results confirm the involvement of vascular ACE in the generation of local AII formation. However, if AII is generated mainly within the extracellular matrix, it may be hydrolyzed or bound to AII receptors in the immediate vicinity, with no indication of its presence in the circulation. The importance of endothelial-derived ACE to the regulation of local AII generation, therefore, may be directly related to the source of AI. Extracellular generation of AI by plasma-derived components may be regulated by this endothelial enzyme. On the other hand, if intracellular AI generation is predominant at the vascular wall (i.e., VSMC), the relative importance of endothelial ACE may be minimal. In summary, local origin of ACE and generation of AII in the vasculature is evident, but it remains to be determined whether ACE is a necessary component for AII generation under all physiological conditions.

AII Generation by Nonrenin Enzymes

In tissues, unlike plasma, proteases other than renin cleave angiotensinogen and directly generate AII, thereby overcoming the need for either renin or ACE. These tissue enzymes, because of their low pH optima, were thought to have little physiological significance until the recent development of effective AII receptor antagonists. For example, AII actions can often be suppressed by receptor antagonists, but not by ACE inhibitors *(55)* indicating AII generation in the absence of ACE. Similarly, ACE inhibition does not always prevent AII generation in tissue, whereas general peptidase inhibitors effectively block AII formation *(52)*. Tonin was the first tissue enzyme in this class reported to directly generate AII from angiotensinogen *(56)*. Direct generation of AII from angiotensinogen by other proteolytic tissue enzymes such as cathepsins *(33)* and from AI by chymases, which are not effected by ACE inhibitors, are undergoing investigation *(57)*. Chronic ACE inhibition stimulates carboxypeptidases, which generate AII from AI via the 1–9 angiotensin intermediate *(58)*. AII can also be generated from synthetic renin substrate (tetradecapeptide) in the perfused rat hindquarter *(59)*. This generation is apparently independent of renin; since no cleavage of angiotensinogen occurs, the renin inhibitor pepstatin does not prevent AI or AII generation, and bilateral nephrectomy does not decrease contraction induced by the synthetic substrate. The physiological relevance of these alternate AII pathways to the overall generation of AII in the vascular wall requires further study.

Potential Functions of the Vascular Tissue Renin System

It is apparent that many fundamental questions remain regarding the presence and biochemistry of a "vascular renin system," despite the fact that vascular tissue has the ability to locally generate AII. Thus, it may be more fruitful to focus on the ability of the vasculature to generate AII, irrespective of the biochemical pathway, and then explore the physiological significance of the system(s).

Isolated tissues (e.g., rat hindquarter) release AII into the perfusion medium *(10,11)*, ACE inhibition leads to an accumulation of AI and suppression of AII *(10)*, indicating that the released AII is not sequestered from the plasma compartment, but is of local origin *(60)*. Local or tissue release of AII is also supported by the finding that long-term bilaterally nephrectomized subjects often exhibit significant levels of plasma AII *(61,62)*, and cardiomyocytes have been reported to generate nanogram quantities of AII from as few as 10^6 cells *(15)*. Opinions range from the idea that the majority of circulating plasma AII is of tissue origin *(63)*, to the opposite that under physiologic conditions, only a small portion of the circulating peptide is derived from the tissue system *(64)*.

Actions of AII at the Plasma Membrane

Support of a functional role for tissue-generated AII comes primarily from in vivo experiments in which plasma renin activity or concentration is either normal or low, and a pathophysiological condition is reversed by either ACE inhibitors or AII receptor antagonists. Examples include blood pressure reduction by ACE inhibitors in the two kidney, one clip Goldblatt model of hypertension *(65)*, and in the spontaneously hypertensive rat (SHR) *(66)*. Similar reductions of blood pressure are not evident in the normal animal when equivalent doses of ACE inhibitors are administered *(67)*. That both of these hypertensive animal models also exhibit elevated levels of aortic renin activity suggests that suppression of nonplasma AII generating systems may be responsible for lowering the blood pressure. Corroborating evidence that elevated tissue renin activity contributes to hypertension is the observation that β-blockers reduce aortic renin activity in the SHR, but only in those animals that respond with a lowering of blood pressure (unpublished results). The importance of tissue renin systems to blood pressure elevation is also seen in another model, where elevation of aortic angiotensinogen levels, induced by administration of rhEPO *(21)*, leads to a parallel increase in blood pressure. Again, no concomitant change in the plasma renin activity is observed, and ACE inhibition prevents the rise in blood pressure. Further support for a functional tissue renin system is gained from the reports that cardiac hypertrophy is reduced by blockade of AII formation with ACE inhibitors under conditions in which blood pressure is not changed, and the activity of the plasma renin system is normal *(68,69)*. That elevated blood pressure in the SHR is reversed by administration of angiotensinogen antisense mRNA *(70)* seems pertinent to the vascular renin system since no concomitant changes in the plasma level of the protein are observed. Probably the most direct evidence for a functional tissue renin system is the transgenic rat model in which an additional mouse renin gene is expressed in a variety of tissues leading to fulminating hypertension *(71)*. Again, plasma renin levels are normal, and the development of hypertension is suppressed by ACE inhibitors.

Since there are no known storage reservoirs for renin system components or AII within the vasculature, functions of AII requiring a rapid response (i.e., vasoconstriction) are probably regulated by the endocrine renin system *(72)*. For example, rapid release of renin from the kidney can fulfill the demand for AngII to prevent a fall in blood pressure in response to hemorrhage. The more chronic requirements for AII may well be regulated via the tissue renin systems *(72)* (e.g., for cellular homeostasis) or development of hypertrophy or hyperplasia. However, whether AII at the cellular level acts solely to regulate these factors indirectly via modulation of gene transcription, or has direct effects is not presently known *(73)*. Alternately, even if tissue-generated AII is merely constitutively released, it may provide the basal or subthreshold level in the vicinity of the receptor and thereby make the vascular AII response significantly more sensitive to modulations in the circulating levels of this hormone. Thus, plasma and locally synthesized AII both acting at the plasma membrane, provide a solution to the enigma that circulating levels of AII alone are generally too low to elicit or sustain a meaningful physiological response *(9)*. Although the relative contributions of plasma-derived and tissue- or intracellular-generated AII to the actions of AII at plasma membrane receptors remains to be established, because of AII's short intracellular half-life *(74)*, and the comparatively large quantities released from vascular tissue both in vitro and in vivo, a significant fraction may well be of local origin.

Intracellular AII Functions

An alternative to the notion that locally synthesized AII performs a supportive function at plasma membrane AII receptors, locally generated AII may regulate more chronic physiological functions via nuclear AII receptors *(75)*. In this case, elevation of intracellular AII may not be apparent from an examination limited to the plasma renin system measurements. Indeed, nuclei isolated from aortic tissue exhibit AII receptors (unpublished data) similar to those reported for hepatocytes *(75)*. In the latter cells, AII binding to nuclear receptors modulates expression of renin and angiotensinogen mRNA in a biphasic manner, stimulation at low ($10^{-9}M$) and suppression at high concentrations of AII ($10^{-5}M$). Thus, tissues including the vasculature are potentially able to regulate local AII production, partially or completely independent of the systemic endocrine RAS. Ability of AII to interact with nuclear receptors to modulate gene expression suggests the presence of an intracrine renin system (*76,77;* unpublished data). Nuclear AII receptors have also been shown to influence a host of mRNAs for growth-related factors (Fig. 2). An action of AII on cardiocyte nuclear regulation of growth factors may help explain the substantial suppression of cardiac hypertrophy by ACE inhibitors *(68,69)*. These observations demand a closer examination of the interrelationship of plasma and nuclear AII receptor populations, since, to date, all AII-related functions have been attributed to the plasma membrane. Studies are now needed to determine the relationship between these various receptors and AII-related functions. A working model for such explorations is illustrated in Fig. 1.

SUMMARY

Although the origin of the individual components of the renin system in the vascular wall are in dispute, vascular tissue has the ability to locally generate and release AII. AII generated in the vasculature may augment and enhance the influence of circulating AII or perform autocrine, paracrine, or intracrine functions either on plasma membrane or nuclear AII receptors. That suppression of local tissue renin systems is often sufficient to prevent expression of AII related functions suggests that tissue renin systems are of major physiological significance. The ubiquitous presence of renin system components in tissues suggests that they may also perform functions in tissues other than those related to blood pressure regulation and growth. For example, ACE is an important constituent of bradykinin metabolism *(67)* and angiotensinogen is a well-established acute phase protein *(78)*. Future studies are required to unravel the relationship between the plasma and vascular renin systems to ascertain whether they act in concert or independently of one another and whether they perform the same or different functions.

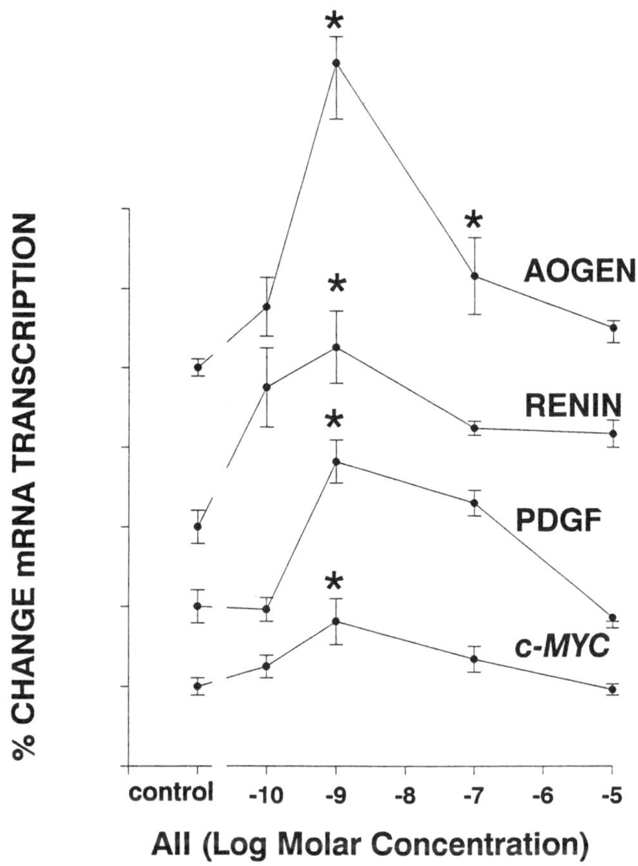

Fig. 2. Effect of AII on the transcription of several mRNA species related to the renin–angiotensin system in isolated hepatic nuclei. The ordinate represents the percent change from control in mRNA transcription of isolated hepatic nuclei. Each hatch mark on the ordinate represents 100%. The maximal increase averaged 80, 200, 280, and in excess of 400% at $1 \times 10^{-9} M$ AII for c-*myc*, platelet-derived growth factor (PDGF), renin, and angiotensinogen, respectively. $*p < 0.05$ as compared to control values.

REFERENCES

1. Barrett PQ, Bollag WB, Rasmussen H. Mechanism of action of angiotensin II. In: Cooke BA, King RJB, van der Molen HJ, eds. Hormones and Their Actions, Part II. Elsevier Science, Amsterdam 1988, pp. 211–229.
2. Naftilan AJ, Pratt RE, Eldridge CS, Lin HC, Dzau VJ. Angiotensin II c-fos expression in smooth muscle via transcriptional control. Hypertension 1989;13:706–711.
3. Phillips MI, Hofman WE. Sensitive sites in the brain for the blood pressure and drinking responses to AII. In: Buckley JP, Ferrario CH, eds. Central Actions of Angiotensin and Related Hormones. Pergamon, New York, 1977, pp. 325–356.
4. Malvin RL, Mouw D, Vander AJ, Gregg C. Hypothalamic stimulation of ADH by angiotensin II. In: Buckley JP, Ferrario CH, eds. Central Actions of Angiotensin and Related Hormones. Pergamon, New York, 1977, pp. 257–267.
5. Schalekamp MA, Derkx FH, van den Meiracker AH. Renin inhibitors, angiotensin converting enzyme inhibitors and angiotensin II receptor antagonists: relationships between blood pressure responses and effects on the renin-angiotensin system. J Hypertens Suppl 1992;10:S157–S164.
6. Swales JD. The renin-angiotensin system as a target for therapeutic intervention. J Cardiovas Pharm 1994;24(Suppl. 2):S1–S5.

7. von Lutterotti N, Catanzaro DF, Sealey JE, Laragh JH. Renin is not synthesized by cardiac and extrarenal vascular tissues. A review of experimental evidence. Circulation 1994;89:458–470.
8. McAreavey D, Robertson JI. Angiotensin converting enzyme inhibitors and moderate hypertension. Drugs 1990;40:326–345.
9. Kalinyak JE, Dorin RI, Hoffman AC, Perlman AJ. Tissue specific regulation of glucocorticoid receptor mRNA by dexamethasone. J Biol Chem 1987;262:460–464.
10. Mizuno K, Tani M, Niimura S, Sanada H, Haga H, Hashimoto S, Watanabe H, Ohtsuki M, Fukuchi S. Losartan, a specific angiotensin II receptor antagonists, increases angiotensin and angiotensin II release from isolated rat hind legs: evidence for locally regulated renin-angiotensin system in vascular tissue. Life Sci 1992;50:209–214.
11. Mizuno K, Niimura S, Tani M, Haga H, Inagami T, Fukuchii S. Direct proof for local generation and release of angiotensin II in peripheral human vascular tissue. Hypertension 1988;11:223–229.
12. Ganong WF. Origin of the angiotensin II secreted by cells. Proc Soc Exp Biol Med 1994;205:213–219.
13. Mulrow PJ, Kusano E, Baba K, Shier D, Doi Y, Franco-Saenz R, Stoner G, Rapp J. Adrenal renin: a possible local hormonal regulator of aldosterone production. Cardiovasc Drugs Ther 1988;2: 463–471.
14. Sawa H. Angiotensinogen: gene expression and protein localization in human tissues. Hokkaido Igaku Zasshi 1990;65:189–199.
15. Dostal DE, Rothblum KN, Conrad KM, Cooper GR, Baker KM. Detection of angiotensin I and II in cultured rat cardiac myocytes and fibroblasts. Am J Physiol 1992;263:C851–C863.
16. Dzau VJ. Molecular and physiological aspects of tissue renin-angiotensin system: emphasis on cardiovascular control. J Hypertens 1988;(Suppl. 6):S7–S12.
17. Dzau VJ. Short and long term determinants of cardiovascular function and therapy: contributions of circulation and tissue renin-angiotensin systems. J Cardiovasc Pharmacol 1989;14:51–55.
18. Dzau VJ, Ingelfinger J, Pratt RE, Ellison KE. Identification of renin and angiotensinogen messenger RNA sequences in mouse and rat brains. Hypertension 1986;8:544–548.
19. Eggena P, Barrett JD, Fredal AM, Morin AM. Stimulation of brain and aortic renin substrate by central administration of steroids in the rat. J Hypertens 1987;(Suppl. 5):S11–S13.
20. Ganten D, Schelling P, Vescsei P, Ganten U. Isorenin of extrarenal origin: "the tissue angiotensinogenase systems." Am J Med 1976;60:760–772.
21. Eggena P, Willesey P, Jamgotchian N, Truckenbrod L, Hu MS, Barrett JD, Eggena MP, Clegg K, Nakoul F, Lee DBN. The influence of recombinant human erythropoietin on blood pressure and tissue renin angiotensin systems of the rat. Am J Physiol 1991;261:E642–E646.
22. Paul M, Wagner J, Dzau V. Gene expression of the renin-angiotensin system in human tissues. Quantitative analysis by polymerase chain reaction. J Clin Invest 1993;91:2058–2064.
23. Yanagawa N, Capprelli AW, Jo OD, Friedal A, Barrett JD, Eggena P. Production of angiotensinogen and renin by renal proximal tubular cells. Kidney Intern 1991;39:938–941.
24. Dzau VJ. Significance of the vascular renin-angiotensin pathway. Hypertension 1986;8:553–559.
25. Asaad MM, Antonaccio MS. Vascular wall renin in spontaneously hypertensive rats: potential relevance to hypertension maintenance and antihypertensive effect of captopril. Hypertension 1982;4:487–493.
26. Rosenthal JH, Pfeifle B, Michanilov ML, Pschoor J, Jacob ICM, Dahlheim H. Investigations of components of the renin angiotensin system in rat vascular tissue. Hypertension 1984;6:383–390.
27. Berka JL, Alcorn D, Ryan GB, Skinner SL, Weaver DA. Renin processing in cultured juxtaglomerular cells of the hydronephrotic mouse kidney. J Histochem Cytochem 1993;41:365–373.
28. Okumura A, Tanaka T, Mori H. Juxtaglomerular cell tumor cell line producing active renin and its precursors. Virchows Arch B Cell Pathol Incl Mol Pathol 1993;64:303–307.
29. Gould LB, Skeggs LT, Kaha JR. Presence of renin activity in blood vessel walls. J Exp Med 1964;119:389,390.
30. Barrett JD, Eggena P, Sambhi MP. A comparison of physical characteristics of renin isolated from aorta and plasma of the rat. In: Sambhi MP, ed. Heterogeneity of Renin and Renin Substrate. American Elsevier, New York, 1981, pp. 317–326.
31. Eggena P, Barrett JD, Sambhi MP, Fredal AM. Renin substrate and the renin–angiotensin system in hog tissues. Biochem Med Metab Biol 1986;36:82–90.
32. Swales JD, Samani NJ. Vascular RAA system. J Hum Hypertens 1993;7(Suppl. 2):S3–S6.
33. Holycross BJ, Saye J, Harrison JK, Peach MJ. Polymerase chain reaction analysis of renin in rat aortic smooth muscle. Hypertension 1992;19:697–701.

34. Rothwell V, Kosowski S, Hadjilambris O, Baska R, Norman J. Glycosylation of active human renin is necessary for secretion: effect of targeted modifications of Asn-5 and Asn-75. DNA Cell Biol 1993;12:291–298.
35. Berka JL, Alcorn D, Ryan GB, Skinner SL. Renin processing studied by immunogold localization of prorenin and renin in granular juxtaglomerular cells in mice treated with enalapril. Cell Tissue Res 1992;268:141–148.
36. Berka JL, Alcorn D, Coghlan JP, Fernley RT, Morgan TO, Ryan GB, Skinner SL, Weaver DA. Granular juxtaglomerular cells and prorenin synthesis in mice treated with enalapril. J Hypertens 1990;8:229–238.
37. Shinagawa T, Do YS, Baxter JD, Carilli C, Schilling J, Hsueh WA. Identification of an enzyme in human kidney that correctly processes prorenin. Proc Natl Acad Sci USA 1990;87:1927–1931.
38. Derkx FH, Deinum J, Lipovski M, Verhaar M, Fischli W, Schalekamp MA. Nonproteolytic "activation" of prorenin by active site-directed renin inhibitors as demonstrated by renin-specific monoclonal antibody. J Biol Chem 1992;267:22,837–22,842.
39. Benjannet S, Reudelhuber T, Mercure C, Rondeau N, Chretien M, Seidah NG. Proprotein conversion is determined by a multiplicity of factors including convertase processing, substrate specificity, and intracellular environment. Cell type-specific processing of human prorenin by the convertase PC1. J Biol Chem 1992;267:11,417–11,423.
40. Iwai N, Matsunaga M, Kita T, Tei M, Kawai C. Regulation of renin-like enzyme in cultured human vascular smooth muscle cells. Jpn Circ J 1988;52:1338–1345.
41. Taddei S, Virdis A, Abdel-Haq B, Giovannetti R, Duranti P, Arena AM, Favilla S, Salvetti A. Indirect evidence for vascular uptake of circulating renin in hypertensive patients. Hypertension 1993;21:852–860.
42. Danser AH, Admiraal PJ, Derkx FH, Lamers JM, Verdouw PD, Saxena PR, Schalekamp MA. Cardiac renin is kidney-derived. J Hypertens 1993;(Suppl. 5):S224,S225.
43. Hilgers KF, Mann JFL. Tissue renin: focus on vascular angiotensin formation. Arzneimittel-Forschung 1993;43:198–201.
44. Campbell DJ, Valentijin AJ. Identification of vascular renin-binding proteins by chemical cross-linking: inhibition of binding of renin by renin inhibitors. J Hypertens 1994;12:879–890.
45. Müller D, Hilgers KF, Bohlender J, Lippoldt A, Wagner J, Fischli W, Ganten D, Mann JFE, Luft FC. Effect of human renin in the vasculature of rats transgenic for human angiotensinogen. Hypertension 1995;26:272–278.
46. Eggena P, Krall JF, Eggena MP, Clegg K, Fittigoff M, Barrett JD. Production of angiotensinogen in rat aortic smooth muscle cells. Clin Exp Hypertens 1990;A12:1175–1189.
47. Kifor I, Dzau VJ. Endothelial renin-angiotensin pathway: evidence for intracellular synthesis and secretion of angiotensins. Circ Res 1987;60:422–428.
48. Rakugi H, Jacob HJ, Krieger JE, Ingelfinger Jr, Pratt RE. Vascular injury induces angiotensinogen gene expression in the media and neointima. Circulation 1993;87:283–290.
49. Frederich PC Jr, Kahn BB, Peach MJ, Flier JS. Tissue-specific nutritional regulation of angiotensinogen in adipose tissue. Hypertension 1992;19:339–344.
50. Naftilan AJ, Zuo WM, Ingelfinger J, Ryan TJ Jr, Pratt RE, Dzau VJ. Localization and differential regulation of angiotensinogen mRNA expression in the vessel wall. J Clin Invest 1991;87: 1300–1331.
51. Sernia C, Shinkel TA, Thomas WG, Ho KK, Lincoln D. Angiotensinogen secretion by single rat pituitary cells: detection by a reverse haemolytic plaque assay and cell identification by immunocytochemistry. Neuroendocrin 1992;55:308 316.
52. Unger T, Gohlke P, Paul M, Rettig R. Tissue renin-angiotensin systems: fact or fiction? J Cardiovasc Pharmacol 1992;2(Suppl. 18):S20–S25.
53. Fishel RS, Eisenberg S, Shai SY, Redden RA, Bernstein KE, Berk BC. Glucocorticoids induce angiotensin-converting enzyme expression in vascular smooth muscle. Hypertension 1995;25:343–349.
54. Ideishi M, Noda K, Sasaguri M, Ikeda M, Arakawa K. Angiotensin II forming activity of vascular endothelial and smooth muscle cells. Artery 1993;20:95–102.
55. Azizi M, Chatellier G, Guyene TT, Murieta-Geoffroy D, Menard J. Additive effects of combined angiotensin-converting enzyme inhibition and angiotensin II antagonism on blood pressure and renin release in sodium-depleted normotensives. Circulation 1995;92:825–834.
56. Boucher R, Asselin J, Genest J. A new enzyme leading to the direct formation of angiotensin II. Circ Res 1974;34/35(Suppl. I):I203–I212.
57. Urata H, Hoffmann S, Ganten D. Tissue angiotensin II system in the human heart. Eur Heart J 1994;Suppl. D:68–78.

58. Drummer OH, Kourtis S, Johnson H. Effect of chronic enalapril treatment on enzymes responsible for the catabolism of angiotensin I and formation of angiotensin II. Biochem Pharmacol 1990;39:513–518.
59. Campbell DJ, Ziogas J, Kladis A. Metabolism of tetradecapeptide, angiotensinogen and angiotensin I and II by isolated perfused rat hindlimbs. Clin Exp Pharmacol Physiol 1990;17:335–350.
60. Sandberg K, Ji H, Catt KJ. Regulation of angiotensin II receptors in rat brain during dietary sodium changes. Hypertension 1994;23(Suppl. 1):I137–I141.
61. Campbell DJ, Kladis A, Skinner SL, Whitworth JA. Characterization of angiotensin peptides in plasma of anephric man. J Hypertens 1991;9:265–274.
62. Eggena P, Barrett JD, Shionoiri H, Sambhi MP. Enzymatic studies with renin substrate. In: Villarreal H, Sambhi P, eds. Topics in Pathophysiology of Hypertension. Martinus Nijhoff, Boston, MA, 1984, pp. 430–439.
63. Admiraal PJJ, Derkx FHM, Danser AHJ, Pieterman H, Schalekamp MADH. Metabolism and production of angiotensin I in different vascular beds in subjects with hypertension. Hypertension 1990;15:44–55.
64. Danser AH, Koning MM, Admiraal PJ, Sassen LM, Derkx FH, Verdouw PD, Schalekamp MA. Production of angiotensins I and II at tissue sites in intact pigs. Am J Physiol 1992;263:H429–H437.
65. Yu H, Rakugi H, Higaki J, Morishita R, Mikami H, Ogihara T. The role of activated vascular angiotensin II generation in vascular hypertrophy in one-kidney one clip hypertensive rats. J Hypertens 1993;11:1347–1355.
66. Oddie CJ, Dilley RJ, Kanellakis P, Bobik A. Chronic angiotensin II type 1 receptor antagonism in genetic hypertension: effects on vascular structure and reactivity. J Hypertens 1993;11:717–724.
67. Kiowski W, Linder L, Kleinbloesem C, van Brummelen P, Buhler FR. Blood pressure control by the renin angiotensin system in normotensive subjects. Assessment by angiotensin converting enzyme and renin inhibition. Circulation 1992;85:1–8.
68. Linz W, Schoelkens BA, Ganten D. Converting enzyme inhibition specifically prevents the development and induces the regression of cardiac hypertrophy in rats. Clin Exp Hypertens 1989;A11:1325–1350.
69. Sneedden W, Fernandex PG, Fernandex D, Vasdev S, Rabin EZ. Correlation of left ventricular hypertrophy and its regression by lisinopril with salt-induced hypertension. Can J Cardiol 1988;4:237–242.
70. Gyurko R, Wielbo D, Phillips MI. Antisense inhibition of AT1 receptor mRNA and angiotensinogen mRNA in the brain of spontaneously hypertensive rats reduces hypertension of neurogenic origin. Reg Peptides 1993;49:167–174.
71. Mullins JJ, Peters J, Ganten D. Fulminant hypertension in transgenic rats harbouring the mouse Ren-2 gene. Nature 1990;344:541–544.
72. Dzau VJ. Local expression and pathophysiological role of renin-angiotensin in the blood vessels and heart. Bas Res Cardiol 1993;88:(Suppl. 1):1–14.
73. Paul M, Ganten D. The molecular basis of cardiovascular hypertrophy: the role of the renin-angiotensin system. J Cardiovasc Pharmacol 1992;19(Suppl. 5):S51–S58.
74. Bianchi C, Gutkowska J, De Lean A, Ballak M, Anand-Srivastava MB, Genest J, Cantin M. Fate of (^{125}I) angiotensin II in adrenal glomerulosa cells. Endocrinology 1986;118:2605–2607.
75. Eggena P, Zhu JH, Clegg K, Barrett JD. Nuclear angiotensin receptors induce transcription of renin and angiotensinogen mRNA. Hypertension 1993;22:496–501.
76. Re RN, Vizard DL, Brown J, Bryan SE. Angiotensin II receptors in chromatin fragments generated by micrococcal nuclease. Biochem Biophys Res Comm 1984;119:220–227.
77. Re R, Parab M. Effect of angiotensin II on RNA synthesis by isolated nuclei. Life Sci 1984;34:647–651.
78. Klett C, Hellmann W, Ganten D, Hackenthal E. Tissue distribution of angiotensinogen mRNA during experimental inflammation. Inflammation 1993;17:183–197.

16 Effects of Insulin on Vascular Smooth Muscle Contraction

Andrew M. Kahn, MD *and Tom Song,* BS

CONTENTS

INTRODUCTION

Many studies have revealed an association between resistance to insulin-induced glucose disposal and high blood pressure. This relationship is present in patients with essential hypertension, obesity, and non-insulin-dependent diabetes mellitus *(1)*. It has been proposed that compensatory hyperinsulinemia increases sympathetic nerve activity and renal Na^+ reabsorption, which could contribute to the genesis of hypertension *(1)*. Despite the effects of hyperinsulinemia on the nervous and renal systems, chronic experimental hyperinsulinemia in dogs *(2)* or insulinoma in humans *(3)* are not associated with hypertension. This may be explicable since insulin infusion causes vasodilation in humans and dogs *(2,4)*. Thus, there exists a balance of insulin's effects to raise blood pressure (stimulation of sympathetic nerve activity and renal Na^+ reabsorption) versus the effect of insulin to lower blood pressure (vasodilation).

In essential hypertension, obesity, and non-insulin-dependent diabetes mellitus, resistance to insulin-induced glucose disposal is associated with resistance to insulin-induced vasodilation *(5,6)*. These studies support the notion that insulin normally inhibits vascular smooth muscle cell (VSMC) contraction, and in conditions where tissues are insensitive to insulin-induced glucose transport, VSMCs are also resistant to insulin's inhibition

From: *Contemporary Endocrinology: Endocrinology of the Vasculature*
Edited by: J. R. Sowers Humana Press Inc., Totowa, NJ

of tonic humoral and neural mediator-induced mechanisms which increase vessel tone. This pathophysiological response would serve to raise arterial tone and contribute to the development of hypertension. We and others have investigated how insulin inhibits VSMC tone in order to explore further the pathophysiology described.

PROPOSED MECHANISMS OF INSULIN-INDUCED INHIBITION OF VSMC CONTRACTION

Agonist-induced VSMC contraction is initiated by a rise in intracellular Ca^{2+} concentration $[Ca^{2+}]_i$ *(1)*. Several investigators have reported that insulin attenuates the agonist-induced $[Ca^{2+}]_i$ transient in cultured VSMC *(7–10)*. It is noteworthy that different laboratories have reported that insulin acutely affects different Ca^{2+} transport mechanisms which could attenuate the $[Ca^{2+}]_i$ transient. Studies in our laboratory have demonstrated that insulin inhibits serotonin (5-HT)-induced Ca^{2+} influx, the Ca_i transient and contraction in primary cultured VSMC from canine femoral arteries *(7,11)*. Moreover, it was shown that insulin did not inhibit Ca^{2+} release from internal stores or stimulate Ca^{2+} efflux from the cell *(11)*. Other investigators observed that insulin inhibited vasopressin-induced and depolarization-induced Ca^{2+} influx in VSMC *(8)*. Others reported that insulin hyperpolarizes retinal capillary pericytes by increasing Ca^{2+} activated K^+ channel activity *(12)*. This would be expected to decrease Ca^{2+} influx via voltage operated Ca^{2+} channels (VOCs). It was reported that insulin attenuated myo-inositol-1,4,5-triphosphate (IP_3)-induced Ca^{2+} mobilization from internal stores in passaged cultured VSMC from rat thoracic aorta *(9)*. It has been reported that insulin increases $^{45}Ca^{2+}$ efflux from rat arterial strips *(13)* and increases plasmalemmal Ca^{2+}-ATPase activity in cultured rat VSMC *(14)*. The aforementioned Ca^{2+} transport studies were performed with different cell preparations, different agonists, and different concentrations of insulin. Nevertheless, it is noteworthy that most of the different effects of insulin on Ca^{2+} transport, which could lower the agonist-induced $[Ca^{2+}]_i$ transient, can be linked to the reported effects of cyclic guanosine 5'-monophosphate (cGMP) on VSMC ion transport. Specifically cGMP or cGMP-dependent protein kinase (cGMP-PK) has been shown to activate Ca^{2+}-activated K^+ channels in VSMC *(15)*, increase the activities of the sarcoplasmic reticular and sarcolemmal Ca^{2+}-ATPase pumps in VSMC *(16,17)*, inhibit IP_3-induced Ca^{2+} release from the sarcoplasmic reticulum (SR) in gastric smooth muscle and VSMC *(9,18)*, and inhibit Ca^{2+} influx via VOCs *(19,20)* and receptor-operated Ca^{2+} channels (ROCs) in VSMC.

ROLE OF NITRIC OXIDE SYNTHASE (NOS)

A unifying hypothesis to explain the pleiotropic effects of insulin on Ca^{2+} transport in VSMC has come from recent studies which suggest that insulin inhibits VSMC contraction by stimulating the synthesis of nitric oxide (NO) in the endothelial and VSMC, which in turn increases the VSMC production of cGMP *(21,22)*. Investigators have reported that the insulin-induced increase in human leg blood flow was inhibited by *N*-mono-methyl-L-arginine (L-NMMA), a specific inhibitor of NOS. They also demonstrated that the augmented blood flow induced by the endothelium-dependent vasodilator, methacholine, was enhanced by hyperinsulinemia, whereas that caused by the endothelium-independent vasodilator, nitroprusside, was not increased by hyperinsulinemia *(21)*. In other studies, L-NMMA inhibited hyperinsulinemia-stimulated human arm blood flow *(22)*. One investigative group reported that insulin acutely increases $[Ca^{2+}]_i$ in intact endothelial

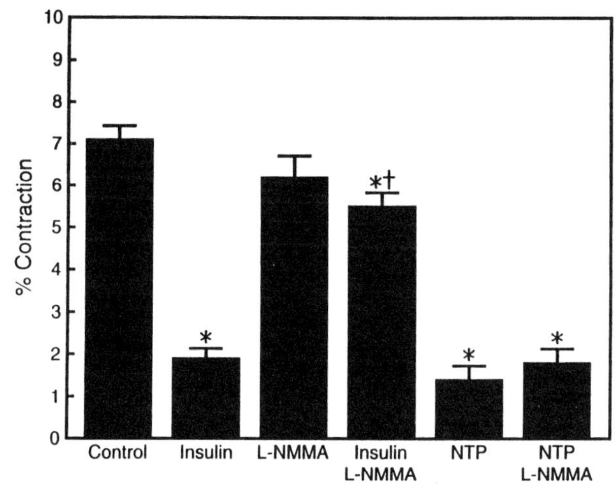

Fig. 1. Effects of L-NMMA on insulin-and nitroprusside (NTP)-inhibited contraction of VSMC. Dishes of cultured VSMC from canine femoral artery were preincubated for 30 min in the absence or presence of 1 n*M* bovine insulin or 0.1 m*M* NTP, with or without 0.1 m*M* L-NMMA. Resting lengths of 6–10 cells/dish were measured by photomicroscopy and the $10^{-5}M$ 5-HT-induced percent contraction at 10 min was determined for each cell.

cells from rat aorta and relaxes the underlying VSMC in an L-NMMA-dependent manner *(23)*. These data suggest that insulin stimulates the activities of the Ca^{2+}- calmodulin-dependent endothelial constitutive NOS (cNOS) and the subsequent production of NO inhibits contraction of the underlying VSMC. The latter occurs by NO-stimulated guanylate cyclase activity with subsequent rises in cGMP and cGMP-PK. Alternatively, NO may directly activate Ca^{2+}-dependent K^+ channels in VSMC, which would indirectly cause decreased Ca^{2+} influx via VOCs *(24)*.

It is not clear how insulin could attenuate the agonist-induced intracellular Ca^{2+} transients and contraction in various cultured VSMC cell preparations, which are devoid of endothelial cells. Preliminary data from our laboratory suggest that insulin inhibits 5-HT-induced contraction of primary cultured canine femoral artery VSMC by stimulating the activity of a putative VSMC NOS *(25)*. As shown in Fig. 1, preincubation of cultured VSMC with insulin for 30 min inhibited 5-HT-induced contraction. This inhibition was reversed by L-NMMA. Nitroprusside, which donates NO independently of NOS, also inhibited 5-HT-stimulated contraction, but the latter effect was not reversed by L-NMMA. It has been reported that L-NMMA partially reverses insulin's inhibition of the angiotensin II-induced $[Ca^{2+}]_i$ transient in cultured VSMC *(9)*. Insulin acutely increases cGMP production by cultured human VSMC *(26)*. Endothelial cells were absent in these cell preparations. In addition, others demonstrated that insulin reduces norepinephrine-stimulated $[Ca^{2+}]_i$ and contraction in intact, endothelium-free rat aortic strips *(23)*. These findings indicate that insulin stimulates an NOS in the VSMC cell itself. This raises the question of how insulin could acutely stimulate VSMC NOS activity, which is generally considered to be the inducible type and is thought not to be acutely regulated *(27)*. The following are possible explanations. First, it has been suggested that gastric smooth muscle *(28)* and VSMC *(29)* contain a cNOS. If insulin initially raises VSMC $[Ca^{2+}]_i$, which could bind calmodulin and stimulate a putative VSMC cNOS, NO production would ensue. In this regard, it is noteworthy that insulin alone transiently increases VSMC $[Ca^{2+}]_i$ via an unknown pathway, but that insulin inhibits the subsequent $[Ca^{2+}]_i$ transient induced by vasoconstrictors *(10)*. These data are consistent with the notion that an insulin-induced $[Ca^{2+}]_i$ spike activates VSMC cNOS, NO production and cGMP production. cGMP-PK would inhibit the subsequent vasoconstrictor-induced $[Ca^{2+}]_i$ increases by affecting one or more of the VSMC Ca^{2+} transport systems described in Proposed Mechanisms of Insulin-Induced Inhibition of VSMC Contraction. Second, several laboratories have reported that inducible NOS (iNOS) can be demonstrated in VSMC which has been treated with certain cytokines *(30,31)*. This occurs over a period of hours as would be expected for a process depending on transcription and translation. It would not be surprising that some VSMC, cultured in the presence of serum, could develop an iNOS. Theoretically, production of NO by a VSMC iNOS could be acutely stimulated by insulin (within minutes) via the provision of intracellular L-arginine or certain cofactors, such as tetrahydrobiopterin or β-nicotinamide-adenine dinucleotide phosphate reduced (NADPH) *(27)*. Third, insulin or high extracellular glucose concentration has been reported to acutely increase protein kinase C activity in VSMC *(32,33)*. Several studies have reported that protein kinase C increases iNOS activity in other cell types *(34–36)*. Thus, insulin, either directly or by increasing glucose influx, could stimulate VSMC protein kinase C and iNOS activities, which could increase the concentration of NO and cGMP.

ROLE OF GLUCOSE TRANSPORT

We have observed that insulin-induced glucose transport is an early event that leads to the inhibition by insulin of 5-HT-induced Ca^{2+} influx, the Ca^{2+} transient, and contraction of cultured VSMC *(37)*. These effects of insulin are dependent on extracellular glucose and are inhibited when glucose uptake is blocked and duplicated when glucose influx is stimulated by a high extracellular glucose concentration in the absence of insulin *(37)*. As shown in Fig. 2, 5-HT-stimulated VSMC contraction is inhibited by insulin in the absence but not presence of phloridzin. This agent inhibits insulin-stimulated glucose uptake in these VSMC *(37)*. As shown in Fig. 3, insulin-inhibited contraction of VSMC in the presence of 5 m*M* extracellular glucose equals that caused by 25 m*M* extracellular glucose in the absence of insulin. Glucose uptake is stimulated equally under both experimental conditions *(37)*. As also shown in Fig. 3, high glucose-induced inhibition of VSMC contraction is not amplified by adding insulin. Taken together, these data demonstrate that insulin-induced glucose uptake initiates insulin-inhibited contraction. In support of this notion, there are preliminary data indicating that the magnitude of insulin-induced vasodilation in the human forearm is directly related to the arterial glucose concentration *(38)*.

At present, we can only speculate how glucose influx leads to inhibition of VSMC contraction. Preliminary data from our laboratory show that insulin acutely acidifies primary cultured VSMC from canine femoral artery *(39)*. Since a substantial portion of transported glucose undergoes aerobic glycolysis in VSMC *(40)*, insulin-stimulated glucose uptake could acidify cells by increasing lactic acid production. We found that insulin-induced cell acidification increases Na^+ influx via the Na^+–H^+ exchanger and increases intracellular Na^+ concentration from 6 to 12 m*M* *(39)*. The latter would be expected to stimulate activity of the Na^+–K^+ pump, which could hyperpolarize the cell,

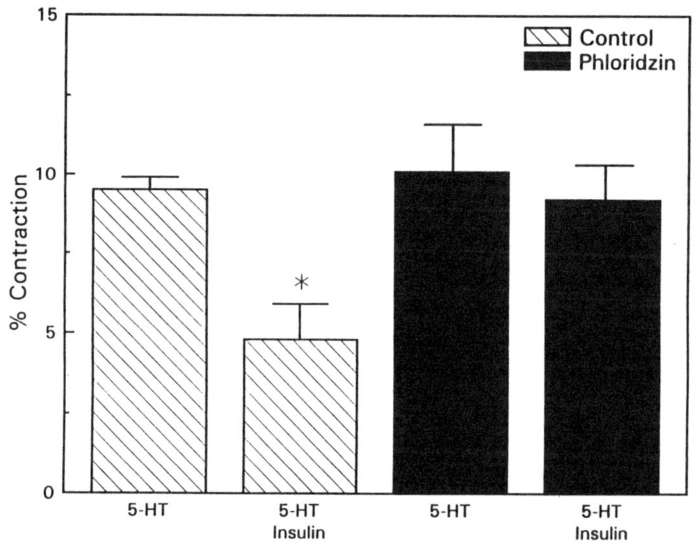

Fig. 2. Effects of insulin and phloridzin on VSMC cell contraction. VSMC were preincubated for 30 min in the presence or absence of 1 n*M* insulin with or without 1 m*M* phloridizin. The percent contraction 10 min after adding 10^{-5}*M* 5-HT was determined as in the legend to Fig. 1.

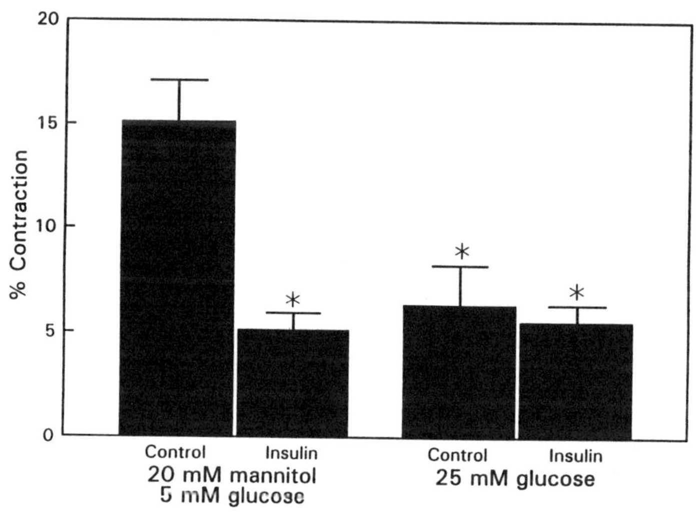

Fig. 3. Effects of high-glucose concentration and insulin on 5-HT-induced contraction of VSMC. Experiments were performed as in Figs. 1 and 2, except preincubation and incubation solutions contained either 20 m*M* mannitol plus 5 m*M* glucose or 25 m*M* glucose, with or without 1 n*M* insulin.

inhibit Ca^{2+} influx via VOCs, and attenuate contraction. In support of this notion, insulin acutely stimulates ouabain-sensitive $^{86}Rb^+$ uptake in these cells *(41)*. Insulin acutely increases Na^+–K^+ ATPase activity in cultured VSMC *(42)*, as well as in skeletal muscle *(43,44)*. In addition, insulin inhibits VSMC contraction in the absence but not presence of either ouabain or verapamil *(7)*. These data support the notion that insulin-inhibited contraction of VSMC involves effects on both the Na^+–K^+ pump and VOCs.

FURTHER SPECULATIONS

A hypothesis which encompasses most of the data published thus far is that insulin stimulates cNOS in the endothelial cell and some undefined NOS in VSMC. The resultant increased NO and/or cGMP concentrations in the VSMC lowers the agonist-induced $[Ca^{2+}]_i$ transient, in part or by inhibiting Ca^{2+} influx. This may be caused by a direct effect on Ca^{2+} channels by hyperpolarization of the cell secondary to increased K^+ channel and/or Na^+–K^+ pump activities. Agonist-induced increases in VSMC $[Ca^{2+}]_i$ would also be attenuated because of inhibition by cGMP of Ca^{2+} release from intracellular stores, stimulation of Ca^{2+} reuptake by those stores, or stimulation of Ca^{2+} efflux from the cell. Insulin probably affects different Ca^{2+} transport systems depending on the source of VSMC and the experimental conditions employed. The resultant blunted contractile agonist-induced increases in VSMC $[Ca^{2+}]_i$ would cause diminished activation of the contractile proteins.

NO and/or cGMP could also directly inhibit VSMC contraction at the level of the contractile proteins. The latter hypothesis is supported by our preliminary data, which demonstrate that insulin inhibits contraction of cultured VSMC that have been permeablized by saponin and contracted by 1.8 m*M* Ca^{2+} *(45)*. Insulin also inhibits the contraction of cells that are exposed to $10^{-5}M$ 5-HT and ionomycin (1.8 m*M* $Ca^{2+}{}_0$). Under both these conditions, $[Ca^{2+}]_i$ is clamped to supraphysiological levels, yet insulin still inhibits contraction. We found that 0.1 m*M* L-NMMA reversed insulin's inhibition of cell contraction under these conditions (unpublished data). These data support the notion that an insulin-mediated increase in NO and/or cGMP concentration inhibits VSMC contraction at the level of the contractile proteins. Consistent with this finding, others reported that cGMP dissociated contraction from myosin light-chain phosphorylation in swine carotid arteries *(46)*, and that cGMP inhibited contraction of rat mesenteric artery where $[Ca^{2+}]_i$ was clamped to a supraphysiological level *(47)*.

As outlined, our data in cultured VSMC from canine femoral artery indicate that insulin-induced glucose uptake is an early step in insulin's inhibition of agonist-induced contraction *(37)*, and that insulin-stimulated NOS activity is part of this process *(25)*. It is unknown how glucose influx into the VSMC cell could stimulate NOS activity. It is possible that glucose could be converted, in part, to diacylglycerol, which activates protein kinase C *(32,33)*. The latter has been reported to increase iNOS activity in various cells, including the VSMC-like mesangial cell *(35)*. Another interesting speculation is that glucose influx stimulates the activity of the pentose monophosphate shunt, thereby increasing NADPH production. The latter is a cofactor for all known types of NOS *(27)*. Thus, insulin-mediated glucose influx might increase VSMC NADPH availability thereby increasing the activities of a VSMC cNOS and/or iNOS. Figure 4 shows a diagram that portrays the proposed mechanisms for inhibition of VSMC contraction by insulin.

CONCLUSION

Insulin is a vasoactive hormone that acutely decreases VSMC tone. The mechanisms for this response are not fully elucidated, but it appears that insulin attenuates the contractile agonist-induced increases in VSMC $[Ca^{2+}]_i$ and may also inhibit contraction at the level of the contractile proteins. Insulin-stimulated glucose uptake in VSMC and insulin-stimulated NOS activity in endothelial and/or VSMC are probably involved in insulin's inhibitory effects on VSMC contraction. Resistance to insulin-induced glucose

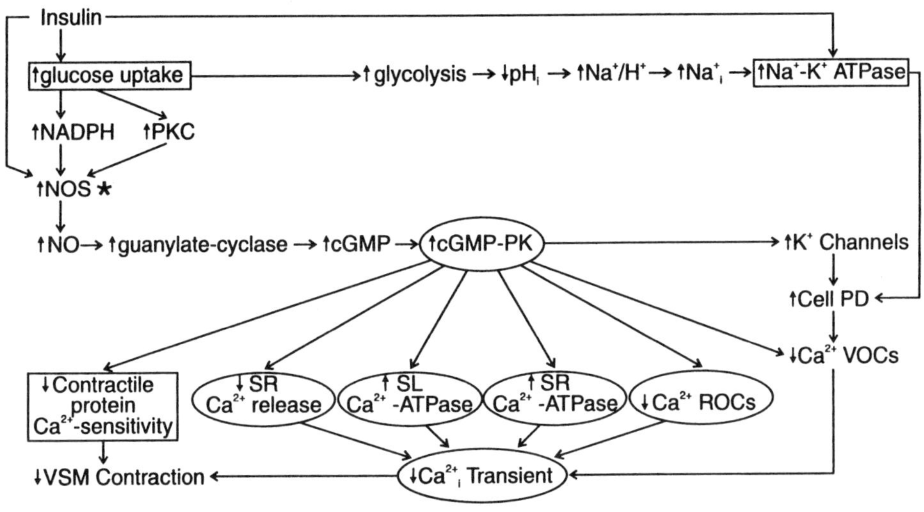

Fig. 4. Proposed mechanisms for the inhibition of VSMC contraction by insulin. *NOS may be endothelial and VSMC cNOS and/or iNOS. Abbreviations are defined in text.

disposal in essential hypertension, obesity, and noninsulin-dependent diabetes mellitus is associated with resistance to insulin-induced vasodilation *(1)*. It is an attractive hypothesis that insulin resistance at the level of the endothelial and/or VSMC cell is partly responsible for the systemic hypertension found in the aforementioned clinical conditions. Further research is needed to test these possibilities.

ACKNOWLEDGMENTS

The authors acknowledge the excellent secretarial assistance of Deborah J. Mumphord and the critical comments of Thomas D. DuBose, Jr. The authors' studies were supported by grants from the National Heart, Lung and Blood Institutes; Diabetes Action Research and Education Foundation; and Astra/Merck Group, Merck and Co., Inc.

REFERENCES

1. Epstein M, Sowers J. Diabetes mellitus and hypertension. Hypertension 1992;19:403–418.
2. Hall JE, Coleman TG, Mizelle HL, Smith MJ Jr. Chronic hyperinsulinemia and blood pressure regulation. Am J Physiol 1990;27:F722–F731.
3. Tsutsu N, Nunoi K, Kodama I, Nomiyama R, Iwase M, Fujishma M. Lack of association between blood pressure and insulin in patients with insulinoma. J Hypertens 1990;8:479–482.
4. Baron AD. Hemodynamic actions of insulin. Am J Physiol 1994;267:E187–E202.
5. Doria A, Fioretto P, Avogaro A, Carraro A, Morocutti A, Trevisan R, Frigato F, Crepaldi G, Viberti G, Nosadini R. Insulin resistance is associated with high sodium-lithium countertransport in essential hypertension. Am J Physiol 1991;261:E684–E691.
6. Laakso M, Edelman SV, Brechtel G, Baron AD. Impaired insulin-mediated skeletal muscle blood flow in patients with NIDDM. Diabetes 1992;41:1076–1083.
7. Kahn AM, Seidel CL, Allen JC, O'Neil RG, Shelat H, Song T. Insulin reduces contraction and intracellular calcium concentration in vascular smooth muscle. Hypertension 1993;22:735–742.
8. Standley PR, Zhang F, Ram JL, Zemel MB, Sowers JR. Insulin attenuates vasopressin-induced calcium transients and a voltage-dependent calcium response in rat vascular smooth muscle cells. J Clin Invest 1991;88:1230–1236.

9. Saito F, Hori MT, Fittingott M, Hino R, Tuck ML. Insulin attenuates agonist-mediated calcium mobilization in cultured rat vascular smooth muscle cells. J Clin Invest 1993;92:1161–1168.
10. Touyz RM, Tolloczko B, Schiffrin EL. Insulin attenuates agonist-evoked calcium transients in vascular smooth muscle cells. Hypertension 1994;23(Suppl. I):I23–I28.
11. Kahn AM, Allen JC, Seidel CL, Song T. Insulin inhibits serotonin-induced Ca^{2+} influx in vascular smooth muscle. Circulation 1994;90:384–390.
12. Berweck S, Hagen T, Lepple-Wienhues A, Helbig H, Wiederholt M. Insulin-induced hyperpolarization in retinal capillary pericytes. Invest Ophthalmol Vis Sci 1993;34:3402–3407.
13. Reddy S, Shehin S, Sowers JR. Aortic calcium-45 flux and blood pressure regulation in streptozotocin-induced diabetic rats. J Vasc Med Biol 1990;2:47–51.
14. Zemel MB, Iannucci A, Moore JW. Role of insulin in regulating vascular smooth muscle Ca^{2+}-ATPase expression. J Vasc Med Biol 1993;4:79–84.
15. Robertson BE, Schubert R, Hescheler J, Nelson MT. cGMP-dependent protein kinase activates Ca-activated K channels in cerebral artery smooth muscle cells. Am J Physiol 1993;265:C299–C303.
16. Twort CHC, van Breemen C. Cyclic guanosine monophosphate-enhanced sequestration of Ca^{2+} by sarcoplasmic reticulum in vascular smooth muscle. Circ Res 1988;62:961–964.
17. Vrolix M, Raeymaekers L, Wuytack F, Hofmann F, Casteels R. Cyclic GMP-dependent protein kinase stimulates the plasma-lemmal Ca^{2+} pump of smooth muscle via phosphorylation of phosphatidylinositol. Biochem J 1988;255:855–863.
18. Murthy KS, Severi C, Grider JR, Makhlouf GM. Inhibition of IP_3 and IP_3-dependent Ca^{2+} mobilization by cyclic nucleotides in isolated gastric muscle cells. Am J Physiol 1993;264:G967–G974.
19. Ishikawa T, Hume JR, Keef KD. Regulation of Ca^{2+} channels by cAMP and cGMP in vascular smooth muscle cells. Circ Res 1993;73:1128–1137.
20. Lorenz JN, Bielefeld DR, Sperelakis N. Regulation of calcium channel current in A7r5 vascular smooth muscle cells by cyclic nucleotides. Am J Physiol 1994;266:C1656–C1663.
21. Steinberg HO, Brechtel G, Johnson A, Fineberg N, Baron AD. Insulin-mediated skeletal muscle vasodilationis nitric oxidedependent. J Clin Invest 1994;94:1172–1179.
22. Scherrer U, Randin D, Vollenweider P, Vollenweider L, Nicod P. Nitric oxide release accounts for insulin's vascular effects in humans. J Clin Invest 1994;94:2511–2515.
23. Han SZ, Ouchi Y, Karaki H, Orimo H. Inhibitory effects of insulin on cytosolic Ca^{2+} level and contraction in the rat aorta. Circ Res 1995;77:673–678.
24. Bolotina VM, Najibl S, Palacino JJ, Pagano PJ, Cohen RA. Nitric oxide directly activates calcium-dependent potassium channels in vascular smooth muscle. Nature 1994;368:850–853.
25. Husid A, Song T, Kahn AM. Insulin-inhibited Ca^{2+} influx and contraction of serotonin-stimulated vascular smooth muscle cells is reversed by N-mono-methyl-L-arginine. Am J Hypertens 1996; 9:129A.
26. Trovati M, Massucco P, Mattiello L, Cavalot F, Mularoni E, Hahn A, Anfossi G. Insulin increases cyclic nucleotide content in human vascular smooth muscle cells: a mechanism potentially involved in insulin-induced modulation of vascular tone. Diabetes 1995;38:936–941.
27. Nathan C, Xie Q. Regulation of biosynthesis of nitric oxide. J Biol Chem 1994;269:13,725–1,3728.
28. Murthy KS, Zhang K-M, Jin J-G, Grider JR, Makhlouf GM. VIP-mediated G protein-coupled Ca^{2+} influx activates a constitutive NOS in dispersed gastric muscle cells. Am J Physiol 1993;265: G660–G671.
29. Wood KS, Buga GM, Byrns RE, Ignarro LJ. Vascular smooth muscle-derived relaxing factor (MDRF) and its close similarity to nitric oxide. Biochem Biophys Res Comm 1990;170:80–88.
30. Busse R, Mülsch A. Induction of nitric oxide synthase by cytokines in vascular smooth muscle cells. FEBS Lett 1990;275:87–90.
31. Beasley D, Schwartz JH, Brenner BM. Interleukin 1 induces prolonged L-arginine-dependent cyclic guanosine monophosphate and nitrite production in rat vascular smooth muscle cells. J Clin Invest 1991;87:602–608.
32. Cooper DR, Khalakdina A, Watson JE. Chronic effects of glucose on insulin signaling in A-10 vascular smooth muscle cells. Arch Biochem Biophys 1993;302:490–498.
33. Williams B, Schrier RW. Characterization of glucose-induced in situ protein kinase C activity in cultured vascular smooth muscle cells. Diabetes 1992;41:1464–1472.
34. Nakane M, Mitchell J, Förstermann U, Murad. Phosphorylation by calcium calmodulin-dependent protein kinase II and protein kinase C modulates the activity of nitric oxide synthase. Biochem Biophys Res Comm 1991;180:1396–1402.

35. Sharma K, Danoff TM, DePiero A, Ziyadeh FN. Enhanced expression of inducible nitric oxide synthase in murine macrophages and glomerular mesangial cells by elevated glucose levels: possible mediation via protein kinase C. Biochem Biophys Res Comm 1995;207:80–88.
36. Bosca L, Laazo PA. Induction of nitric oxide release by MRC OX-44 (anti-CD53) through a protein kinase C-dependent pathway in rat macrophages. J Exp Med 1994;179:1119–1126.
37. Kahn AM, Lichtenberg RA, Allen JC, Seidel CL, Song T. Insulin-stimulated glucose transport inhibits Ca^{2+} influx and contraction in vascular smooth muscle. Circulation 1995;2:1597–1603.
38. Ueda S, Petrie JR, Elliott HL, Connell MC. Insulin mediated vasodilatation is dependent on local glucose concentrations. Hypertension 1995;26:561 (abstract).
39. Kahn AM, Song T. Insulin-induced intracellular lactic acid production in vascular smooth muscle (VSMC) cells lowers pH_i which raises Na^+_i by stimulating the activity of the Na^+–H^+ exchanger. J Invest Med 1995;43:213A.
40. Lynch RM, Paul RJ. Compartmentation of glycolysis and glycogenolysis in vascular smooth muscle. Science 1983;222:1344–1346.
41. Kahn AM, Song T. Insulin inhibits dog vascular smooth muscle contraction and lowers Ca^{2+}_i by inhibiting Ca^{2+} influx. J Nutr 1995;125:1732S–1737S.
42. Tirupattur PR, Ram JL, Standley PR, Sowers JR. Regulation of Na^+, K^+-ATPase gene expression by insulin in vascular smooth muscle cells. Am J Hypertens 1993;6:626–629.
43. Rosic NK, Standaert ML, Pollet RJ. The mechanism of insulin stimulation of (Na^+, K^+)-ATPase transport activity in muscle. J Biol Chem 1985;260:6206–6212.
44. Hundal HS, Marette A, Mitsumoto Y, Ramlal T, Blostein T, Klip A. Insulin induces translocation of the $\alpha 2$ and $\beta 1$ subunits of the Na^+/K^+-ATPase from intracellular compartments to the plasma membrane in mammalian skeletal muscle. J Biol Chem 1992;267:5040–5043.
45. Kahn AM, Song T. The inhibition of vascular smooth muscle (VSMC) contraction by insulin is independent of effects on intracellular Ca^{2+} concentration (Ca^{2+}_i). J Am Soc Nephrol 1995;6:661 (abstract).
46. McDaniel NL, Chen X, Singer HA, Murphy RA, Rembold CM. Nitrovasodilators relax arterial smooth muscle by decreasing $[Ca^{2+}]_i$ and uncoupling stress from myosin phosphorylation. Am J Physiol 1992;263:C461–C467.
47. Nishimura J, van Breemen C. Direct regulation of smooth muscle contractile elements by second messengers. Biochem Biophys Res Comm 1989;163:929–935.

17 Sex Hormones and the Vasculature

Suzanne Oparil, MD,
Ronald L. Levine, MD, MS,
and Yiu-Fai Chen, PHD

CONTENTS

INTRODUCTION

Epidemiological studies have defined a sexually dimorphic pattern in the development of atherosclerotic vascular disease in humans *(1)*. The incidence of cardiovascular disease is lower in premenopausal women than in age-matched men, but rises steadily after menopause *(2)*. Postmenopausal women on estrogen replacement therapy have less severe coronary artery disease and a lower risk for cardiovascular mortality than women without hormone treatment *(3)*. Thus, estrogens inhibit the development of atherosclerotic cardiovascular disease in women *(4)*. The mechanism of this vasoprotective effect is complex and involves alterations in lipid metabolism, endothelial function, vascular smooth muscle cell (VSMC) proliferation and associated extracellular matrix formation, and vascular reactivity. Evidence that other sex hormones, including androgens and progestogens, can also alter these processes is emerging. This chapter reviews effects of sex hormones on the vasculature with emphasis on the processes that influence the progression of atherosclerosis and thus alter cardiovascular risk. Effects of postmenopausal hormone replacement on cardiovascular risk are reviewed.

From: *Contemporary Endocrinology: Endocrinology of the Vasculature*
Edited by: J. R. Sowers Humana Press Inc., Totowa, NJ

LIPID METABOLISM

Approximately 25–50% of the antiatherosclerotic effect of estrogens in humans has been attributed to alterations in plasma lipid and lipoprotein levels *(5,6)*. Estrogen supplementation increases serum high-density lipoprotein (HDL) cholesterol, HDL_2, HDL_3, apolipoprotein A-1, and triglycerides and decreases total and low-density lipoprotein (LDL) cholesterol, apolipoprotein B, and lipoprotein (a) *(7)*. HDL is increased and LDL is decreased by 10–15% during estrogen administration in both sexes *(8,9)*. Each of these estrogen effects is mediated by a different mechanism. Estrogen increases HDL cholesterol levels by suppressing hepatic lipoprotein lipase, resulting in decreased conversion of HDL_2 to HDL_3, as well as by increasing synthesis of apolipoprotein A-1. It decreases LDL cholesterol by upregulating hepatic LDL receptor expression. Estrogen also induces increased hepatic synthesis of very low density lipoprotein (VLDL), resulting in elevated triglyceride levels *(10)*. Progestin reduces the favorable effects of estrogen on lipid metabolism, causing decreases in HDL cholesterol and triglycerides and increases in LDL cholesterol *(10)*. Interestingly, animal studies suggest that addition of progestin to an estrogen regimen does not attenuate the antiatherosclerotic effect of the estrogen and that retardation in arterial lesion development can occur in response to estrogen treatment in the absence of alterations in serum cholesterol levels *(11,12)*. These findings support the notion that changes in lipid and lipoprotein concentrations account for only a portion of the vasoprotective effects of estrogen use. The remaining vasoprotective effects relate to direct, presumably receptor-mediated, effects on the vasculature.

EXPRESSION OF SEX STEROID HORMONE RECEPTORS ON THE BLOOD VESSEL WALL

Steroid hormones function through the action of specific receptors that belong to the same superfamily of proteins *(13,14)*. Receptors for estrogen *(15)*, androgen *(16)*, and progesterone *(17)* have been characterized by biochemical and molecular biological methods. Ligand binding and molecular biological studies have identified and characterized at least two separate estrogen receptors for 17β-estradiol estrogen and estriol *(13)*, two molecular forms of progesterone receptors (A and B subtypes) *(14,18)*, and also two androgen receptors for dihydrotestosterone (DHT) and testosterone *(19)*. The relative proportion of estrogen, androgen, and progesterone preceptor subtypes varies among tissues and species *(14,18)*. In target tissues, most of the biological effects of steroid hormones are mediated through their intracellular receptors that act as ligand-activated signal transducers and transcription factors. In the presence of steroid hormones, the cytosolic ligand–receptor complex translocates into nucleus and binds in a highly specific fashion to DNA containing a *cis*-acting transcriptional regulatory element, resulting in an altered pattern of gene expression *(13,14,20,21)*.

ESTROGEN RECEPTORS

Endothelial and VSMC are the major cell types in vascular tissue that play a role in the pathogenesis of atherosclerosis and restenosis following balloon injury. Estrogen binds specifically to vascular walls in several species *(22–29)*, including humans *(28,29)*. Autoradiographic studies demonstrate that the [^{3}H]-17β-estradiol is taken up uniformly by a variety of cell types in the pig coronary artery *(25)*. In human vessels, immunohistochemical staining for the estrogen receptor demonstrates positive-stained cells adjacent to the internal elastic lamina that also stain positively for human VSMC α-actin, suggesting that these receptors are located primarily on VSMCs *(29)*. Further, demonstrated estrogen receptor expression has been shown in both soluble and nuclear compartments of human aorta *(28)*. Thus, the vascular wall is a target tissue of estrogen.

In vitro ligand binding studies have also demonstrated estrogen receptors in cultured endothelial cells from human aorta *(30)* and VSMCs from rat and bovine aorta *(31–33)*, canine coronary artery *(34)*, and human saphenous vein and mammary artery *(35)*. Recent studies *(35,36)* also demonstrate the expression of estrogen receptor mRNA in human and rat VSMCs by Northern blot analysis, RNase protection, and reverse transcription-polymerase chain reaction (RT-PCR) methods. Further, immunoblotting and immunocytochemical localization with monoclonal anti-estrogen receptor antibody demonstrate estrogen receptor protein in cultured human and rat VSMC. Immunostaining for estrogen receptors is distributed predominantly in the perinuclear region of the cytoplasm, but is also seen in the nuclei *(35,37)*. Addition of estrogen to the culture medium increases the resting membrane potential (hyperpolarization) *(34)*, stimulates the biosynthesis of prostacyclin *(33)*, inhibits cell proliferation *(38,39)*, and inhibits collagen production *(32)* in cultured VSMC. These data support the hypothesis that estrogen can regulate the growth, differentiation, and function of VSMCs through its own receptor present in these cells.

Heterogeneity of estrogen receptor distribution has been reported among various vascular beds, between male and female animals, and between normal and atherosclerotic vessels *(23,25,28,29,40)*. Priming with 17β-estradiol causes an increase in estrogen binding in the male rabbit aorta, but has no effect on estrogen binding in the female rabbit aorta *(23)*. Binding of [^{3}H]-17β-estradiol is higher in coronary arteries from sexually mature female pigs than in arteries from castrated males *(25)*. In baboons, the estrogen receptor content of cytoplasmic extracts of aortic arch and thoracic aorta of intact males is indistinguishable from that of proestrus females, whereas estrogen receptor content of cytoplasmic extracts of abdominal aorta of proestrus females is greater than that of males *(40)*. In humans, atherosclerotic coronary arteries of premenopausal women demonstrate distinctly diminished expression of estrogen receptors compared with normal arteries of premenopausal women *(29)*. These results indicate an association between the absence of estrogen receptors and the presence of atherosclerosis and suggest that the restenosis- and athero-protective effects of estrogen are in part mediated by a receptor-mediated effect of estrogen on endothelial cells and VSMCs.

ANDROGEN RECEPTORS

Androgen receptors also have been described in blood vessel walls and cultured VSMCs. Autoradiographic and biochemical analyses of the hearts of rhesus monkeys, baboons *(41)*, and rats *(42)* indicate that atrial and ventricular myocardial cells contain androgen receptors. Specific binding sites for [^{3}H]-testosterone and [^{3}H]-DHT have been detected in the cytosolic fraction of the aorta from male and female rabbits primed with testosterone and estrogen *(23)*. In canine aorta, the majority of the androgen receptors (measured by the [^{3}H]-R1881-19-nor-androgen binding) are found in the media and adventitia, and not in the endothelium or in the fibrous tissue elements of the intima *(24)*.

Androgen receptor levels are greatly reduced in veins compared to aorta, reaching undetectable levels in veins of male dogs *(24)*. Testosterone inhibits prostacyclin production by rat aortic VSMC in culture *(31)* and exacerbates the development of atherosclerosis in rabbits fed an atherogenic diet *(43)*. Androgen receptor mRNA in rat aortic VSMC has recently been detected using the RT-PCR technique *(44)*.

Ligand binding studies identify a single class of binding sites for testosterone and DHT in rat VSMC. Testosterone and DHT have similar B_{max} in VSMC and the affinity of binding of DHT is greater than that of testosterone. To access the direct effect of androgens on cell growth and proliferation, effects of testosterone and DHT on DNA synthesis of the VSMC as measured by [^{3}H]-thymidine incorporation indicate both DHT and testosterone stimulate DNA synthesis in growing VSMC, but that DHT has a more robust effect than unreduced testosterone. In many androgen target tissues, DHT is the active form of androgen and testosterone is reduced to DHT by the enzyme 5α-reductase before binding to the androgen receptor *(45)*. Significant 5α-reductase activity has been found in rat VSMC *(44)*. It is possible that in VSMC testosterone is converted to DHT which produces androgenic effects in the vasculature. These data suggest that androgen may act directly on the blood vessel wall to accelerate atherosclerosis and restenosis by simulating the proliferation of VSMC.

PROGESTERONE RECEPTORS

Progesterone receptors have been identified in baboon aorta and myocardium using radioligand techniques *(46)* and in human aorta, coronary and internal carotid artery, and heart, using immunocytochemical techniques with a highly specific monoclonal antibody against primate progesterone receptors *(47)*. In the aorta, progesterone receptors have been described in the nuclei of VSMCs and endothelial cells of intima, media, and adventitia. In the myocardium, progesterone receptors are localized in the nuclei of the myocytes. In internal carotid and coronary arteries, progesterone receptors have been described in the nuclei of endothelial cells, and in vascular channels within atherosclerotic plaques. In cardiovascular tissues, expression of progesterone receptors can be induced in response to estrogen acting through estrogen receptors *(24)*. Several putative estrogen response elements have been identified on the 5'-flanking untranslated region and on the first exon in the rat progesterone receptor gene, which can form a strong estrogen-responsive enhancer when linked together *(48)*. Progesterone binding is not present in aorta of the ovariectomized dogs, but progesterone receptors are induced in these animals by 1 wk of treatment with physiological doses of estrogen, suggesting that both estrogen and progesterone receptors are present and functional in cardiovascular tissues *(24)*.

ENDOTHELIAL FUNCTION

Many of the direct vasoprotective effects of estrogen are mediated by the endothelium. These include enhancement of endothelial degradation of LDL cholesterol, suppression of collagen and elastin synthesis, and restoration of endothelium-dependent vasodilator mechanisms postinjury *(43,49–53)*. Estrogens also interfere with the oxidation of deposited LDL particles *(53)*, thus limiting the progression of atherosclerosis.

The endothelium plays a central role in the control of vascular tone and the growth of the blood vessel wall, mainly through synthesis and release of endothelium-derived relaxing factor (EDRF), which has been shown to be nitric oxide (NO) *(54)*. NO is both a vasorelaxant and an antimitogen for VSMCs. Release of EDRF in response to infused acetylcholine, the standard test for assessing endothelium-dependent vascular tone, has been shown to be responsive to acute and chronic estrogen administration. Paradoxical vasoconstrictor responses to acetylcholine infusion have been demonstrated in the coronary arteries of ovariectomized monkeys fed an atherogenic diet; normal vasodilator responses were restored following either chronic (3 mo) *(53)* or short-term (20 min) *(55)* estrogen administration. Similar restitution of normal coronary vasomotor responses to acetylcholine have been reported in postmenopausal women following short-term administration of ethinyl estradiol *(56)*.

Mechanisms by which chronic estrogen administration mediates its vasorelaxant effect may involve upregulation of the genes involved in the biosynthesis of prostacyclin (PGI_2) and NO, prostacyclin synthetase, cyclo-oxygenase, and NO synthase (NOS) *(57)*. Basal release of NO from endothelium-intact vascular rings, calcium-dependent NOS (eNOS) activity, and eNOS mRNA levels are increased in response to increased levels of exogenous and endogenous estrogens *(58,59)*. In contrast, the acute vasodilator effect of infused estrogen is too rapid to be accounted for by increased gene transcription. Potential mechanisms for the immediate vasomotor effects of estrogen, include increased NO release *(60)*, antagonism of vasoconstrictor responses to endothelin *(61)*, direct hyperpolarization of resting VSMCs *(34)*, and antagonism of VSMC calcium channels *(62)*. Although most of these putative mechanisms require an intact endothelium, some involve direct effects of estrogen on VSMCs.

SEX HORMONES AND VSMC FUNCTION

VSMC proliferation is an integral part of the atherosclerotic process. Atherosclerosis appears to be initiated by injury to the vessel wall *(63)*. Vascular injury can be caused by a variety of factors, including hyperlipidemia, oxidative stress, hypertension, vessel disruption owing to bypass surgery, or balloon catheters. VSMCs, which normally have a contractile phenotype, change to a secretory phenotype after injury. In the secretory phase, the VSMCs manufacture and secrete extracellular matrix (collagen and elastin), which reduces the effective lumen of the vessel involved. Estrogen inhibits atherosclerosis, in part by inhibiting the growth and proliferation of VSMCs. Estrogen inhibits atherosclerosis in cholesterol-fed chicks *(64)*, inhibits the growth of VSMCs in culture *(25,39)*, and the proliferation of VSMCs in atherosclerotic lesions *(65–68)*. These early studies, although provocative, were flawed by the use of supraphysiologic doses of estrogen, atherogenic diets and/or failure to measure levels of circulating estrogen.

Recently, animal models of vascular injury have been used to examine the effect of estrogen on VSMC proliferation in vivo *(69–73)*. In these models, endothelial denudation induces a highly reproducible intimal migration/proliferation of VSMCs over the entire length of the affected vessel, mimicking the early injury phase of atherosclerosis. These studies have provided evidence that estrogen inhibits VSMC proliferation after balloon injury of an artery. Estrogen has been shown to inhibit neointimal formation (VSMC proliferation and extracellular matrix formation) after balloon injury of the common and external iliac arteries of rabbits *(69)*. Myointimal proliferation after balloon injury of the carotid artery is reduced in intact female Sprague-Dawley rats compared to age-matched

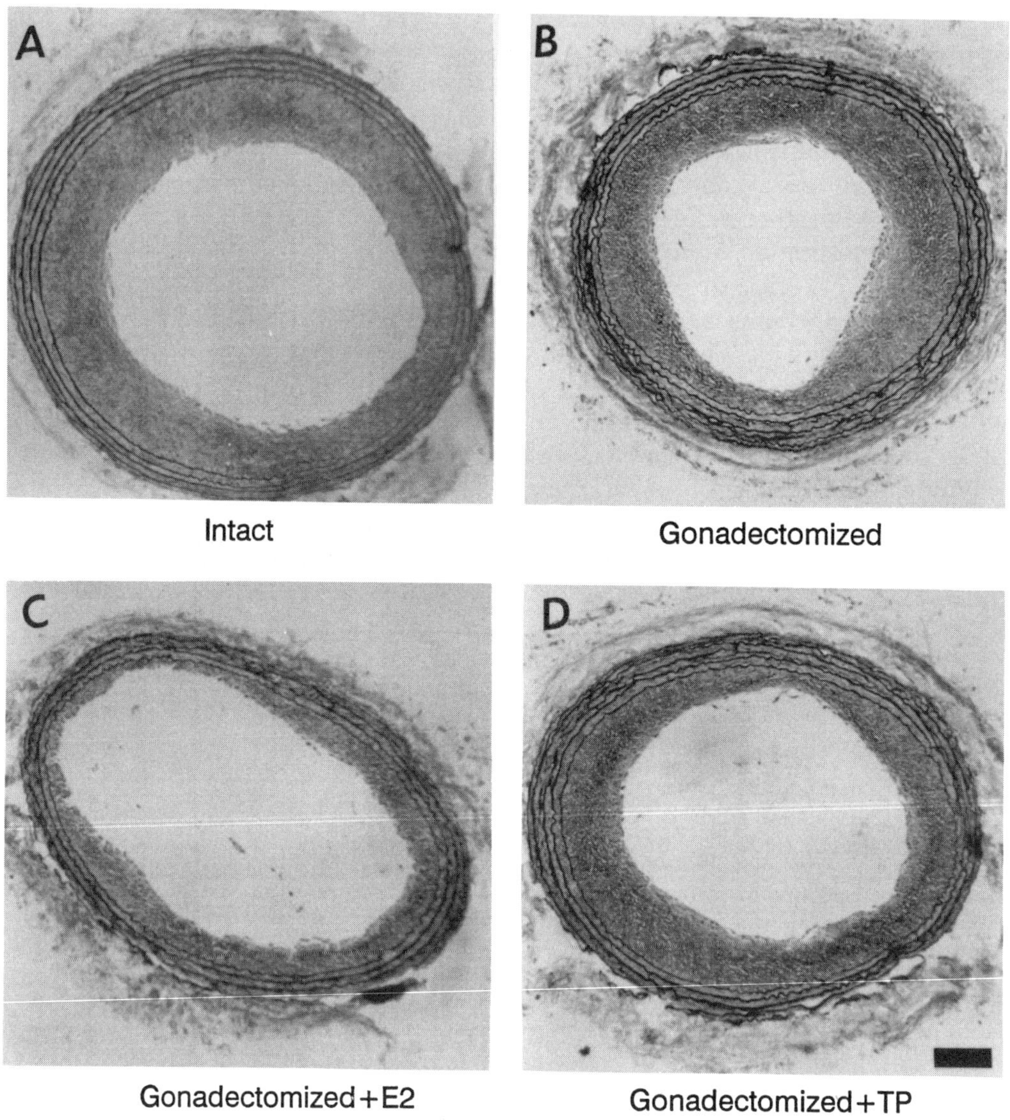

Fig. 1. Representative light micrographs of right common carotid arteries from male Sprague-Dawley rats 14 d after balloon injury. Balloon-injured right carotid arteries from an intact male rat **(A)**, a gonadectomized male rat **(B)**, a gonadectomized + 17β-estradiol-treated male rat **(C)**, and a gonadectomized + testosterone-treated male rat **(D)** (magnification ×100, bar = 100 μm). Reproduced with permission from ref. *70*.

males and that this sexual dimorphism is dependent on estrogen rather than testosterone *(70)*. This study further showed that physiologic levels of exogenous estrogen can prevent neointima formation in damaged vessels of gonadectomized rats of both sexes (Figs. 1 and 2). Estrogen inhibited the myointimal response to balloon injury by ~60%, an effect comparable to results observed with a variety of other proliferative agents in the rat carotid injury model. In contrast, neither endogenous nor exogenous testosterone at physiologic levels affected neointima formation in this model.

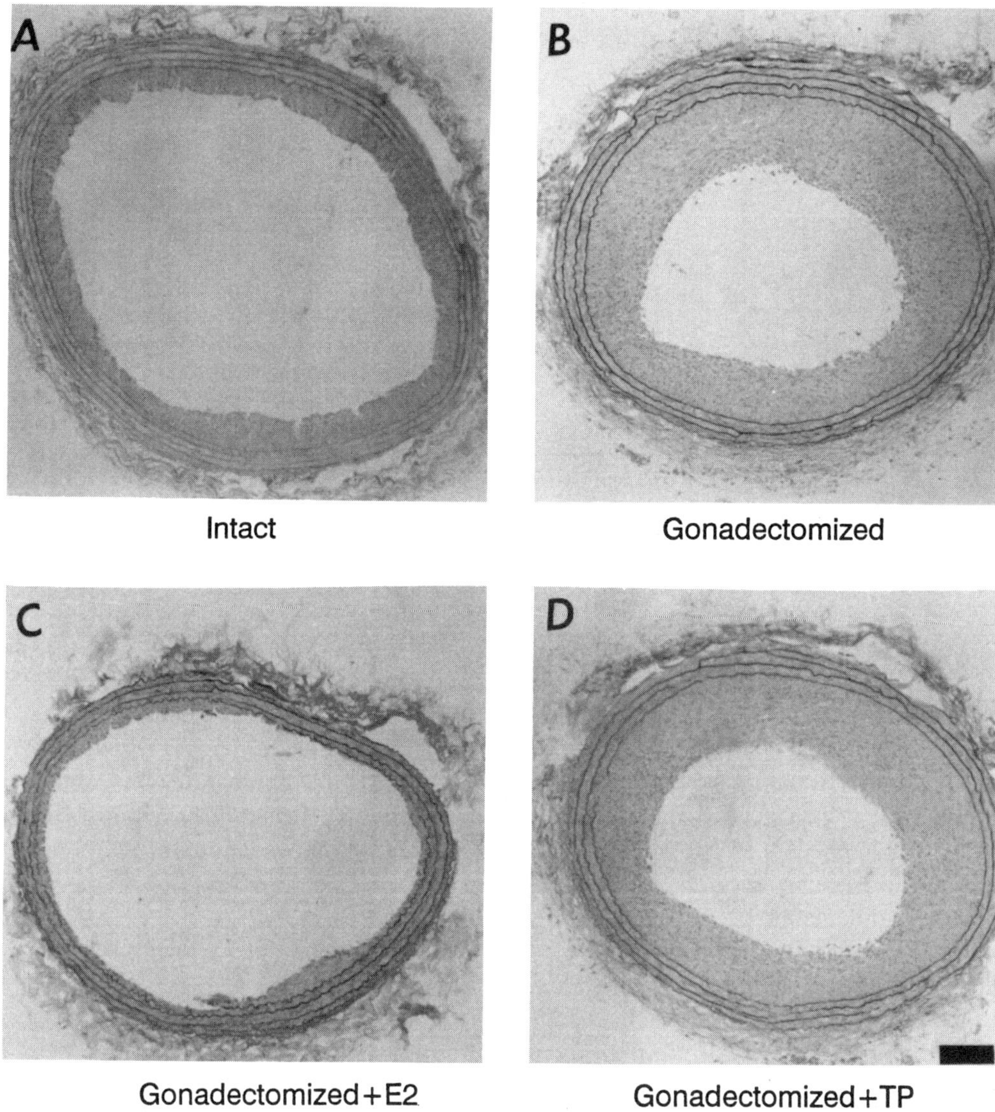

Fig. 2. Representative light micrographs of right common carotid arteries from female Sprague-Dawley rats 14 d after balloon injury. Balloon-injured right carotid arteries from an intact female rat **(A)**, a gonadectomized female rat **(B)**, a gonadectomized + 17β-estradiol-treated female rat **(C)**, and a gonadectomized + testosterone-treated female rat **(D)** (magnification ×100, bar = 100 μm). Reproduced with permission from ref. *70*.

The c-*myc* transcript levels, used as indices of early response gene expression, are lower in the undamaged carotid artery of intact female rats than in intact males, suggesting a reduced level of baseline mitotic activity in the artery of the female rat. These c-*myc* levels increase dramatically within 1 hr of balloon injury in male rats; the c-*myc* response in females was both delayed and attenuated in magnitude (Fig. 3). This suggests that estrogen reduces the expression of c-*myc* in VSMCs in vivo in response to injury. This is directly opposite to the effects of estrogen on breast cancer cells, where major increases

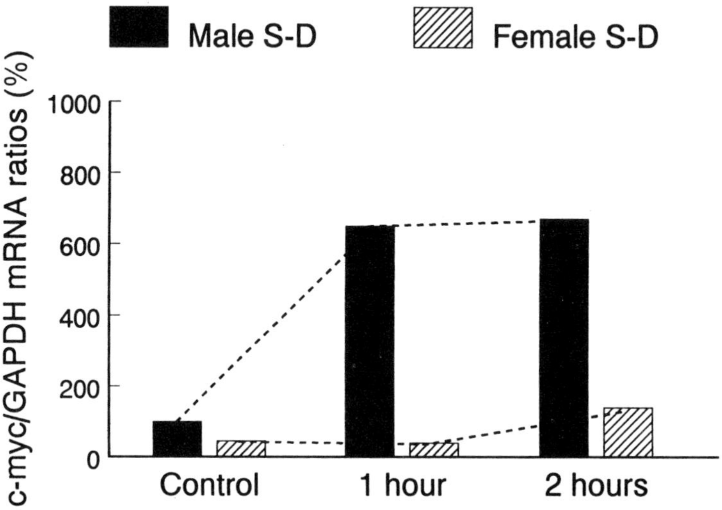

Fig. 3. Effects of sexual dimorphism on c-*myc* mRNA levels in balloon-injured right common carotid artery of male and female Sprague-Dawley rats at 1 and 2 h after injury. Results are presented as means ± SE. Each bar represents a single experiment carried out with RNA isolated from six injured carotid arteries and pooled. Reproduced with permission from ref. *70*.

in c-*myc* expression are seen in response to estrogen exposure. The dichotomy in these regulatory mechanisms of estrogen in different cell types merits further investigation. We are currently evaluating the effects of progestins, alone and in combination with estrogen, on neointima formation in the rat carotid injury model. Preliminary data suggest that progestins reduces the beneficial effects of 17β-estradiol on neointima formation after balloon injury, but have no independent effect on the hyperproliferative response to endothelial denudation *(71)*.

Using the mouse carotid injury model *(74)*, gonadectomy has been shown to enhance, and physiologic levels of 17β-estradiol replacement to suppress, subintimal hyperproliferation in vessels damaged by repetitive passage of angioplasty wires in female mice *(72)*. In this study, cellular proliferation in injured vessels, as assessed by bromodeoxyuridine (Brd U) labeling, was increased 20-fold following ovariectomy but was markedly attenuated by estrogen replacement. The effects of estrogen on the response to injury observed in this study may have been related to direct actions on VSMC proliferation, as suggested by previous studies, inhibition of the synthesis, and/or deposition of vascular matrix elements that contribute to lesion growth in injured vessels; an altered rate of re-endothelialization after injury; and/or inhibition of the inflammatory response in the injured vessel wall.

The swine model of coronary artery injury by balloon dilation offers advantages over rodent models of vascular injury in that the coronary anatomy, lipid metabolism, vascular cell biology, and coagulation profile of the pig are similar to the human *(75,76)*. We are currently examining the effects of exogenous estrogen on neointima formation after balloon injury of swine coronary arteries. Preliminary results indicate that 17β-estradiol administered sc from sustained release pellets reduces neointima formation in both male and female pigs *(73)*, and that the magnitude of this effect is related to circulating estrogen levels.

ESTROGENS, PROGESTINS, AND CARDIOVASCULAR RISK

Early studies of the effects of estrogens on cardiovascular risk were based on findings associated with oral contraceptive use. They suggested that estrogen use increased cardiovascular risk *(77,78)*. This was further supported by the Coronary Drug Project, a study in which men with an established history of cardiovascular disease were given Premarin® 5, 2.5 mg, or placebo and followed longitudinally *(79)*. The high-dose arm was stopped at 18 mo because of an increased incidence of myocardial infarction, thromboembolism, and stroke; the low-dose arm was stopped at 56 mo because of a statistically nonsignificant trend toward increased mortality in the treatment group. This trial has been criticized because of the high dose of estrogen used, equivalent to eight times the dose that is commonly used for estrogen replacement in postmenopausal women.

After the results of the Coronary Drug Project were reported, observational studies appeared suggesting that estrogen had protective effects against cardiovascular disease *(80,81)*. These studies examined outcomes in postmenopausal women receiving estrogen replacement. A meta-analysis of 31 studies of the association between coronary heart disease and the use of estrogen according to study design resulted in a calculated relative risk of myocardial infarction of 0.56 (95% CI 0.50–0.61) for estrogen users *(82)*. The discrepancy between the early and later data has been attributed to dose differences. Typical oral contraceptive doses of estrogen are considerably higher than postmenopausal replacement doses, and although higher doses of estrogen promote thrombosis *(83,84)*, lower doses tend to reduce atherosclerosis *(80,81)*.

Relative risks reported in the literature were used in a decision analysis to assess the value of estrogen replacement on a hypothetical cohort of 10,000 women assumed to be age 50 *(85)*. Health outcomes were extrapolated to age 75. According to this analysis, estrogen use for 25 yr should decrease fatal cardiac events by 48% (567 cases), decrease deaths from hip fracture by 49% (75 cases), and increase deaths from breast and endometrial cancer by 21% (39 cases) and 207% (29 cases), respectively. Twenty-five years of estrogen replacement in a cohort of 10,000 women could be expected to prevent 574 deaths and add 3951 quality-adjusted life years compared to women not using estrogen.

The 50% reduction in heart disease risk in postmenopausal women taking estrogen replacement therapy suggested by meta-analyses *(86)* may be misleading since observational studies have the severe limitation of treatment selection bias. In this case, women who are taking postmenopausal hormone replacement therapy tend to be healthier, better educated, and more attentive to lifestyle modification strategies for reducing cardiovascular risk and to have better health care *(87)*. Accordingly, prospective, randomized trials are needed to assess the impact of postmenopausal hormone replacement therapy on cardiovascular risk factors and event rates. The Postmenopausal Estrogen/Progestin Interventions (PEPI) Trial is a prospective, randomized, double-blind, placebo-controlled trial that is assessing differences between placebo, unopposed estrogen, and each of three estrogen/progestin regimens on selected heart disease risk factors in healthy postmenopausal women *(88)*. Primary endpoints are systolic blood pressure, HDL cholesterol, serum insulin, and fibrinogen. At 3 yr of followup, estrogen alone and in combination with progestin increased HDL and lowered LDL cholesterol and fibrinogen levels. Unopposed estrogen was the optimal regimen, but was associated with a high rate of endometrial hyperplasia and of hysterectomy (35 and 6%, respectively over 3 yr of followup), restricting its use to women without a uterus. In women with a uterus, conjugated equine estrogen combined with micronized progesterone had the most favorable effect on HDL cholesterol with no excess risk of endometrial hyperplasia. Systolic blood pressure increased in parallel with weight gain in all treatment groups, whereas diastolic blood pressure remained close to baseline levels. There was no treatment effect on blood pressure. These findings give strong evidence that estrogen alone or combined with progestin has a cardioprotective effect in postmenopausal women, particularly those with preexisting coronary disease or at high risk for developing coronary disease *(86,88)*. Whether these beneficial effects on cardiovascular risk factors translate into a reduced incidence of heart disease and reduced cardiovascular mortality rates awaits the results of large-scale, multicenter, long-term randomized trials, as are in progress in the Women's Health Initiative.

In considering whether or not to use postmenopausal hormone replacement therapy, women and their physicians must weigh its beneficial effects on risk of heart disease and osteoporosis against its adverse effects on risk of breast and uterine cancer *(86)*. Because heart disease is so much more common than breast cancer, the impact of postmenopausal hormone replacement therapy on lives saved by decreasing fatal heart attack rates is far greater than on lives lost by increasing breast cancer rates. However, relative risks of cardiovascular disease vs breast cancer vary greatly among women, so decisions about postmenopausal hormone replacement therapy should be individualized *(86)*.

REFERENCES

1. Godsland IF, Wynn V, Crook D, Miller NE. Sex, plasma lipoproteins, and atherosclerosis: prevailing assumptions and outstanding questions. Am Heart J 1987;114:1467–1503.
2. Bush TL, Barrett-Connor E. Noncontraceptive estrogen use and cardiovascular disease. Epidemiol Rev 1985;7:89–104.
3. Knopp RH. The effects of postmenopausal estrogen therapy on the incidence of arteriosclerotic vascular disease. Obstet Gynecol 1988;72:23S–30S.
4. Riedel M, Rafflenbeul W, Lichtlen P. Ovarian sex steroids and atherosclerosis. Clin Invest 1993;71:406–412.
5. Bush TL, Barrett-Conner E, Cowan LD, Criqui MH, Wallace RB, Suchindran CM, Tyroler HA, Rifkind BM. Cardiovascular mortality and non contraceptive use of estrogen in women: results from the Lipid Research Clinics Program Follow-up Study. Circulation 1987;75:1102–1109.
6. Gruchow HW, Anderson AJ, Barboriak JJ, Sobocinski KA. Postmenopausal use of estrogen and occlusion of coronary arteries. Am Heart J 1988;115:954–963.
7. Nabulsi AA, Folsom AR, White A, Patsch W, Heiss G, Wu KK, Szklo M. Association of hormone-replacement therapy with various cardiovascular risk factors in postmenopausal women. The Atherosclerosis Risk in Communities Study Investigators. N Engl J Med 1993;28:1069–1075.
8. Cauley JA, LaPorte RE, Kuller LH, Bates M, Sandler RB. Menopausal estrogen use, high density lipoprotein cholesterol subfractions and liver function. Atherosclerosis 1983;49:31–39.
9. Wallentin L, Varenhorst E. Plasma lipoproteins during anti-androgen treatment by estrogens or orchidectomy in men with prostatic carcinoma. Horm Metab Res 1981;13:293–297.
10. Tikkanen MJ. Role of lipoproteins in the pathogenesis of atherosclerotic disease with special reference to sex hormone effects. Am J Obstet Gynecol 1990;163:296–304.
11. Clarkson TB, Shively CA, Morgan TM, Koritnik DR, Adams MR, Kaplan JR. Oral contraceptives and coronary artery atherosclerosis of cynomolgus monkeys. Obstet Gynecol 1990;75:217–222.
12. Adams MR, Kaplan JR, Manuck SB, Koritnik DR, Parks JS, Wolfe MS, Clarkson TB. Inhibition of coronary artery atherosclerosis by 17-beta estradiol in ovariectomized monkeys. Lack of an effect of added progesterone. Arteriosclerosis 1990;10:1051–1057.
13. Evans RM. The steroid and thyroid hormone receptor superfamily. Science 1988;240:889–895.
14. Carson-Jurica MA, Schrader WT, O'Malley BW. Steroid receptor family: structure and functions. Endocr Rev 1990;11:201–220.
15. Koike S, Sakai M, Muramatsu M. Molecular cloning and characterization of rat estrogen receptor cDNA. Nucleic Acids Res 1987;15:2499–2513.

16. Kuiper G, Faber GJM, van Rooij HCJ, van der Korput JAGM, Ris-Stalpers C, Klaassen P, Trapman J, Brinkmann AO. Structural organization of the human androgen receptor gene. J Mol Endocrinol 1989;2:R1–R4.
17. Schott DR, Shyamala G, Schneider W, Parry G. Molecular cloning, sequence analyses, and expression of complementary DNA encoding murine progesterone receptor. Biochemistry 1991;30:7014–7020.
18. Kato J, Hirata S, Norzawa A, Yamada-Mouri N. Gene expression of progesterone receptor isoforms in the rat brain. Horm Behav 1994;28:454–463.
19. Mooradian AD, Morley JE, Korenman SG. Biological actions of androgens. Endocr Rev 1987;8:1–28.
20. Beato M. Gene regulation by steroid hormones. Cell 1989;56:335–344.
21. Smith DF, Toft DO. Steroid receptors and their associated proteins. Mol Endocrinol 1993;7:4–11.
22. Lin AL, Shain SA. Estrogen-mediated cytoplasmic and nuclear distribution of rat cardiovascular estrogen receptors. Arteriosclerosis 1985;5:668–677.
23. Tamaya T, Misao R, Nakagawa M, Itoh T, Wada K, Fujimoto J, Imai A. Estrogen and androgen receptors in aorta of the rabbit and regulation by estrogen and androgen. Res Commun Chem Pathol Pharmacol 1993;82:3–11.
24. Horwitz KB, Horwitz LD. Canine vascular tissues are targets for androgens, estrogens, progestins, and glucocorticoids. J Clin Invest 1982;69:750–758.
25. Vargas R, Wroblewska B, Rego A, Hatch J, Ramwell PW. Oestradiol inhibits smooth muscle cell proliferation of pig coronary artery. Br J Pharmacol 1993;109:612–617.
26. McGill HC Jr, Sheridan PJ. Nuclear uptake of sex steroid hormones in the cardiovascular system of the baboon. Circ Res 1981;48:238–244.
27. Lin AL, Gonzalez R, Carey KD, Shain SA. Estradiol-17β affects estrogen receptor distribution and elevates progesterone receptor content in baboon aorta. Arteriosclerosis 1986;6:495–504.
28. Campisi D, Cutolo M, Carruba G, Casto ML, Comito L, Granata OM, Valentino B, King RJB, Castagnetta L. Evidence for soluble and nuclear site I binding of estrogens in human aorta. Atherosclerosis 1993;103:267–277.
29. Losordo DW, Kearney M, Kim EA, Jekanowski J, Isner JM. Variable expression of the estrogen receptor in normal and atherosclerotic coronary arteries of premenopausal women. Circulation 1994;89:1501–1510.
30. Colburn P, Buonassisi V. Estrogen-binding sites in endothelial cell cultures. Science 1978;201:817–819.
31. Nakao J, Chang WC, Murota SI, Orimo H. Estradiol-binding sites in rat aortic smooth muscle cells in culture. Atherosclerosis 1981;38:75–80.
32. Beldekas JC, Smith B, Gerstenfeld LC, Sonenshein GE, Franzblau C. Effects of 17β-estradiol on the biosynthesis of collagen in cultured bovine aortic smooth muscle cells. Biochemistry 1981;20:2162–2167.
33. Chang WC, Nakao J, Orimo H, Murota S. Stimulation of prostacyclin biosynthesis activity by estradiol in rat aortic smooth muscle cells in culture. Biochem Biophys Acta 1980;619:107–118.
34. Harder DR, Coulson PB. Estrogen receptors and effects of estrogen on membrane electrical properties of coronary vascular smooth muscle. J Cell Physiol 1979;100:375–382.
35. Karas RH, Patterson BL, Mendelsohn ME. Human vascular smooth muscle cells contain functional estrogen receptor. Circulation 1994;89:1943–1950.
36. Orimo A, Inoue S, Ouchi Y, Orimo H. Vascular smooth muscle cells possess estrogen receptor and respond to estrogen. Ann NY Acad Sci 1995;748:592–594.
37. Orimo A, Inoue S, Ikegami A, Hosoi T, Akishita M, Ouchi Y, Muramatsu M, Orimo H. Vascular smooth muscle cells as target for estrogen. Biochem Biophys Res Commun 1993;195:730–736.
38. Karas RH, Baur W, Tassi L, Mendelsohn ME. Inhibition of vascular smooth muscle cell growth by estrogen. Circulation 1993;88:I-325 (abstract)
39. Fischer-Dzoga K, Wissler RW, Vesselinovitch D. The effect of estradiol on the proliferation of rabbit aortic medial tissue culture cells induced by hyperlipemic serum. Exp Mol Pathol 1983;39:355–363.
40. Lin AL, Gonzalez R, Carey KD, Shain SA. Gender and baboon aortic steroid hormone receptors. Arteriosclerosis 1987;7:248–255.
41. McGill HC Jr, Anselmo VC, Buchanan JM, Sheridan PJ. The heart is a target organ for androgen. Science 1980;207:775–777.
42. Krieg M, Smith K, Elvers B. Androgen receptor translocation from cytosol of rat heart muscle, bulbocavernosus/levator ani muscle and prostate into heart muscle nuclei. J Steroid Biochem 1980;13:577–587.
43. Fischer GM, Bashey RI, Rosenbaum H, Lyttle CR. A possible mechanism in arterial wall for mediation of sex difference in atherosclerosis. Exp Mol Pathol 1985;43:288–296.

44. Fujimoto R, Morimoto I, Morita E, Sugimoto H, Ito Y, Eto S. Androgen receptors, 5 alpha-reductase activity and androgen-dependent proliferation of vascular smooth muscle cells. J Steroid Biochem Mol Biol 1994;50:169–174.
45. Wilson J. Metabolism of testicular androgen. In: Greep RO, Astwood EB, eds. Handbook of Physiology, vol. 5. American Physiological Society, Washington, DC, 1975, p. 491.
46. Lin AL, McGill HC, Shain SA. Hormone receptors of the baboon cardiovascular system: biochemical characterization of aortic and myocardial cytoplasmic progesterone receptors. Circ Res 1982;50:610–616.
47. Ingegno MD, Money SR, Thelmo W, Greene GL, Davidian M, Jaffe BM, Pertschuk LP. Progesterone receptors in the human heart and great vessels. Lab Invest 1988;59:353–356.
48. Kraus WL, Montano MM, Katzenellenbogen BS. Identification of multiple, widely spaced estrogen-responsive regions in the rat progesterone receptor gene. Mol Endocrinol 1994;8:952–969.
49. Alexander JJ, Hoenig M, Graham D, Imbembo AL. The effect of estrogen on low-density lipoprotein binding kinetics in aortic endothelial cells. Surgery 1989;106:386–391.
50. Rifici VA, Khachadurian AK. The inhibition of low-density lipoprotein oxidation by 17-β estradiol. Metabolism 1992;41:1110–1114.
51. Gilligan DM, Quyyumi AA, Cannon RO, III. Effects of physiological levels of estrogen on coronary vasomotor function in postmenopausal women. Circulation 1994;89:2545–2551.
52. Keaney JF Jr, Shwaery GT, Xu A, Nicolosi RJ, Loscalzo J, Foxall TL, Vita JA. 17β-estradiol preserves endothelial vasodilator function and limits low-density lipoprotein oxidation in hypercholesterolemic swine. Circulation 1994;89:2251–2259.
53. Williams JK, Adams MR, Klopfenstein HS. Estrogen modulates responses of atherosclerotic coronary arteries. Circulation 1990;81:1680–1687.
54. Palmer RMJ, Ferrige AG, Moncada S. Nitric oxide release accounts for the biological activity of endothelium-derived relaxing factor. Nature 1987;327:524–526.
55. Williams JK, Adams MR, Herrington DM, Clarkson TB. Short-term administration of estrogen and vascular responses of atherosclerotic coronary arteries. J Am Coll Cardiol 1992;20:452–457.
56. Reis SE, Gloth ST, Blumenthal RS, Resar JR, Zacur HA, Gerstenblith G, Brinker JA. Ethinyl estradiol acutely attenuates abnormal coronary vasomotor responses to acetylcholine in postmenopausal women. Circulation 1994;89:52–60.
57. Chang WC, Nakao J, Orimo H, Murota SI. Stimulation of prostaglandin cyclooxygenase and prostacyclin synthetase activities by estradiol in rat aortic smooth muscle cells. Biochim Biophys Acta 1980;620:472.
58. Hayashi T, Fukuto JM, Ignarro LJ, Chaudhuri G. Basal release of nitric oxide from aortic rings is greater in female rabbits than in male rabbits: implications for atherosclerosis. Proc Natl Acad Sci USA 1992;89:11259–11263.
59. Weiner CP, Lizasoain I, Baylis SA, Knowles RG, Charles IG, Moncada S. Indication of calcium-dependent nitric oxide synthases by sex hormones. Proc Natl Acad Sci USA 1994;91:5212.
60. Mendelsohn ME, Karas RH. Estrogen and the blood vessel wall. Curr Opin Cardiol 1994;9:619–626.
61. Jiang C, Sarrel PM, Poole-Wilson PA, Collins P. Acute effect of 17β-estradiol on rabbit coronary artery contractile responses to endothelin-1. Am J Physiol 1992;263:H271–H275.
62. Zhang F, Ram JL, Standley PR, Sowers JR. 17β-estradiol attenuates voltage-dependent Ca^{2+} currents in A7r5 vascular smooth muscle cell line. Am J Physiol 1994;266:C975–C980.
63. Ross R. The pathogenesis of atherosclerosis: a perspective for the 1990s. Nature 1993;362:801–809.
64. Stamler J, Pick R, Katz LN. Prevention of coronary atherosclerosis by estrogen-androgen administration in the cholesterol-fed chick. Circ Res 1953;1:94–98.
65. Moskowitz MS, Moskowitz AA, Bradford WL, Wissler RW. Changes in serum lipids and coronary arteries of the rat in response to estrogens. Arch Pathol 1956;61:245–263.
66. Constantinides P, Gutmann-Auersperg N, Hospes D, Williams K. Estradiol and prednisone in rabbit atherosclerosis. Arch Pathol 1962;73:277–280.
67. Rhee CY, Spaet TH, Temerman MB, Lajam F, Shiang HH. Estrogen suppression of surgically induced vascular intimal hyperplasia in rabbits. J Lab Clin Med 1977;90:77–84.
68. Foegh ML, Khirabadi BS, Nakanishi T, Vargas R, Ramwell PW. Estradiol protects against experimental cardiac transplant atherosclerosis. Transplant 1987;19:90–95.
69. Foegh M, Asotra S, Howell M, Ramwell P. Estradiol inhibition of arterial neointimal hyperplasia after balloon injury. J Vasc Surg 1994;19:722–726.
70. Chen SJ, Li H, Durand J, Oparil S, Chen YF. Estrogen reduces myointimal proliferation after balloon injury of rat carotid artery. Circulation 1996;93:577–584.

71. Levine RL, Chen SJ, Durand J, Chen YF, Oparil S. 17β-estradiol but not medroxyprogesterone inhibits neointima formation after balloon injury of rat carotid arteries. J Invest Med 1996;44:26A.
72. Sullivan TR Jr, Karas RH, Aronovitz M, Faller GT, Ziar JP, Smith JJ, O'Donnell TF, Mendelsohn ME. Estrogen inhibits the response-to-injury in a mouse carotid artery model. J Clin Invest 1995;96(5): 2482–2488.
73. Levine RL, Anderson PG, Lyle K, Yadav SS, Oparil S, Roubin GS. 17β-estradiol inhibits restenosis after coronary angioplasty in pigs. J Invest Med 1996;44:26A.
74. Lindner V, Fingerle J, Reidy MA. Mouse model of arterial injury. Circ Res 1993;73:792–796.
75. Schwartz RS, Murphy JG, Edwards WD, Camrud AR, Vliestra RE, Holmes DR. Restenosis after balloon angioplasty. A practical proliferative model in porcine coronary arteries. Circulation 1990;82:2190–2200.
76. Steele PM, Chesebro JH, Stanson AW, Holmes DR Jr, Dewanjee MK, Badimon L, Fuster V. Balloon angioplasty. Natural history of the pathophysiological response to injury in a pig model. Circ Res 1985;57:105–112.
77. Mann JI, Inman WHW. Oral contraceptives and death from myocardial infarction. Br Med J 1975;2:245–248.
78. Shapiro S, Slone D, Rosenberg L, Kaufman DW, Stolley PD, Miettinen OS. Oral contraceptive use in relation to myocardial infarction. Lancet 1979;1:743–747.
79. The Coronary Drug Project Research Group. The Coronary Drug Project: initial findings leading to modifications of its research protocol. JAMA 1970;214:1303–1313.
80. Rosenberg L, Slone D, Shapiro S, Kaufman D, Stolley PD, Miettinen OS. Noncontraceptive estrogens and myocardial infarction in young women. JAMA 1980;244:339–342.
81. Stampfer MJ, Willett WC, Colditz GA, Rosner B, Speizer FE, Hennekens CH. A prospective study of postmenopausal estrogen therapy and coronary heart disease. N Engl J Med 1985;313:1044–1049.
82. Stampfer MJ, Colditz GA. Estrogen replacement and coronary heart disease: a quantitative assessment of the epidemiologic evidence. Prev Med 1991;20:47–63.
83. Meade TW. Oral contraceptives, clotting factors and thrombosis. Am J Obstet Gynecol 1982;142(Part 2):758–761.
84. Bottiger LE, Boman G, Eklund G, Westerholm B. Oral contraceptives and thromboembolic disease: effects of lowering oestrogen content. Lancet 1980;1:1097–1101.
85. Gorsky RD, Koplan JP, Peterson HB, Thacker SB. Relative risks and benefits of long term estrogen replacement therapy: a decision analysis. Obstet Gynecol 1994;83:161–166.
86. Grady D, Rubin SM, Petitti DB, Fox CS, Black D, Ettinger B, Ernster VL, Cummings SR. Hormone therapy to prevent disease and prolong life in postmenopausal women. Ann Intern Med 1992;117:1016–1037.
87. Barrett-Connor E. Postmenopausal estrogen and prevention. Ann Intern Med 1991;115:455,456.
88. PEPI Trial Writing Group. Effects of estrogen or estrogen/progestin regimens on heart disease risk factors in postmenopausal women. The Postmenopausal Estrogen/Progestin Interventions (PEPI) trial. JAMA 1995;3:199–208.

18 Vitamin D and the Vessel Wall

Richard D. Bukoski, PHD

CONTENTS

INTRODUCTION

The purpose of this chapter is to review the actions of vitamin D_3 on the vessel wall. The discussion starts with an outline of basic vascular considerations, including an overview of the physiological chemistry of vitamin D_3, and the role of the steroid in the regulation of whole animal Ca^{2+} homeostasis. The focus then turns to vascular actions of 1,25 $(OH)_2$ vitamin D_3 and discusses the cellular mechanisms of action of this hormone, its role in normal and pathophysiologic states, and the potential cardiovascular applications of recently developed structural analogs. The discussion then moves to a body of work that describes vessel wall pathology induced by pharmacologic concentrations of vitamin D_3, and the use of the sterol in the production of a model for the study of calcifying arteriosclerotic disease. Data that implicates excess vitamin D_3 intake in human cardiovascular disease is also considered. Although this chapter provides a thorough review of the known vascular actions of vitamin D_3 and its metabolites, it cannot be comprehensive in the areas of vascular smooth muscle physiology, vitamin D_3 chemistry, or Ca^{2+} metabolism. For in-depth analysis of these areas, the reader is referred to other material *(1–6)*.

Vascular Considerations

When discussing the vascular actions of any hormone it must be recognized that the vasculature is a complex network of multiple cell types *(7)*. Blood vessels are comprised of three strata:

1. The intima consisting of a single layer of endothelial cells;
2. The muscular media consisting of vascular smooth muscle cells embedded in a connective tissue matrix; and
3. An outer adventitial layer made of connective tissue and varying degrees of innervation by sympathetic, parasympathetic, and sensory nerve fibers.

From: *Contemporary Endocrinology: Endocrinology of the Vasculature*
Edited by: J. R. Sowers Humana Press Inc., Totowa, NJ

The relative contribution of each of these components varies along the vascular tree such that conduit arteries are highly elastic, and smaller arteries that contribute to vascular resistance are significantly more muscular and can be densely innervated. Thus, there can be considerable regional heterogeneity in the vascular response to any stimulus.

It is well understood that the vasculature undergoes dynamic changes throughout the life of an organism and that the major human vascular disease processes, e.g., atherosclerosis *(8)* and essential hypertension *(9,10)*, develop over periods of years to decades. It is somewhat surprising, therefore, that much of the research that is performed in the area of vascular function is focused on the mechanisms by which acute effectors of the vasculature act. For example, volumes have been written about the vascular actions and pharmacology of neurotransmitters including catecholamines and vasoactive peptides, and about modulation of vascular function by derivatives of the endothelial cell, including nitric oxide and the prostanoids *(11,12)*. In contrast, little is known about the long-term effects of endocrine factors on the development, function, and health of the vessel wall. We anticipate that the study of the vascular actions of vitamin D_3, its metabolites, and analogs will serve as a model system for identifying the mechanisms by which local and humoral factors modulate the function and health of the vasculature over long periods of time, and for understanding how disturbances in these systems may contribute to disease processes.

Physiological Chemistry of Vitamin D_3

The pathways by which vitamin D_3 arises in the body are illustrated in Fig. 1. In the presence of ultraviolet radiation, 7-dehydrocholesterol (provitamin D_3) in the skin is converted to the 9,10 secosteroid previtamin D_3. Previtamin D_3 in the skin then slowly converts to vitamin D_3 by a temperature-dependent process. In addition to production in the dermis, vitamin D_3 also enters the body via ingestion of food and vitamin supplements. After absorption from the skin or the intestine, vitamin D_3 is carried through the blood by a specific transport protein to the liver where it undergoes hydroxylation at the 25 position. 25 (OH) vitamin D_3 is then hydroxylated at the 1-α position in the proximal renal epithelia forming 1,25 $(OH)_2$ vitamin D_3, which biologically is the most potent metabolite of the steroid. In addition to these main products, the hormone undergoes a number of chemical modifications and the biologic actions of these resulting metabolites for the most part remain to be delineated.

As noted, vitamin D_3 and its metabolites are carried through the serum by a specific vitamin D_3 binding protein which is also known as human group-specific component (G_C) *(13)*. This protein, which is synthesized by the liver, is a member of the albumin family of proteins, and in addition to its high-affinity binding sites for vitamin D_3, also binds actin. G_C is highly polymorphic in the human; three common alleles and more

Fig. 1. *(opposite page)* Physiological chemistry of vitamin D. **(A)** Numbering scheme of the 1,25 vitamin D backbone. **(B)** In the presence of ultraviolet radiation, 7-dehydrocholesterol (provitamin D_3) is converted to the 9,10 secosteroid previtamin D_3 and then to vitamin D_3. Vitamin D_3 also enters the body via an oral route. After absorption from the skin or the intestine, vitamin D is carried by a specific transport protein to the liver where it is hydroxylated to form 25-OH-vitamin D_3 position, then carried to the kidney where 1-α hydroxylation catalyzed by 1-α hydroxylase occurs. 1,25 $(OH)_2$ vitamin D_3 is then carried through the blood on a specific vitamin D binding protein. Adapted from ref. *5* with permission.

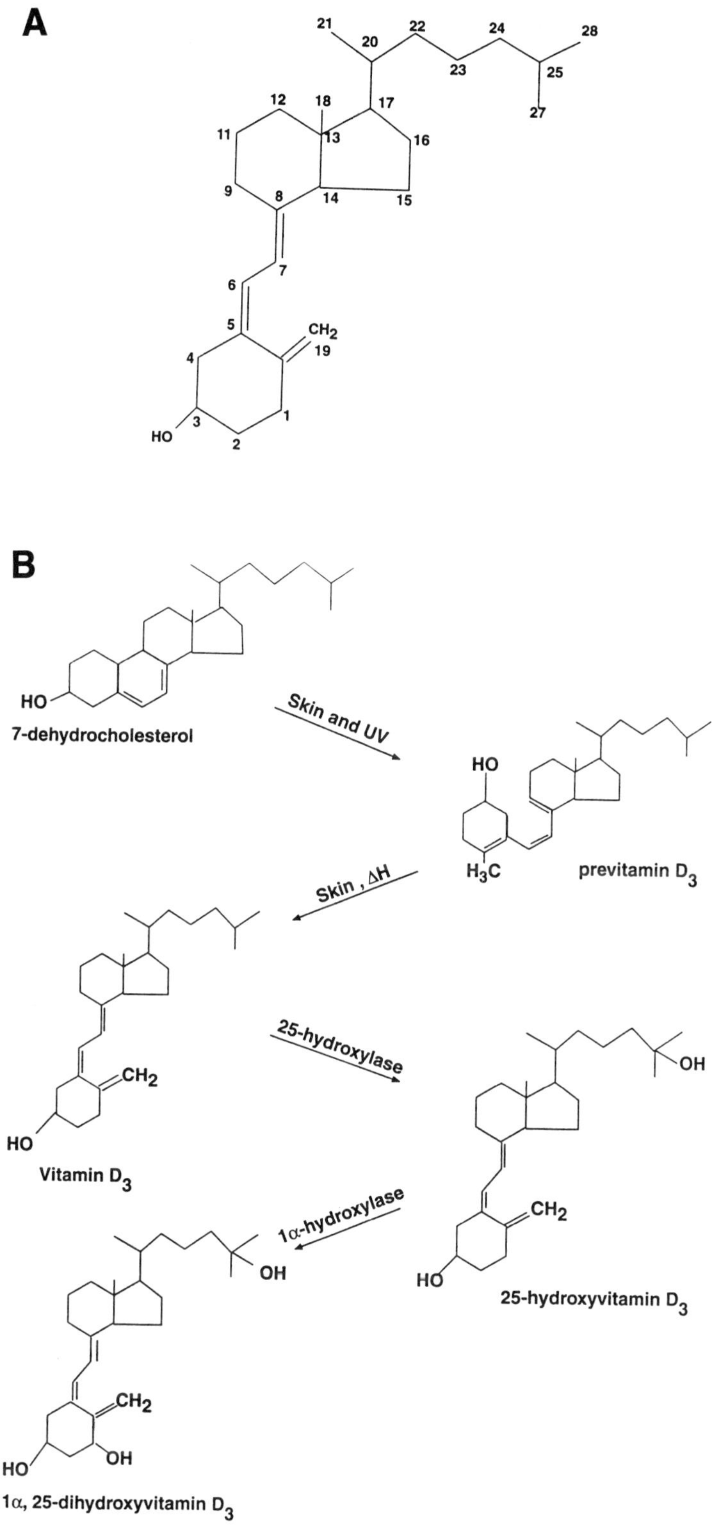
A
B
HO
7-dehydrocholesterol
Skin and UV
HO
H_3C
previtamin D_3
Skin, ΔH
CH_2
HO
Vitamin D_3
25-hydroxylase
OH
CH_2
HO
25-hydroxyvitamin D_3
1α-hydroxylase
OH
CH_2
HO
OH
1α, 25-dihydroxyvitamin D_3

Fig. 1.

than 120 variants have been described *(14,15)*. Thus far, however, it does not appear that these polymorphisms alter the affinity of the protein for vitamin D_3. Moreover, there is no evidence for allosteric modulation of the affinity of the D_3 binding protein for vitamin D_3, or for preferred transfer of the hormone into cells mediated by an interaction of the protein with the cell membrane. Nonetheless, the concentration of bioavailable 1,25 $(OH)_2$ vitamin D_3 in blood is a function of the total amount of 25 (OH) and 1,25 $(OH)_2$ vitamin D_3 and related metabolites, the concentration of vitamin D binding protein, and the affinity of the vitamin D binding protein relative to other high-affinity binding sites *(16)*.

At target tissues, 1,25 $(OH)_2$ vitamin D_3 enters the cell and binds to a specific steroid receptor which then translocates to the nucleus where it initiates cellular processes through a genomic mechanism that is characteristic of steroid hormones *(17)*. Although our understanding of the molecular events by which 1,25 $(OH)_2$ vitamin D_3 and other steroids modulate cell function has become increasingly sophisticated, for the purpose of this review it is sufficient to know that the hormone has multiple genomic actions including the ability to initiate synthesis of mRNA via transcriptional regulation and to both stimulate cell growth and induce differentiation *(18)*. In addition to genomic effects, there is also evidence which supports the postulate that 1,25 $(OH)_2$ vitamin D_3 modulates cell function by a rapid nongenomic effects that may be mediated by activation of a cell membrane receptor *(19)*. The most thoroughly studied example of this effect is the stimulation of Ca^{2+} uptake across the intestine of the chick by administration of 1,25 $(OH)_2$ vitamin D_3 to the blood. This effect, which is termed transcaltachia, is inhibited by Ca^{2+} channel antagonists (blockers of protein kinase C), is associated with a rise in intracellular cAMP, and has been proposed to be linked with a specific cell membrane receptor *(20)*. Whether this effect is present in mammalian species remains to be established.

1,25 $(OH)_2$ Vitamin D_3 and Ca^{2+} Homeostasis

A rise or fall of ionized Ca^{2+} in the serum elicits a series of endocrine responses that restore Ca^{2+} to a level that is normal for a given individual, i.e., 1.15–1.35 mmol/L. For example, a decrease in serum ionized Ca^{2+} stimulates the release of parathyroid hormone (PTH) from the parathyroid gland through an action mediated by the extracellular Ca^{2+} receptor *(21,22)*. PTH acts to restore serum Ca^{2+} by mobilizing Ca^{2+} from bone via stimulation of osteoclasts and osteocytes and by enhancing renal tubular reabsorption of Ca^{2+}. PTH is also a powerful stimulus at the renal tubule cell for the conversion of 25 (OH) vitamin D_3 to 1,25 $(OH)_2$ vitamin D_3. In intestinal and renal epithelial cells 1,25 $(OH)_2$ vitamin D_3 increases the synthesis of vitamin D-dependent Ca^{2+} binding proteins which facilitate intestinal absorption and renal reabsorption of the cation. In contrast to PTH and 1,25 $(OH)_2$ vitamin D_3, calcitonin acts as a Ca^{2+} lowering agent by inhibiting osteoclast activity and preventing the mobilization of Ca^{2+} from bone. Although release of this peptide is apparently mediated by the extracellular Ca^{2+} receptor, it is regulated in a manner that is opposite to PTH, such that a fall in serum ionized Ca^{2+} decreases release of the peptide. The net effect of this orchestrated series of events is the maintenance of serum ionized Ca^{2+} at the preset level.

When considering 1,25 $(OH)_2$ vitamin D_3 production, it is important to note that in addition to production by the kidney, 1,25 $(OH)_2$ vitamin D_3 is also produced by hematopoietic cells *(23)*, sarcoid tissue *(24)*, and the vascular endothelium *(25)*. The total amount of 1,25 $(OH)_2$ vitamin D_3 in the serum therefore increases and decreases according to the Ca^{2+} status of the animal, and in certain microenvironments may be significantly different from that which is present in the mixed venous plasma.

VASCULAR ACTIONS OF 1,25 $(OH)_2$ VITAMIN D_3

It is now well established that 1,25 $(OH)_2$ vitamin D_3 significantly modulates Ca^{2+} metabolism, contractile activity, and growth of the vascular smooth muscle cell *(26)*. The groundwork for studies on vascular smooth muscle lies in two separate areas. One was the search for actions of 1,25 $(OH)_2$ vitamin D_3 on nonclassic target tissues including cardiac and skeletal muscle *(27,28)*. The second was work that was directed toward understanding the mechanism by which manipulation of dietary Ca^{2+} intake modulates blood pressure and vascular reactivity by testing the hypothesis that the hormones of the vitamin D PTH axis mediate the actions of Ca^{2+} supplied to the gut *(29)*. Among the earliest findings were simultaneous reports that appeared in 1987 demonstrating that receptors specific for 1,25 $(OH)_2$ vitamin D_3 are present in the A7r5 cell line derived from vascular smooth muscle and in cultured aortic smooth muscle cells *(30,31)*. Shortly thereafter, our laboratory and others initiated studies to determine whether 1,25 $(OH)_2$ vitamin D_3 modulates vascular smooth muscle function.

1,25 $(OH)_2$ Vitamin D_3 and Vascular Contractility

An important piece of the puzzle was provided by our demonstration that injection of the rat with 1,25 $(OH)_2$ vitamin D_3 in an amount that raises serum levels by 50–75%, enhances contractile force generation by subsequently isolated mesenteric resistance arteries *(32)*. The fact that the force response was normalized to cross-sectional area of the media eliminated the possibility that the enhanced force was the result of medial hypertrophy. Resistance arteries of 1,25 $(OH)_2$ vitamin D_3-treated rats have since been shown to exhibit an increased force response to norepinephrine, arginine vasopressin, serotonin, and K^+ depolarization; a pattern that is consistent with a postreceptor site of action. Analysis of the time-course over which the inotropic action of 1,25 $(OH)_2$ vitamin D_3 occurs showed that more than 24 h is required for the response to be detected and that it persists for up at least up to 24 d with continued administration of the hormone *(33,34)*. We have also observed that a single injection of 1,25 $(OH)_2$ vitamin D_3 induces an increase in force generation in vessels isolated from the animals 4 d later *(35)*. These data have been interpreted to indicate that the inotropic effect of 1,25 $(OH)_2$ vitamin D_3 is mediated by a genomic action of the hormone.

The observation that 1,25 $(OH)_2$ vitamin D_3 enhances vascular reactivity has been confirmed by Hatton et al. *(36)* using rat aorta, and by Roca-Cusachs et al. *(37)* and Shimosawa et al. *(38)* using in vivo preparations. Figure 2 outlines the pathways by which activation of the smooth muscle cell leads to contraction and is provided as a means of illustrating the hypothetical mechanisms of action that have been studied. We and others have thus far considered the possibilities that 1,25 $(OH)_2$ vitamin D_3:

1. Modulates Ca^{2+} handling, including both transmembrane influx and intracellular Ca^{2+} mobilization;
2. Alters phosphorylation of the myosin regulatory light chain; and
3. Alters expression of contractile proteins.

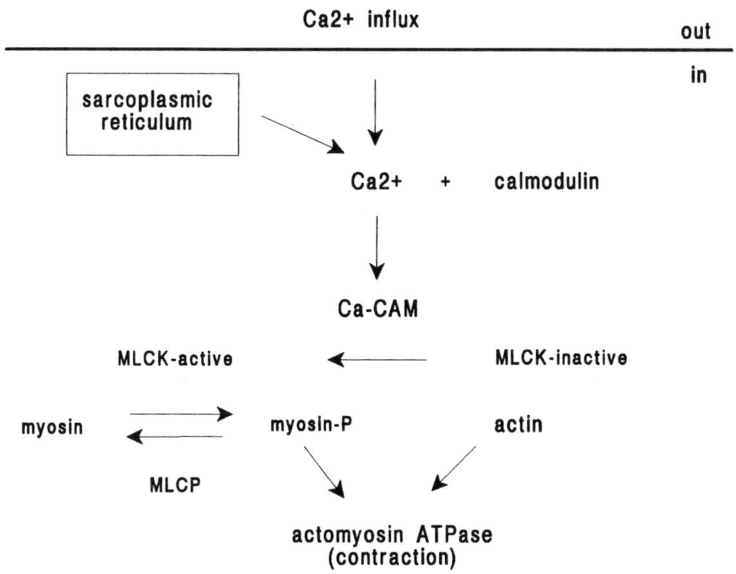

Fig. 2. Putative genomic mechanisms by which 1,25 $(OH)_2$ vitamin D_3 may enhance contractile force generation by vascular smooth muscle. Ca^{2+} enters the smooth muscle through voltage-sensitive or other types of Ca^{2+} channels, and can be released from internal stores denoted as sarcoplasmic reticulum. Intracellular Ca^{2+} then binds to calmodulin (CAM) which activates myosin light-chain kinase (MLCK) which in turn phosphorylates the regulatory light chain of myosin. Phosphorylation of the light chain results in activation of actomyosin ATPase and force generation by the smooth muscle cell. Effects of 1,25 $(OH)_2$ vitamin D_3 have thus far been demonstrated on ^{45}Ca influx *(39–41)*, L-type Ca^{2+} channel activity *(35,42)*, basal Ca^{2+} and agonist-induced intracellular Ca^{2+} mobilization *(35)*, myosin light-chain phosphorylation *(35)*, and myosin heavy-chain and regulatory light-chain content *(43,44)*.

1,25 $(OH)_2$ Vitamin D_3 and Vascular Ca^{2+} Handling

Shortly after the first reports that vascular smooth muscle expresses a high-affinity receptor for 1,25 $(OH)_2$ vitamin D_3, our laboratory reported that 1,25 $(OH)_2$ vitamin D_3 enhances ^{45}Ca uptake by primary cultures of aortic myocytes of spontaneously hypertensive (SHR) and normotensive Wistar Kyoto rats *(39)*. Inoue and Kawashima *(40)* confirmed these results and provided evidence suggesting that in the A7r5 cell line, the stimulation of ^{45}Ca uptake is dependent on protein synthesis and is selective for the 1,25 $(OH)_2$ metabolite of vitamin D_3. We demonstrated subsequently that 1,25 $(OH)_2$ vitamin D_3 differentially stimulates ^{45}Ca uptake by subcultured mesenteric artery myocytes *(41)*. The action occurs over a physiologic concentration range, depends on the synthesis of intracellular protein, and exhibits a time-course that is consistent with a genomic mechanism of action. Although Kawashima *(45)* subsequently showed that Ca^{2+}-ATPase activity is enhanced in microsomes prepared from A7r5 cells treated with 1,25 $(OH)_2$ vitamin D_3, the significance of this observation in terms of vascular Ca^{2+} handling has not been delineated.

Although these early data were consistent with a calciotropic action of the steroid on vascular smooth muscle, they did not provide information about its effect on the level of free intracellular Ca^{2+} or the magnitude of Ca^{2+} mobilization in response to contractile agonists. It was not until methods for measurement of intracellular Ca^{2+} in intact vessels were developed that was it possible to assess these parameters *(46)*. A recent report from our laboratory that employed fura-2-based technology has provided insight into the mechanisms by which 1,25 $(OH)_2$ vitamin D_3 modulates smooth muscle force generating capacity *(35)*. It was observed that ip injection of 1,25 $(OH)_2$ vitamin D_3 (30 ng/100 g body weight) into the Wistar rat significantly modulates mesenteric resistance artery Ca^{2+} handling. Under resting conditions there was both an increase in the basal level of free intracellular Ca^{2+} and in the level of myosin regulatory light-chain phosphorylation in tissue of 1,25 $(OH)_2$ vitamin D_3-treated rats. Moreover, during activation with norepinephrine, we observed enhanced force generation and an increase in intracellular Ca^{2+} mobilization both of which were inhibited by the Ca^{2+} channel antagonist verapamil. These results have led to the hypothesis that treatment with 1,25 $(OH)_2$ vitamin D_3 enhances either Ca^{2+} channel density in the cell membrane or activity of the channel such that opening probability is increased. These changes would then be responsible for the observed increase in basal Ca^{2+} which would drive basal myosin light-chain phosphorylation, and for the increase in agonist-induced Ca^{2+} mobilization which would lead to enhanced force generation.

The results of our experiments assessing intracellular Ca^{2+} confirm and extend the report of Shan and colleagues *(42)* in which it was observed that treatment of primary cultures of aortic smooth muscle cells of the rat with pharmacologic concentrations of 1,25 $(OH)_2$ vitamin D_3 results in an opening of L-type Ca^{2+} channels and an increase in intracellular Ca^{2+}. However, their experiments showed that this calciotropic effect occurs after only a 20-min delay and that a similar concentration of 1,25 $(OH)_2$ vitamin D_3 applied acutely is without effect on force generation in an isolated vessel preparation. Thus, this rapid action may be part of the signaling process through which 1,25 $(OH)_2$ vitamin D_3 initiates genomic activity.

1,25 $(OH)_2$ Vitamin D_3 and Contractile Protein Expression

As illustrated in Fig. 2, another potential mechanism by which 1,25 vitamin D_3 might modulate vascular force generation is by altering synthesis of contractile proteins. To address this possibility we tested the hypothesis that treatment of the rat with 1,25 $(OH)_2$ vitamin D_3 enhances vascular smooth muscle myosin light-chain and heavy-chain expression. Wistar rats were injected with 1,25 $(OH)_2$ vitamin D_3 (30 ng/100 g body weight) for 3 consecutive days and on the 4th day aorta, superior mesenteric artery, and mesenteric resistance arteries were isolated and protein was extracted and analyzed by polyacrylamide gel electrophoresis *(43)*. Aortas of rats receiving 1,25 $(OH)_2$ vitamin D_3 exhibited an increase in total myosin heavy-chain and light-chain content. Furthermore, the increase in regulatory light-chain content was the result of a selective increase in expression of the smooth muscle isoform of this protein. In contrast, no differences in myosin heavy-chain or light-chain content or myosin light-chain isoforms were seen in the mesenteric resistance artery which is the tissue in which force generation has been shown to be enhanced *(32–35)*. These data indicate that there is regionally specific activity of 1,25 $(OH)_2$ vitamin D_3 along the vascular tree, i.e., a promyosin effect in the aorta, but not in the resistance artery.

Recent work carried out in our laboratory using a cultured organ preparation has extended the observation that myosin isoform expression is selectively modulated by 1,25 $(OH)_2$ vitamin D_3. In previous studies using a cell culture model, we observed that incubation of the mesenteric resistance artery for a 48 hr period results in a significant loss of force generating capacity *(47)*. We have now found that the 48-hr incubation results in a decline in myosin heavy-chain content that is the result of a specific loss of the SM-2 isoform of the heavy chain *(44)*. Moreover, supplementation of the culture medium with 1,25 $(OH)_2$ vitamin D_3 (300 pg/mL) prevents the loss of the SM-2 isoform and fully preserves force generating capacity. These latter data have been interpreted to indicate that 1,25 $(OH)_2$ vitamin D_3 exerts a significant effect on myosin heavy-chain isoform content which results in maintenance of the contractile phenotype. These data, in combination with the fact that 1,25 $(OH)_2$ vitamin D_3 enhances myosin expression in the intact aorta and Ca^{2+} channel-dependent Ca^{2+} mobilization in the resistance artery have led to our hypothesis that 1,25 $(OH)_2$ vitamin D_3 exerts a differentiating action on the smooth muscle cell. Moreover, we suggest that the steroid modulates the expression of a cassette of genes that encode proteins that establish the contractile phenotype of the smooth muscle cell.

1,25 $(OH)_2$ Vitamin D_3 and Smooth Muscle Proliferation

The effects of 1,25 $(OH)_2$ vitamin D_3 on growth of cultured vascular smooth muscle cells has been examined by several laboratories. In the experiments in which we assessed the effect of 1,25 $(OH)_2$ vitamin D_3 on ^{45}Ca uptake by cultured mesenteric artery myocytes, we found that the hormone stimulates vascular smooth muscle growth with an apparent requirement for a low concentration of fetal calf serum *(48)*. It is now clear that 1,25 $(OH)_2$ vitamin D_3 exerts significant growth regulatory actions on the smooth muscle cell. Koh et al. *(49)* using cultured rat aortic smooth muscle cells showed that in the presence of 10% fetal calf serum, 1,25 $(OH)_2$ vitamin D_3 stimulates ^3H-thymidine uptake over a concentration range of 0.1–100 nmol/L and the effect is specific for the 1,25 dihydroxy form of vitamin D_3. Subsequently, the same group reported that in the absence of fetal calf serum 1,25 $(OH)_2$ vitamin D_3 (1 pmol/L–10 nmol/L) stimulates aortic smooth muscle cell growth and inhibits glycosaminoglycan production *(50)*. In contrast to these results, MacCarthy and colleagues *(51)* reported that 1,25 $(OH)_2$ vitamin D_3 inhibits thc growth of cultured aortic smooth muscle cells between 0.1 and 100 nmol/L both in the absence of a growth stimulus and in the presence of epidermal growth factor. Growth inhibitory actions of the hormone have also been reported for mesangial cells cultured from both the mouse and the human *(52,53)*.

In 1991 Mitsuhashi et al. *(54)* further documented the complexity of the effect of 1,25 $(OH)_2$ vitamin D_3 on smooth muscle growth when they showed that the hormone stimulates growth of cultured aortic smooth muscle cells if added to preparations that were previously made quiescent by serum deprivation, and potentiates the growth response to thrombin or platelet-derived growth factor (PDGF). In contrast, when added to cells that were not made completely quiescent, 1,25 $(OH)_2$ vitamin D_3 depresses the growth response to either thrombin or PDGF. Thus, the growth response of vascular smooth muscle to 1,25 $(OH)_2$ vitamin D_3 is dependent on the position of the cell in the cell cycle at the time of its addition. Tu-Yu et al. *(55)* further assessed the effect of the hormone on early response genes in cultured smooth muscle cells and found that 1,25 $(OH)_2$ vitamin D_3 added with thrombin causes a fivefold increase in c-*jun* expression whereas pretreatment with 1,25 $(OH)_2$ vitamin D_3 for 48 h reduces the c-*jun* response to thrombin by 75%. Expression of c-*fos* was unaffected by the sterol with the result that the c-*jun*:c-*fos* ratio was markedly altered. Tu-Yu and colleagues *(55)* suggested that the effects of 1,25 $(OH)_2$ vitamin D_3 on c-*jun* and c-*fos* expression and their and subsequent interaction at the AP-1 transcription site may be a central component of the growth modulatory action of the hormone.

1,25 $(OH)_2$ Vitamin D_3 and Vascular Pathophysiology

Given these significant vascular actions of 1,25 $(OH)_2$ vitamin D_3, one must raise the question of whether pathophysiologic changes in the serum levels of the hormone contribute to human vascular disease. Serum 1,25 $(OH)_2$ vitamin D_3 is elevated in a variety of human conditions including primary hyperparathyroidism *(56)*, sarcoidosis *(24)*, patients with end stage renal disease receiving calcitriol supplements *(57)*, the third trimester of pregnancy *(58)*, and postmenopausal women receiving estrogen supplements for osteoporosis *(59)*. The hormone therefore has the potential to modulate the course of either etiologically associated, or naturally occurring vascular disease. As an example, the normal rise of 1,25 $(OH)_2$ vitamin D_3 during the third trimester of pregnancy might contribute to vascular pathology of gestational hypertension in that the vascular calciotropic actions of 1,25 $(OH)_2$ vitamin D_3 could contribute to the elevated peripheral resistance of this condition. Moreover, in the case of end stage renal disease, administration of 1,25 $(OH)_2$ vitamin D_3 supplements induces phasic increases of the hormone to pharmacologic levels with the result that the patient undergoes periodic activation of the vascular wall during the course of their therapy.

With regard to the question of vascular pathophysiology, however, it must be noted that at the present time, no clear linkage has been established between elevated serum levels of 1,25 $(OH)_2$ vitamin D_3 and any cardiovascular disease. Nevertheless, it is important to remember that changes in vitamin D binding protein content may occur *(16)* which could alter the amount of bioavailable 1,25 $(OH)_2$ vitamin D_3 and that significant local production of the 1,25 dihydroxy metabolite may occur and could result in elevated levels of 1,25 $(OH)_2$ vitamin D_3 in regional compartments *(23)*.

The Promise of 1,25 $(OH)_2$ Vitamin D_3 Analogs

The potent and significant effects of 1,25 $(OH)_2$ vitamin D_3 on the growth and state of differentiation of a multiple types of cells including leukemia *(60)* and solid tumor cell lines *(61)* and the dermal epithelium *(62)* has been viewed as an opportunity to use the steroid in an effort to develop new therapeutic strategies *(63)*. A major limitation of using 1,25 $(OH)_2$ vitamin D_3 as a pharmacologic agent, however, is the narrow therapeutic window that results from its potent hypercalcemic actions. Fortunately, chemical modification of the 1,25 $(OH)_2$ vitamin D_3 molecule has provided compounds with potent differentiating actions and minimal calciotropic effects *(64–66)*. One common characteristic of many of these analogs is a low affinity for the vitamin D binding protein. Thus, the analogs reach very high concentrations in the blood, exert genomic effects, suppress endogenous 1,25 $(OH)_2$ vitamin D_3 production, and are rapidly cleared from the circulation.

1,25 $(OH)_2$ vitamin D_3 analogs are currently in clinical trials for the treatment of psoriasis and development is underway for treatment of metabolic bone disease and cancer. There are at least two reports that one analog, 22-oxa-calcitriol (22-OCT), exerts significant vascular actions. One is an effect to increase peripheral vascular resistance *(38)*, the second is an ability to increase prostacyclin production *(67)*. We anticipate, therefore, that as the mechanisms of the vascular actions of 1,25 $(OH)_2$ vitamin D_3 become better understood, analogs with selectivity for smooth muscle will be identified and targeted toward treatment of cardiovascular pathologies such as atherosclerosis and restenosis after balloon angioplasty.

VASCULAR ACTIONS OF VITAMIN D_3

A body of data has accumulated over the past two decades which demonstrates that vitamin D_3 has deleterious actions on the vascular wall which are apparently independent of the effects of the 1,25-dihydroxy metabolite which are described earlier. Among the first indications that vitamin D_3 alters vessel wall morphology were studies which showed that hypervitaminosis D is associated with calcification of multiple organs *(68–70)*. The primary effects of vitamin D_3 on the vessel wall are degeneration of smooth muscle cells, deposition of lipid material, and formation of calcium deposits both in the area of degenerate smooth muscle cells and along elastic fibers *(71)*. A number of laboratories have viewed the response of the arterial wall to high doses of vitamin D_3 as an opportunity to develop an experimental model for nonatheromatous arteriosclerosis.

Vitamin D_3-Induced Arteriosclerosis

To fairly assess the potential of using vitamin D_3-induced changes in the vessel wall as a model of nonatheromatous arteriosclerosis, it is useful to consider the pathology of the atherosclerotic disease process which is the leading cause of death in the United States. Atherosclerosis is characterized in early stages by fatty streaks along the intimal surface that contain cholesterol esters, macrophages, and smooth muscle cells. In later stages fibrous plaques develop that have a core of extracellular lipid material and debris from necrotic tissue, and are covered by fibrous tissue made of proliferating smooth muscle cells, macrophages, and connective tissue *(8)*. The fibrous plaque can progress to a complicated lesion containing various degrees of necrosis, thrombosis, and ulceration. In the latter instance, rupture of the fibrous cap releases thrombogenic material that can lead to blockage of the artery and subsequent tissue infarction.

With this progression in mind, it will be seen that vitamin D-induced arteriosclerosis reflects the human condition to varying degrees and this heterogeneity may be dependent on both the dose of vitamin D and the animal species being studied. For example, Taura et al. *(72)* showed that coronary arteriosclerosis develops in normolipemic swine fed diets supplemented with vitamin D_3 ranging from 31,250–125,000 U/kg of diet over a 3-mo period. Calcified lesions were characterized by fibromuscular intimal thickening which in some cases exhibited abundant lipid, cholesterol crystals, foam cell formation, necrosis, and fibroelastosis. Similar results were obtained by the same group using swine fed vitamin D_3 at 100,000–4,000,000 U/ton of diet for a 4-mo period *(73,74)*. In addition to swine, rats also respond to excess vitamin D_3 with atherosclerotic-like lesions. Takeo et al. *(75)* showed that rats given a single injection of 500,000 U of vitamin D_3/kg develop lesions along the aorta with massive accumulation of calcium in the media. Other models, including those produced by combined treatment with vitamin D_3 and nicotine *(76)* or cholesterol, cholic acid, and thiouracil *(77)* induce similar arterial changes. Among the functional consequences of vitamin D_3-induced calcifying arteriosclerosis are a decrease force generating capacity of subsequently isolated arteries *(75,78)* and a decrease in the elasticity of the vessel wall with a secondary increase in pulse pressure *(76)*.

One use of the vitamin D_3-induced models of arteriosclerosis has been the study of pharmacologic or physiologic means of preventing development of the calcifying plaque. A number of studies initiated by Fleckenstein and colleagues *(79–82)* have examined the effect of pretreatment of animals with Ca^{2+} channel blockers as inhibitors of the vitamin

D_3-induced arterial changes. These compounds, as a class, are generally effective at preventing the changes *(83,84)*. In addition, Ito and colleagues *(85,86)* showed that Mg^{2+} restriction enhances the arteriosclerotic effect of vitamin D_3 whereas supplementation with Mg^{2+} suppresses vitamin D_3-induced arterial changes. Although these observations have been reproduced, few if any mechanistically oriented experiments have been carried out to provide insight into cellular mechanisms of action.

Mechanism of Vitamin D's Vascular Actions

It is generally believed that vitamin D_3 induces the characteristic arterial changes through a complex series of interrelated effects. One response of the organism to vitamin D_3 is an elevation in serum Ca^{2+} *(72,73,76,77,85,86)*. The availability of excess extracellular Ca^{2+} would then be likely to contribute to the increase in arterial wall Ca^{2+} content and play a role in intracellular calcification, possibly secondary to enhanced permeability of the smooth muscle cell to Ca^{2+}. Although not proven, it is also possible that the cellular degeneration that has been reported is the result of this intracellular Ca^{2+} overload. The changes in lipid content of the arterial wall may be related to changes in lipid metabolism that can result from vitamin D_3 excess. For example, Kummerow and colleagues *(73)* suggested that 25-hydroxy vitamin D_3 is metabolized and esterified in a manner similar to 25-hydroxy cholesterol.

In the context of this chapter, we must also ask the question of whether the effects of vitamin D_3 overload are mediated in any way by conversion of the parent molecule to 1,25 $(OH)_2$ vitamin D_3 which then acts by the classic steroid-like mechanism described. Although none of the articles that were reviewed reported measurements of serum 1,25 $(OH)_2$ vitamin D_3 after vitamin D_3 administration, consistent increases in serum Ca^{2+} were observed *(72,73,76,77,85,86)*. Whether this increase is the result of an increase in intestinal absorption and renal reabsorption of Ca^{2+}, or another action, is not clear. Indirect evidence that these actions of vitamin D_3 are not mediated by increased levels of 1,25 $(OH)_2$ vitamin D_3 is the finding that when vascular contractility is assessed in vessels of vitamin D_3 supplemented animals, it is depressed *(75,78)*. This contrasts with the observed inotropic effects of the 1,25 $(OH)_2$ metabolite *(32–35)*.

Implications of Vitamin D's Vascular Actions

Although the effects of vitamin D_3 on the vascular wall are obviously deleterious and provide a model for the study of calcifying arteriosclerosis, they are of interest for another reason which relates to the controversy regarding the recommended requirements for vitamin D_3 intake in the human population. It has been proposed that supplementation of the human diet with vitamin D_3, either through direct treatment of food or through supplementation of the diets of precursor sources including farm animals, has resulted in excess intake of vitamin D_3 in humans *(87–89)*. Moreover, it has been argued that the rise in arteriosclerosis and related Ca^{2+} metabolic diseases has reached epidemic proportions and the advent of this onset began during the period of time when wholesale supplementation of food with vitamin D_3 occurred *(88)*. Although many cogent arguments can be raised against retrospective historical analysis, the fact remains that vitamin D_3 is a fat soluble vitamin which can be stored in human tissues, and when present in excess amounts in swine and rodents, induces rapid calcification, deterioration of the medial layer, and intimal thickening of muscular arteries. Additional work along these lines is thus needed to clarify these issues.

SUMMARY AND CONCLUSIONS

The actions of vitamin D_3 and its primary active metabolite 1,25 $(OH)_2$ vitamin D_3 have been reviewed. It is now established that the 1,25 dihydroxy metabolite exerts significant vascular actions including modification of vascular smooth muscle cell growth, Ca^{2+} handling, contractile protein expression, and force generation. These findings have led to the hypothesis that 1,25 $(OH)_2$ vitamin D_3 exerts a differentiating action in the vascular smooth muscle cell. The possibility that 1,25 $(OH)_2$ vitamin D_3 analogs with specific cardiovascular actions is highly promising. In contrast with these effects of the dihydroxy metabolite, administration of high doses of vitamin D_3 results in the development of calcifying arteriosclerotic lesions in a variety of mammalian species. These models have been used to establish that Ca^{2+} channel antagonists and dietary Mg^{2+} intake can modulate the development of calcifying arteriosclerosis and in part support the hypothesis that excess vitamin D_3 intake in the human may contribute to atherosclerotic vascular disease.

ACKNOWLEDGMENTS

We acknowledge the expert secretarial assistance of Wilma Frye. Original work was supported by grants from the National Institutes of Health, R29-HL41816 and RO1-HL54901, and from the John Sealy Memorial Foundation.

REFERENCES

1. Somlyo AP, Somlyo AV. Signal transduction and regulation in smooth muscle. Nature 1994;372:231–236.
2. Missiaen L, De Smedt, Droogmans G, Himpens B, Casteels R. Calcium ion homeostasis in smooth muscle. Pharmacol Ther 1992;56:191–231.
3. Stull JT, Gallagher PJ, Herring P, Kamm KE. Vascular smooth muscle contractile elements. Hypertension 1991;17:723–732.
4. Murphy RA. Do the cytoplasmic and muscle-specific isoforms of actin and myosin heavy and light chains serve different functions in smooth muscle? Jpn J Pharmacol 1992;58(Suppl. 2):67P–74P.
5. Holick MF, Potts JT. Vitamin D: In: Petersdorf RG, Adams RD, Braunwald E, Isselbacher KJ, Martin JB, Wilson JD, eds. Harrison's Principles of Internal Medicine. McGraw-Hill, New York, 1983, pp. 1944–1949.
6. Civiletti R, Avioli LV. The biochemistry and function of calciotropic hormones. In: Crass W, Avioli L, eds. Calcium-Regulating Hormones and Cardiovascular Function. CRC Press, Boca Raton, FL, 1995, pp. 1–44.
7. Schwartz SM, Heimark RL, Majesky MW. Developmental mechanisms underlying pathology of arteries. Physiol Rev 1990;70:1177–1209.
8. Bierman EL, Ross R. Aging and atherosclerosis. In: Paoletti R, Gotto AM Jr, eds. Atherosclerosis Reviews. Raven, New York, 1977, pp. 79–111.
9. Cowley AW Jr. Long-term control of arterial blood pressure. Physiol Rev 1992;72:231–300.
10. Folkow B. Physiology of cardiovascular aging. Physiol Rev 1993;73:725–764.
11. Burnstock G, Ralevic V. New insights into the local regulation of blood flow by perivascular nerves and endothelium. Br J Anesthesiol 1994;47:527–543.
12. Moncada S. Nitric oxide. J Hypertens 1994;12:S35–S39.
13. Bishop JE, Collins ED, Okamura WH, Norman AW. Profile of ligand specificity of the vitamin D binding protein for 1α,25-dihydroxyvitamin D_3 and its analogs. J Bone Min Res 1994;9:1277–1288.
14. Kofler A, Braun A, Jenkins T, Serjeantson SW, Cleve H. Characterization of mutants of the vitamin-D-binding protein/group Specific Component: GC aborigine (1A1) from Australian aborigines and South African Blacks, and 2A9 from South Germany. Vox Sang 1995;68:50–54.
15. Yuasa I, Kofler A, Braun A, Umetsu K, Bichlmaier R, Kammerer S, Cleve H. Characterization of mutants of the vitamin D-binding protein/group-specific component: molecular evolution of GC$*$1A2 and GC$*$1A3, common in some Asian populations. Hum Genet 1995;95:507–512.

16. Vieth R. Simple method for determining specific binding capacity of vitamin D-binding protein and its use to calculate the concentration of "free" 1,25-dihydroxyvitamin D. Clin Chem 1994;40: 435–441.
17. Minghetti PP, Norman AW. 1,25 $(OH)_2$-vitamin D_3 receptors: gene regulation and genetic circuitry. FASEB J 1988;2:3043–3053.
18. Carlberg C, Bendik I, Wyss A, Meier E, Sturzenbecker LJ, Grippo JF, Hunziker W. Two nuclear pathways for vitamin D. Nature 1993;361:657–660.
19. Nemere I, Zhou LX, Norman, AW. Nontranscriptional effects of steroid hormones. Receptor 1993;3:277–291.
20. Nemere I, Dormanen MC, Hammond MW, Okamura WH, Norman AW. Identification of a specific binding protein for 1α,25-dihydroxyvitamin D_3 in basal-lateral membranes of chick intestinal epithelium and relationship to transcaltachia. J Biol Chem 1994;269:23,750–23,756.
21. Brown EM, Gamba G, Riccardi D, Lombardi M, Butters R, Kifor O, Sun A, Hediger MA, Jytton J, Hebert SC. Cloning and characterization of an extracellular Ca^{2+}-sensing receptor from bovine parathyroid. Nature 1993;366:575–580.
22. Garrett JE, Capuano IV, Hammerland LG, Hung BCP, Brown EM, Hebert SC, Nemeth EF, Fuller F. Molecular cloning and functional expression of human parathyroid calcium receptor cDNAs. J Biol Chem 1995;270:12,919–12,925.
23. Dusso A, Brown A, Slatopolsky E. Extrarenal production of calcitriol. Sem Nephrol 1994;14:144–155.
24. Bell NH, Stern PH, Pantzer E, Sinha TK, DeLuca HF. Evidence that increased circulating 1α,25-dihydroxyvitamin D is the probable cause for abnormal calcium metabolism in sarcoidosis. J Clin Invest 1979;64:218–225.
25. Merke J, Milde P, Lewicka S, Hügel U, Klaus G, Mangelsdorf DJ, Haussler MR, Rauterberg EW, Ritz E. Identification and regulation of 1,25-dihydroxyvitamin D_3 receptor activity and biosynthesis of 1,25-dihydroxyvitamin D_3. J Clin Invest 1989;83:1903–1915.
26. Bukoski RD, Ishibashi K, Bian K. Vascular actions of the calcium regulating hormones. Sem Nephrol 1995;15(6)536–549.
27. Boland AR, Boland R. Suppression of 1,25-dihydroxy-vitamin D_3-dependent calcium transport by protein synthesis inhibitors and changes in phospholipids in skeletal muscle. Biochim Biophys Acta 1985;845:237–241.
28. Walters MR, Ilenchuk T, Claycomb WC. 1,25-dihydroxyvitamin D_3 stimulates $^{45}Ca^{2+}$ uptake by cultured adult rat ventricular cardiac muscle cells. J Biol Chem 1987;262:2536–2541.
29. McCarron DA. Calcium metabolism and hypertension. Kidney Int 1989;35:717–736.
30. Kawashima H. Receptor for 1,25 dihydroxyvitamin D in a vascular cell line derived from rat aorta. Biochem Biophys Res Comm 1987;146:1–6.
31. Merke J, Hofmann D, Goldschmidt H. Demonstration of 1,25 $(OH)_2$ vitamin D_3 receptors and actions in vascular smooth muscle in vitro. Calcif Tiss Int 1987;41:112–114.
32. Bukoski RD, Wagman DW, Wang DH. Injection of 1,25 vitamin D enhances resistance artery contractile properties. Hypertension 1990;16:523–531.
33. Bukoski RD, Xue H. On the vascular inotropic action of calcitriol. Am J Hypertens 1993;6:388–396.
34. Bukoski RD, Li J, Bo J. Effect of long-term administration of calcitriol on blood pressure and resistance artery contractility in the hypertensive rat. Am J Hypertens 1993;6:944–950.
35. Bian K, Ishibashi K, Bukoski RD. Effect of 1,25 $(OH)_2$ vitamin D_3 on resistance artery intracellular Ca^{2+} and force generation. Am J Physiol (Heart) 1995;270(39):H230–H237.
36. Hatton DC, Xue H, DeMerritt J, McCarron DA. 1,25 $(OH)_2$ vitamin D_3-induced alterations in vascular reactivity in the spontaneously hypertensive rat. Am J Med Sci 1994;307(Suppl. 1):S154–S158.
37. Roca-Cusachs A, DiPette DJ, Carson J, Graham GA, Holland OB. Systemic and regional hemodynamic effects of 1,25 vitamin D_3 administration. J Hypertension 1992;10:939–947.
38. Shimosawa T, Ando K, Fujita T. Enhancement of vasoconstrictor responses by a noncalcemic analogue of vitamin D_3. Hypertension 1993;21:253–258.
39. Bukoski RD, Xue H, McCarron DA. Effect of 1,25 $(OH)_2$ vitamin D_3 and ionized Ca^{2+} on ^{45}Ca uptake by primary cultures of aortic myocytes of spontaneously hypertensive and Wistar-Kyoto normotensive rats. Biochem Biophys Res Comm 1987;146:1330–1335.
40. Inoue T, Kawashima H. 1,25-dihydroxyvitamin D_3 stimulates ^{45}Ca-uptake by cultured VSMCs derived from rat aorta. Biochem Biophys Res Comm 1988;152:1388–1394.
41. Xue H, McCarron DA, Bukoski RD. 1,25 $(OH)_2$ vitamin D_3 and ^{45}Ca uptake by vascular myocytes of hypertensive and normotensive rats. Life Sci 1991;49:651–659.

42. Shan J, Resnick LM, Lewanczuk R, Karpinski E., Li B, Pang PKT. 1,25-Dihydroxyvitamin D as a cardiovascular hormone. Effects on calcium current and cytosolic free calcium in VSMCs. Am J Hypertens 1993;6:983–988.
43. Ishibashi K, Evans A, Shingu T, Bian K, Bukoski RD. Differential distribution and steroid responsiveness of myosin regulatory light chain in the arterial tree. Am J Physiol (Cell) 1995;38: C443–C450.
44. Ishibashi K, Bukoski RD. Myosin isoform content determines force generation in cultured resistance arteries: effect of 1,25 vitamin D and insulin. Hypertension 1995;26:578.
45. Kawashima H. 1,25-dihydroxyvitamin D_3 stimulates Ca-ATPase in VSMC line. Biochem Biophys Res Comm 1988;150:1138–1143.
46. Bukoski RD, Bergmann C, Gairard A, Stoclet JC. Intracellular Ca^{2+} and force determined simultaneously in isolated resistance arteries. Am J Physiol (Heart) 1989;257:H1728–H1735.
47. Xue H, McCarron DA, Bukoski RD. 1,25 $(OH)_2$ vitamin D_3 attenuates the loss of resistance artery contractile function associated with incubation in culture media. Biochem Biophys Res Comm 1991;174:11–17.
48. Bukoski RD, DeWan P, McCarron DA. 1,25 $(OH)_2$ vitamin D_3 modifies growth and contractile function of vascular smooth muscle of spontaneously hypertensive rats. Am J Hypertens 1989;2:533–556.
49. Koh E, Morimoto S, Fukuo K, Itoh K, Hironaka T, Shiraishi T, Onishi T, Kumahara Y. 1,25-Dihydroxyvitamin D_3 binds specifically to rat VSMCs and stimulates their proliferation in vitro. Life Sci 1988;42:215–223.
50. Koh E, Morimoto S, Nabata T, Takamoto S, Kitano S, Ogihara T. Effects of 1,25-dihydroxyvitamin D_3 on the synthesis of DNA and glycosaminoglycans by rat aortic smooth muscle cells in vitro. Life Sci 1990;46:1545–1551.
51. MacCarthy EP, Yamashita W, Hsu A, Ooi BS. Modulating effect of 1,25-dihydroxyvitamin D_3 ($1,25D_3$) on rat VSMC (VSMC) growth. Hypertension 1988;13:954–959.
52. Hariharan S, Hong SY, Hsu A, MacCarthy EP, Gartside PS, Ooi BS. Effect of 1,25-dihydroxyvitamin D_3 on mesangial cell proliferation. J Lab Clin Med 1991;117:423–429.
53. Weinreich T, Merke J, Schönermark M, Reichel H, Diebold M, Hänsch GM, Ritz E. Actions of 1,25-dihydroxyvitamin D_3 on human mesangial cells. Am J Kidney Dis 1991;XVIII:359–366.
54. Mitsuhashi T, Morris RC, Ives HE. 1,25-dihydroxyvitamin D_3 modulates growth of VSMCs. J Clin Invest 1991;87:1889–1895.
55. Tu-Yu A, Morris C, Ives HE. Differential modulation of fos and jun gene expression by 1,25-dihydroxyvitamin D_3. Biochem Biophys Res Comm 1993;193:161–166.
56. Broadus AE, Horst RL, Lang R, Littledike ET, Rasmussen H. The importance of circulating 1,25-dihydroxyvitamin D in the pathogenesis of hypercalcemia and renal-stone formation in primary hyperparathyroidism. N Engl J Med 1980;302:421–426.
57. Coburn JW, Salusky IB, Norris KC, Goodman WG. Oral and parenteral calcitriol for the management of end-stage renal disease. Contrib Nephrol 1990;90:166–182.
58. Verhaeghe J, Bouillon R. Calciotropic hormones during reproduction. J Ster Biochem Mol Biol 1992;41:469–477.
59. Bikle DD, Halloran BP, Harris ST, Portale AA. Progestin antagonism of estrogen stimulated 1,25-dihydroxyvitamin D levels. J Clin Endocr Metab 1993;72:519–523.
60. Shiina Y, Abe E, Miyaura C, Tanaka H, Yamada S, Ohmori M, Nakayama K, Takayama H, Matsunaga I, Nishii Y, DeLuca HF, Suda T. Biological activity of 24,25-difluoro-1 alpha, 25-dihydroxyvitamin D_3 and 1 alpha, 25-dihydroxyvitamin D_3-26,23 lactone in inducing differentiation of human myeloid leukemia cells. Arch Biochem Biophys 1983;220(1):90–94.
61. Frampton RJ, Osmand SA, Eisman JA. Inhibition of human cancer cell growth by 1,25-dihydroxyvitamin D_3 metabolites. Cancer Res 1983;43:4443–4447.
62. Bikle DD, Pillai S. Vitamin D, calcium and epidermal differentiation. Endocr Rev 1993;14:3–19.
63. Bikle DD. Clinical counterpoint: vitamin D: new actions, new analogs, new therapeutic potential. Endocr Rev 1992;13:765–784.
64. Zhou JY, Norman AW, Lubbert M, Collins ED, Uskokovich MR, Koeffler HP. Novel vitamin D analogs that modulate leukemic cell growth and differentiation with little effect on either intestinal calcium absorption or bone calcium mobilization. Blood 1989;74:82–93.
65. Kobayashi T, Tsugawa N, Okano T, Masuda S, Takeuchi A, Kubodera N, Nishii Y. The binding properties with blood proteins, and tissue distribution of 22-oxa-1α,25-dihydroxyvitamin D_3, a noncalcemic analog of 1α,25-dihydroxyvitamin D_3 in rats. J Biochem 1994;115:373–380.

66. Bouillin R, Allewaert K, Xiang DZ, Tan BK, Van Baelen H. Vitamin D analogs with low affinity for the vitamin D binding protein: enhanced in vitro and decreased in vivo activity. J Bone Min Res 1991;6(10):1051–1057.
67. Inoue M, Wakasugi M, Wakao R, Gan N, Tawata M, Nishii Y, Onaya T. A synthetic analog of vitamin D_3, 22-oxa-1,25-dihydroxy-vitamin D_3, stimulates the production of prostacyclin by vascular tissues. Life Sci 1992;51:1105–1112.
68. Danowski TS, Winkler AW, Peters JP. Tissue calcification and renal failure produced by massive dose vitamin D therapy of arthritis. Ann Intern Med 1945;23:22–29.
69. Hass GM, Trueheart RE, Taylor CB, Stumple M. An experimental histologic study of hypervitaminosis D. Am J Pathol 1958;34:395–422.
70. Kent SP, Vawter GF, Domben RM, Benson RE. Hypervitaminosis D in monkeys—a clinical and pathological study. Am J Pathol 1958;34:37–59.
71. Taura S, Taura M, Imai H, Kummerow FA, Tokuyasu K, Cho SB. Ultrastructure of cardiovascular lesions induced by hypervitaminosis D and its withdrawal. Paroi Arterielle 1978;4:245–249.
72. Taura S, Taura M, Kamio A, Kummerow FA. Vitamin D-induced coronary atherosclerosis in normolipemic swine: comparison with human disease. Tohoku J Exp Med 1979;129:9–16.
73. Toda T, Ito M, Smith T, Kummerow F. Angiotoxicity in swine of a moderate excess of dietary vitamin D_3. Food Chem Toxic 1985;23:585–592.
74. Toda T, Toda Y, Kummerow FA. Coronary arterial lesions in piglets from sows fed moderate excesses of vitamin D. Tohoku J Exp Med 1985;145:303–310.
75. Takeo S, Anan M, Fujioka K, Kajihara T, Hiraga S, Miyake K, Tanonaka K, Minematsu R, Mori H, Taniguchi Y. Functional changes of aorta with massive accumulation of calcium. Atherosclerosis 1989;77:175–181.
76. Atkinson J, Poitevin P, Chillon JM, Lartaud I, Levy B. Vascular Ca overload produced by vitamin D_3 plus nicotine diminishes arterial distensibility in rats. Am J Physiol 1994;266:H540–H547.
77. Kamio A, Taguchi T, Shiraishi M, Shitama K, Fukushima K, Takebayashi S. Vitamin D sclerosis in rats. Acta Path Jpn 1979;29(4):545–562.
78. Kitagawa S, Yamaguchi Y, Kunitomo M, Imaizumi N, Fujiwara. Altered vasoconstrictor responsiveness in vitamin D-induced arteriosclerotic rat aortas. Jpn J Pharmacol 1993;61:283–289.
79. Fleckenstein A, Frey M, Zorn J, Fleckenstein-Grün G. Experimental basis of the long-term therapy of arterial hypertension with calcium antagonists. Am J Cardiol 1985;56:3H–14H.
80. Fleckenstein A, Fleckenstein-Grün G. Mechanism of action of calcium antagonists in heart and vascular smooth muscle. Eur Heart J 1988;9(Suppl. H):95–99.
81. Fleckenstein-Grün G, Frey M, Thimm F, Luley C, Czirfusz A, Fleckenstein A. Differentiation between calcium- and cholesterol-dominated types of arteriosclerotic lesions: antiarteriosclerotic aspects of calcium antagonists. J Cardiovasc Pharmacol 1991;18(Suppl. 6):S1–S9.
82. Fleckenstein-Grün G, Thimm F, Frey M, Czirfusz A. Role of calcium in arteriosclerosis—experimental evaluation of antiarteriosclerotic potencies of Ca antagonists. Basic Res Cardiol 1994;89(Suppl. 1):145–159.
83. Holzgreve H, Bürkle B. Anti-atherosclerotic effects of calcium antagonists. J Hypertens 1993;11(Suppl. 1):S55–S59.
84. Makki T, Lartaud I, Bray-des Boscs L, Capdeville-Atkinson C, Chillon JM, Hoffman M, Nicolas JP, Atkinson J. Haemodynamic effects of a new dihydropyridine calcium entry blocker, S-12968-(—), in rat model of cardiovascular calcium overload. Br J Pharmacol 1992;106:79–84.
85. Ito M, Sekine I, Kummerow FA. Dietary magnesium effect on swine coronary atherosclerosis induced by hypervitaminosis D. Acta Pathol Jpn 1987;37(6):955–964.
86. Ito M, Cho BHS, Kummerow FA. Effects of a dietary magnesium deficiency and excess vitamin D_3 on swine coronary arteries. J Am Coll Nutr 1990;9(2):155–163.
87. Holmes RP, Kummerrow FA. The relationship of adequate and excessive intake of vitamin D to health and disease. J Am Coll Nutr 1983;2:173–199.
88. Davies H. Coronary heart disease: the significance of coronary pathology in infancy and the role of mitogens such as vitamin D. Med Hypoth 1989;30:179–185.
89. Moon J, Bandy B, Davison AJ. Hypothesis: etiology of atherosclerosis and osteoporosis: are imbalances in the calciferol endocrine system implicated? J Am Coll Nutr 1992;11;567–583.

19 Vascular Action Natriuretic Peptide Receptors

Kailash N. Pandey, PHD

Contents

INTRODUCTION

Discovery of structurally related natriuretic peptide hormones: atrial natriuretic peptide (ANP), brain natriuretic peptide (BNP), and C-type natriuretic peptide (CNP) suggests that their role in control of body fluid and blood pressure homeostasis is complex. This complexity is further enhanced by the existence of at least three types of natriuretic peptide receptors, designated as Npra (GC-A), Nprb (GC-B), and Nprc (clearance receptor) *(1–3)*. Although these three natriuretic peptides have highly homologous structure, they also have distinct sites of synthesis, bind to specific receptors, and probably elicit discrete biological functions *(1–3)*. Both Npra and Nprb belong to the members of receptor guanylyl cyclase (GC) family, which produce their own second messenger cyclic guanosine monophosphate (cGMP). Production of cGMP in response to natriuretic peptides results from their binding to the extracellular domain of Npra or Nprb, which probably allosterically regulates an increased activity of the intracellular GC catalytic domain *(3,4)*. The extracellular domain of Npra and Nprb is homologous to Nprc which apparently does not contain a GC catalytic domain. ANP and BNP bind to Npra and CNP binds to Nprb; however, all three natriuretic peptides indiscriminately bind to Nprc *(4)*. CNP is a natural ligand for Nprb and is the prominent cGMP-generating and the biologically active receptor in vascular smooth muscle cells (VSMC). CNP and its specific receptor Nprb are expressed in vasculature and, therefore, CNP/Nprb might emerge as an important natriuretic peptide-receptor system in vasorelaxation and preventing vas-

From: *Contemporary Endocrinology: Endocrinology of the Vasculature*
Edited by: J. R. Sowers Humana Press Inc., Totowa, NJ

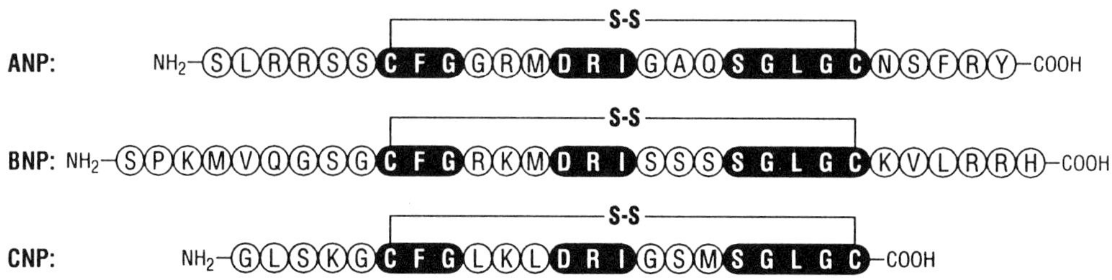

Fig. 1. Structure of human natriuretic peptides. The sequence comparison of the mature human ANP, BNP, and CNP conserved residues represented by darkened boxes. The line between the two cysteine residues in each peptide indicates a disulfide bridge. Reproduced with permission from ref. *4*.

cular injury. VSMCs contain a high density of Nprc that functions to remove natriuretic peptides from the circulation *(2)*. The full implication of the structure–activity relationship of the natriuretic peptides and their receptors in target tissues, including VSMC, is not yet completely understood. The aim of this chapter is to summarize the roles of natriuretic peptides and their receptors with particular emphasis of cellular and physiological function(s) in vasculature.

GENERAL BACKGROUND, NOMENCLATURE, AND SIGNALING OF NATRIURETIC PEPTIDES AND THEIR RECEPTORS

Extracts of atria were discovered to provoke a marked natriuresis, diuresis, and hypotension when injected into rats, and the active substance was given the name "atrial natriuretic factor" (ANF or ANP) *(5)*. It was soon recognized that specific granules in the atria were the storage sites for ANP and that these granules resemble the secretory granules of endocrine cells, suggesting that the heart via secretion of ANP has an endocrine role in regulation of extracellular fluid volume and blood pressure *(6)*. Two other natriuretic peptides have been identified and isolated with molecular and biochemical characteristics similar to ANP, but each is derived from separate genes *(7)*. The nomenclatures of these peptides are referred to as type-A natriuretic peptide (ANP), primarily synthesized in the granules of heart atrium; type-B natriuretic peptide (BNP) initially isolated from brain, but located predominantly in the heart and displaying the most variability in primary structure; and C-type natriuretic peptide (CNP), isolated from porcine brain, is highly conserved among the species.

ANP is synthesized first as the 152-amino acid prepro-ANP that contained sequences of active peptides in its carboxy-terminal region, and the major form of circulatory ANP is a 28-residue molecule. Different lengths of sequences of ANP were synthesized for studies of structure–activity relationship, and results indicate that the ring conformation of the ANP molecule is comprised of 17-amino acid residues and a disulfide-bonded loop essential for biological activities. The carboxy terminal sequence extending from the ring structure to Asn-Phe-Arg-Tyr is required for activity *(1,8)*. Circulating ANP elicits multiple physiological responses, largely directed to the reduction of blood pressure and fluid volume.

BNP and CNP are also synthesized from large precursor proteins and the mature active peptides contain a 17-residues disulfide loop (Fig. 1). Human natriuretic peptides contain 11 identical residues in the disulfide loop, whereas the amino- and carboxy-terminal ends are variable. BNP was initially discovered in porcine brain *(9)* and subsequently was found to be more abundant in cardiac atria than in the central nervous system *(10)*. BNP is secreted by the heart, circulates in plasma, and has similar biological actions and potency to ANP and is therefore a true cardiac hormone. CNP, originally identified from porcine brain *(11)*, is structurally homologous to ANP and BNP, which are largely synthesized in the heart and circulate in plasma. ANP expression has also been found in the lung, aortic arch, kidney, pituitary, adrenal medulla, testis, and central nervous system *(1,7,12)*. Sites of CNP production are also thought to be multiple, including brain, vascular endothelium, kidney, and monocytes *(13–16)*. Circulating or locally formed CNP has vascular effects such as decreases in blood pressure *(17,18)* and inhibition of vascular hypertrophy and VSMC proliferation *(19,20)*.

The cellular responsiveness of natriuretic peptides are manifested through binding to specific cell surface receptors in different target tissues. Initial crosslinking and photoaffinity labeling studies showed the existence of ANP receptors of the 65–70- and 120–180-kDa proteins *(1,2,8)*. High-affinity binding sites for ANP were copurified with particulate GC activity, which indicated that both ANP binding and GC activity resides in the 120–180-kDa receptor molecules *(21–24)*. A 70-kDa protein also was isolated and did not have GC activity *(25,26)*. Initially, ANP receptors were characterized based on the differential binding characteristics and abilities to generate cGMP in response to various lengths of ANP peptides, truncated at the amino and/or carboxy terminal of 28-residues ANP *(27,28)*. Full length ANP (28-residues) provides the structural framework, whose specificity is defined by the unique amino acid sequences of Asn-Phe-Arg-Tyr at the carboxyl terminus of ANP molecule. Lack of these residues markedly reduces the binding of the truncated peptide (atriopeptin I [API]) to the 135-kDa ANP receptor, as well as the natriuretic and vasorelaxant activities of ANP *(28)*. Based on the biological activity of different ANP analogs, ANP receptors were classified as biologically active and clearance or silent receptors *(29)*. Different subtypes of ANP receptor appear to be specific to different target cell types *(30–32)*.

There are two specific binding sites in rat thoracic aortic VSMC *(32,33)*. These include a larger M_r receptor of the 140 kDa and a smaller M_r receptor of 66–70 kDa. Under reducing conditions, there is a marked shift to the 66–70-kDa band (Fig. 2) with a diminution and sometimes almost complete disappearance of the 135–140-kDa band. The unlabeled full length $ANP_{(103–123)}$, inhibits the labeling of both the 140- and 66–70-kDa bands in a dose-dependent manner. Truncated $ANP_{(103–123)}$ (API) also inhibits labeling of both the 140- and 66–70-kDa band in a dose-dependent manner *(30,32,33)*. Affinity labeling of whole kidney extracts or cultured kidney tubular epithelial (MDCK) cells also yield high M_r (120 kDa) and low M_r (66–70 kDa) receptor bands. Full length $ANP_{(99–126)}$ inhibits labeling of both the 120- and 66–70-kDa bands. Truncated $ANP_{(103–123)}$ almost completely inhibits the labeling of the 66–68-kDa band, but only minimally the labeling of the higher M_r receptor corresponding to the 120-kDa band. Cultured endothelial cells also display two distinct bands of 66- and 133-kDa proteins *(27)*. $ANP_{(99–126)}$ blocks the labeling of both the 66- and 130-kDa bands, whereas $ANP_{(103–123)}$ fails to completely block the labeling of 130-kDa receptor band. Endothelial cells appear to possess similar high M_r ANP receptor to MDCK or adrenal glomerulosa cells *(26,30)*.

In cultured VSMC, >90% and in some instances up to 95%, of the total population of ANP receptor consists of ANP-clearance receptors *(25,30–32)*. In adrenal glomerulosa, kidney tubular epithelium (MDCK), and endothelial cells, the nonreducible 120–180-kDa

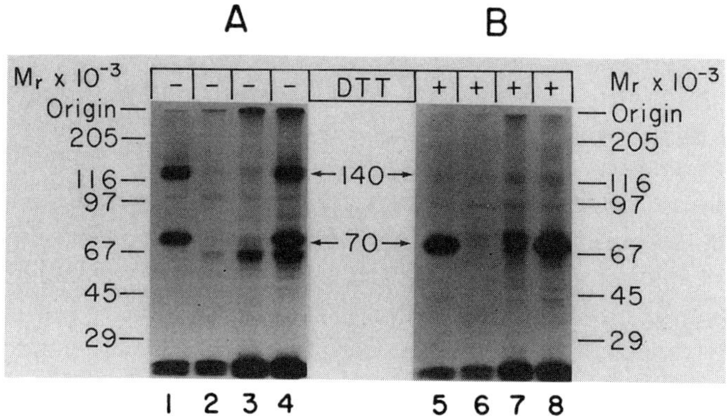

Fig. 2. Autoradiograms showing the specificity of 140-kDa disulfide-linked and 70-kDa disulfide-unlinked (monomer) Nprc in VSMC. Cells were labeled with azidobenzoyl-^{125}I-ANP (AZB-^{125}I-ANP) in the absence (lane 1) or presence of ANP (lane 2), ANP$_{(103-123)}$ (lane 3), angiotensin II or adrenocorticotropic hormone (ACTH) (lane 4). Samples were electrophoresed under unreduced (lanes 1–4) and reduced (lanes 5–8) conditions and radiolabeled bands were visualized by autoradiography. Arrows indicate the position and M_r of 140-kDa disulfide-linked and 70-kDa disulfide-unlinked (monomer) Nprc radiolabeled bands. Reproduced with permission from ref. *30*.

receptor exhibits similar biochemical and pharmacological properties. Variation between the 120- and 180-kDa mass of the single chain disulfide-unlinked receptor in these cells may be explained by differences in the carbohydrate moieties of the proteins owing to culture conditions. In VSMC, proteolytic cleavage produces multiple smaller distinct bands (52, 38, 26, and 14 kDa). After tryptic treatments of photoaffinity-labeled VSMC, the 70-kDa ANP receptor is persistent; however, the 140-kDa receptor band is completely abolished. It is not clear whether smaller tryptic fragments are generated from the 140- or 70-kDa receptor bands, since the apparent persistence of the 70-kDa band may be caused by the reappearance of tryptic products from the 140-kDa band.

Molecular Cloning and Structural Determination of Natriuretic Peptide Receptors

Biological actions of natriuretic peptides are mediated by membrane-bound GC receptors. Membrane-bound forms of GC represent biologically active natriuretic peptide receptors (Nprs) cloned and sequenced *(34)*. Thus cGMP is considered a second messenger of the natriuretic peptide family *(3)*. Cloning and expression of cDNAs have identified two different forms of natriuretic peptide-specific GC receptors, which have been designated as Npra and Nprb, also referred to as GC-A and GC-B, respectively. Both ANP and BNP selectively stimulate Npra, whereas CNP has been shown to stimulate primarily Nprb *(35)*. The structure and homology of these natriuretic peptide receptors together with their putative physiological ligands, ANP, BNP and CNP, are shown in Fig. 3. The general topological structure of the GC receptor family is consistent with at least four distinct domains. The entire coding region of both Npra and Nprb is separated by a single transmembrane spanning region into extracellular ligand-binding domain and intracellular protein kinase (PK)-like and GC catalytic domains. The extracellular domains of Npra and Nprb have approx 44% sequence identity. The intracellular regions of both

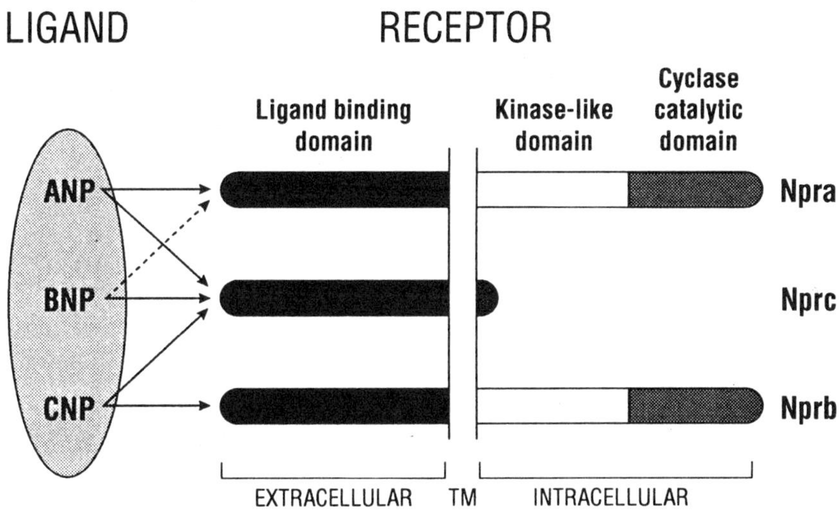

Fig. 3. Ligand specificity for the natriuretic peptide receptors. A schematic representation of the ability of the natriuretic peptides to specifically activate the natriuretic peptide receptors Npra, Nprb, and Nprc. The solid lines connect the receptors with their preferred ligand. The ambiguity of BNP's role in activation of Npra is represented by a dashed line. TM, transmembrane domain. Reproduced with permission from ref. *35*.

receptors can be divided into two domains: the approx 250 amino acid residues of the C-terminal portion of Npra and Nprb is the GC catalytic domain. The PK-like domain is approx 280 amino acids that immediately follow the transmembrane spanning region of these receptor proteins. The GC catalytic region has the highest sequence similarity (88%) between Npra and Nprb. The PK-like domain, also known as kinase homology domain (KHD), has only 60% sequence identity between Npra and Nprb. Although, >80% of the conserved amino acid residues that have been found in all PKs *(36)* are considered to be present in Npra and Nprb *(3)*, the functional significance of this homology of PKs, has not been established. Whether Npra and Nprb contain intrinsic kinase activity for autophosphorylation or to phosphorylate other cellular proteins, also is not known.

Comparison of the amino acid sequences indicates 62% identity among Npra and Nprb. Intracellular regions appear more highly conserved than the extracellular domain of these two receptors (78 vs 43%); however, unlike Npra, the intracellular regions of Nprb do not contain any putative glycosylation sites and cysteine residues. Five of the six cysteine residues found in the extracellular domains of both Npra and Nprb are located in the same relative position, but only two of the seven potential *N*-linked glycosylation sites found in both receptors are conserved *(3)*. The sequence in the kinase domain is less conserved between Npra and Nprb than sequence in the cyclase catalytic domain.

The third member of the natriuretic peptide receptor family is Nprc, which is found in abundant quantity in VSMCs. Nprc was isolated from cultured aortic VSMC and a partial amino acid sequence of the purified receptor was determined *(25)*. The Nprc cDNA has been cloned and nucleotide sequence determined *(37)*. The mature receptor has 496 amino acids with a large extracellular domain, a single transmembrane domain, and a very short 37-amino acid cytoplasmic tail that bears no homology to the intracellular domain of any other known receptor protein. The extracellular region of Nprc is approx 30% identical to Npra and Nprb. Ligand–receptor binding studies have demonstrated that Nprc has a much less stringent specificity for structural variants of ANP than does Npra or Nprb *(38)*. The extracellular domain possesses two pairs of cysteine residues along with one isolated cysteine near the transmembrane domain, three potential signals for *N*-glycosylation and several serines and threonines for *O*-linked glycosylation sites *(37)*. Nprc may function as a clearance receptor to remove natriuretic peptides from the circulation *(29)*. Its abundance in vascular tissues may provide protection against onset of hypotension caused by a sudden surge of ANP and overproduction of cGMP. Nprc may also mediate the biological effects of ANP through second messengers other than cGMP. Analogs of ANP, which are known to interact with Nprc, have been shown to inhibit the adenylyl cyclase and to reduce the level of intracellular cAMP *(38)* or to activate the phosphoinositol pathway in VSMC *(39)*.

Natriuretic Peptide Receptors and Transmembrane Signal Transduction

In intact aortic rings or in cultured VSMC there is an elevation of cGMP in response to ANP, BNP, or CNP, suggesting that cGMP mediates dilator responses to these peptide hormones. However, there is evidence against cGMP being the second messenger of these vasodilatory responses. $ANP_{(103-123)}$ relaxes rabbit aortic rings without stimulating GC activity *(32)*. Certain ANP analogs stimulate GC activity but cause little relaxation of aortic rings. Furthermore, the GC inhibitor, LY83583 prevents the GC response to ANP but not its vasodilatory effect *(40)*. Similarly, the Npra antagonist A74186 also inhibits the activation of GC activity but not the vasorelaxation response to infused ANP *(41)*. Another Npra antagonist HS142-1 also fails to prevent the majority of hypotensive effect caused by infused ANP *(42)*. However, in VSMC and renal mesangial cells, ANP as well as exogenous cGMP have been found to reduce the agonist or depolarization-induced increases in cytosolic $[Ca^{2+}]_i$ *(43,44)*. cGMP may activate sarcolemmal Ca^{2+}-ATPase and this mechanism may be important in the ANP-induced decrease in VSMC $[Ca^{2+}]_i$ *(45,46)*. The ultimate effect of cGMP in VSMC may be the result of activation of cGMP-dependent PKs *(47)*. Obviously, more work is needed to provide a firm mechanistic interpretation of any of the known biological action of cGMP, which is stimulated by natriuretic peptide hormone family in VSMC.

ANP appears to inhibit adenylyl cyclase and reduce the intracellular levels of cAMP in many tissues, including VSMC *(48)*. The precise role of ANP-mediated decrease in the intracellular cAMP in VSMC is not clear, as neither pertussin toxin nor Nprc-specific peptides affect the dilatory responses to ANP *(49,50)*. ANP stimulates the phospholipase C activity and increased the rate of IP_3 accumulation in cultured VSMC *(39,48)*. However, ANP inhibits phospholipase C activity after stimulation by vasoconstrictor agonists such as angiotensin II (AII) *(51)*. Similarly, the increase in vascular PKC activity caused by AII is also inhibited by ANP *(52)*. The significance of ANP-mediated effects on cAMP and IP_3 systems in VSMC remains to be investigated in greater detail.

ANP and BNP may act synergistically in the vasculature; however, the higher levels of structural diversity of CNP and its ability to activate Nprb suggest the possibility of CNP-specific mechanisms that may cause structural diversity and signaling of Nprb in VSMC *(53,54)*. The restricted presence of its receptors in brain and VSMC strongly suggests that CNP may signal, in a coordinated fashion in brain and vasculature, to control the interactive role of central and peripheral aspects of vascular tone and body fluid homeostasis *(54)*.

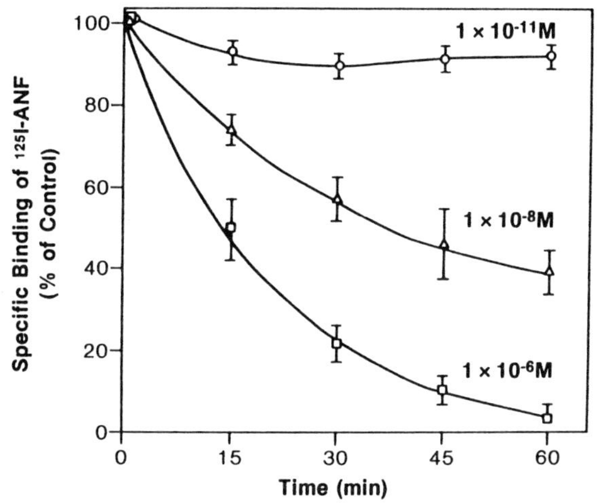

Fig. 4. Time- and dose-dependent downregulation of ANP-binding in rat thoracic aortic vascular smooth muscle (RTASM) cells: Confluent cells in 6 cm^2 dishes were exposed to various concentrations of ANP for the indicated times. Cells were then washed with acid buffer to remove any surface-bound ANP and assayed for specific ^{125}I-ANP binding. The concentrations of ANP used were 10 pm (○), 10 n*M* (Δ), and 1 μ*M* (□). Reproduced with permission from ref. *59*.

Internalization, Metabolism, and Turnover of Natriuretic Peptide Receptors in VSMC

Despite extensive cellular, biochemical, and molecular-biological studies, the mechanisms and physiological significance of natriuretic peptide receptor translocation after ligand binding is not completely clear. Binding of hormones to target cells seems to be highly regulated by several mechanisms including the ligand itself. After exposure of cultured VSMC to ANP, there is a decrease in ^{125}I-ANP binding *(55–59)*. In particular, exposure of rat VSMC to ANP (10 n*M*) caused a substantial decrease (50–60%) in total receptor number (Fig. 4). Internalization of ANP receptor complexes in VSMC has been documented *(59,60)*; however, the interrelationships between the endocytotic mechanisms, intracellular sequestration of ANP receptor complexes, and ANP-dependent downregulation have not been resolved. Based on ^{125}I-ANP binding method, VSMC have been suggested to contain 90–95% Nprc. Therefore, these largely mirror the metabolic turnover of Nprc in VSMC. Homeostatic regulation of receptor and cellular sensitivity of ligand may be dependent on a dynamic equilibrium and reutilization of the ligand–receptor complexes from cell surface to cell interior. Therefore, to understand the dynamics of the interrelationship between these processes, the events that occur after binding in target cells need to be investigated. ^{125}I-ANP binds to VSMC cell-surface receptors, enters through the process of receptor-mediated endocytosis and is delivered to the intracellular compartments *(59)*. The majority of ^{125}I-ANP is degraded and rapidly released into culture media *(59,60)*. The distribution of ^{125}I-ANP radioactivity between the cell surface, intracellular compartments, and culture medium provided a dynamic equilibrium between the rates of ^{125}I-ANP uptake and its degradation and extrusion by VSMC.

The rate of both uptake and breakdown of ^{125}I-ANP is markedly decreased in the presence of metabolic inhibitors such as chloroquine and low temperature, which suggests that the processing pathway of ^{125}I-ANP in VSMC is, in part, lysosomal *(59,60)*.

Indeed, a major portion of VSMC internalized ^{125}I-ANP is released into the culture media as both degraded products and intact ^{125}I-ANP *(59)*. Approximately 80–85% of the released ^{125}I-radioactivity constituted degraded products and about 15–20% is intact ligand. These observations suggest that the majority of VSMC internalized ^{125}I-ANP is processed through the degradative compartments. An alternative mechanism also seems to exist for the release of intact ligand in the VSMC. Release of degraded ligand is blocked to a great extent by the lysosomotropic agent chloroquine; however, this agent is only partially effective in blocking the release of intact ligand. Dual pathways for intracellular processing of peptide hormones have been described, suggesting the release of intact ligand through retroendocytosis and release of degraded products through simple diffusion in the culture medium *(61)*. It also is conceivable that retroendocytosis of certain ligand could be the result of recycling of ligand–receptor complexes leading to the dissociation of the ligand from receptor at the plasma membranes. Internalization, recycling, and metabolic degradation of Npra have been found to occur rapidly in MA-10 cells *(62)*. However, studies on the internalization and metabolic turnover of ^{125}I-CNP and Nprb either in VSMC or other cell systems have not been carried out.

ANTIMITOGENIC ACTIVITY OF NATRIURETIC PEPTIDES IN VSMC

Natriuretic peptides act not only as vasodilators but also as growth inhibitors in a variety of tissue and cell types, including the endothelial and VSMC *(19,20,63–67)*. Both ANP and CNP exert antimitogenic effects via elevation of cGMP, yet the effect of CNP on the inhibition of serum- and mitogen-induced DNA synthesis is more pronounced than ANP in cultured VSMC *(20,68)*. cGMP analogs mimic the antiproliferative action of both ANP and CNP, providing further evidence that natriuretic peptides elicit their antimitogenic action through the second messenger cGMP *(19,64)*. CNP is produced and secreted in endothelial cells and this production/secretion is markedly augmented by transforming growth factor β (TGFβ) and vasoconstrictors such as AII and endothelin *(68)*. Indeed, CNP may act as a local regulator in vascular beds, inducing relaxation and/or growth inhibition of VSMC in a paracrine manner and modulate endothelial cell proliferation and/or its function by autocrine mechanisms.

NATRIURETIC PEPTIDES AND VASCULAR MEDIATION

The stimulatory effect of CNP on cGMP production in cultured VSMC has been reported to be more potent than that of ANP or BNP *(19,20,69)*. Thus, CNP is considered to be a local regulator of vascular tone and growth. CNP inhibits the development of intimal lesions induced by balloon injury in the carotid artery of rabbit *(70)*. This CNP action in VSMC is caused by intracellular accumulation of cGMP and inhibition of DNA synthesis *(71)*. Thus, CNP provides a new tool for investigating the role of Nprb in vascular injury. CNP has been found to be produced in the endothelial cells where its secretion can be regulated by cytokines, growth factors, and even by other members of natriuretic peptide family, ANP and BNP *(14,68,72)*. Because CNP is found at low levels in plasma, any vascular actions of CNP are likely to be of autocrine and/or paracrine in nature *(14,18)*. Since CNP is a potent vasodilator and inhibitor of VSMC hyperplasia *(20)*, the endothelial synthesis of CNP is likely an important mediator of VSMC function. Recently, it has also been shown that renal mesangial cells are highly responsive and sensitive to CNP as compared to ANP, whereas renal epithelial cells respond to both ANP and CNP *(73)*. Immunoreactive CNP, as well as its mRNA, has been demonstrated in rat, mouse, and human kidney *(16,74)*, suggesting autocrine and/or paracrine roles of CNP in the kidney, probably similar to that in vasculature.

CNP and its specific receptor Nprb are expressed at the site of vascular injury, and CNP is considered to be important in preventing the progression of restenosis caused by intimal thickening after coronary angioplasty. A recent study showed that in the intact aorta, Nprb mRNA levels were found to be 10-fold higher than Npra mRNA *(75)*. This dominance is further amplified (1000-fold) in long-term culture (10–15 passages) of aortic VSMC. An increase in Nprb expression from contractile to proliferative phenotype of cultured aortic VSMC may play an important role in pathophysiology of hypertension. VSMC proliferation with accompanying vascular growth and remodeling is considered to be a critical factor contributing to the increased peripheral vascular resistance in hypertension.

The physiological and clinical implication of the phenotype-related alterations in the expression of natriuretic peptide receptors in VSMC is not immediately clear. As described, in cultured VSMC, the density of Npra is decreased and the density of Nprb increased dramatically *(76)*. A recent study also indicates that VSMC contained predominantly the 130-kDa Npra in vivo and that Nprc found in cultured VSMC is induced from the cell culturing process in vitro *(77)*. VSMC are less sensitive to ANP and BNP as compared to CNP for vasorelaxation and also for growth inhibition. Since Nprc does not contain GC activity, the increase in the expression of Nprc is unlikely to contribute to the growth inhibition or relaxation of VSMC. A recent study in human patients with congestive heart failure also has shown that CNP attenuated the peripheral forearm resistance in a manner distinct from ANP *(78)*. CNP is a highly potent stimulus to produce cGMP and to relax contracted aorta involving Nprb, suggesting that CNP-dependent activation of Nprb is intimately associated with vascular relaxation and VSMC metabolic function *(79)*.

SUMMARY AND CONCLUSIONS

Investigation of Npra, Nprb, and Nprc shows that the field of the natriuretic peptides and their receptors has advanced tremendously in the last 5 yr. Biochemical, pharmacological, and molecular characterization of the receptors for the natriuretic peptide hormone family have provided the impetus to delineate the functional efficacy of ANP, BNP, and CNP in target tissues, including vasculature. The knowledge and experimental tools generated in the last 4 yr have provided new evidence that CNP/Nprb system seem to play the central role in the VSMC function. The Nprc is the most abundant and most widely distributed receptor subtype in VSMC across the species. Although it does not contain GC activity, it binds to all three natriuretic peptides (ANP, BNP, and CNP) and may function as a clearance receptor to protect against dangerously low blood pressure. The ultimate role(s) of natriuretic peptide receptors and their signaling mechanisms in vasculature awaits further investigation.

ACKNOWLEDGMENTS

The research of the author's laboratory has been supported by the National Institutes of Health Grant HD25527 and the American Heart Association Established Investigatorship Award (900260) and Grant-in-Aid (920-1011).

REFERENCES

1. Brenner BM, Ballerman BJ, Gunning ME, Zeidel MD. Diverse biological actions of atrial natriuretic peptide. Physiol Rev 1990;70:665–699.
2. Macck T. Receptors for atrial natriuretic factor. Ann Rev Physiol 1992;54:11–27.
3. Garbers DL. GC receptors and their endocrine paracrine and autocrine ligands. Cell 1992;71:1–4.
4. Koller KJ, Goeddel DV. Molecular biology of the natriuretic peptides and their receptors. Circulation 1992;86:1081–1088.
5. de Bold AJ, Borenstein HB, Veress AT, Sonnenberg H. A rapid and potent natriuretic response to intravenous injection of atrial myocardial extract in rats. Life Sci 1981;28:89–94.
6. de Bold AJ. Atrial natriuretic factor: a hormone produced by the heart. Science 1985;230:767–770.
7. Rosenzveig A, Seidman CE. Atrial natriuretic factor and related peptide hormones. Annu Rev Biochem 1991;60:229–255.
8. Inagami T. Atrial natriuretic factor. J Biol Chem 1989;264:3043–3046.
9. Sudoh T, Kangawa K, Minamino N, Matsuo H. A new natriuretic peptide in porcine brain. Nature 1988;332:78–81.
10. Saito Y, Nakao K, Arai H, Nishimura K, Okamura K, Obata K, Takemura G, Fujiwara H, Sugawara A, Yamada T, Itoh H, Mukoyama M, Hosoda K, Kawai C, Ban T, Yasue H, Imura H. Augmented expression of atrial natriuretic polypeptide gene in ventricle of human failing heart. J Clin Invest 1989;89:298–305.
11. Sudoh T, Minamino N, Kangawa K, Matsuo H. C-type natriuretic peptide (CNP): a new member of natriuretic peptide family identified in porcine brain. Biochem Biophys Res Commun 1990;168:863–870.
12. Gardner DG, Deschepper CF, Ganong WF, Home S, Fidds J, Baxter JD, Lewicki J. Extra-atrial expression of the gene for atrial natriuretic factor. Proc Natl Acad Sci USA 1986;83:6697–6701.
13. Komatsu KJ, Nakao K, Suga S, Ogawa Y, Mukoyama M, Arai H, Shirakami G, Hosoda K, Nakagawa O, Hama N. C-type natriuretic peptide in rats and human. Endocrinology 1991;129:1104–1106.
14. Stingo AJ, Clavell AL, Heublein DM, Wei CM, Pittelkom MR, Burnett JC Jr. Presence of C-type natriuretic peptide in cultured human endothelial cells and plasma. Am J Physiol 1992;263:H1318–H1321.
15. Ishizaka Y, Kangawa K, Minamino N, Ishi K, Takano S, Eto T, Matsuo H. Isolation and identification of C-type natriuretic peptide in human monocytic cell line THP. Biochem Biophys Res Commun 1992;189:697–704.
16. Suzuki E, Hirarta Y, Hayakawa H, Omata M, Kojma M, Kangawa K, Minamino M, Matsuo H. Evidence for C-type natriuretic peptide production in the rat kidney. Biochem Biophys Res Commun 1993;192:532–538.
17. Charles CJ, Richards AM, Espiner EA. Central C-type natriuretic peptide but not atrial natriuretic factor lowers the blood pressure and adrenocortical secretion in normal conscious sheep. Endocrinology 1992;131:1721–1726.
18. Clavell AL, Stingo AJ, Wei GM, Heublein DM, Burnett JC Jr. C-type natriuretic peptide: a selective cardiovascular peptide. Am J Physiol 1993;264:R290–R295.
19. Furuya M, Yoshida M, Hayashi Y, Ohnuma N, Minamino N, Kangawa K, Matsuo H. C-type natriuretic peptide is a growth inhibitor of rat VSMC. Biochem Biophys Res Commun 1991;177:927–931.
20. Porter JG, Catalano R, McEnroe G, Lewicki JA, Protter A. C-type natriuretic peptide inhibits growth factor-dependent DNA synthesis in smooth muscle cells. Am J Physiol 1992;263:C1001–C1006.
21. Kuno T, Andresen JW, Kamisaki Y, Waldman SA, Chang LY, Saheki S, Leitman DC, Nakane M, Murad F. Co-purification of an atrial natriuretic factor receptor and particulate GC from rat lung. J Biol Chem 1986;261:5817–5823.
22. Paul AK, Marala RB, Jaiswal RK, Sharma RK. Co-existence of guanylate cyclase and atrial natriuretic factor receptor in 180 kDa protein. Science 1987;235:1224–1227.
23. Takayanagi R, Snajdar RM, Imada T, Tamura M, Pandey KN, Misono KS, Inagami T. Purification and characterization of two types of atrial natriuretic factor receptors from bovine adrenal cortex: guanylate cyclase-linked and cyclase-free receptors. Biochem Biophys Res Commun 1987;144:244–250.
24. Meloche S, McNicoll N, Liu B, Ong H, DeLean A. Atrial natriuretic factor R1 receptor from bovine adrenal glomerulosa: purification characterization and modulation by amiloride. Biochemistry 1988;27:8151–8158.
25. Schenk DB, Phelps MN, Porter JG, Fuller F, Cordell B, Lewicki JA. Purification and subunit composition of atrial natriuretic peptide receptor. Proc Natl Acad USA 1987;84:5121–5125.
26. Takayanagi R, Inagami T, Snajdar RM, Imada T, Tamura M, Misono KS. Two distinct forms of receptors for atrial natriuretic factor in bovine adrenocortical cells. Purification ligand binding and peptide mapping. J Biol Chem 1987;262:12,104–12,113.

27. Leitman DC, Andresen LW, Kuno T, Kamisaki Y, Chang JK, Murad F. Identification of multiple binding sites for atrial natriuretic factor by affinity cross-linking in cultured endothelial cells. J Biol Chem 1986;261:11,650–11,655.
28. Scarborough RM, McEnroe GA, Arfsten A, Kang LL, Schwartz K, Lewicki JA. D-amino acid-substituted atrial natriuretic peptide analogs reveal novel receptor recognition requirements. J Biol Chem 1988;263:16,818–16,822.
29. Maack T, Suzuki M, Almeida FA, Nussenzveig D, Scarborough RM, McEnroe GA, Lewicki JA. Physiological role of silent receptors of atrial natriuretic factor. Science 1987;238:675–678.
30. Pandey KN, Pavlou SN, Inagami T. Identification and characterization of three distinct atrial natriuretic factor receptors. Evidence for tissue-specific heterogeneity of receptor subtypes in vascular smooth muscle, kidney tubular epithelium and Leydig tumor cells by ligand binding, photoaffinity labeling and tryptic proteolysis. J Biol Chem 1988;263:13,406–13,413.
31. Leitman DC, Andresen JW, Catalano RM, Waldman SA, Tuan JJ, Murad F. Atrial natriuretic peptide binding cross-linking and stimulation of cyclic GMP accumulation and particulate guanylate cyclase activity in cultured cells. J Biol Chem 1988;263:3720–3728.
32. Budzik GP, Firestone SL, Bush EN, Connally PJ, Rockway TW, Sarin VK, Holleman WH. Divergence of ANF analogs in smooth muscle cell cGMP response and aorta vasorelaxation. Evidence for receptor subtypes. Biochem Biophys Res Commun 1987;144:422–431.
33. Pandey KN, Inagami T, Misono KS. Three distinct forms of atrial natriuretic factor receptors: kidney tubular epithelium cells and VSMC contain different types of receptors. Biochem Biophys Res Commun 1987;148:589–595.
34. Pandey KN, Singh S. Molecular cloning and expression of murine guanylate cyclase/atrial natriuretic factor receptor cDNA. J Biol Chem 1990;265:12,342–12,348.
35. Koller KJ, Lowe DG, Bennett GL, Minamino N, Kangawa K, Matsuo H, Goeddel DV. Selective activation of the B natriuretic peptide receptor by C-type natriuretic peptide (CNP). Science 1991;252:120–123.
36. Hanks SK, Quinn AM, Hunter T. The protein kinase C family Conserved features and deduced phylogeny of the catalytic domains. Science 1988;241:42–52.
37. Fuller F, Porter JG, Arfsten AE, Miller J, Schilling JW, Scarborough RM, Lewicki JA, Schenk DB. Atrial natriuretic peptide clearance receptor. Complete sequence and functional expression of cDNA clones. J Biol Chem 1988;263:9395–9401.
38. Anand-Srivastava MB, Trachte GJ. Atrial natriuretic factor receptor and signal transduction mechanisms. Pharmacol Rev 1993;45:455–497.
39. Hirata M, Chang CH, Murad F. Stimulatory effects of atrial natriuretic factor on phosphoinositide hydrolysis in cultured bovine aortic smooth muscle cells. Biochim Biophys Acta 1989;1010: 346–351.
40. Gupta S, Cragoe EJ Jr, Deth RC. Influence of atrial natriuretic factor on 5-(*N*-ethyl-*N*-isopropyl) amiloride-sensitive[22] Na uptake in rabbit aorta. J Pharmacol Exp Ther 1989;248:991–996.
41. von Geldern TW, Budzik GP, Dillan TP, Holleman WH, Holst MA, Kiso Y, Novosad EI, Opgenorth TJ, Rockway TW, Thomas AM, Yeh S. Atrial natriuretic peptide antagonists: biochemical evaluation and structural correlations. Mol Pharmacol 1990;38:771–778.
42. Sano T, Morishita Y, Matsuda Y, Yamada K. Pharmacological profile of HS-142-1 a novel nonpeptide atrial natriuretic peptide antagonist of microbial origin. I Selective inhibition of the actions of natriuretic peptides in anesthetized rats. J Pharmacol Exp Ther 1992;260:825–831.
43. Hassid A. Atriopeptin II decreases cytosolic free Ca^{2+} in cultured VSMC. Am J Physiol 1986;251: C681–C686.
44. Hassid A. Atriopeptins decrease resting and hormone-elevated cytosolic Ca^{2+} in cultured mesangial cells. Am J Physiol 1987;253:F1077–F1082.
45. Popescu LM, Panoiu C, Hinescu M, Nutu O. The mechanism of cGMP-induced relaxation in vascular smooth muscle. Eur J Pharmacol 1985;107:393,394.
46. Rashatwar SS, Cornwell TL, Lincoln TM. Effects of 8-bromo cGMP on calcium levels in VSMC. Possible regulation of calcium ATPase by cGMP-dependent protein kinase. Proc Natl Acad Sci USA 1987;83:5685–5691.
47. Cornwell TL, Lincoln TM. Regulation of Ca^{2+} levels in cultured VSMC. Reduction of Ca^{2+} by atriopeptin and 8-bromo cGMP is mediated by cyclic-GMP-dependent protein kinase. J Biol Chem 1989;264:1146–1155.
48. Resink TJ, Scott-Burden T, Jones CR, Baur U, Jones CK, Buhler FR. Atrial natriuretic peptide induces breakdown of phosphatidylinositol phosphates in cultured VSMC. Eur J Biochem 1987;172:499–505.

49. Ljusegren ME, Axelsson BR, Friedman RL. Effects of pertussis-toxin on vasodilation and cyclic-GMP in bovine mesenteric arteries and demonstration of a 40 kDa soluble protein ribosylation substrate for pertussis toxin. Life Sci 1990;46:543–552.
50. Elmquist BJ, Trachte GJ. Atrial natriuretic factor vasodilation is independent of R1 (GC-coupled) receptors. FASEB J 1992;6:A1010 (abstracts).
51. Winquist RJ, Hintze TH. Mechanisms of atrial natriuretic factor-induced vasodilation. Pharmacol Ther 1990;48:417–426.
52. Tamm C, Lang U, Vallottan NB. Effects of atrial natriuretic factor on angiotensin II and phorbol ester-stimulated protein kinase C and prostacyclin production in cultured rat aortic smooth muscle cells. Endocrinology 1990;126:658–663.
53. Mukoyama M, Nakao K, Hosoda K, Suga S, Saito Y, Ogawa Y, Shirakami G, Jougasaki M, Obata K, Yasue H, Kambayashi Y, Inoye K, Imura H. Brain natriuretic peptide as a novel cardiac hormone in humans: evidence for an exquisite dual natriuretic peptide system ANP and BNP. J Clin Invest 1991;87:1402–1412.
54. Yoshimura M, Yasue H, Morita E, Sakaino N, Jougasaki M, Kurose M, Mukoyama M, Saito Y, Nakao K, Imura H. Hemodynamic renal and hormonal responses to brain natriuretic peptide infusion in patients with congestive heart failure. Circulation 1991;84:1581–1588.
55. Roupert P, Lanchampt MO, Chabrier PE, Plas P, Goulin J, Braquet P. Down-regulation of atrial natriuretic factor receptors and correlation with cGMP stimulation in rat cultured VSMC. Biochem Biophys Res Commun 1987;148:61–67.
56. Bellemann P, Neuser D. Modulation of ANP receptor-mediated cGMP accumulation by atrial natriuretic peptides and vasopressin in A10 VSMC. J Receptor Res 1988;8:407–417.
57. Hamet P, Hadrava V, Kruppa U, Trembley J. VSMC hyperresponsiveness to growth factors in hypertension. J Hypertens 1988;(Suppl. 6):536–539.
58. Cahill PA, Redmond EM, Keenan AK. Vascular atrial natriuretic factor receptor subtypes are not independently regulated by atrial peptides. J Biol Chem 1990;265:21,896–21,906.
59. Pandey KN. Kinetic analysis of internalization, recycling and redistribution of atrial natriuretic factor receptor complex in cultured VSMC. Biochem J 1992;288:55–61.
60. Nussenzveig DR, Lewicki JA, Maack T. Cellular mechanisms of the clearance function of type C receptors of atrial natriuretic factor. J Biol Chem 1990;265:20,952–20,958.
61. Marshall S. Dual pathways for the intracellular processing of insulin: relationship between retroendocytosis of intact hormone and the recycling of insulin receptors. J Biol Chem 1985;260:13,524–13,531.
62. Pandey KN. Stoichiometric analysis of internalization, recycling and redistribution of photoaffinity-labeled guanylate cyclase/atrial natriuretic factor receptors in cultured murine Leydig tumor cells. J Biol Chem 1993;268:4382–4390.
63. Johnson A, Lermioglu F, Garg UC, Morgan-Boyd R, Hassid A. A novel biological effect of atrial natriuretic hormone: inhibition of mesangial cell mitogenesis. Biochem Biophys Res Commun 1988;152:893–897.
64. Itoh H, Pratt RE, Dzau V. Atrial natriuretic polypeptide inhibits hypertrophy of VSMC. J Clin Invest 1990;86:1690–1697.
65. Levin E, Frank H. Natriuretic peptides inhibit rat astroglial proliferation: mediation by C-receptor. Am J Physiol 1991;261:R453–R457.
66. Itoh H, Pratt RE, Ohno M, Dzau VJ. Atrial natriuretic polypeptides as a novel antigrowth factor of endothelial cells. Hypertension 1992;19:758–761.
67. Hagiwara H, Sakaguchi H, Itakura M, Yoshimoto T, Furuya M, Tanaka S, Hirose S. Autocrine regulation of rat chondrocyte proliferation by natriuretic peptide C and its receptor natriuretic peptide receptor-B. J Biol Chem 1994;269:10,729–10,733.
68. Suga S, Nakao K, Itoh H, Komatsu Y, Ogawa Y, Hama N, Imura H. Endothelial production of C-type natriuretic peptide and its marked augmentation by transforming growth factor-β. J Clin Invest 1992;90:1145–1149.
69. Fethiere J, Graihle R, DeLean A. Identification of the atrial natriuretic factor-R_{1C} receptor subtype (B-clone) in cultured rat aortic smooth muscle cells. FEBS Lett 1992;305:77–88.
70. Shinomiya M, Tashiro J, Saito Y, Yoshida S, Furuya M, Oka N, Tanaka S, Kangawa K, Matsuo H. C-type natriuretic peptide inhibits intimal thickening of rabbit carotid artery after balloon catheter injury. Biochem Biophys Res Commun 1994;205:1051–1056.
71. Furuya M, Aisaka K, Miyazaki T, Hanbou N, Kowashima K, Ohno T, Tanaka S, Minamino N, Kangawa K, Matsuo H. C-type natriuretic peptide inhibits intimal thickening after vascular injury. Biochem Biophys Res Commun 1993;193:248–253.

72. Nazario B, Hu R-M, Pedram A, Prins B, Levin E. Atrial and brain natriuretic peptides stimulate the production and secretion of C-type natriuretic peptide from bovine aortic endothelial cells. J Clin Invest 1995;261:R453–R457.
73. Zhao J, Ardaillou N, Lu C-Y, Placier S, Pham P, Badre L, Cambar J, Ardaillou R. Characterization of C-type natriuretic peptide receptors in human mesangial cells. Kidney Inter 1994;46:717–725.
74. Dean AD, Vehaskari VM, Greenwald JE. Synthesis and localization of C-type natriuretic peptide in mammalian kidney. Am J Physiol 1994;266:F491–F496.
75. Fujio N, Garrard F, Bayard F, Tremblay J. Regulation of natriuretic peptide receptor A and B expression by transforming growth factor-β1 in cultured aortic smooth muscle cells. Hypertension 1994;23:908–913.
76. Suga S, Nakao K, Kishimoto I, Hosoda K, Mukoyama M, Arai H, Shirakami G, Ogawa Y, Komatsu Y, Nakogawa O, Hama N, Imura H. Phenotype related alteration in expression of natriuretic peptide receptors in aortic smooth muscle cells. Cir Res 1992;71:34–39.
77. Abe T, Nishiyama K, Snajdar R, He X, Misono KS. Aortic smooth muscle contains guanylate cyclase-coupled 130 kDa atrial natriuretic factor receptor as predominant receptor from spontaneous switching to 60 kDa C-receptor upon cell culturing. Eur J Biochem 1993;217:295–304.
78. Nakamura M, Arakawa N, Yoshida H, Makita S, Hiramori K. Vasodilatory effects of C-type natriuretic peptide on forearm resistance vessels are distinct from those of atrial natriuretic peptide in chronic heart failure. Circulation 1994;90:1210–1214.
79. Drewett JG, Fendly BM, Garbers DL, Lowe DG. Natriuretic peptide receptor-B (GC-B) mediates C-type natriuretic peptide relaxation of precontracted rat aorta. J Biol Chem 1995;270:4668–4674.

20 A Novel Vascular Hormone

Adrenomedullin

Willis K. Samson, PhD

Contents

THE ENDOTHELIAL–VASCULAR SMOOTH MUSCLE INTERFACE

The close apposition of the endothelial elements of the vasculature to the smooth muscle provides the anatomic framework for what has been called by some the largest endocrine gland of the body *(1)*. Indeed it is now clear *(2,3)* that an endothelial cell (EC) not only responds to circulating vasoactive substances, but also produces and releases vasoactive factors adluminally into the blood and abluminally into the adjacent tissue space communicating with vascular smooth muscle cells (VSMC). These factors may act as classical hormones when released into the circulation or more significantly as local paracrine or autocrine agents that control vascular permeability and tone. Peptides, prostaglandins, and even bioactive gases make up this buffet of locally generated agents, and recent evidence suggests profound interactions of these multiple vasoactive factors describing the control of vascular function. Numerous reviews *(4–6)* and this entire book categorize and detail the multiple agents that belong to the recently recognized class of vasoactive hormones. Their characterization has led to the development of a new subdiscipline in endocrinology, the endocrinology of the vasculature.

In elucidating the interactive effects of vascular paracrine and autocrine hormones, it has become clear that the vasodilatory agents not only antagonize the pressor effects of vasoconstrictors, but also antagonize in some cases the mitogenic effects of those substances as well *(5)*. This may in fact be one of the most clinically relevant aspects of the cardiovascular hormones since vascular growth and remodeling accounts for a significant portion of cardiovascular disease. In the early 1980s it was realized that the heart produced and released into the circulation a hormone (atrial natriuretic factor) that not

From: *Contemporary Endocrinology: Endocrinology of the Vasculature*
Edited by: J. R. Sowers Humana Press Inc., Totowa, NJ

only exerted renal actions, thus controlling fluid and electrolyte homeostasis, but also vasodilatory effects in certain vascular beds. It is now clear that the first cardiac hormone discovered is a member of a family of "natriuretic peptides," and that at least one member of the family (C-type natriuretic peptide) is produced in the vasculature where it exerts potent actions on vessel tone and permeability *(2)*. Later in that same decade the identity of the vascular-derived pressor agent *(7,8)* became known *(9)* and the interactive effects of the prorelaxant natriuretic peptides and the proconstrictive endothelins became a major target of cellular and molecular inquiry. At a time when the pressor actions of the angiotensins were well established *(10)*, the field of cardiovascular endocrinology became engulfed in a race to characterize the multiple interactive effects of these numerous vasoactive agents. But peptides were not the only players on the stage and a strong cast of nonpeptidergic factors were being established as significant regulators of vascular biology. The prostaglandins were known to affect permeability and muscle contraction *(11)* and by the end of the decade a gas revolutionized our thinking about the cellular basis for the maintenance of vascular reactivity *(12)*. That a soluble gas could be used for intercellular communication came as a surprise to many; however, it is now recognized that nitric oxide (NO) serves as intracellular (autocrine) signal and is utilized for cell–cell (paracrine) communication across short intercellular distances. In some cases the actions of vasoactive peptides are dependent on the generation of this potent molecule.

But why speak of these other factors when the topic of this chapter is adrenomedullin (AM)? It is because of the lessons we have learned from the discovery of those other vasoactive substances and the elucidation of their physiologic effects that this potent vasorelaxant peptide was identified *(13)*, and that we have learned in just two short years since its discovery so much about its production, release, and biologic effects. The templates of discovery imprinted during the characterization of the effects of the natriuretic peptides, the endothelins, and NO are being utilized now in the early stages of discovery as the physiological relevance of AM begins to emerge.

THE DISCOVERY OF AM

Using a bioassay system to monitor the elevation of cAMP levels in platelets, Kitamura and colleagues *(13)* in 1993 reported in extracts of a human pheochromocytoma a peptide that exerted profound hypotensive effects when injected intravenously into anesthetized rats. In that initial report the plasma levels of this peptide, named AM, were reported to be similar to those of other vasoactive peptides and its presence was detected by radioimmunoassay in normal tissues. Although the ability of AM to elevate cyclic adenosine monophosphate (cAMP) levels in platelets was the initial bioassay, now the gold standard bioassay for AM is its vasorelaxant effect *(14)*.

Structure and Bioassay

When first identified to be a 52 amino acid peptide in humans, the structural similarity between AM and calcitonin gene-related peptide (CGRP), also a potent vasodilator, was recognized and the bioassays utilized responded approximately equally to both peptides *(15)*. Cloning revealed AM to be processed from a 185 amino acid precursor (Fig. 1), which also contains a biologically active fragment in the N-terminal region of the prohormone *(16)*. This 20 amino acid fragment, which exerts some actions similar to AM and some unique effects *(16–18)*, was designated proadrenomedullin N-terminal 20

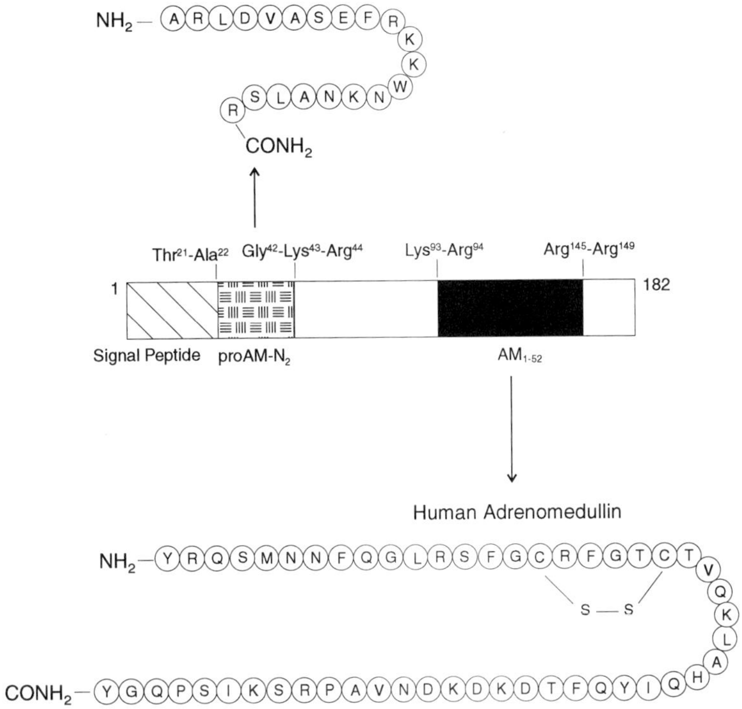

Fig. 1. Structure of human preproadrenomedullin and the amino acid sequences of human adrenomedullin and the C-terminal peptide PAMP.

peptide (PAMP). Maximal hypotensive actions of AM are achieved with doses approx 3 nmol/kg, whereas similar depression of blood pressure is obtained with an injection of 50 nmol/kg PAMP *(16)*. A further difference in the biologic activities of AM and PAMP is the duration of action. The hypotensive effect *(13)* of intravenously administered AM lasts a remarkable 30–50 min, while that of PAMP abates within 5–10 min, suggesting (vide infra) differing mechanisms of action. Cloning of the rat cDNA for AM revealed a homologous peptide precursor that similarly contained PAMP in the N-terminus *(19)*. Rat AM differs from the human peptide in that it is only 50 amino acids in length, and demonstrates 6 amino acid residue substitutions. Rat PAMP differs from that in human by only 3 amino acids. Similar interspecies homology also has been reported in the pig. Porcine AM differs from human in only one amino acid, with a glycine for asparagine substitution at residue 40 *(20)*.

Molecular Biology of Adrenomedullin

Sites of Production

The initial report *(21)* describing the cloning of the AM gene also indicated that AM mRNA could be detected by RNA blot analysis in extracts of human adrenal medulla, lung, ventricle, and kidney. At the level of resolution employed, AM mRNA was not detected in brain, liver, pancreas, intestine, or spleen. In the rat *(22)*, AM mRNA has been identified in adrenal gland, lung, kidney, heart, and spleen. Low levels of mRNA have been detected in duodenum and submandibular glands and a faint band appears to have been detected in pancreas and brain. Similarly some AM mRNA was detected by blot analysis in the brain of the pig *(20)*, although the relative amounts of message detected were minor in comparison to that present in similar concentrations of extracts from adrenal glands, lung, and kidney.

Using immunologic detection methods, a broader distribution of AM has been identified. In human tissue, the highest concentration (47 fmol/mg wet tissue) of AM-like immunoreactivity (henceforth simply referred to as AM) was detected in acid extracts of adrenal medulla *(22)*. Fortyfold lower amounts were detected in extracts of atrium, pancreas, small intestine, and lung. Hundredfold lower levels than in adrenal medulla were detected in heart ventricle, aorta, kidney, liver, spleen, brain cortex, and thyroid gland. Plasma levels were reported to be approx 17 pg/mL. Other investigators *(23)* extended the initial findings of AM in brain extracts (where mRNA had not originally been detected) to demonstrate regional distribution of AM with highest concentration present in extracts of human thalamus and hypothalamus (1.3–1.4 pmol/g wet weight) and lower amounts in frontal cortex, cerebellum, pons, and medulla. These levels compared favorably with determinations of AM content in human adrenal gland, which contained approx 12–13 pmol/g wet weight of tissue. High levels of AM detected in ganglioblastomas and neuroblastomas by this group may represent the extensive vascularization of these tumors, since (vide infra) AM is produced in both the endothelial and muscular components of the vasculature *(24,25)*. It has been reported that the distribution of immunoreactive AM in the rat is wider than that identified by Northern analysis *(22)*. In this species approximately equivalent amounts of AM (9–13 fmol/mg wet tissue) were detected in extracts of lung, adrenal gland, and cardiac atrium. Significantly, for the first time the presence of AM in pituitary gland was reported, with levels similar to those in thyroid gland extracts, both approximately 10-fold lower than concentration present in adrenal gland. Lower levels of AM have been measured in extracts of rat brain, submandibular gland, aorta, kidney, spleen, duodenum, pancreas, liver, testis, and muscle. Plasma levels *(22)* have been reported to be similar to those reported in humans *(13,26,27)*.

Immunohistochemical studies have localized AM to the adrenal medulla, but not cortex, in humans, rats, and pigs *(28)*. Similarly, AM staining has been observed in all three species in the stomach, pancreatic islet, small intestine, colon, and choroid plexus. Staining is absent from the interstitium of the cerebellum and cerebrum, and also surprisingly absent from the heart, lung, kidney, and thyroid gland. Immunoreactive AM has been observed in the anterior, but not posterior, pituitary gland in humans and pig. Others *(29)* have observed AM immunoreactivity in the canine myocardium, aorta, and importantly, in the kidney. Positive immunoreactivity has been localized to the glomeruli, cortical distal tubule, and medullary collecting ducts. Recently, investigators *(30)* have reported that renal arterial VSMC express AM mRNA, providing the evidence for an autocrine effect of AM in the regulation of renal vascular tone. This may explain the effects of exogenous AM on renal blood flow observed by several groups in whole animal models *(31–34)*.

The anatomic framework for the potent hypotensive effects of AM in whole animals *(14,15,22,35,36)* and the ability of the peptide to relax smooth muscle strips in vitro *(30,37)* is provided by the description of AM gene transcripts in both ECs *(38)* and VSMC *(25)*. Thus, AM may act in a paracrine or autocrine fashion in the vasculature and the existence of cell lines in which gene transcription can be studied has lead to insight into the interactive role the peptide may play in the physiologic control of vascular tone and also the potential for its recruitment in shock *(39)*. AM is produced in and released from

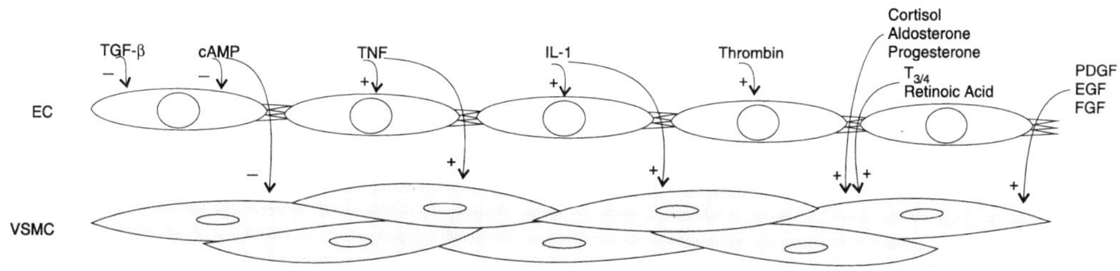

Fig. 2. Control of vascular production of adrenomedullin as determined by mRNA and peptides levels in both ECs and VSMCs. cAMP, cyclic adenosine monophosphate; EGF, epidermal growth factor; FGF, fibroblast growth factor; IL, interleukin; PDGF, platelet-derived growth factor; TGF, transforming growth factor; TNF, tumor necrosis factor.

cultured human ECs *(24)* at a rate similar to the production of another vasoactive agent, endothelin. Production of AM in endothelial cells and VSMC (Fig. 2) is potently stimulated by tumor necrosis factor-alpha (TNF-α), a cytokine that also stimulates AM release *(38)*. Similarly, interleukin-1 beta (IL-1β) and lipopolysaccharide (LPS) also increased AM production. Other agents demonstrated to stimulate AM production in ECs include thrombin, cortisol, and aldosterone. Inhibitory agents include transforming growth factor-beta (TGF-β), 8 bromo-cAMP, and high-dose phobol ester. The observation of in vivo release of AM in response to LPS challenge has led to the speculation that AM's vasorelaxant effect may underlie the hypotension of endotoxin shock *(38)*.

Cytokines and growth factors also significantly affect AM production in and release from cultured VSMC *(25)*. The most potent stimulators of AM gene transcription are IL-1α and IL-Iβ, and LPS. Production of AM peptide is driven by these cytokines and by several growth factors including fibroblast, epidermal, and platelet-derived growth factors (Fig. 3). As was the case in ECs, hormones stimulate AM production in VSMCs *(25,38,40,41)*. Although less potent than the cytokines, dexamethasone, hydrocortisone, and aldosterone enhance AM production, and lesser effects of retinoic acid and thyroid hormones have been demonstrated. Cycloheximide increases AM mRNA levels under basal and stimulated conditions, as it does for mRNAs encoding various cytokines and NO synthase (NOS), indicating that mRNA for AM is extremely labile. Actinomycin D treatment rapidly decreases AM mRNA levels indicating rapid turnover of the message. Both findings suggest that under in vivo conditions, the AM gene is transcribed and protein produced rapidly in response to pathophysiologic stimuli *(25)*. Other circulating factors may significantly affect AM gene transcription and hormone production. Agents that elevate cAMP levels in the VSMC inhibit AM production *(40)*. Thus thrombin, vasoactive intestinal peptide, and interferon-γ inhibit AM production. This is surprising because of reports of a cAMP response element (enhancer) in the 5'-upstream region of the human AM gene *(42)*.

In the adrenal gland, both AM and PAMP immunoreactivity have been localized to the medulla *(17,43)*. Calcium-dependent cosecretion of AM, PAMP, and catecholamines has been observed in response to nicotinic agents *(17,43)*. Whether AM secreted by the adrenal medulla is largely responsible for plasma levels of the peptide is yet to be determined; however, clearance studies do not support that possibility *(27)*. The lungs are a major site of AM clearance from the circulation *(27)*. It is possible that locally produced AM/PAMP played a significant autocrine role in the gland, since addition of exogenous

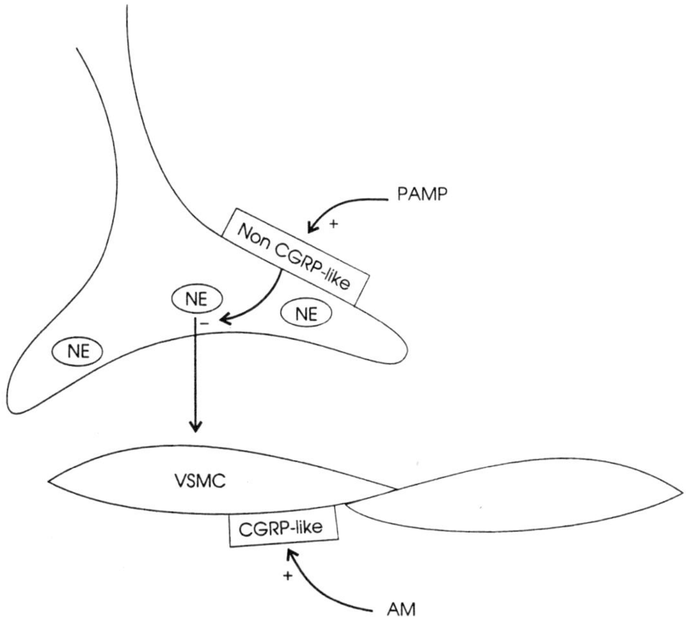

Fig. 3. Effects of PAMP on blood pressure are exerted via a non-CGRP-like receptor on sympathetic nerve terminals innervating the vasculature, resulting in decreased norepinephrine (NE) release to nerve stimulation. The effect of adrenomedullin is directly on the vascular smooth muscle via a CGRP-like receptor.

PAMP to cultures of bovine adrenal medullary cells inhibited the ability of nicotinic agents to induce sodium influx, ultimately reducing calcium entry via voltage-dependent calcium channels *(43)*. This presynaptic, antinicotinic effect (Fig. 3) may explain the hypotensive actions of PAMP *(16)*.

BIOLOGY OF AM

In Vivo Effects

Although the most impressive and readily recognized action of AM is its potent, long-lasting hypotensive effect, the peptide exerts multiple pharmacologic effects in a variety of tissues and all seem related to the regulation of vascular homeostasis *(44)*. Although the physiologic relevance of some of these multiple actions remains obscure except in one case *(45,46)*, there still remain many questions to be answered and it is in the vasculature that most current work finds focus.

Vascular Actions

Already in 1993, the ability of exogenous AM to decrease blood pressure in anesthetized rats was identified *(13)* and, using rat mesenteric vascular bed perfusion techniques, it was reported that AM's noncholinergic and nonadrenergic vasodilatory effects were blocked by the calcitonin gene-related peptide antagonist CGRP 8-37, suggesting vascular actions through an endogenous CGRP receptor *(15)*. Hindquarter vascular perfusion pressure was decreased in a dose-dependent fashion by AM, in both the cat *(36)* and rat *(14)*, and the half-life of the effect (1–2 min) was much shorter than the duration of hypotensive action when the peptide is given systemically, 20–30 min. Additionally, although AM and CGRP have similar potency in the hindlimb preparation, at least in the rat, the effects of AM on perfusion pressure are blocked by inhibition of NOS, with the false substrate *N*-omega-nitro-L-arginine methyl ester (L-NAME), whereas the effects of CGRP are not *(14)*. Cyclo-oxygenase inhibition has no effect on the fall in perfusion pressure to either peptide. Decreases in pulmonary vascular bed perfusion pressure also are observed subsequent to AM infusion *(47)*, and in intact-chest models where left atrial pressure and pulmonary blood flow are held constant *(48–50)*, the effect of AM has been reported to be caused by a decrease in pulmonary vascular resistance. Both AM and CGRP exert this action and it is clear that the six-membered ring structure of AM is necessary for biologic activity *(50)*. In conscious rats, iv infusion of human or rat AM elicited dose-dependent hypotension and tachycardia *(33)*. The tachycardia observed may not simply be a reflex-mediated phenomenon since direct cardiostimulatory effects of AM have been demonstrated in sheep *(51)*.

More recently the unique actions of AM, not expressed via the CGRP receptor, have been cataloged *(52)*. In conscious rats, AM infusion significantly elevates blood flow in the renal, mesenteric, and hindquarter circulations (reflecting increased vascular conductance), whereas CGRP only affects hindquarter blood flow *(33)*. The effect of CGRP, but not those of AM, were antagonized by GRP 8-37. Another dissociation of the AM and the CGRP effects is observed in the presence of a false substrate for NOS, which partially blocks the effects of AM alone. Similarly in the inactin-anesthetized rat, the dose-dependent increases in renal blood flow and arterial conductance, as well as the increases in glomerular filtration rate, urine flow, and urinary sodium excretion observed following renal artery infusion of AM are not attenuated by CGRP 8-37 *(32)*. The mechanism of the renal vasodilatory effect of AM has been examined in rats and dogs. In anesthetized dogs the increase in renal blood flow is dependent on NO production and not dependent on the glibenclamide-sensitive potassium channel *(53)*. In the rat, AM infusion increases the release of NO and the decrease in renal vascular resistance to the peptide is blocked by pretreatment with false substrates for NOS *(54)*. Video-based analysis of renal arteriolar diameter revealed a dilatory effect of AM in both the afferent and efferent arterioles. AM exerts less of an effect on renal vascular resistance in DOCA-salt hypertensive rats, a model with documented endothelial damage. Thus it is likely that AM exerts at least some of its actions via NO generation in endothelial cells, a concept that is supported by data from endothelium intact and denuded vessel preparations *(55)*.

Nonvascular Actions

Intravenous infusion of AM results, in the face of significant peripheral hypotension, in increases in renal blood flow *(34)*. In addition there exist unique, direct tubular actions of this peptide that persist even when the renal blood flow response has been blocked by pretreatment with N^G-monomethyl-L-arginine (L-NMMA) *(56)*. We have observed that the diuretic and natriuretic effects of AM are accentuated when renal blood flow is controlled by blocking NOS *(56)*. These data suggest a direct tubular action of the peptide, and data from another lab *(57)* supports this notion. That group *(57)* identified local production of AM in the tubule, and observed an increase in fractional sodium excretion and a decrease in distal tubular sodium reabsorption that was restricted to the kidney into which the peptide was infused. These effects are not exerted via the CGRP receptor, since in the rat, CGRP 8-37 does not reverse the increases in fractional sodium excretion in response to AM infusion. Thus, in addition to unloading the pressure of the vascular tree via peripheral vasodilation, AM can unload the vasculature further by stimulating sodium and water excretion into the urine.

These volume regulatory effects of AM are mirrored by similar actions in other tissues as well. In the adrenal gland, AM inhibits angiotensin II and potassium-stimulated aldosterone secretion *(58)*. In the anterior pituitary gland, dose-dependent inhibition of basal and corticotropin releasing factor (CRH)-stimulated adrenocorticotropin (ACTH) secretion has been reported *(59)*. Additionally, the peripheral actions of AM are complemented by central nervous system (CNS) action to inhibit both water drinking *(45)* and salt appetite *(46)*. The effect on salt appetite has physiological relevance since passive immunoneutralization of endogenous AM results in an exaggerated, abnormal thirst for salt. Whether AM can act within the brain to affect the releases of volume regulatory hormones such as vasopressin and the natriuretic peptides remains to be determined; however, the potent volume regulatory effects of AM are exerted within the CNS and those effects seem well coordinated to the peripheral actions on volume and electrolyte homeostasis. One mismatch does possibly exist. Although we and others *(45,51)* have failed to observe significant effects of centrally administered AM, one group has reported dose-dependent increases in peripheral blood pressure in urethane anesthetized rats *(60)*. More work is needed to clarify potential autonomic effects of the peptide in a variety of CNS sites. Direct neuronal actions have been demonstrated in brain sites known to be important in the control of autonomic function *(61)*, so it will not be surprising if sympathetic activity is affected by central administration of AM.

In Vitro Effects

The second messengers systems employed by AM in signaling are not all dependent on activation of adenylate cyclase (Fig. 4). In most tissues AM stimulates cAMP accumulation *(62)*; however, the transduction of its effect in intact vasculature may be more related to its ability to mobilize calcium (Ca^{2+}) into endothelial cells with a resultant stimulation of NOS *(63)*. That mobilization of Ca^{2+} has two components, a thapsigargin-sensitive recruitment of $[Ca^{2+}]_i$ and a delayed but longer lasting increase in Ca^{2+} entry into the cell. The cAMP elevation can be dissociated from the Ca^{2+}-dependent events. In renal arterial VSMCs, on the other hand, AM decreases $[Ca^{2+}]_i$ and VSMC contractility *(30)*. This is also the case in cultured porcine coronary VSMC *(37)*. AM not only decreases Ca^{2+} mobilization into VSMC *(30)*; it also decreases the production of the vasoconstrictor endothelin in these cells *(54)*. Thus, effects of AM on vascular tone may be mediated by rapid effects via decreases in $[Ca^{2+}]_i$, intermediate effects via NO activation of guanylyl cyclase, or longer effects via reduction of endothelin production *(64)*. This effect of AM on endothelin production predicts antimitogenic effects of the peptide will be discovered, similar to those of the natriuretic peptides *(5)*.

Like the VSMC, adrenal glomerulosa cells respond to AM with decreased Ca^{2+} mobilization to the ionophore A23187 *(58)*. This blockade of aldosterone secretion to the secretagog is dependent on cAMP formation. AM's inhibitory effects have recently been demonstrated in mesangial cells to occur by an action distal to activation of protein kinase C, probably via an inactivation of mitogen-activated protein kinase activity *(65)*. This may as well describe the ability of AM to inhibit basal and CRH-stimulated ACTH secretion in anterior pituitary cell cultures; however, a nonadenylate cyclase intermediate step must be envisioned since AM failed to elevate cAMP levels in those cells and did not antagonize the ability of CRH itself to stimulate adenylate cyclase *(59)*.

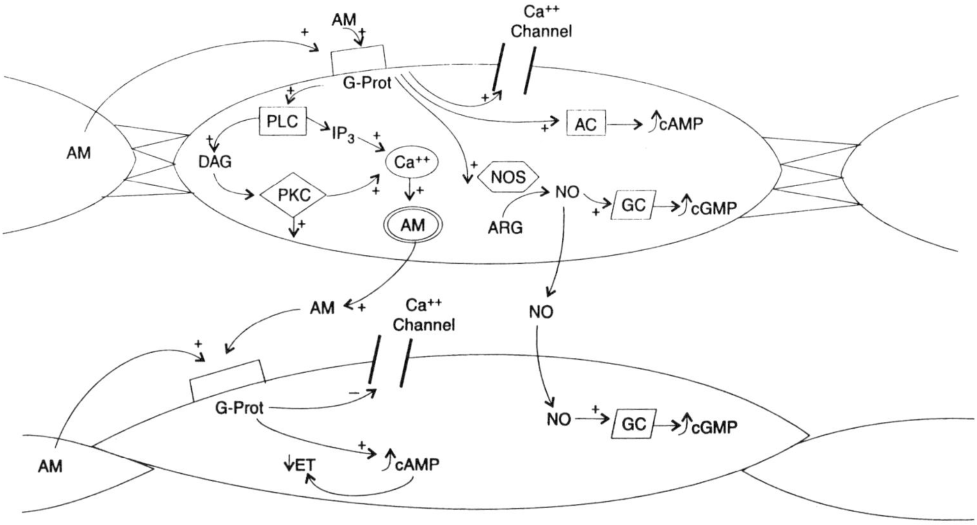

Fig. 4. Multiple signaling pathways for adrenomedullin in the vasculature. AC, adenylate cyclase; ARG, arginine; cAMP, cyclic adenosine monophosphate; cGMP, cyclic guanosine monophosphate; DAG, diacylglycerol; ET, endothelin; GC, guanylyl cyclase; G-Prot, G protein; IP_3, inositol triphosphate; NO, nitric oxide; NOS, nitric oxide synthase; PKC, protein kinase C; PLC, phospholipase C.

It is clear that multiple receptors for AM may exist, if not solely from the results of effects with the CGRP antagonist CGRP 8-37. The receptors may be G-protein linked, as has been demonstrated in coronary artery smooth muscle cells *(37)*, and they may be directly linked to ion channels in the membrane. Indeed, the presynaptic effects of PAMP on sympathetic neurons in perfused mesenteric arteries and in medulla chromaffin cells may be the result of direct effects on sodium channels *(18)*. Perhaps some of the initial confusion over receptor subtypes for AM is created by the interaction of the peptide with CGRP-like receptors *(52)*. Specific binding sites for AM have been identified *(66)*. Cross-linking analysis has revealed two forms of the AM receptor. The first form has a molecular weight of 83,000, which is most abundant in lung, diaphragm, spleen, and liver. Binding of AM to this receptor is not effectively competed for by islet amyloid polypeptide (IAPP) or CGRP. The second form of AM has an approximate molecular weight of 94,000, and predominates in heart and skeletal muscle. Binding of labeled AM to this receptor can be reduced by excess CGRP and IAPP. Indeed, this suggests that at least two molecular forms of AM receptor exist. Investigators *(52)* reported the presence of two isoforms of AM receptors; however, in their VSMC preparations CGRP competes for binding at both sites. In ECs, there may be a dissociation, since the effects of CGRP on cAMP formation are blocked by the CGRP antagonist, whereas those of AM are not *(67)*.

Very recently, investigators *(68)* reported the cloning and expression of a rat AM receptor cDNA. The clone was originally isolated from rat lung and encodes a 352 residue polypeptide that is a member of the seven transmembrane domain super family of G-protein-linked receptors. When expressed in COS-7 cells, the receptor mediates a stimulation of cAMP by AM and the binding of the peptide is saturable with a K_D of $8.2 \times 10^{-9} M$ *(68)*. The receptor gene expresses several species of mRNA that are detected in lung, adrenal, ovary, spleen, heart, and central nervous system. This landmark advance in the study of the physiology of AM promises to facilitate the further elucidation of the relevance of the peptide. Armed with the knowledge of receptor structure, the specificity of AM can be established and physiologically based studies can now characterize the peptide's role in normal vascular function.

PATHOPHYSIOLOGIC SIGNIFICANCE OF AM

A peptide with such potent in vivo effects on cardiovascular and renal function as AM creates a great deal of excitement in the early phases of discovery. Indeed, the potent diuretic and natriuretic effects have predicted its potential therapeutic role in renal failure and the hypotensive actions suggest a physiologic role in the maintenance of normal vascular tone. Thus it is not surprising that attention has been focused on plasma levels of the hormone in pathologic states. However, this agent appears, like endothelin, to be better suited for local paracrine or autocrine effects and as a result circulating levels may only be indicative of spill-over from the tissue of production and action. Just the same, increased plasma AM levels have been described in congestive heart failure (CHF), and the progression of disease is paralleled by the increase in plasma hormone levels *(39)*. Since the peptide is produced in the myocardium, it may play a role in the physiologic adaptation that characterizes the early phases of CHF *(69)*, just like the other cardiac hormone, atrial natriuretic peptide. Increases in plasma AM levels have also been reported in patients with renal failure *(70,71)* and hypertension *(70,72)*. This may reflect tissue damage or perhaps a physiologic attempt by the vasculature to compensate by secreting a hormone that will improve renal function and protect against vascular damage of hypertension. These remain important questions to be addressed by both molecular and integrative approaches. Similarly, it is imperative to determine if CNS actions of AM exert physiologic control over vascular status. It is already clear that at least one effect of AM in brain, its ability to inhibit salt appetite, does have physiological relevance. Thus we return to the beginning. Just as the lessons we have learned in the study of the pathophysiologic relevance of the endothelins and the natriuretic peptides provided templates on which to study the actions of this novel hypotensive peptide, now what we are learning about AM forms the framework for the elucidation of the interactive mechanisms by which numerous vasoactive hormones control vascular homeostasis. Not only in states of cardiovascular and renal dysfunction, but also in normal physiology, important interactive effects must determine the integrated mechanisms by which fluid and electrolyte homeostasis and cardiovascular competence are maintained.

ACKNOWLEDGMENTS

The author acknowledges the continued generous support of the American Heart Association and Phoenix Pharmaceuticals for his work on the endocrinology of cardiovascular hormones.

REFERENCES

1. Anggard EE. The endothelium—the body's largest endocrine gland? J Endocrinol 1990;127:371–375.
2. Inagami T, Naruse M, Hoover R. Endothelium as an endocrine organ. Annu Rev Physiol 1995;57:171–189.
3. Luscher TF. Imbalance of endothelium-derived relaxing and contracting factors. A new concept in hypertension? Am J Hypertens 1990;3:317–330.

4. Dzau VJ, Gibbons GH, Morishita R, Pratt RE. New perspectives in hypertension research. Potentials of vascular biology. Hypertension 1994;23:1132–1140.
5. Levin ER. Endothelins. N Engl J Med 1995;333:356–363.
6. Samson WK. Cardiovascular hormones. In: Conn PM, Melmed S, eds. The Scientific Basis of Endocrinology: Fundamental and Clinical Principals. Humana, Totowa, NJ, 1996, in press.
7. Hickey KA, Rubyani GM, Paul RJ, Highsmith RF. Characterization of a coronary vasoconstrictor produced by cultured endothelial cells. Am J Physiol 1985;248:C550–C556.
8. Rubyani GM, Vanhoutte PM. Hypoxia releases a vasoconstrictor substance from the canine vascular endothelium. J Physiol (Lond) 1985;364:45–56.
9. Yanagisawa M, Kurihara H, Kimura S, Tomobe Y, Kobayashi M, Mitsui Y, Yazaki Y, Goto K, Masaki T. A novel potent vasoconstrictor peptide produced by vascular endothelial cells. Nature 1988;332:411–415.
10. Dzau VJ. Significance of the vascular renin-angiotensin pathway. Hypertension 1986;8:553–559.
11. Moncada S, Vane JR. Pharmacology and endogenous role of prostaglandin endoperoxides, thromboxane A_2, and prostacyclin. Pharmacol Rev 1979;30:293–331.
12. Moncada S, Palmer R, Higgs E. Nitric oxide: physiology, pathophysiology, and pharmacology. Pharmacol Rev 1991;43:109–142.
13. Kitamura K, Kangawa K, Kawamoto M, Ichiki Y, Nkamura S, Matsuo H, Eto T. Adrenomedullin: a novel hypotensive peptide isolated from human pheochromocytoma. Biochem Biophys Res Commun 1993;192:553–560.
14. Feng CJ, Kang B, Kaye AD, Kadowitz PJ, Nossaman BD. L-NAME modulates responses to adrenomedullin in the hindquarters vascular bed of the rat. Life Sci 1994;55:433–438.
15. Nuki C, Kawasaki H, Kitamura K, Takenaga M, Kangawa K, Eto T, Wada A. Vasodilator effect of adrenomedullin and calcitonin gene related peptide receptors in rat mesenteric vascular beds. Biochem Biophys Res Commun 1993;196:245–251.
16. Kitamura K, Kangawa K, Ishiyama Y, Washimine H, Ichiki Y, Kawamoto M, Minamino N, Matsuo H, Eto T. Identification and hypotensive activity of proadrenomedullin N-terminal 20 peptide (PAMP). FEBS Lett 1994;351:35–37.
17. Katoh F, Kitamura K, Niina H, Yamamoto R, Washimine H, Kangawa K, Yamamoto Y, Kobayashi H, Eto T, Wada A. Proadrenomedullin N-terminal 20 peptide (PAMP), an endogenous anticholinergic peptide: its exocytotic secretion and inhibition of catecholamine secretion in adrenal medulla. J Neurochem 1995;64:459–461.
18. Shimosawa T, Ito Y, Ando K, Kitamura K, Kangawa K, Fujita T. Proadrenomedullin NH_2-terminal 20 peptide, a new product of the adrenomedullin gene, inhibits norepinephrine overflow from nerve endings. J Clin Invest 1995;96:1672–1676.
19. Sakata J, Shimokubo T, Kitamura K, Nakamura S, Kangawa K, Matsuo H, Eto T. Molecular cloning and biological activities of rat adrenomedullin, a hypotensive peptide. Biochem Biophys Res Commun 1993;195:921–927.
20. Kitamura K, Kangawa K, Kojima M, Ichiki Y, Maysuo H, Eto T. Complete amino acid sequence of porcine adrenomedullin and cloning of cDNA encoding its precursor. FEBS Lett 1994;338:306–310.
21. Kitamura K, Sakata J, Kangawa K, Kojima M, Matsuo H, Eto T. Cloning and characterization of cDNA encoding a precursor for human adrenomedullin. Biochem Biophys Res Commun 1993;194:720–725.
22. Sakata J, Shimokubo T, Kitamura K, Nishizono M, Iehiki Y, Kangawa K, Matsuo H, Eto T. Distribution and characterization of immunoreactive rat adrenomedullin in tissue and plasma. FEBS Lett 1994;352:105–108.
23. Satoh F, Takahashi K, Murakami O, Totsune K, Sone M, Ohneda M, Abe K, Miura Y, Hyashi Y, Sasano H, Mouri T. Adrenomedullin in human brain, adrenal glands and tumor tissues of pheochromocytoma, ganglioneuroblastoma and neuroblastoma. J Clin Endocrinol Metab 1995;80:1750–1752.
24. Sugo S, Minamino N, Kangawa K, Miyamoto K, Kitamura K, Sakata J, Eto T, Matsuo H. Endothelial cells actively synthesize and secrete adrenomedullin. Biochem Biophys Res Commun 1994;201:1160–1166.
25. Minamino N, Shoji H, Sugo S, Kangawa K, Matsuo H. Adrenocortical steroids, thyroid hormones and retinoic acid augment the production of adrenomedullin in vascular smooth muscle cells. Biochem Biophys Res Commun 1995;211:686–693.
26. Ichiki Y, Kitamura K, Kangawa K, Kawamoto M, Matsuo H, Eto T. Distribution and characterization of immunoreactive adrenomedullin in human tissue and plasma. FEBS Lett 1994;338:6–10.
27. Nishikimi T, Kitamura K, Saito Y, Shimada K, Ishimitsu T, Takamiya M, Kangawa K, Matsuo H, Eto T, Omae T, Matsuoka H. Clinical studies on the sites of production and clearance of circulating adrenomedullin in human subjects. Hypertension 1994;24:600–604.

28. Washimine H, Asada Y, Kitamura K, Ichiki Y, Hara S, Yamamoto Y, Kangawa K, Sumiyoshi T, Eto T. Immunohistochemical identification of adrenomedullin in human, rat, and porcine tissue. Histochem Cell Biol 1995;103:251–254.
29. Jougasaki M, Wei CM, Heublein DM, Sandberg SM, Burnett JC. Immunohistochemical localization of adrenomedullin in canine heart and aorta. Peptides 1995;16:773–775.
30. Seguchi H, Nishimura J, Kobayashi S, Kumazawa J, Kanaide H. Autocrine regulation of the renal arterial tone by adrenomedullin. Biochem Biophys Res Commun 1995;215:619–625.
31. Ebara T, Miura K, Okumura M, Matsuura T, Kim S, Yukimura T, Iwao H. Effect of adrenomedullin on renal hemodynamics and functions in dogs. Eur J Pharmacol 1994;263:69–73.
32. Haynes JM, Cooper ME. Adrenomedullin and calcitonin gene-related peptide in the rat isolated kidney and in the anesthetized rat: in vitro and in vivo effects. Eur J Pharmacol 1995;280:91–94.
33. Gardiner SM, Kemp PA, March JE, Bennett T. Regional hemodynamic effects of human and rat adrenomedullin in conscious rats. Br J Pharmacol 1995;114:584–591.
34. Vari RC, Adkins SD, Samson WK. Adrenomedullin increases renal plasma flow and sodium excretion. Proc Soc Exp Biol Med 1996;211:178–183.
35. Ishiyama Y, Kitamura K, Ichiki Y, Nakamura S, Kida O, Kangawa K, Eto T. Hemodynamic effects of a novel hypotensive peptide, human adrenomedullin, in rats. Eur J Pharmacol 1993;41:271–273.
36. Santiago JA, Garrison EA, Ventura VL, Coy DH, Bitar K, Murphy WA, McNamara DB, Kadowitz PJ. Synthetic human adrenomedullin and adrenomedullin 15–52 have potent short-lived vasodilator activity in the hindlimb vascular bed of the cat. Life Sci 1994;55:85–90.
37. Kureishi Y, Kobayashi S, Nishimura J, Nakano T, Kanaide H. Adrenomedullin decreases both cytosolic Ca^{2+} concentration and Ca^{2+}-sensitivity in pig coronary arterial smooth muscle. Biochem Biophys Res Commun 1995;212:572–579.
38. Sugo S, Minamino N, Shoji H, Kangawa K, Kitamura K, Eto T, Matsuo H. Production and secretion of adrenomedullin from vascular smooth muscle cells: augmented production by tumor necrosis factor alpha. Biochem Biophys Res Commun 1994;203:719–726.
39. Kitamura K, Kangawa K, Matsuo H, Eto T. Adrenomedullin: implications for hypertension research. Drugs 1995;49:485–495.
40. Sugo S, Minamino N, Shoji H, Kangawa K, Matsuo H. Effects of vasoactive substances and cAMP related compounds on adrenomedullin production in cultured vascular smooth muscle cells. FEBS Lett 1995;369:311–314.
41. Sugo S, Minamino N, Shoji H, Kangawa K, Kitamura K, Eto T, Matsuo H. Interleukin-1, tumor necrosis factor and lipopolysaccharide additively stimulate production of adrenomedullin in vascular smooth muscle cells. Biochem Biophys Res Commun 1995;207:25–32.
42. Ishimitsu T, Kojima M, Kangawa K, Hino J, Matsuoka H, Kitamura K, Eto T, Matsuo H. Genomic structure of human adrenomedullin gene. Biochem Biophys Res Commun 1994;203:631–639.
43. Katoh F, Niina H, Kitamura K, Ichiki Y, Yamamoto Y, Kangawa K, Eto T, Wada A. Calcium-dependent cosecretion of adrenomedullin and catecholamines mediated by nicotinic receptors in bovine cultured adrenal medullary cells. FEBS Lett 1994;348:61–64.
44. Schell DA, Vari RC, Samson WK. Adrenomedullin: a newly discovered hormone controlling fluid and electrolyte homeostasis. Trends Endocrinol Metab 1996;7:7–13.
45. Murphy TC, Samson WK. The novel vasoactive hormone, adrenomedullin, inhibits water drinking in the rat. Endocrinology 1995;136:2459–2463.
46. Murphy TC, Samson WK. Adrenomedullin is a potent suppressor of salt appetite in the rat. Soc Neurosci 1995;21:459, (abstract #188.3).
47. Nossaman BD, Feng CJ, Cheng DY, Dewitt BJ, Coy DH, Murphy WA, Kadowitz PJ. Comparative effects of adrenomedullin, an adrenomedullin analog, and CGRP in the pulmonary vascular bed of the cat and rat. Life Sci 1995;56:63–66.
48. Cheng DY, DeWitt BJ, Wegmann MJ, Coy DH, Bitar K, Murphy WA, Kadowitz PH. Synthetic human adrenomedullin and ADM 15–52 have potent short-lasting vasodilator activity in the pulmonary vascular bed of the cat. Life Sci 1994;55:251–256.
49. DeWitt BJ, Cheng DY, Caminiti GN, Nossaman BD, Coy DH, Murphy WA, Kadowitz PJ. Comparison of responses to adrenomedullin and calcitonin gene-related peptide in the pulmonary vascular bed of the cat. Eur J Pharmacol 1994;257:303–306.
50. Lippton H, Chang JK, Hao Q, Summer W, Hyman AL. Adrenomedullin dilates the pulmonary vascular bed in vivo. J Appl Physiol 1994;76:2154–2156.
51. Parkes DG. Cardiovascular actions of adrenomedullin in conscious sheep. Am J Physiol 1995;268: H2574–H2578.

52. Eguchi S, Hirata Y, Kano H, Sato Y, Watanabe Y, Matanabe TX, Nakajima K, Sakakibara S, Marumo F. Specific receptors for adrenomedullin in cultured rat vascular smooth muscle cells. FEBS Lett 1994;340:226–230.
53. Miura K, Ebara T, Okumura M, Matsuura T, Kim S, Yukimura T, Iwao H. Attenuation of adrenomedullin-induced renal vasodilatation by N^{G}-nitro L-arginine but not glibenclamide. Br J Pharmacol 1995;115: 917–924.
54. Hirata Y, Hayakawa H, Suzuki Y, Suzuki E, Ikenouchi H, Kohmoto O, Kimura K, Eto T, Kangawa K, Matsuo H, Omata M. Mechanisms of adrenomedullin-induced vasodilation in the rat kidney. Hypertension 1995;25:790–795.
55. Nakamura K, Toda H, Terasako K, Kakuyama M, Hatano Y, Mori K, Kangawa K. Vasodilative effect of adrenomedullin in isolated arteries of the dog. Jpn J Pharmacol 1995;67:259–262.
56. Vari RC, Adkins SD, Samson WK. Role of nitric oxide in the renal responses to adrenomedullin in the rat. J Am Soc Nephrol 1995;6:749 (abstract).
57. Jougasaki M, Wei CM, Aarhus LL, Heublein DM, Sandberg SM, Burnett JC. Renal localization and actions of adrenomedullin: a natriuretic peptide. Am J Physiol 1995;268:F657–F663.
58. Yamaguchi T, Baba K, Doi Y, Yano K. Effect of adrenomedullin on aldosterone secretion by dispersed rat adrenal zona glomerulosa cells. Life Sci 1995;56:379–387.
59. Samson WK, Murphy TC, Schell DA. A novel vasoactive peptide, adrenomedullin, inhibits pituitary adrenocorticotropin release. Endocrinology 1995;136:2349–2352.
60. Takahashi H, Watanabe T, Nishimura M, Nakanishi T, Sakamoto M, Yoshimura M, Komiyama Y, Masuda M, Murakami T. Centrally induced vasopressor and sympathetic responses to a novel endogenous peptide, adrenomedullin, in anesthetized rats. Am J Hypertension 1994;7:478–482.
61. Allen MA, Sun K, Ferguson AV. In vitro recordings from area postrema neurons demonstrate responsiveness to adrenomedullin, a newly discovered vasoactive peptide. Soc Neurosci 1995;21:889 (abstract #353.16).
62. Ishizaka Y, Ishizaka Y, Tanaka M, Kitamura K, Kangawa K, Minamino N, Matsuo H, Eto T. Adrenomedullin stimulates cyclic AMP formation in rat vascular smooth muscle cells. Biochem Biophys Res Commun 1994;200:642–646.
63. Shimekake Y, Nagata K, Ohta S, Kambayashi Y, Teraoka H, Kitamura K, Eto T, Kangawa K, Matsuo H. Adrenomedullin stimulates two signal transduction pathways, cAMP accumulation and calcium mobilization, in bovine aortic endothelial cells. J Biol Chem 1995;270:4412–4417.
64. Kohno M, Kano H, Horio T, Yokokawa K, Yasunari K, Takeda T. Inhibition of endothelin production by adrenomedullin in vascular smooth muscle cells. Hypertension 1995;25:1185–1190.
65. Kusaka I, Ishikawa S, Saito T. Inhibition by adrenomedullin of arginine vasopressin-induced mitogen activated protein kinase in cultured rat glomerular mesangial cells [abstract P1-630]. 77th Annual Meeting of the Endocrine Society, Washington, DC. The Endocrine Society, Bethesda, MD, 1995.
66. Owji AA, Smith DM, Coppock HA, Morgan DGA, Bhogal R, Ghatei MA, Bloom SR. An abundant and specific binding site for the novel vasodilator adrenomedullin in the rat. Endocrinology 1995;136:2127–2134.
67. Kato J, Kitamura K, Kangawa K, Eto T. Receptors for adrenomedullin in human vascular endothelial cells. Eur J Pharmacol 1995;289:383–385.
68. Kapas S, Catt KJ, Clark AJL. Cloning and expression of cDNA encoding a rat adrenomedullin receptor. J Biol Chem 1995;27:25,344–25,347.
69. Jougasaki M, Wei CM, McKinley LJ, Burnett JC. Elevation of circulating and ventricular adrenomedullin in human congestive heart failure. Circulation 1995;92:286–289.
70. Ishimitsu T, Nishikimi T, Saito Y, Kitamura K, Eto T, Kangawa K, Matsuo H, Omae T, Matsuoka H. Plasma levels of adrenomedullin, a newly identified hypotensive peptide, in patients with hypertension and renal failure. J Clin Invest 1994;94:2158–2161.
71. Sato K, Hirata Y, Imai T, Iwashina M, Marumo F. Characterization of immunoreactive adrenomedullin in human plasma and urine. Life Sci 1995;57:189–194.
72. Kitamura K, Ichiki Y, Tanaka M, Kawamoto M, Emura J, Sakakibara S, Kangawa K, Matsuo H, Eto T. Immunoreactive adrenomedullin in human plasma. FEBS Lett 1994;341:288–290.

21 Calcium and Magnesium in the Regulation of Smooth Muscle Function and Blood Pressure

The Ionic Hypothesis of Cardiovascular and Metabolic Diseases and Vascular Aging

Mario Barbagallo, MD,
and Lawrence M. Resnick, MD

CONTENTS

INTRACELLULAR REGULATION OF CONTRACTION BY CALCIUM AND MAGNESIUM

Calcium (Ca^{2+}) is a unique cellular ion having a large intra- vs extracellular gradient (1:10,000) and playing a key role in mediating stimulus-contraction coupling in cardiac, skeletal, and vascular smooth muscle (VSM), as well as stimulus-secretion coupling in endocrine, neural, and renal tissues *(1–8)*. Mechanistically, increasing myoplasmic free Ca^{2+} concentrations $[Ca^{2+}]_i$, initiates contraction by binding to calmodulin, altering its

From: *Contemporary Endocrinology: Endocrinology of the Vasculature*
Edited by: J. R. Sowers Humana Press Inc., Totowa, NJ

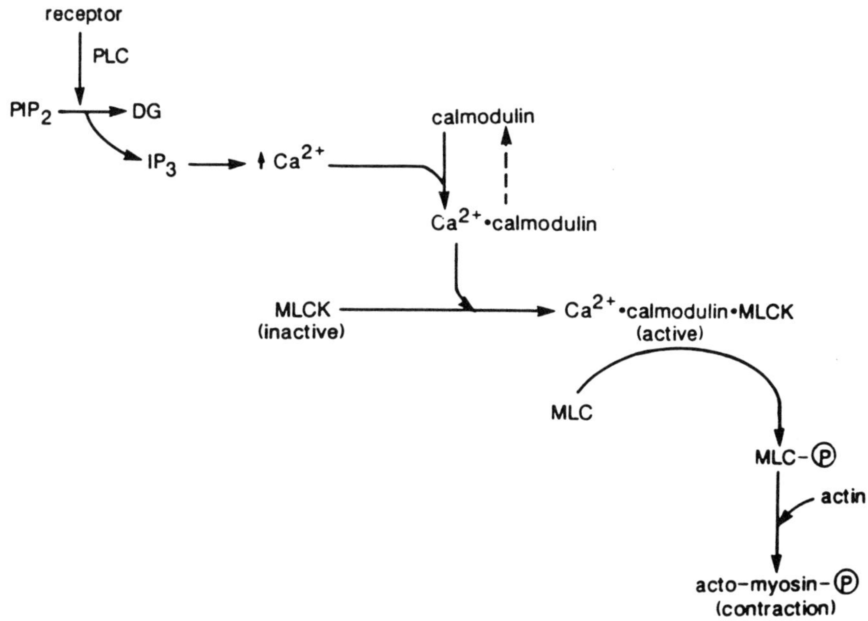

Fig. 1. Cascade of enzymatic reactions leading to contraction in VSM. The initial increase in intracellular Ca^{2+} initiates a cascade of kinase activation, ultimately resulting in actin-myosin interaction and contraction. MLC, Myosin light chain; MLCK, MLC kinase *(9)*.

tertiary structure, and promoting its binding to myosin light chain kinase (MLCK) *(2)*, thereby removing the normal autoinhibition of this enzyme. Activation of MLCK begins a cascade of molecular rearrangements leading to myofilament shortening and contraction. Activated MLCK phosphorylates the light chain of myosin, stimulating its binding to actin filaments, resulting in fiber shortening and consequent contraction *(3)* (Fig. 1). This $[Ca^{2+}]_i$-initiated process is important in both depolarization-mediated and agonist-mediated contraction.

Mechanisms by which $[Ca^{2+}]_i$ becomes available for initiation of contraction vary (Fig. 2). Thus, changes in membrane potential activate L-type Ca^{2+}-channel current, inducing Ca^{2+}-influx and subsequent contraction (electromechanical coupling) *(4)*. Circulating pressor molecules also can increase or decrease VSM tension, in part by regulating Ca^{2+} influx through receptor-mediated Ca^{2+} channels or through other second messenger-operated systems. In addition to Ca^{2+} entering vascular smooth muscle cells (VSMC) across the plasma membrane, smooth muscle agonists may also trigger a rise in $[Ca^{2+}]_i$ by release of Ca^{2+} from intracellular stores. This involves agonist receptor-mediated activation of G-protein-coupled phospholipase C (PLC). PLC catalyzes the hydrolysis of phosphatidylinositol 4,5 bisphosphate to form inositol 1,4,5 triphosphate (IP_3) and diacylglycerol (DAG) (Figs. 1 and 2), and IP_3 releases Ca^{2+} from sarcoplasmic reticulum (SR) via IP_3-specific receptors *(5)*. DAG is also a second messenger, increasing the affinity of protein kinase C (PKC) for Ca^{2+}. In the presence of DAG and Ca^{2+}, activated PKC subsequently phosphorylates a number of cellular proteins *(6)*. PKC activates plasma membrane Na^+–Ca^{2+} exchange and thereby modulates intracellular pH and $[Ca^{2+}]_i$. In VSMC, PKC also activates Ca^{2+}–ATPase *(7)* and MLCK *(8)*, affecting

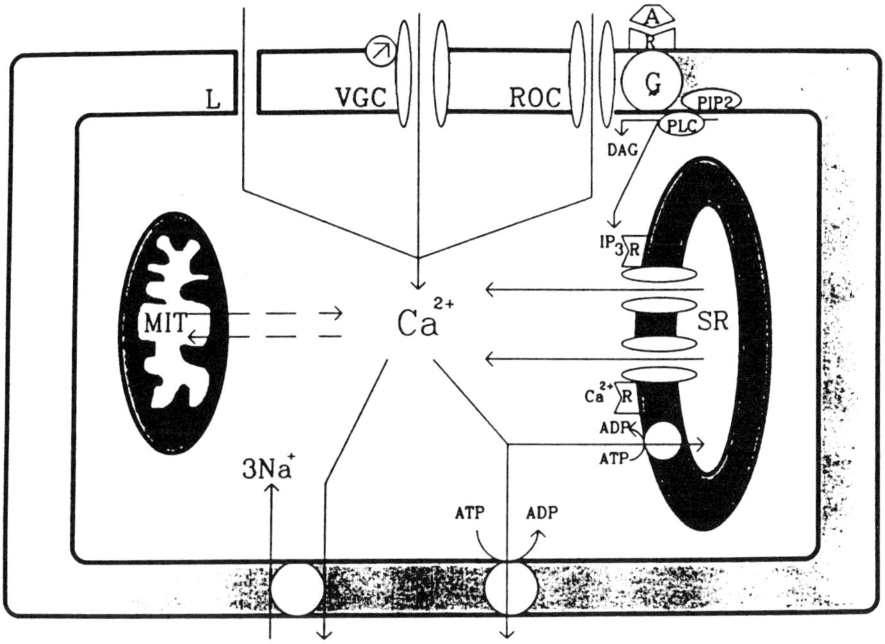

Fig. 2. Ca^{2+} mobilizing and Ca^{2+} homeostatic mechanisms in VSM. Extracellular Ca^{2+} enters the cell through the passive Ca^{2+} leak (L), receptor-operated Ca^{2+} channels (ROC), and voltage-gated Ca^{2+} channels (VGC). Intracellular Ca^{2+} stores in the SR are released in response to IP_3 or to Ca^{2+}. The increased intracellular Ca^{2+} is taken up by the Ca^{2+} pump or extruded by the plasmalemmal Ca^{2+} pump. At high concentrations of Ca^{2+}, the Na^+-Ca^{2+} exchanger and the mitochondria (MIT) may also play a role in Ca^{2+} homeostasis *(10)*.

both $[Ca^{2+}]_i$ and VSMC tone. Thus, these intracellular pathways translating depolarization and/or agonist-dependent signals into a mechanical event are all dependent on and contribute to $[Ca^{2+}]_i$ homeostasis.

Also important in determining VSMC tone are factors facilitating relaxation, generally thought to be associated with a fall in the $[Ca^{2+}]_i$. Three primary mechanisms appear to be involved (Fig. 2). Two utilize active pumps (ATP-dependent Ca^{2+}-transport or Ca^{2+}–ATPases) that use energy derived from ATP to move Ca^{2+} out of the cytosol against concentration gradients. VSMC have at least two different Ca^{2+}–ATPases, one for outward transport of Ca^{2+} across the plasma membrane and the other for storage into the SR *(11)*. The third Ca^{2+} lowering mechanism is Na^+–Ca^{2+} exchange *(12)*, a lower affinity, higher capacity system, utilizing steady-state Ca^{2+} and sodium (Na^+) gradients to couple extrusion of Ca^{2+} with movement of Na^+ into VSMC. Net VSMC tone is thus a balance between contractile and relaxant factors, each critically involving alterations of $[Ca^{2+}]_i$.

Lastly, the role of $[Ca^{2+}]_i$ in stimulus-contraction coupling and relaxation is itself dependent on intracellular steady-state activities of other mineral ions, such as magnesium ($[Mg^{2+}]_i$), potassium ($[K^+]_i$), and hydrogen (pHi). In particular, it is now clear that $[Mg^{2+}]_i$ modulates VSMC tone and contractility by affecting $[Ca^{2+}]_i$ and Ca^{2+} availability at critical sites (e.g., on calmodulin in VSMC). By stimulating Ca^{2+}-dependent K^+ channels, competitively inhibiting Ca^{2+} binding to calmodulin, stimulating both plasma membrane and SR Ca^{2+}–ATPases, and by activating the membrane Na^+, K^+, ATPase pump, $[Mg^{2+}]_i$ serves to actively promote relaxation, offset Ca^{2+}-related excitation-contraction coupling, and decrease cellular responsiveness to depolarizing stimuli *(13–16)*. Consistent with the aforementioned, Ca^{2+}-induced VSMC contraction is not only sensitive to changes in $[Mg^{2+}]_i$ *(13–15)*, but direct reduction of extracellular Mg^{2+} raises VSMC $[Ca^{2+}]_i$, whereas elevations in Mg^{2+} reciprocally lower Ca^{2+} content in VSMC *(17)*.

EXTRACELLULAR REGULATION OF INTRACELLULAR DIVALENT CATIONS

$[Ca^{2+}]_i$ and $[Mg^{2+}]_i$ are not only involved in regulating cardiac and VSMC contractile function, but are critical to cellular responses to a wide variety of external stimuli, including stimulus-secretion coupling in endocrine cells, neurotransmitter release from nerve terminals, and renal function *(18)*. As such, endocrine, neural, and renal aspects of blood pressure homeostasis, as well as cardiac and VSMC function are all determined, at least in part, by the steady-state $[Ca^{2+}]_i$ and $[Mg^{2+}]_i$. Recent research demonstrates a common pattern of altered intracellular cation content, characterized by excess $[Ca^{2+}]_i$ and/or reciprocally suppressed $[Mg^{2+}]_i$ in subjects with the accelerated atherosclerosis and vascular "aging" resulting from essential hypertension, obesity, and type II diabetes mellitus *(19)*. What is responsible for these abnormalities of cellular cation content in hypertension and associated metabolic conditions? Although genetic mechanisms and other intracellular control mechanisms (e.g., altered membrane pump activities, phosphorylating and dephosphorylating enzyme cascades, and intracellular regulating factors such as G-proteins, phospholipases, etc.) may be involved, our group has focused on the potential contribution of dietary and hormonal factors. We suggest that alterations of $[Ca^{2+}]_i$ and $[Mg^{2+}]_i$ homeostasis mediate the influence of diverse environmental and hormonal factors such as glucose, insulin, dietary salt, etc. on blood pressure and vascular disease.

Role of Glucose and Insulin in Regulating Intracellular Cations in VSMC

The cellular ionic environment is also influenced by dietary nutrients and their regulating hormones. Glucose appears to contribute to cellular cation homeostasis independently of insulin. We reported the effects of hyperglycemia on the $[Ca^{2+}]_i$ content in cultured VSMC, where glucose in a specific, concentration-, and time-dependent manner, at concentrations often observed clinically, and independent of insulin, increased VSMC $[Ca^{2+}]_i$ *(20)* (Fig. 3), suggesting a mechanism for the increased vasoconstriction associated with diabetes. These results paralleled work in peripheral erythrocytes, in which hyperglycemia elevated Ca^{2+} and reciprocally lowered Mg^{2+} *(21)*. These ionic effects of glucose were blunted in cells from hypertensive subjects; the greater the basal Ca^{2+}, or the lower the basal Mg^{2+}, the less responsive were the cells to glucose. Thus, ambient glucose levels affect intracellular cation content, and cellular cation content may also influence cell responsiveness to glucose. This ionic dependence of cellular responsiveness may be an example of a more general property of cells also observed with insulin.

The mechanism by which glucose modulates intracellular divalent cation content remains unclear. Osmotic or other nonspecific effects are ruled out by the failure of equiosmolar amounts of L-glucose or mannitol to reproduce the D-glucose effect (Fig. 3B). Davis et al. *(22)* demonstrated a direct inhibitory effect of hyperglycemia on plasma membrane Ca^{2+}–ATPase, possibly mediated by nonenzymatic glycosylation *(23)*. This

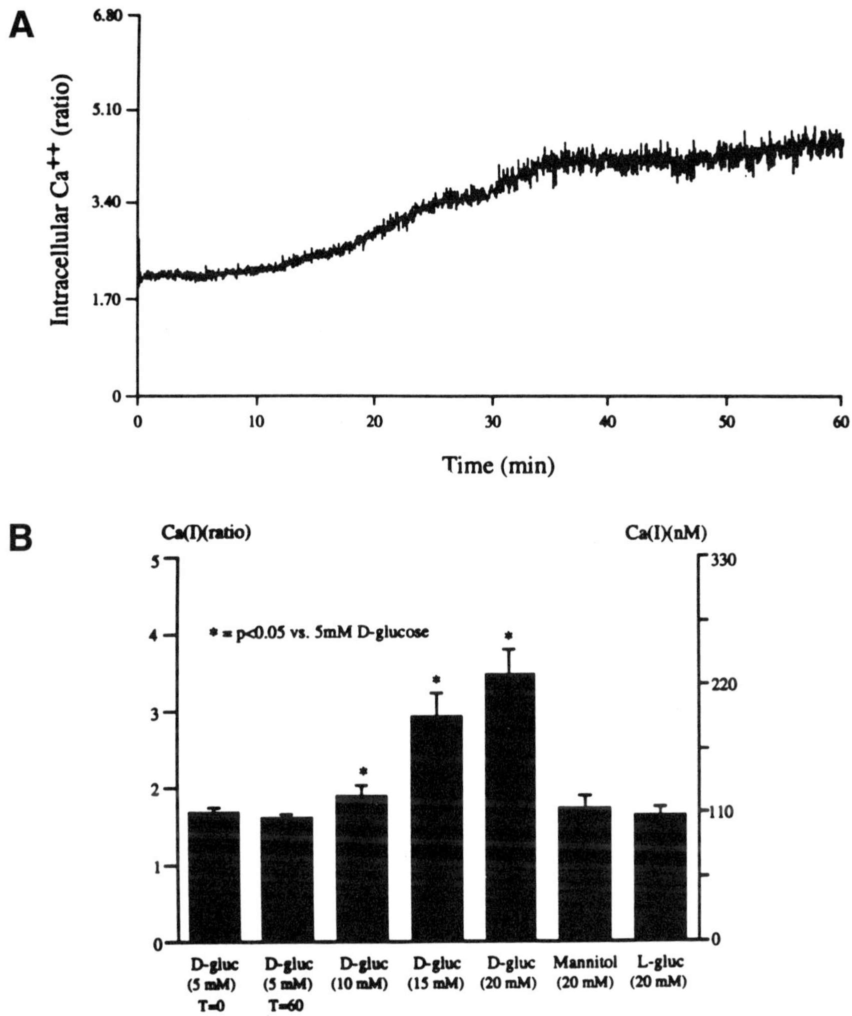

Fig. 3. (A) Continuous tracing of intracellular $[Ca^{2+}]_i$ concentrations in isolated VSMC exposed to 20 m*M* D-glucose (D-gluc) over the course of 60 min *(20)*. **(B)** Effect of D-gluc at 5 m*M* (before $T = 0$) and after 1 h of incubation ($T = 60$) at 5, 10, 15, and 20 m*M*; effect of L-glucose (L-gluc at 20 m*M*) and of mannitol (at 20 m*M*) on intracellular-free Ca^{2+} concentrations ($[Ca^{2+}]_i$, n*M*) in primary cultures of VSMC *(20)*.

would promote $[Ca^{2+}]_i$ accumulation from the extracellular space by retarding Ca^{2+} efflux. A second potential mechanism involves glucose-induced stimulation of PKC *(24)*, with its potential for recruiting Ca^{2+} from intracellular storage sites via IP_3 formation. However, this mechanism cannot be primary since red blood cells, devoid of intracellular organelles, also display the same behavior *(21)*. Moreover, the effect of glucose seems to be dependent on extracellular Ca^{2+}, since glucose has no effects on $[Ca^{2+}]_i$ in a Ca^{2+}-free medium *(20)*. Another possible third mechanism involves activation of glycolysis by increased cellular glucose uptake, and increased organic acid formation, since a decrease in pH may increase $[Ca^{2+}]_i$ *(24,25)*. The importance of changes in pH is also suggested by the failure of glucose to increase $[Ca^{2+}]_i$ in VSMC exposed to an acid environment *(20)*. This glucose-induced stimulation of VSMC $[Ca^{2+}]_i$ may be clinically significant occurring at a threshold concentration of 10 m*M*, which is observed in individuals with impaired glucose tolerance and clinical diabetes mellitus, and thus may help explain the increased incidence of hypertension in these conditions.

Insulin may also regulate both $[Ca^{2+}]_i$ and $[Mg^{2+}]_i$ in a variety of cells *(26–28)*. This is a specific, dose-related action, independent of cellular glucose uptake *(26–28)*. Furthermore, it appears that these effects of insulin are blunted in cells from hypertensive individuals *(27,29)*. As is the case for glucose, the higher the basal Ca^{2+}, and/or the lower the Mg^{2+}, the less responsive is the cell to insulin stimulation. These data have led to the notion that the "insulin resistance" of hypertension, currently defined by measurements of tissue glucose uptake, might equally well be defined on the basis of altered VSMC divalent cation metabolism. Furthermore, this "ionic" insulin resistance is probably not specific for insulin, but may rather be one tissue manifestation of a general property of cells in which steady-state $[Ca^{2+}]_i$ and/or $[Mg^{2+}]_i$ level may determine cell responsiveness to insulin, glucose, depolarizing stimuli, and so on, that depend on cell Ca^{2+} uptake from the extracellular space.

Role of Ca^{2+}-Regulating Hormones and Steroids in the Modulation of Vascular Tone

Several hormones responsible for body Ca^{2+} homeostasis are also vasoactive hormones, modulating $[Ca^{2+}]_i$ metabolism and force generating capacity in cardiovascular tissues. Peptide hormones, such as parathyroid hormone (PTH), calcitonin and calcitonin gene-related peptide (CGRP), and parathyroid hypertensive factor (PHF), may all affect the intra- and extracellular distribution of Ca^{2+}. Additionally, many steroid hormones such as 1,25 dehydroxyvitamin D ($1,25[OH]_2D_3$), estradiol, and progesterone, and the adrenal steroid dihydroepiandrosterone sulfate (DHEAS) have all been demonstrated to directly influence contractile tone and intracellular Ca^{2+} metabolism in VSM.

PTH

Over 70 yr ago, investigators observed the vasodilatory effects of PTH *(30)*, which when confirmed by others *(31)*, suggested that PTH functions physiologically as a vasodilator to regulate peripheral vascular tone. However, chronic excess PTH levels seen in hyperparathyroidism are often associated with elevations of blood pressure *(32,33)*. A similar paradox is also present at the cellular level. Despite evidence that PTH can increase myocyte Ca^{2+} influx and $[Ca^{2+}]_i$ *(34)*, electrophysiological patch clamp studies and direct cellular measurement of $[Ca^{2+}]_i$ also reveal PTH to possess Ca^{2+} channel-blocking properties in VSM *(35)*. Although an unresolved issue, the different physiologic actions of PTH at target organs depend on and may, in turn, be mediated by its binding to one or more receptor subtypes associated with activation of either adenyl cyclase-dependent or $[Ca^{2+}]_i$-dependent transduction systems *(36,37)*. The cyclic adenosine monophosphate (cAMP)-dependent actions of PTH are presumably mediated by the activation of PKA and subsequent protein phosphorylation. Since direct and indirect stimulation of cAMP generation in vascular tissue is associated with vasodilatation, the acute vasodilatory effects of PTH are presumably consequent to and depend on cAMP stimulation *(37)*.

Other documented postreceptor effects of PTH also may have vascular consequences, either vasodilatory or vasoconstrictive in nature. Thus, PTH has been observed to either stimulate or inhibit Na, K-ATPase *(38,39)* and to inhibit Na^+–H^+ exchange *(40)*. A variety of tissue and organ responses occur as a result of these various adenyl cyclase-dependent and cellular ionic actions of PTH. In vascular tissues in vitro and in vivo, PTH induces acute vasodilation within 1–3 min, with resolution over 5–20 min *(41)*. These effects correspond to the time-course of PTH stimulation of cAMP, independently of changes in circulating Ca^{2+} itself. In contrast, longer term vascular effects of PTH may relate more to its cellular cationic action and its peripheral hypercalcemic action. Since hypercalcemia itself causes peripheral and renal vasoconstriction *(42)*, it remains unclear what role if any PTH has in vascular homeostasis. It appears more likely that PTH-related peptide (PTH-RP), present in endothelial tissues, may have more of a role to play in regulating vascular tone *(43)*.

PHF

A bioassayable factor of parathyroid origin, parathyroid hypertensive factor (PHF), is present in the plasma of spontaneously hypertensive rats (SHR) and DOCA-NaCl but not of normotensive rats *(44,45)*, induces a slow rise in blood pressure and stimulates arterial ^{45}Ca uptake by increasing the opening of L-type Ca^{2+} channels in VSMC *(46)*. This factor also exists in humans, among predominantly low renin and salt-sensitive hypertensive subjects *(47)*. Circulating PHF activity may account for much of the ability of hypertensive serum to increase intracellular-free Ca^{2+} levels as measured by nuclear magnetic resonance spectroscopy *(48)*. Furthermore, dietary salt loading elevates circulating PHF activity, and blood pressure elevations following high salt diets are directly related to the ambient PHF level *(47)*. Lastly, PHF may be responsible for the hypertension associated with primary hyperparathyroidism, since elevated PHF levels, but not levels of Ca^{2+}, PTH, renal function, or other factors predict blood pressure following parathyroidectomy *(49,50)*.

Calcitonin and CGRP

Calcitonin is a peptide secreted from perifollicular C cells of the thyroid, with actions on bone and Ca^{2+} metabolism in other tissues. In the liver, calcitonin increases Ca^{2+} uptake in a specific, apparently L-channel-dependent manner *(51)*. Calcitonin also suppresses in vitro renal renin secretion, an effect blocked by a calcium antagonist *(52)*. These findings indicate that calcitonin may increase $[Ca^{2+}]_i$ accumulation through specific, voltage-dependent L-channels. However, in other situations calcitonin appears to have vasodilatory effects *(53)*. The vascular effects of calcitonin must also be distinguished from possible overlap effects mediated by cross-binding of calcitonin to CGRP receptors. CGRP, a 37 amino acid neuropeptide, is a potent vasodilator, mainly located in the central nervous system, perivascularly in peripheral sympathetic and parasympathetic ganglia, in cardiac atria, and the mesenteric vasculature *(54)*. Activation of receptors specific for CGRP present on the VSMC membrane leads to cAMP accumulation and vasodilatation, both in vivo and in vitro *(55–57)*.

1,25 $(OH)_2D_3$

$1,25(OH)_2D_3$ is the hormonally active form of vitamin D derived from inactive steroid precursors in the diet and from the skin following UV irradiation of 7-dehydrocholesterol. There are now data consistent with an action of vitamin D both on the Ca^{2+} metabolism and contractile activity of VSMC. Specific intracellular 1,25 $(OH)_2D_3$ receptors have been identified in both cardiac *(58)* and VSMC *(59,60)*. In the vasculature, $1,25(OH)_2D_3$

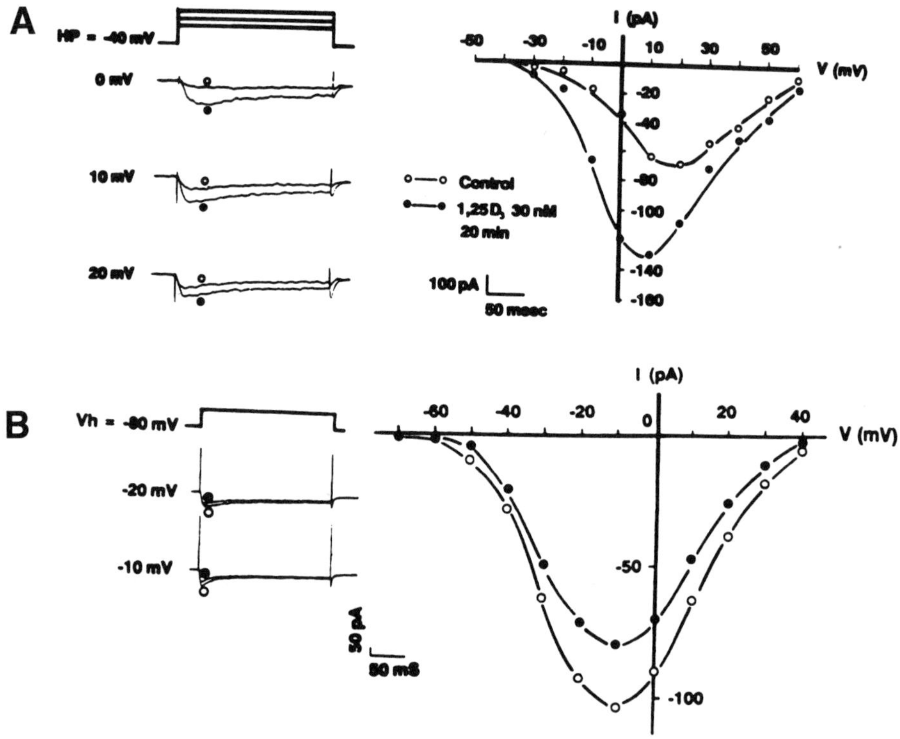

Fig. 4. (A) Effect of $1,25(OH)D_2$ on L-type calcium channel current in isolated vascular smooth muscle cells *(61)*. **(B)** Effect of 17-β estradiol on L-type Ca^{2+} channel current in isolated VSMC *(74)*.

potentiates contractile responses to norepinephrine (NE), vasopressin, and angiotensin *(61,62)*. The cellular basis of these vascular effects of $1,25(OH)_2D_3$ remains incompletely understood. Aside from actions determined by classic cytosolic receptor-mediated nuclear transcription, other presumably nongenomic effects have been documented. Utilizing whole-cell patch clamp, our group has shown that $1,25(OH)_2D_3$ activates L-type Ca^{2+}-channel current and in parallel, increases VSMC $[Ca^{2+}]_i$ *(63)* (Fig. 4A). $1,25(OH)_2D_3$ also stimulates $^{45}Ca^{2+}$ uptake into primary cultures of aortic myocytes from both SHR as well as normotensive Wistar-Kyoto (WKY) rats *(64)*. Vascular effects of $1,25(OH)_2D_3$ are more extensively reviewed in Chapter 18.

Sex Steroid Hormones

The involvement of sex steroid hormones in the regulation of cardiovascular function and vascular tone is suggested by the findings of specific receptors for both estrogen (βE_2) and progesterone (P) located in the heart and in the vasculature *(65–70)*. In isolated rabbit heart, βE_2 may directly reduce myocardial contractility while causing coronary vasodilatation *(71)*, and inhibitory actions of βE_2 and P on vascular contractile tone have also been shown in other vascular beds as well *(72,73)*. Despite an increasing number of studies describing the effects of sex steroids on the cardiovascular system, underlying mechanisms remain unclear. Recently, we investigated the effect of βE_2 and P on blood pressure in vivo, on rat tail artery tension in vitro, and on $[Ca^{2+}]_i$ concentrations and Ca^{2+} channel current activity in cultured VSMC *(74)*. Administration of βE_2s did not affect

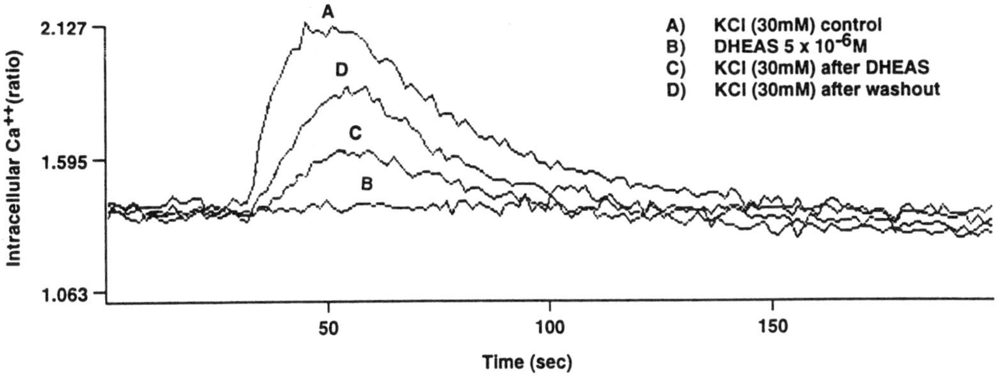

Fig. 5. Actual tracing of the effect of DHEAS ($5 \times 10^{-6} M$) on KCl (30 m*M*)-induced stimulation of intracellular-free Ca^{2+} (Ca^{2+}) in VSMC *(90)*.

basal blood pressure but inhibited pressor responses to NE. In rat tail artery helical strips, βE_2 (10^{-6} to $10^{-4} M$) inhibited contractile responses to KCl, vasopressin, and NE. These effects of βE_2 may be partially explained by reductions in $[Ca^{2+}]_i$, since βE_2 decreases L-type Ca^{2+} channel current *(74,75)* (Fig. 4B), and concurrently blunts the rise in $[Ca^{2+}]_i$ induced by depolarizing stimuli in cultured VSMC *(74,75)*. P has similar effects on VSMC $[Ca^{2+}]_i$, blunting the Ca^{2+} increment induced by KCl and decreasing L-type Ca^{2+} currents in VSMC *(76)*. These Ca^{2+}-inhibitory actions of female sex steroid hormones are also specific, since other steroids hormones, such as $1,25(OH)_2D_3$, increase both L-type Ca^{2+} channel currents and VSMC $[Ca^{2+}]_i$ (Fig. 5) *(63)*. Similarly, testosterone also potentiates KCl-induced elevations of $[Ca^{2+}]_i$ as well as vasoconstriction *(77)*, while glucorticoids have no demonstrated effects on Ca^{2+} transients *(78)*.

Mechanistically, the aforementioned vascular and Ca^{2+}-related effects produced by βE_2s and P cannot easily be attributed to a genomic effect, since this presupposes a significant latency period. Rather, because of their rapid VSMC actions, sex steroid hormones appear to exert vascular effects by modulating plasma membrane-dependent, Ca^{2+}-related transduction mechanisms *(66,71,73–77)*. Since activation of L-type Ca^{2+} channel activity and/or increases in VSMC $[Ca^{2+}]_i$ links electrical excitation to subsequent vascular contraction, the inhibition of these Ca^{2+}-related events by sex steroids may underlie female sex hormone-induced vasodilatation.

DHEAS

Dehydroepiandrosterone (DHEA) is the most abundantly produced adrenal steroid, and serum concentrations of its sulfate ester, DHEAS, are approx 20-fold higher than those of any other circulating steroid hormone *(79)*. The remarkable age-related decline in circulating DHEAS levels *(79,80)* has been linked to the increased incidence of atherosclerotic disease with age *(81)*, whereas high plasma DHEAS levels have been associated with a reduction of mortality and cardiovascular diseases *(82)*. These observations and animal studies have led to the notion that DHEAS may participate in the pathophysiology of vascular diseases associated with atherosclerosis and aging. A reduction in aortic atherosclerosis in rabbits fed a high cholesterol diet was seen following supplementation with DHEA *(83,84)*, and chronic DHEA administration also significantly

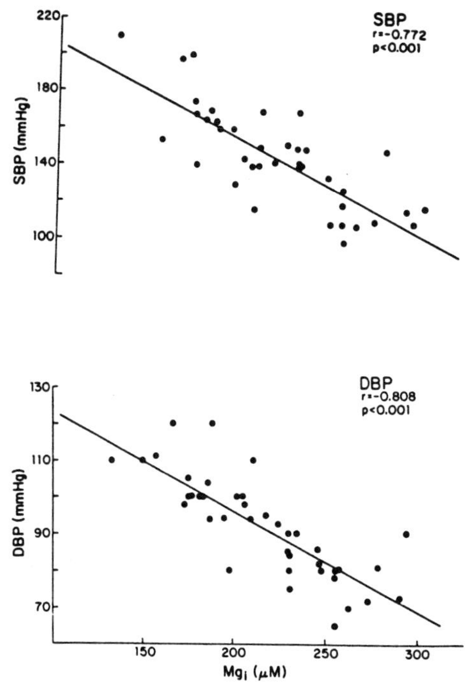

Fig. 6. Relation of systolic (SBP) and diastolic (DBP) blood pressures to basal fasting intracellular-free Mg^{2+} concentrations ($[Mg^{2+}]_i$) in peripheral red blood cells of normal and hypertensive subjects *(92)*.

retards progression of accelerated coronary atherosclerosis in the transplanted heart of a hypercholesterolemic rabbit model *(85)*.

Although its mechanism of action is unknown, direct vascular effects of DHEAS have also been suggested. Administration of DHEAS blunts in a dose-related fashion, both corticosteroid-induced hypertension *(86)* and the development of atherosclerosis *(83–85)*. We have recently confirmed that DHEAS, in doses reflecting circulating levels of the hormone in vivo *(79)*, exerts direct Ca^{2+}-related effects on the vasculature *(87)*. At the tissue level, DHEAS modulates the vasoconstrictor response to depolarizing stimuli and to specific endogenous agonists, such as NE and vasopressin. In a parallel fashion, at the cellular level, DHEAS blunts depolarization-induced increases in VSMC $[Ca^{2+}]_i$ (Fig. 5). Thus, DHEAS may function endogenously to physiologically buffer vascular Ca^{2+}-dependent responses to various electrophysiologic and hormonal stimuli. This may be one mechanism by which the progressive decline of DHEAS with age contributes to atherosclerotic disease in the elderly.

INTRACELLULAR CATIONS, CLINICAL HYPERTENSION, AND INSULIN RESISTANCE

The previous discussion suggests a critical role for dietary and hormonal factors in the regulation of intracellular cations in VSMC and thus of vascular tone. Clinically, intracellular-free Mg^{2+} levels in peripheral erythrocytes from normotensive, hypertensive, and diabetic subjects are closely, continuously, and inversely related to the levels of blood pressure (Fig. 6), fasting blood glucose values, and to the hyperinsulinemic response to

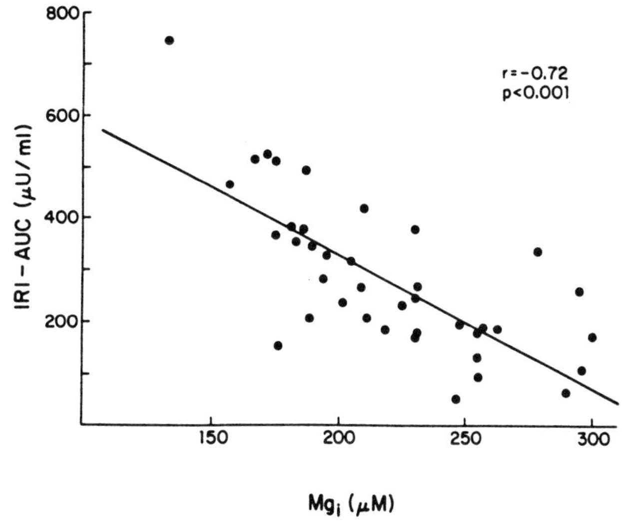

Fig. 7. Relation of the integrated insulinemic response to oral glucose loading (IRI-AUC) to basal fasting intracellular-free Mg^{2+} concentrations ($[Mg^{2+}]_i$) in normal and hypertensive subjects *(92)*.

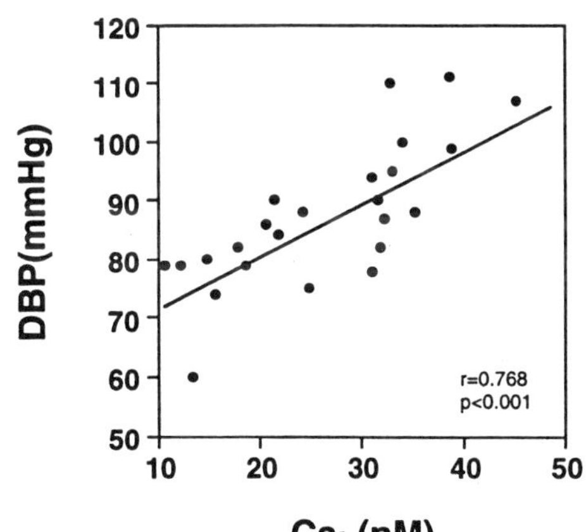

Fig. 8. Relation of DBP to basal fasting cytosolic-free calcium concentrations (Ca_i) in peripheral red blood cells of normal and hypertensive subjects.

oral glucose loading. The lower the free Mg^{2+}, the greater the blood pressure, the higher the fasting blood glucose, the greater the peripheral insulin resistance (Figs. 6 and 7) *(88,89)*. These relations are continuous at all blood pressure and blood sugar values. These observations are also consistent with studies demonstrating that reductions in $[Mg^{2+}]_i$ enhance Ca^{2+}-mediated vasoconstriction *(90)*, decrease cellular glucose utilization, and thus promote peripheral insulin resistance *(91)*. Conversely, $[Ca^{2+}]_i$ levels in normotensive, hypertensive, and diabetic subjects are directly and positively related to blood pressure (Fig. 8), fasting blood glucose values, and the hyperinsulinemic response to glucose loading (i.e., the higher the basal fasting $[Ca^{2+}]_i$, the greater the amount of insulin required to metabolize glucose), indicating decreased insulin sensitivity *(19)*.

Results also extend to structural indices of the cardiovascular system as well, with these same intracellular erythrocyte measurements of $[Ca^{2+}]_i$ and $[Mg^{2+}]_i$ being predictive of the degree of cardiac hypertrophy, as assessed by echocardiographic determination of left ventricular mass index *(92)*. Although these data suggest that cellular cation content may determine clinically relevant biologic outcomes such as blood pressure, cardiac mass, and cellular insulin responsiveness *(93)*, it is also true that factors such as glucose and insulin may in turn, alter $[Ca^{2+}]_i$ and $[Mg^{2+}]_i$ *(26)*. Definitive experiments have not been performed to distinguish the "chicken" from the "egg," i.e., the extent to which the cation abnormalities present in these conditions represent a primary defect causing altered insulin secretion and/or cellular insulin responsiveness, or rather being secondary to insulin resistance of other etiologies.

CLINICAL ROLE OF SALT AND SUGAR IN REGULATION OF INTRACELLULAR CATIONS

Measuring $[Ca^{2+}]_i$ and $[Mg^{2+}]_i$ after dietary salt or sugar loading has been used to assess the role of different dietary circumstances in regulating blood pressure and cellular cation metabolism. Hypertensive subjects were studied on low (<50 mq/d) and high (>200 mq/d) NaCl diets for 1 mo each *(94)*. The ability of dietary salt to elevate blood pressure in some "salt-sensitive" hypertensive subjects was dependent on salt-induced cellular Ca^{2+} accumulation from the extracellular space with reciprocal suppression of Mg^{2+} levels in these subjects. The relation of salt-induced pressure and cation changes was continuous for all subjects (i.e., the greater the salt-induced rise in Ca^{2+} and the greater the fall in Mg^{2+}, the more blood pressure rose). Furthermore, the efficacy of Ca^{2+} channel blockade to reverse salt-induced hypertension was closely related to its ability to reverse these ionic effects of salt loading *(94)*. Hence, in "salt-sensitive" subjects, dietary salt intake may be one determinant of cellular cation levels and thereby, of blood pressure.

Elevations of blood sugar may also contribute to cell cation abnormalities, and thus may directly contribute to the hypertension and vascular disease of diabetes. Specifically, the transient hyperglycemia of oral glucose loading reproduces in normal subjects the same altered ionic profile of increased $[Ca^{2+}]_i$ and decreased $[Mg^{2+}]_i$ that occurs chronically in diabetics *(95)*. The longer term clinical significance of these glucose-induced ionic changes is indicated by a close, positive relation of $HbA1_c$ levels to fasting $[Ca^{2+}]_i$, observed even among nondiabetic, normotensive, and essential hypertensive individuals *(19)*. This glucose-mediated effect is presumably independent of insulin action, since hyperglycemia induces these changes not only in VSMC, but also in red cells, where glucose transport is unaffected by insulin *(24,26)*. Hence, it appears that circulating glucose concentrations, even within the "normal" range, may be another physiologic determinant of basal VSMC $[Ca^{2+}]_i$, and thus of vascular tone.

THE IONIC HYPOTHESIS OF CARDIOVASCULAR AND METABOLIC DISEASE

Altogether, we suggest a critical role for the abnormal cellular ion "profile" described previously in explaining the shared pathophysiologic characteristics of hypertension and diabetic vascular disease (Fig. 9). Thus, rather than hyperinsulinemia and insulin resis-

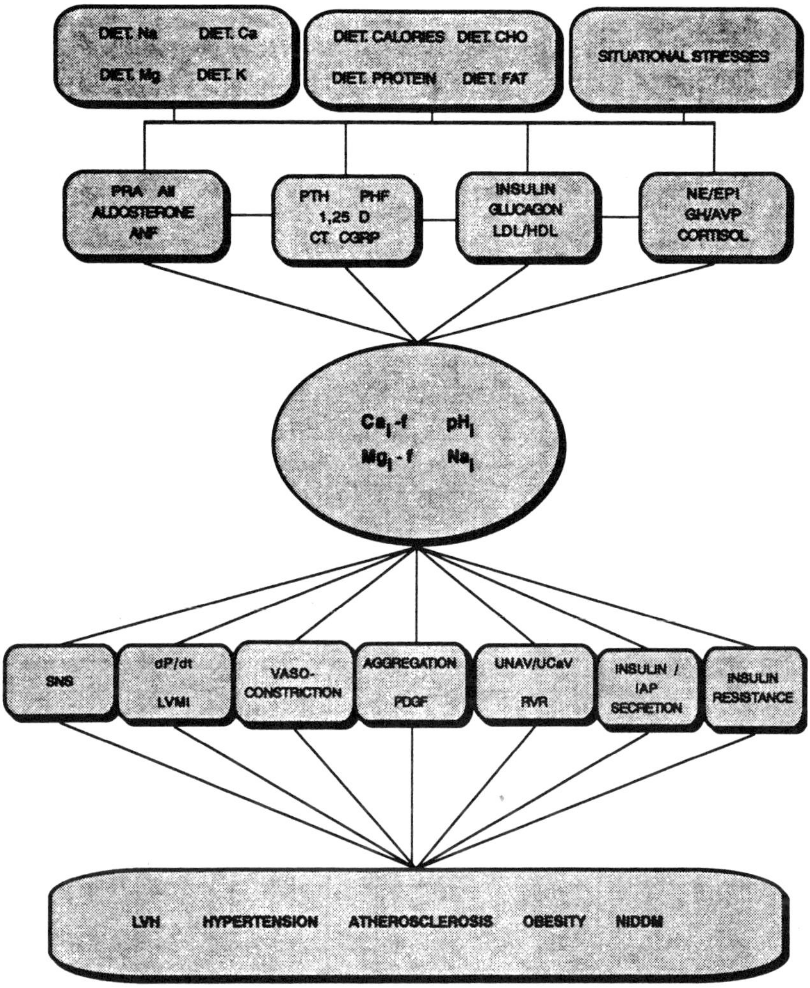

Fig. 9. Ionic hypothesis of cardiovascular and metabolic disease, in which the different clinical components (bottom) represent different clinical manifestations of shared cellular ion abnormalities (top) expressed differently in different organ systems (middle).

tance causing hypertension, or elevated blood pressure causing insulin resistance, it is more reasonable to suggest that both phenomena derive from and are different tissue expressions of the same cellular cation abnormality.

According to this "ionic hypothesis," in VSMC, increased $[Ca^{2+}]_i$ and deficient $[Mg^{2+}]_i$ predispose to vasoconstriction and/or elevated blood pressure. In skeletal muscle and fat tissue, insulin resistance would be the expected outcome of increased $[Ca^{2+}]_i$ and suppressed $[Mg^{2+}]_i$, *(27,89–93,96)*. In pancreatic β-cells, and in neural cells, since $[Ca^{2+}]_i$ also mediates stimulus-secretion coupling, increased $[Ca^{2+}]_i$ would promote hyperinsulinemia and the increased sympathetic tone often observed in hypertension and associated metabolic conditions *(96)*. Similarly, altered cellular divalent cation content would necessarily alter renal cation excretion, resulting in the exaggerated Ca^{2+} excretion and/or Na^+ retention common to hypertension and chronic hyperglycemic states *(97,98)*. Increased platelet $[Ca^{2+}]_i$ and suppressed $[Mg^{2+}]_i$

increases aggregability and thus promotes thrombosis, and in the heart, causes increasing myocardial contractility, thus explaining the "supernormal" ejection fraction often present early in hypertensive disease, ultimately resulting in cardiac hypertrophy. Thus, the ionic hypothesis explains the onset of elevated blood pressure, left ventricular hypertrophy, dysmetabolic states such as insulin resistance and type II noninsulin-dependent diabetes mellitus (NIDDM), and thus accelerated atherosclerotic vascular disease in a unified manner *(19)* (Fig. 9).

VASCULAR "AGING," ATHEROSCLEROSIS, AND INTRACELLULAR IONS

The aforementioned cellular cation-based approach to cardiovascular disease suggests: The critical importance of Ca^{2+} and/or Mg^{2+} metabolism in regulating vascular tone, blood pressure homeostasis, and various other cardiovascular and metabolic processes; the ability of environmental factors such as dietary nutrient sugar and mineral content to alter the set point of steady-state cell ion activity in all or at least some individuals; and common defects of divalent cellular cation metabolism, consisting in part of $[Ca^{2+}]_i$ excess and $[Mg^{2+}]_i$ deficiency, are present in and may help to explain why many disease states predispose to and/or are characterized by accelerated atherosclerosis. Consistent with this concept, aging itself is another biological process epidemiologically linked to an increased incidence of both impaired glucose tolerance and hypertension, and associated with parallel elevations of $[Ca^{2+}]_i$ and a reciprocal fall in cytosolic free Mg^{2+} levels *(99)*. These alterations are indistinguishable from those present in essential hypertension or NIDDM, independently of age *(99)* and might therefore help to explain the age-related increased incidence of these diseases. Hypertension and NIDDM are thus literally diseases of accelerated vascular aging, since both of these diseases display premature ionic changes of "aging." Thus, having these conditions is "ionically," the same as getting older (e.g., a 48-yr-old diabetic having cellular ionic alterations indistinguishable from a healthy 84 yr old).

Furthermore, atherosclerosis in general may thus be explained as a vascular consequence of altered $[Ca^{2+}]_i$ and/or $[Mg^{2+}]_i$ homeostasis *(95,96,99)*. Indeed, increased Ca^{2+} influx into endothelial cells is associated with, and may be induced by plasma components (mainly oxidized low-density lipoprotein) *(100)*, with enhanced release of chemotactic and growth factors that promote leukocyte and macrophage infiltration into the vessel wall and VSMC proliferation, thereby initiating the atherosclerotic lesion *(101)*. Moreover, the accumulation of VSMC $[Ca^{2+}]_i$ may trigger the transition from a contractile state to a proliferative state during which proliferation and migration to the media/lumen may occur. Cholesterol-fed rabbits that develop atherosclerosis have increased free Ca^{2+} in their aortic wall cells and an increased Ca^{2+} influx into the VSMC *(101)*. Indeed, cholesterol itself has been shown to increase Ca^{2+} currents and Ca^{2+} influx into VSMC *(102)*. As for smooth muscle contractile function, Mg^{2+} deficiency may potentiate these cholesterol-induced, Ca^{2+}-related vascular atherosclerotic changes; indeed, increased availability of Mg^{2+} may protect against induction of atherosclerosis *(103)*. Aging and atherosclerosis are thus both characterized by a parallel accumulation of Ca^{2+} and cholesterol in the arterial wall, a process that is accelerated in hypertension and diabetes, supporting the underlying ionic basis for these clinically linked syndromes.

REFERENCES

1. Ringer S. A third contribution regarding the infusion of the inorganic constituents of the blood on the ventricular contraction. J Physiol 1883;22:2–5.
2. Means AR, VanBerkum MFA, Bagchi I, Lu KP, Rasmussen CD. Regulatory functions of calmodulin. Pharmacol Ther 1991;50:255–270.
3. Hai CM, Murphy RA. Ca^{2+}, crossbridge phosphorylation, and contraction. Annu Rev Physiol 1989;51:285–298.
4. Hermsmeyer K, Sturek M, Rush NJ. Ca^{2+} channel modulation by dihidropyridines in VSM. Ann NY Acad Sci 1988;522:25–31.
5. Kitazawa T, Kobayashy S, Horiuty K, Somlyo AV, Somlyo AP. Receptor-coupled, permeabilized smooth muscle: role of phosphatidylinositol cascade, G-proteins, and modulation of the contractile response to Ca^{2+}. J Biol Chem 1989;264:5339–5342.
6. Nishizuka Y. Studies and perspectives of protein kinase C. Science 1986;233:305–312.
7. Iwasa Y, Hosey MM. Phosphorylation of cardiac sarcolemma proteins by the Ca^{2+} activated phospholipid dependent protein kinase. J Biol Chem 1984;259:534–540.
8. Nishikawa M, Hidaka H, Adelstein RS. Phosphorylation of smooth muscle heavy meromyosin by Ca^{2+} activated, phospholipid dependent protein kinase. J Biol Chem 1983;258:14,069–14,072.
9. Griendling KK, Alexander RW. Angiotensin, other pressor, and the transduction of vascular smooth muscle contraction. In: Laragh JH, Brenner BM, eds. Hypertension, Pathophysiology, Diagnosis and Management, 2nd ed. Raven, New York, 1995, pp. 541–556.
10. Khalil RA, van Breeman C. Mechanisms of calcium mobilization and homeostasis in vascular smooth muscle and their relevance to hypertension. In: Laragh JH, Brenner BM, eds. Hypertension, Pathophysiology, Diagnosis and Management, 2nd ed. Raven, New York, 1995, pp. 523–539.
11. Eggermont JA, Vrolix M, Raeymaekers L, Wuytack F, Casteels R. Ca^{2+} transport ATPases of VSM. Circ Res 1988;62:266–278.
12. Nabel EG, Berk BC, Brock TA, Smith TW. Na^{+}–Ca^{2+} exchange in cultured VSM cells. Circ Res 1988;62:486–489.
13. Altura BM, Altura BT. Mg^{2+} ions and contractions on VSMs: relationship to some vascular diseases. Fed Proc 1981;40:2672–2679.
14. Altura BM, Altura BT, Carella A, Turlapaty PDMV. Ca^{2+} coupling in VSM: Mg^{2+} and buffer effects on contractility and membrane Ca^{2+} movements. Can J Physiol 1982;60:459–482.
15. Altura BM, Altura BT. Mg^{2+} and contractions of arterial smooth muscle. Microvasc Res 1974;7: 145–155.
16. Woods WT, Katholi RE, Urthaler F, James TN. Electrophysiological effects of Mg^{2+} on cells in the canine sinus node and false tendon. Circ Res 1979;44:182–188.
17. Turlapaty PDMV, Altura BM. Extracellular Mg^{2+} ions control Ca^{2+} exchange and content of VSM. Eur J Pharmacol 1978;52:421–423.
18. Rubin RP. The role of Ca^{2+} in the release of neurotransmitter substances and hormones. Pharmacol Rev 1970;22:389–427.
19. Resnick LM. Ionic basis of hypertension, insulin resistance, vascular disease and related disorders. The mechanism of "Syndrome X." Am J Hypertens 1993;6:123S–134S.
20. Barbagallo M, Shan J, Pang PKT, Resnick LM. Glucose-induced alterations of $[Ca^{2+}]_i$ in cultured rat tail artery VSM cells. J Clin Invest 1995;95:763–767.
21. Resnick LM, Barbagallo M, Gupta RK, Laragh JH. Ionic basis of hypertension in diabetes mellitus: role of hyperglycemia. Am J Hypertens 1992;5:296–301.
22. Davis FB, Davis PJ, Gerard N, Blas S, MacGillivray S, Gutman S, Feldman J. The effect of in vivo glucose administration on human Ca-ATPase activity and on enzyme responsiveness in vitro to thyroid hormone and calmodulin. Diabetes 1985;34:639–646.
23. Deziel MR, Safeer RS, Blas S, Davis FB, Davis PJ. Hexose-specific inhibition in vitro of human red cell Ca^{2+}-ATPase-ATP-ase activity. Biochem Biophys Acta 1992;1110:119–122.
24. Draznin B, Leitner W, Sussman KE, Sherman N. Insulin and glucose modulate protein kinase C in rat adipocytes. Biochem Biophys Res Commun 1988;156:570–575.
25. Vaugham-Jones RD, Lederer WJ, Eisner DA. Ca^{2+} ions can affect intracellular pH in mammalian cardiac cells. Nature 1983;301:522–524.
26. Barbagallo M, Gupta RK, Resnick LM. Cellular ionic effects of insulin in normal human red cells: a nuclear magnetic resonance study. Diabetologia 1993;36:146–149.

27. Kuriyama S, Nakamura K, Horiguchi M, Uchida H, Sakai O. Decreased insulin-sensitive Ca^{++} transport in cultured vascular smooth muscle cells from spontaneously hypertensive rats. Am J Hypertens 1992;5:892–895.
28. Standley PR, Zhang F, Ram JL, Zemel MB, Sowers JR. Insulin attenuates vasopressin-induced Ca^{2+} transient and a voltage-dependent Ca^{2+} response in rat VSM cells. J Clin Invest 1991;88:1230–1236.
29. Resnick LM, Barbagallo M, Gupta RK, Laragh JH. Ionic effects of insulin in normal and hypertensive cells: an ionic definition of insulin resistance? Am J Hypertens 1994;7:61 (abstract).
30. Collip JB, Clark EP. Further studies on the physiological action of a parathyroid hormone. J Biol Chem 1925;64:485–491.
31. Charbon GA, Brummer F, Reneman RS. Diuretic and vascular action of parathyroid extracts in animals and in man. Arch Int Pharmacodyn Ther 1968;171:1–11.
32. Rosenthal FD, Roy S. Hypertension and hyperparathyroidism. Br Med J 1972;4:396,397.
33. Massry SG, Iseky K, Campese VM. Serum Ca^{2+}, parathyroid hormone and blood pressure. Am J Nephrol 1986;6:19–28.
34. Bogin E, Massey SG, Harary L. Effect of parathyroid hormone on rat heart cells. J Clin Invest 1981;67:1215–1227.
35. Pang PKT, Yang MCM, Shan J. Parathyroid hormone and Ca^{2+} entry blockade in vascular tissue. Life Sci 1988;42:1395–1400.
36. Herrmann-Erlee MPM, Nijiweide PJ, Van der Meer JM, Ooms MA. Action of BPTH and bPTH-fragments on embryonic bone in vitro: dissociation of the cyclic AMP and bone resorbing response. Calcif Tissue Int 1983;35:70–77.
37. Nickols GA. Increased cAMP in cultured VSM cells and relaxation of aortic strips by parathyroid hormone. Eur J Pharmacol 1985;116:137–144.
38. Acceto R, Weder AB. Parathyroid hormone and verapamil inhibit Na^+–K^+ pump in human erythrocytes. Clin Res 1987;35:437A.
39. De Luise M, Harker M. Parathyroid hormone stimulation of the Na^+–K^+ pump in rat clonal osteosarcoma cells. J Endocrinol 1986;111:61–66.
40. Kahn AM, Zimmer RA, Navran SS. Parathyroid hormone inhibits Na^+-H^+ exchange in cultured VSM cells. Kidney Intl 1988;33:298A.
41. Pang PKT, Yang MCM, Shew R, Tenner TE Jr. The vasorelaxant action of parathyroid hormone fragments on isolated rat tail artery. Blood Vessels 1985;22:57–64.
42. Benabe JE, Martinez-Maldonado M. Hypercalcemic nephropathy. Arch Intern Med 1978;138:777–779.
43. Ogino K, Burkhoff D, Bilezekian JP. The hemodynamic basis for the cardiac effects of parathyroid hormone (PTH) and PTH-related protein. Endocrinology 1995;136(7):3024–3030.
44. Lewanczuk RZ, Wang J, Zhang ZR, Pang PKT. Effects of spontaneously hypertensive rat plasma on blood pressure and tail artery Ca^{2+} uptake in normotensive rats. Am J Hypertens 1989;2:26–31.
45. Pang PKT, Lewanczuk RZ. Parathyroid origin of a new circulating hypertensive factor in spontaneously hypertensive rats. Am J Hypertens 1989;2:898–902.
46. Shan J, Benishin CG, Lewanczuk RZ, Pang PKT. The mechanism of the vascular action of parathyroid hypertensive factor. J Cardiovasc Pharmacol 1994;23(Suppl. 2):S1.
47. Resnick LM, Lewanczuk RZ, Laragh JH, Pang PKT. Parathyroid hypertensive factor-like activity in human essential hypertension: relationship to plasma renin activity and dietary salt sensitivity. J Hypertens 1993;11:1235–1241.
48. Barbagallo M, Gupta RK, Lewanczuk RZ, Pang PKT, Resnick LM. Serum mediated intracellular Ca^{2+} changes in normotensive and hypertensive red blood cells: role of parathyroid hypertensive factor (PHF). J Cardiovasc Pharmacol 1994;23(Suppl. 2):S14–S17.
49. Lewanczuk RZ, Pang PKT. Expression of parathyroid hormone in hypertensive primary hyperparathyroid patients. Blood Pressure 1993;2:22–27.
50. Lind L, Ljunghall S. Hypertension, primary hyperparathyroidism and the parathyroid hypertensive factor. Blood Pressure 1993;2:4,5.
51. Yamaguchi M, Yoshida H. Participation of Ca^{2+} channel in liver regulation by calcitonin in rats. Acta Endocrinol 1985;110:239–243.
52. Resnick LM, Churchill PC, Churchill M, Laragh JH, Orlowsky R. The effects of calcitonin, calcitonin analogs, and calcitonin gene related peptide on basal, in vitro, renin secretion. Am J Hypertens 1989;2:453–457.
53. Resnick LM, Muller FB, Nicholson JP, Laragh JH. Calcitonin is a vasoactive hormone in hypertensive man. Clin Res 1984;32:523A.

54. Uddman R, Edvinsson L, Ekblad E, Hakanson Sundler F. Calcitonin gene-related peptide (CGRP): perivascular distribution and vasodilatory effects. Regul Pept 1986;15:1–23.
55. Gennari C, Fisher JA. Cardiovascular actions of calcitonin gene related peptide in humans. Calcif Tissue Int, 1985;37:581–584.
56. Kline L, Pang PKT. Calcitonin gene-related peptide relaxed rat tail artery helical strips in vitro an intracellular Ca^{2+}-dependent manner. Eur J Pharmacol 1988;150:233–823.
57. Hirata Y, Tagagi Y, Takata S, Fukuda Y, Yoshima H, Fujiita T. Calcitonin gene-related peptide receptor in cultured VSM and endothelial cells. Biochem Biophys Res Commun 1988;151:1113–1121.
58. Walters MR, Wicker DC, Riggle PC. 1,25 Dihydroxyvitamin D_3 receptors identified in the rat heart. J Mol Cell Cardiol 1986;18:67–72.
59. Merke J, Hoffman D, Goldschmidt H. Demonstration of 1,25 (OH) vitamin D receptors and action in VSM in vitro. Calc Tissue Int 1987;41:112–114.
60. Kawashima H. Receptor for 1,25 dihydroxyvitamin D in a vascular cell line derived from rat aorta. Biochem Biophys Res Commun 1987;146:1–6.
61. Bukosky RD, Xue H. On the vascular inotropic action of 1,25 $(OH)_2$ vitamin D_3. Am J Hypertens 1993;6(5 Part 1):388–396.
62. Shimosawa T, Ando K, Fujiita T. Enhancement of vasoconstrictor response by a noncalcemic analogue of vitamin D_3. Hypertension 1993;21:253–258.
63. Shan J, Resnick LM, Lewanczuk RZ, Karpinsky E, Pang PKT. 1,25 Dihydroxyvitamin D as a cardiovascular hormone: effects on Ca^{2+} current and $[Ca^{2+}]_i$ in VSM cells. Am J Hypertens 1993;6: 983–988.
64. Bukosky RD, Xue H, McCarron DA. Effect of 1,25 $(OH)_2$ vitamin D_3 and ionized Ca^{2+}, on ^{45}Ca uptake by primary cultures of aortic myocites of spontaneously hypertensive and Wistar-Kyoto normotensive rats. Biochem Biophys Res Commun 1988;152:1388–1394.
65. Stumpf WE, Sar M, Amuller G. The heart a target organ for estradiol. Science 1977;196:319–321.
66. Hardner DR, Coulson PB. BE_2 receptors and effect of βE_2 on membrane electrical properties of coronary VSM. J Cell Physiol 1979;100:375–382.
67. Nakao J, Chang WC, Murota SI, Orimo H. Estradiol binding sites in rat aortic smooth muscle cells in culture. Atherosclerosis 1981;38:75–80.
68. McGill HC, Sheridan PJ. Nuclear uptake of sex steroid hormones in the cardiovascular system of the baboon. Circ Res 1982;48:234–244.
69. Lin AL, Mc Gill HC, Shain SA. Hormone receptors of the baboon cardiovascular system. Biochemical characterization of aortic and myocardial cytoplasmic P receptors. Circ Res 1982;50:610–616.
70. Horowitz KB, Horowitz LD. Canine vascular tissues are targets for androgens, βE_2s, progestins and glucocorticoids. J Clin Invest 1982;69:750–758.
71. Raddino R, Poli E, Pela G, Manca C. Action of steroid sex hormones on the isolated rabbit heart. Pharmacology 1989;38:185–190.
72. McCalden TA. The inhibitory action of estradiol 17β and P on venous smooth muscle. Br J Pharmacol 1975;53:183–192.
73. Altura BM, Altura BT. Influence of sex hormones, oral contraceptives and pregnancy on vascular muscle and its reactivity. In: Carrier O, Shibata S, eds. Factors Influencing Vascular Reactivity. Igaku-Shoin, New York, 1977, pp. 221–254.
74. Shan J, Resnick LM, Liu Q, Wu X, Barbagallo M, Pang PKT. Vascular effect of 17β estradiol in male SD rats. Am J Physiol 1994;266:H967–H973.
75. Zhang F, Ram JL, Standley PR, Sowers JR. 17β-estradiol attenuates voltage-dependent Ca^{2+} current in rat vascular smooth muscle cell. Am J Physiol 1994;6:C1–C6.
76. Barbagallo M, Shan J, Pang PKT, Resnick LM. Vascular effects of P: role intracellular Ca^{2+} metabolism. Am J Hypertens 1995;8(Part 2):66A.
77. Peuler JD, Ravi J, Boggaram B, Sowers JR. Insulin blocks accentuation of adrenergic tone by dihydrotestosterone. Am J Hypertens 1995;8(4):54 (abstract).
78. Clark TP, Kemppainen RJ. Glucocorticoid do not affect intracellular Ca^{2+} transients in corticotrophs: evidence supporting effect distal to Ca^{2+} influx. Neuroendocrinology 1994;60:273–282.
79. Orentreich N, Brind JL, Rizer RL, Vogelamn JH. Age changes and sex differences in serum dehydroepiandrosterone sulfate concentrations throughout adulthood. J Clin Endocrinol Metab 1984;59:551–555.
80. Yamaji T, Ibayashi H. Plasma dehydroepiandrosterone sulfate in normal and pathological conditions. J Clin Endocrinol Metab 1969;29:273–278.

81. Marmoston J, Griffith GC, Geller PJ, Fishman EL, Welsch F, Weiner JM. Urinary steroids in the measurement of aging and atherosclerosis. J Am Geriatr Soc 1975;23:481–492.
82. Barret-Connor E, Khaw KT, Yen SSC. A prospective study of dehydroepiandrosterone sulfate, mortality and cardiovascular disease. N Engl J Med 1986;315:1519–1524.
83. Gordon GB, Bush DE, Weishman HF. Reduction of atherosclerosis by administration of dehydroepiandrosterone. J Clin Invest 1988;82:712–720.
84. Arad Y, Badimon JO, Hembrec W, Ginsberg HN. Dehydroepiandrosterone feedings prevents aortic fatty stream formation and cholesterol accumulation in cholesterol-fed rabbit. Arteriosclerosis 1989;9:159–166.
85. Eich DM, Nestler JE, Johson DE, Dworkin GH, Daijin K, Wechsler, Hess ML. Inhibition of accelerated coronary atherosclerosis with dehydroepiandrosterone in the heterotopic rabbit model of cardiac transplantation. Circulation 1993;87:261–269.
86. Shafagoj Y, Opoku J, Quereshi D, Regelson W, Kalimi M. Dehydroepiandrosterone prevents dexamethasone-induced hypertension in rats. Am J Physiol 1992;203:E210-E213.
87. Barbagallo M, Shan J, Pang PKT, Resnick LM. Effects of dehydroepiandrosterone sulfate on cellular calcium responsiveness and vascular contractility. Hypertension 1995;26:1065–1069.
88. Resnick LM, Gupta RK, Bhargava KK, Gruenspan H, Alderman MH, Laragh JH. Cellular ions in hypertension, diabetes, and obesity: a nuclear magnetic resonance spectroscopic study. Hypertension 1991;17:951–957.
89. Resnick LM, Gupta RK, Gruenspan H, Alderman MH, Laragh JH. Hypertension and peripheral insulin resistance: mediating role of intracellular free Mg^{2+}. Am J Hypertens 1990;3:373–379.
90. Altura BM, Altura BT. Mg^{2+} deficiency and hypertension: correlation between Mg^{2+}-deficient diets and microcirculatory changes in situ. Science 1984;223:1315–1317.
91. Nadler JL, Buchanan T, Natarajan R, Antonipillai I, Bergman R, Rude R. Mg^{2+} deficiency produces insulin resistance and increased tromboxane synthesis. Hypertension 1993;21:1024–1029.
92. Barbagallo M, Gupta RK, Resnick LM. Cellular ion in diabetic hypertension: relation to hyperglycemia and cardiac hypertrophy. Hypertension 1995;25:1358.
93. Draznin B, Sussman KE, Eckel R, Kao M, Yost T, Sherman NA. Possible role of $[Ca^{2+}]_i$ concentration in mediating insulin resistance of obesity and hyperinsulinemia. J Clin Invest 1988;82:1848–1852.
94. Resnick LM, Gupta RK, Di Fabio B, Barbagallo M, Marion R, Laragh JH. Intracellular ionic consequences of dietary salt loading in essential hypertension. J Clin Invest 1994;94:1269–1276.
95. Resnick LM, Gupta RK, Gruenspan H, Laragh JH. Intracellular ion response to glucose tolerance: Relation of hypertension, obesity and insulin resistance. Circulation 1988;78(Suppl. II):II–570.
96. Levy J, Gavin J Jr III, Sowers JR. Diabetes mellitus: a disease of abnormal cellular calcium metabolism? Am J Med 1994;96:260–273.
97. Barbagallo M, Resnick LM, Sosa RE, Corbett ML, Laragh JH. Renal divalent cation excretion in secondary hypertension. Clin Sci 1992;83:561–565.
98. McCarron DA, Pingree PA, Rubin RJ, Gaucher SM, Molitch M, Krutzik S. Enhanced parathyroid function in essential hypertension: a homeostatic response to a urinary Ca^{2+} leak. Hypertension 1980;2:162–168.
99. Barbagallo M, Gupta RK, Resnick LM. Effect of aging on cellular divalent cations: relation to hypertension and diabetes. J Invest Med 1995;43(Suppl. 2):300A.
100. Sachidinis A, Mengden T, Locher R, Brunner C, Vetter W. Novel cellular activities for low density lipoprotein in VSM cells. Hypertension 1990;15:704–711.
101. Orimo H, Ouchi Y. The role of Ca^{2+} and Mg^{2+} in the development of atherosclerosis. Experimental and clinical evidence. Ann NY Acad Sci 1990;598:444–457.
102. Sen L, Biasecky RA, Smith E, Smith TW, Colucci W. Cholesterol increases the L-type voltage-sensitive Ca^{2+} channel current in arterial smooth muscle cells. Circ Res 1992;71:1008–1014.
103. Altura BT, Brust M, Bloom S, Barbour RL, Stempack JG, Altura BM. Mg^{2+} dietary intake modulates blood lipid levels and atherogenesis. Proc Natl Acad Sci USA 1990;87:1840–1844.

22 Regulation of Intracellular pH and the Na⁺/H⁺ Antiporter in Vascular Smooth Muscle

Michael S. LaPointe, PHD
and Daniel Batlle, MD

CONTENTS

OVERVIEW OF INTRACELLULAR pH REGULATION

The hydrogen ion concentration, usually expressed as pH, is highly regulated in both the intracellular and extracellular environments *(1,2)*. Although the body has developed multiple systems to maintain pH homeostasis, changes in the pH of the extracellular and intracellular environments can occur under pathophysiological conditions. It has also become apparent in recent years that transient changes in intracellular pH (pH_i) are part of the vascular smooth muscle cell (VSMC) response to physiologic stimuli.

Study of pH_i regulation has been facilitated by technical advances that allow accurate, noninvasive measurement *(2)*. In most mammalian cells the pH_i is maintained at about 7.2, which is slightly more acidic than the extracellular (pH 7.4) environment. Steady-state pH_i reflects the balance between cellular acid loading and acid removal systems. The major means of cell acidification are cellular acid production and entry of H^+ and organic

From: *Contemporary Endocrinology: Endocrinology of the Vasculature*
Edited by: J. R. Sowers Humana Press Inc., Totowa, NJ

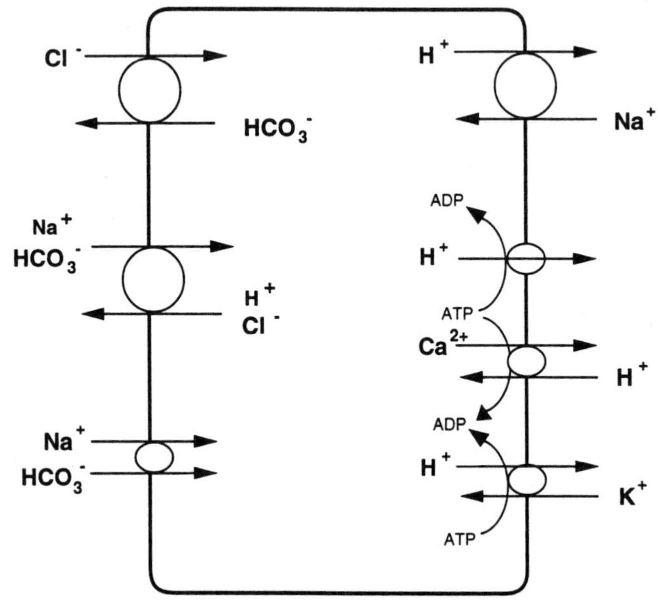

Fig. 1. Plasma membrane transporters involved in pH_i homeostasis. These include (in order top to bottom) the Na^+/H^+ antiporter (NHE-1 isoform), an electrogenic H^+–ATPase, a Ca^{2+}–ATPase, and an H^+/K^+–ATPase. HCO_3^-/CO_2-dependent transporters are shown on the left side. These include the Na^+-independent Cl^-/HCO_3^- exchanger (band 3 protein), the Na^+-dependent Cl^-/HCO_3^- exchanger, and an Na^+, HCO_3^- symporter. The three major transporters are shown as large circles, whereas the transporters that, in VSMC, play a minor role in pH_i homeostasis are shown as small circles.

acids into the cell across the cell membrane. Acid production by the cell is the result of cell metabolism. Utilization of glucose for energy and the hydrolysis of ATP results in the production of CO_2 and organic acids such as lactate and pyruvate *(1)*. Removal of cellular HCO_3^-, by a membrane transport protein, the sodium (Na^+)-independent Cl^-/HCO_3^- exchanger, also contributes to acid loading of the cell *(3)*. These acid loading mechanisms are balanced by the removal of acid from the cytosol. Most cells, including VSMC, accomplish this by the activity of two transporters in the cell membrane, the Na^+/H^+ antiporter and a Na^+-dependent Cl^-/HCO_3^- exchanger. In addition to these three major pH_i homeostatic transport proteins, other transporters also may be present in VSMC and contribute to the maintenance of a steady-state pH_i, as summarized in Fig. 1.

An electrical potential across the cell membrane (–60 to –90 mV depending on the cell type examined) provides a large electrical driving force for the entry of permeable cations such as Na^+ and H^+ and organic acids that carry a net positive charge. Na^+ entry is further facilitated by the large chemical gradient of Na^+ across the cell membrane (Na^+_i 10 vs Na^+_o 140 m*M*) that is maintained by the Na^+ pump. The large electrochemical gradient for Na^+ is used by cells as the energy force to drive other Na^+-dependent transport systems such as Na^+/H^+ exchange. The large electrical potential across the cell membrane also favors diffusion of H^+ down its electrical gradient into the cell despite the chemical gradient, which should result in H^+ extrusion from the cell (H^+_i 63 n*M* [pH_i 7.2] vs H^+_o 40 n*M*, pH_i 7.4). Calculations with the Nernst equation, assuming a membrane potential of about –60 mV and an external pH of 7.4, predict an equilibrium pH_i for most mammalian cells between 6.4 and 6.2 *(4,5)*. The resting pH_i, however, is maintained at a much more alkaline range (7.1–7.3) predicted based on the H^+ electrochemical gradient. This higher pH_i reflects the concerted effort of the membrane transporters that actively extrude acid equivalents.

The first and immediate line of pH_i defense against acute acid or base perturbations is the intracellular H^+ buffering power *(2)*. Buffering power is the capacity of the intracellular milieu to reduce the magnitude of change produced by sudden acid/base alterations. The greater the cellular buffering power, the more acid or base that is required to effect a change in pH. Three types of processes contribute to intracellular H^+ buffering: titration of weak acids and bases, biochemical reactions, and organellar buffering. Most buffering in the physiologic pH_i range is thought to be done by weak acids and bases *(1,2)*, including organic acids and bases as well as proteins and other components of the cell. Organellar buffering involves the sequestration of acids or bases from the cytosol, into subcellular organelles, such as lysosomes *(6)*.

Na^+/H^+ ANTIPORTER (NHE-1)

General Features

Na^+/H^+ exchange (NHE) activity has been found in virtually all mammalian cells including VSMC. The Na^+/H^+ antiporter translocates extracellular Na^+ across the cell membrane down its electrochemical gradient in exchange for intracellular H^+ (Fig. 1). The Na^+/H^+ antiporter is involved in intracellular pH regulation, regulation of intracellular Na^+, and volume, and may be involved in vascular growth and in the cellular signaling by various hormones and growth factors. Under normal physiologic conditions the antiporter cannot be reversed. However, experimentally the antiporter is reversible if dramatic alterations in the ion gradients are employed. Although the antiporter is reversible, it is not a symmetric exchanger. The antiporter is regulated by an internal allosteric binding site that is sensitive to the H^+ concentration inside the cell. Binding of H^+ to the allosteric modification site alters antiporter activity by increasing the affinity of H^+ to the substrate binding site *(7)*.

A major breakthrough in the study of the Na^+/H^+ antiporter occurred when the first human Na^+/H^+ exchange gene in mutant cell lines that lacked NHE activity was isolated and functionally expressed *(8–10)*. This was followed by the molecular cloning and sequencing of a human Na^+/H^+ antiporter *(11)*. Creation of mutant cell lines that lack antiporter activity was done by what is referred to as the "H^+ suicide technique." In this technique, cells are initially loaded with Li^+ by exposing the cells to an acute acid load and allowing them to recover in a Na^+-free, Li^+-containing media. The cells are then exposed to a Na^+ and Li^+-free media at an acidic pH (~5.5). Under these conditions the cells with the highest rate of NHE activity quickly die as a consequence of the rapid uptake of H^+. Cells with little or no Na^+/H^+ exchange activity survive the "suicide" process. Surviving cells are then regrown and the process repeated, until a homogeneous population of mutant cells devoid of antiporter activity remains *(10)*. Using this technique, transfected cells overexpressing the human NHE-1 gene were selected in the opposite manner as the suicide technique. Cells were acidified using the NH_4Cl technique and the pH_i was allowed to recover under conditions of reduced NHE activity, i.e., either in the presence of reduced extracellular Na^+ or in the presence of an antiporter inhibitor. Cells with the greatest levels of antiporter activity survived the process, whereas cells with low levels of expressed antiporter died *(8,10)*.

There are various isoforms of the Na^+/H^+ antiporter that show a high degree of homology *(11–13)* and each isoform is a separate gene product. The NHE-1 isoform has been isolated and cloned *(11)* and is ubiquitous and relatively sensitive to inhibition by amiloride analogs. In polarized epithelium, NHE-1 is usually associated with the basolateral membrane. It is activated by growth factors, peptide hormones, and other agents that stimulate protein kinase C (PKC) activity *(14,15)*. NHE-1 functions to maintain pH_i homeostasis, regulate cell volume, and may be involved in regulation of growth in VSMC and other cells *(14–16)*.

Isoform Expression and Genetics

NHE in mammalian cells consists of numerous isozymes from a family of genes that have been cloned and sequenced *(11,15,17–23)*. These isozymes are numbered for the order in which they were discovered (NHE-1, 2, 3, and 4). Recently, another NHE isoform, NHE-5, has been reported *(24)*. All NHE isoform cDNAs code for proteins containing 700–900 amino acids and a molecular mass of 80–95 kDa *(5,12)*. There is considerable homology between the different NHE isoforms within the same species and an extremely high level of conservation for each isoform between species *(12,25)*. Overall homology between different isoforms is about 40%. The cytosolic tail shows about 25–35% homology whereas the transmembrane domain exhibits an overall homology of 45–65% *(12)*. Some transmembrane domains are highly conserved with the homology reaching 95% *(12)*. A comparison of the human and rat NHE-1 protein sequence database reveals an overall identity of 85% between the two species. The majority of the difference between the two species is caused by the addition of about 75 amino acids at the C-terminal end of the human sequence. If the terminal portion of the protein is excluded the level of identity becomes 93% (754 identical amino acids of 812 total amino acids).

Thc human NHE-1 gene, also known as APNH, is located on chromosome 1, locus p34–36 *(26)*. It spans 70 kb and is divided into 12 exons and 11 introns. The promoter region of the gene consists of 1377 base pairs in the 5' flanking region of the gene and contains a number of consensus sequences for known transcription factors including a TATA box, three GC boxes, two CAT boxes, three AP-1 sites, as well as other DNA binding sites of known transcription factors *(27,28)*. In the rat, the NHE-1 gene has recently been shown to lie on chromosome 5, extending the homology with that chromosome and the human chromosome 1p *(29)*. The level of expression of NHE-1 protein is relatively low *(5,13,30,31)*. Even in tissues that express large amounts of NHE-1 protein, the level of expression is much lower than that of other membrane proteins such as the Na^+/K^+ ATPase *(13)*. Despite its relatively low level of expression, transport capacity of the antiporter is extremely high and can exceed the transport capacity of the Na^+/K^+ ATPase *(13)*. The low level of NHE-1 protein expression may be the result of the structure of the 5' untranslated region of the message. This region contains up to three minicistrons that are out of frame with the initiating sequence of the main open reading frame. Such a structure can be inhibitory to translational efficiency, or can cause failure to recognize the major initiating sequence of the NHE-1 message *(13)*. This is exemplified by the fact that removal of most of the 5' untranslated region of the message results in an increase in Na^+/H^+ exchange activity *(22)*.

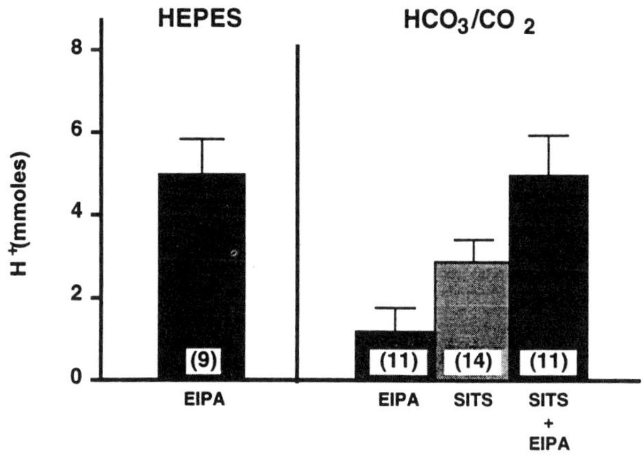

Fig. 2. Net H^+ accumulation 10 min after addition of each inhibitor. In the absence of HCO_3^-/CO_2, inhibition of Na^+/H^+ exchange with EIPA caused a progressive increase in H^+ accumulation (decline in steady-state pH_i). In the presence of HCO_3^-/CO_2, EIPA only had a marginal effect on H^+ accumulation. The addition of EIPA and SITS together, however, was additive indicating that the Na^+/H^+ antiporter was active both in the absence and in the presence of HCO_3^-/CO_2. The number of experiments is shown in parentheses (LaPointe and Batlle, unpublished observations, 1991).

NHE-1 IN VSMC

Demonstration of NHE in primary cultures of VSMC and VSMC-like cell lines and the activation of the antiporter by intracellular acidification is well established. In VSMC, there is an amiloride-sensitive entry of Na^+ that is hormonally stimulated *(32,33)*. Platelet-derived growth factor (PDGF) stimulates Na^+ influx into VSMC, suggesting activation of NHE *(34)*. Characterization of the antiporter in both cultured VSMC and rat aortic segments indicates that up to 80% of the Na^+ entry into VSMC is through the Na^+/H^+ antiporter *(35–38)*. As in other cell types, NHE in VSMC is active near steady-state pH_i and is stimulated by decreasing pH_i *(36,37)*. These studies, however, were performed in the absence of HCO_3/CO_2 in the media. LaPointe and colleagues *(38,39)* examined the activity of the NHE in VSMC both in the presence and absence of HCO_3/CO_2 *(38,39)*. In the absence of HCO_3/CO_2, inhibition of the Na^+/H^+ antiporter with the amiloride analog, EIPA, caused a progressive decrease in pH_i, indicating that in cultured VSMC the Na^+/H^+ antiporter is active at steady-state pH_i (Fig. 2). This is in contrast to other cell types, such as fibroblasts, in which inhibition of the antiporter has little effect on the steady-state pH_i *(40,41)*. In the presence of HCO_3/CO_2, the effect of EIPA on steady-state pH_i in VSMC is not as great as in its absence (Fig. 2) *(42)*. HCO_3-dependent mechanisms probably mask the ability to detect the activity of the antiporter by stabilizing the pH_i *(39)*. Indeed, addition of EIPA in the presence of the stilbene derivative, SITS, to block HCO_3-dependent transporters results in a greater fall in pH_i than the addition of SITS alone, indicating that the antiporter is also active in the presence of HCO_3/CO_2 (Fig. 2) *(42)*.

Activity of the Na^+/H^+ antiporter can be stimulated by acute cell acidification both in the presence and in the absence of HCO_3/CO_2. In the absence of HCO_3/CO_2, almost the entire pH_i recovery from an acute cell acidification can be inhibited by the addition of EIPA, or by removal of external Na^+ (replacement with either choline or *n*-methyl-D-glucamine). In the presence of HCO_3/CO_2, the Na^+/H^+ antiporter accounts for almost the

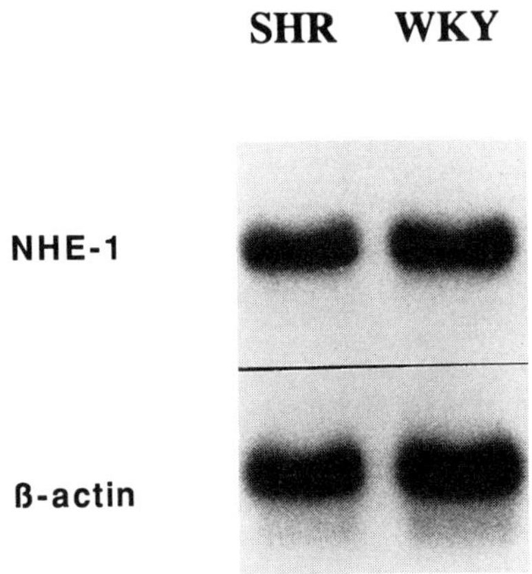

Fig. 3. Na^+/H^+ antiporter mRNA levels in VSMC from SHR and WKY rats. There was no difference in Na^+/H^+ antiporter mRNA levels in VSMC from SHR and WKY rats by Northern blot analysis using the human Na^+/H^+ c28 cDNA (NHE-1 isoform). β-actin levels were used as a control. Data from ref. *39* with permission.

entire pH_i recovery when the pH_i is relatively low (~6.5). Thereafter, only about 50% of the pH_i recovery is due to Na^+/H^+ exchange activity and the remainder is due to a Na^+- and HCO_3^--dependent transporter(s) that are inhibited by SITS *(38,39)*.

Cultured VSMC from rat aorta possess abundant mRNA for the NHE-1 isoform of the Na^+/H^+ antiporter *(43)*. Likewise, we also have demonstrated the presence of abundant NHE-1 mRNA in cultured aortic VSMC derived from the spontaneously hypertensive rat (SHR) and from cells derived from Wistar-Kyoto rats (WKY) (Fig. 3) *(39)*. Other NHE isoforms are not expressed in cultured VSMC *(44)* although expression of mRNA for NHE-2 has been demonstrated in trachea and skeletal muscle *(17)* and a recently discovered isoform, NHE-5, has been reported to be expressed in low amounts in skeletal muscle *(24)*.

PRIMARY AND SECONDARY STRUCTURE OF NHE-1

The human NHE-1 isoform sequence is now believed to contain 893 amino acids, whereas in the rat, NHE-1 protein consists of 820 amino acids. Based on the hydropathy plot of its amino acid sequence, the Na^+/H^+ antiporter can be divided into two major domains: an N-terminal domain consisting of 10–12 membrane-spanning units, and a large cytosolic domain at the C-terminal end of the protein. In this chapter, the different membrane spanning regions are named in order (M1–M10) beginning with the N-terminus *(15)*. Two additional transmembrane regions may lie between M5 and M6. These have been named M5a and M5b *(15)*. The membrane-spanning region consists of approx 500 amino acids, whereas the cytosolic tail consists of approx 300 amino acids *(15)*. Only the membrane-spanning domain is necessary for Na^+ and H^+ transport, since deletion of the cytoplasmic tail did not prevent antiporter activity *(22)*. The cytoplasmic tail, on the other hand, likely contains many of the regulatory sites that control the activity of the antiporter *(22,45)*.

The cDNA for NHE-1 codes for a protein with a molecular mass of about 85 kDa. However, determination of the molecular mass from immunoblots of NHE-1 protein results in a molecular mass of the protein of about 110 kDa (Fig. 4). The additional mass is owing to *N*-linked and *O*-linked glycosylation *(15)*. Treatment of NHE-1 with neuramidase and endoglycosidase F but not endoglycosidase H resulted in a reduction of

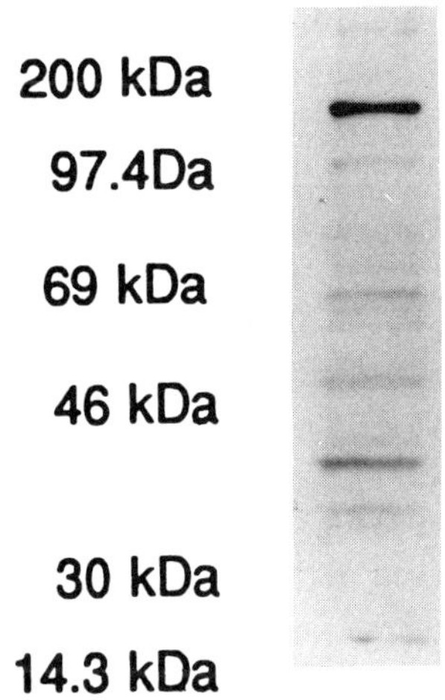

Fig. 4. Western Blot of NHE-1 from cultured VSMC. Protein was extracted from cultured VSMC and probed for NHE-1. The anti-NHE-1 antibody recognized a major protein band at 110 kDa (LaPointe and Batlle, unpublished observations, 1995).

the molecular mass to 90 kDa, the calculated molecular weight based on the primary amino acid sequence of the protein. Glycosylation of NHE-1 protein occurs in the M2 membrane-spanning region *(12,15)*. There is a second putative *N*-linked glycosylation site in region M7 of the protein *(15)*. In mammalian cells, the non-glycosylated form of NHE-1 is not transported to the cell membrane *(15)*. However, transfection of NHE-1 into Sf9 cells, an insect cell line that is not capable of glycosylating the protein, showed that glycosylation was not essential for the expression of functional NHE-1. Moreover, mutation of aspartamine 75 to alanine to prevent glycosylation does not alter the K_i for amiloride or the K_m for Na^+ *(12)*. Treatment of renal brush border membranes (which contain NHE-3) with endoglycodase F but not endoglycosidase H, however, partially decreased the V_{max} of the NHE for external Na^+, suggesting that glycosylation may be important for the full activation of the Na^+/H^+ antiporter *(15)*.

Recent studies have suggested that the Na^+/H^+ antiporter may be present as a functional dimer *(5,46,47)*. In concordance with this data is the unpublished observation by our laboratory, and others *(31)*, that immunoblots of NHE protein often show a protein band ~200 kDa, approximately twice the reported molecular mass of the NHE-1 protein, even in denaturing conditions. There is evidence that the NHE-1 and NHE-3 isoforms of the antiporter form stable homodimers in vivo, although it appears that each subunit of the oligomer functions independently *(30)*. Domains responsible for the dimerization lie in the transmembrane region of the protein, since deletion of the entire cytosolic tail does not prevent dimerization from occurring. Cotransfection of both isoforms into the same cell line did not lead to the formation of heterodimers, indicating that there is isoform specificity for dimerization *(30)*.

SUBSTRATE AND AMILORIDE BINDING SITES

Competitive binding studies favor the ping-pong theory of action for the Na^+/H^+ antiporter, with sequential binding of the substrates to one binding site. Binding of the second substrate (i.e., H^+) cannot occur until the first substrate (i.e., Na^+) has been translocated to the opposite side of the membrane and released *(15)*. The substrate binding site for the antiporter has not been located, though it is in the transmembrane domain of the protein since deletion of the cytoplasmic tail does not inhibit antiporter activity *(22,30)*. There is a strong possibility that the substrate binding site lies within the putative transmembrane regions M5a and M5b. These regions are the most highly conserved regions among the NHE isoforms with a homology reaching 95% *(12)*. Moreover, mutation of glutamate 262 in the M5b region to isoleucine completely inhibits NHE *(30)*.

Binding of H^+ to an internal allosteric modification site greatly enhances Na^+/H^+ antiporter activity *(7)*. There is strong evidence that the allosteric modification site lies in the membrane-spanning region of the protein since deletion of the entire cytoplasmic tail does not curtail allosteric modification *(12,22)*. The cytoplasmic tail is, however, crucial for determining the set point of the "H^+ sensor" *(31,45)*. Likely candidates for the allosteric modification site include areas containing a histidine residue since this residue is capable of protonation in the physiological pH range *(12)*. One of the distinguishing features about the different Na^+/H^+ antiporter isoforms is their sensitivity to inhibition by amiloride and its five *N*-substituted analogs *(12)*. On the basis of amiloride sensitivity, it was predicted that at least two forms of the NHE existed *(48)*. The different NHE isoforms have different sensitivities to amiloride and its analogs, and generally, the order of sensitivity of the NHE isoforms to amiloride and its five *N*-substituted analogs is NHE-1 > NHE-2 >> NHE-3 *(12)*. Amiloride acts as a competitive inhibitor for Na^+ on the extracellular side of the protein, and the site of amiloride binding to NHE-1 appears to be in the M4 region of the protein, another highly conserved region between the different NHE isoforms *(12)*. Mutations of NHE-1 at tyrosine 165 or leucine 167 greatly increase the IC_{50} for amiloride and MPA *(49)*. The M4 region of NHE-2 and NHE-3 also appear to be involved in amiloride sensitivity of these isoforms *(12)*. The M4 region is not, however, the only region involved in amiloride binding. Substitution of the M4 region of NHE-1 with the M4 region of NHE-3 does not induce the same level of amiloride resistance as is seen in native NHE-3 *(12)*. The other region(s) of amiloride binding lie between M4 and M7 of the protein *(12,15)*, and further determination of the other amiloride binding sites should help in elucidating the tertiary structure of the protein in the plasma membrane.

NHE-1 PHOSPHORYLATION

The mechanism by which NHE-1 activity is regulated by mitogens and other hormones is quite complex. NHE-1 is a constitutively phosphorylated protein and there is evidence to suggest that this phosphorylation may be necessary for the full activation of the protein. NHE-1 activation is greatly diminished in ATP-depleted cells, which would suggest that ATP depletion decreases the level of phosphorylation of the protein *(16,50,51)*. However, there is no difference in either the phosphorylation level, or the pattern of phosphorylated peptides after enzymatic digestion of the NHE-1 protein in control and ATP-depleted cells *(50)*. Thus, ATP depletion inhibits the antiporter in a manner different from the direct inhibition of NHE-1 phosphorylation. Phosphorylation of NHE-1 occurs strictly on serine residues in the cytosolic tail *(50,52,53)*. Activation of the antiporter is associated with an increase in the level of phosphorylation, but not the pattern of NHE-1 residue phosphorylation *(22,31,52,53)*. This is surprising, since NHE-1 is activated by a number of different substances, including tyrosine kinases and GTP-dependent kinases that phosphorylate tyrosine and threonine residues *(12,15,52,53)*. Phosphorylation of the cytosolic tail is not the only mechanism by which mitogenic stimulation works, however, since truncated NHE-1 proteins in which all the phosphorylation sites are removed can still be activated by mitogens, although to a lesser extent than the native protein *(5)*. Moreover, mutagenic deletion of individual phosphorylated serine residues has no effect on mitogenic stimulation *(15,54)*. This phosphorylation-independent pathway may involve the direct binding of Ca^{2+}-calmodulin to the protein *(55,56)*. Ca^{2+}-calmodulin binds to NHE-1 between residues 636 and 656. This sequence of amino acids exerts a chronic inhibitory effect on the protein. Deletion mutations of the region or binding of Ca^{2+}-calmodulin to the region in wild-type NHE-1 removes this inhibition and thus increases NHE activity *(55,56)*.

Examination of the primary sequence of NHE-1 reveals that the protein contains multiple recognition motifs for kinase activation in both the transmembrane region and the cytosolic tail *(5)*. NHE-1 has ideal recognition motifs for the binding of calmodulin-dependent protein kinase II (CaM kinase II) and for the MAP kinases, but it does not have a recognition motif for protein kinase A or an ideal consensus sequence PKC binding *(5)*. Lack of an ideal consensus sequence for the binding of PKC is surprising, since hormonal activation of PKC or activation of PKC by phorbol esters is known to increase the level of NHE-1 phosphorylation. A potential phosphorylation site for PKC has been identified at serine 652 *(25)*. The possibility also exists that PKC is binding NHE-1 at another unidentified site, or that it is acting through an intermediary kinase. That a vast array of mitogens and agonists that activate NHE-1 result in a similar pattern of protein phosphorylation has lead to the proposal that there is a common pathway through which NHE-1 is activated *(12,15)*. The point of convergence may be a kinase cascade, similar to the MAP kinase cascade, or it may simply involve a regulatory phosphoprotein that binds to NHE-1 *(12)*.

KINETIC REGULATION OF NHE-1 ACTIVITY IN VSMC

Activity of the Na^+/H^+ antiporter is dependent on the net concentrations of Na^+ and H^+ across the cell membrane, and under normal physiologic conditions there is a net inward Na^+ gradient of about one order of magnitude and a mild net outward H^+ gradient. This results in the electroneutral exchange of internal H^+ for external Na^+. Because the Na^+/H^+ antiporter is an electroneutral exchanger, it is unaffected by the electrical potential across the cell membrane. The antiporter is, however, inhibited to some degree by conditions that lower the external pH (e.g., ischemia and acidosis) *(5,35)*. Although the antiporter can be experimentally driven in either the forward or reverse mode, the antiporter is not a symmetric transporter. Na^+/H^+ antiporter activity is modulated by increases in internal H^+ concentration, beyond that of simple substrate activation. In addition to the substrate binding site, the Na^+/H^+ antiporter has another internal H^+-binding site that allosterically modifies activity of the antiporter *(7,57)*. Binding of H^+ to the allosteric modifier site results in a steep pH_i dependence in activity beyond simple first order kinetics that results from substrate activation at the transport site. External pH dependence of the antiporter, on the other hand, indicates that the Na^+/H^+ antiporter follows simple first order kinetics for external H^+ *(57)*. In renal brush border vesicles, the NHE-1 isoform of the antiporter expressed in VSMC is not the isoform that is responsible for the luminal NHE in the renal proximal tubule. The internal allosteric modification site, however, has been reported to be present in all NHE isoforms and in all cells examined *(12)*.

In VSMC, as in most other cells, the V_{max} occurs at a very low pH_i (~6.0) that is never seen under nonexperimental conditions. At the other extreme, the zero set point (pH 0.01), the pH_i at which the activity of the antiporter is only 1% of V_{max} *(45)*, is between 7.3 and 7.5 *(39)*. The Hill coefficient for NHE-1 in VSMC (<3.0) is higher than what is observed in most cells such as lymphocytes *(5,58)*, but are similar to what is reported in myocardial cells *(5)*. The large Hill coefficients of the antiporter in myocardium and VSMC may be necessary to maintain the pH_i in a very tight range despite fluctuations in cell metabolism during contractile cycling. The tight control on pH_i may facilitate the normal functions of these cells since fluctuations in pH_i could have adverse effects on the contractile force generated *(5)*. Alterations in external Na^+ concentrations in the physiologic range are not involved in the regulation of antiporter activity, since antiporter activity is near maximal at Na^+ concentrations around 100 m*M*. Hormonal stimulation, however, can regulate the antiporter in such a manner that the external Na^+ kinetics are altered. Stimulation of cultured VSMC with angiotensin II (AII) causes an increased affinity of the antiporter for external Na^+ *(59,60)*.

Examination of the kinetic parameters of the antiporter reveals valuable information about the normal physiologic function of the protein, and also allows one to explore differences in the function of the antiporter under various pathologic conditions *(61)*. We have examined the kinetics of the Na^+/H^+ antiporter in cultured VSMC from SHR and WKY rats *(39)*. VSMC were acutely acidified and then allowed to spontaneously recover, and the rates of H^+ efflux were then plotted against the prevailing pH_i (converted to H^+ concentration, Fig. 5) and the kinetic parameters of the Na^+/H^+ antiporter were calculated using nonlinear regression analysis of the Hill equation. We showed that the maximal activity of the antiporter, the V_{max}, was greater in VSMC derived from the SHR than those derived from WKY rats *(39)*. The increase in the V_{max} in cells derived from the SHR may be the result of an increase in the amount of NHE-1 protein in these cells *(62)*.

REGULATION OF NHE-1 BY VASOACTIVE HORMONES AND GROWTH FACTORS

That numerous growth factors *(40,63–65)* and vasoactive substances such as arginine vasopressin (AVP), *(66–68)* AII, *(59,68–70)* thromboxane, and PGF2 *(71)* stimulate NHE-1 activity has lead to the suggestion that activation of NHE may be an integral component in VSMC physiologic responses to these factors *(14,16,60)*. Mitogens stimulate antiporter activity through a phosphorylation-induced conformational change in the antiporter, thus changing the affinity of the allosteric H^+ modification site *(66–68,79,90)*. Stimulation by PDGF *(34)* and AII *(32,33,73)* is associated with increased $^{22}Na^+$ influx in VSMC. The enhanced Na^+ uptake secondarily stimulates Na^+/K^+ ATPase activity as measured by ^{86}Rb influx *(74)*. Total cellular Na^+ remains increased at 4 and 8 h after AII stimulation and then returns to control levels by 24 h *(74)*. We have shown that acute stimulation with AII rapidly increased free cytosolic Na^+ and that this effect is mediated by activation of the Na^+/H^+ antiporter via the type I Ang II receptor *(69)*.

In quiescent VSMC, the stimulation of NHE activity by AII is greatly attenuated by downregulation of PKC activity after a 24-h incubation with the phorbol ester (PMA) *(59)*, but was unaffected by removal of external Ca^{2+} or blockade of Ca^{2+} channels *(75)*. In serum-stimulated cells, AII appears to act via a PKC-independent pathway *(59,76)*. AII reduces the K_m of the antiporter for external Na^+, but does not affect the V_{max} *(59,73)*

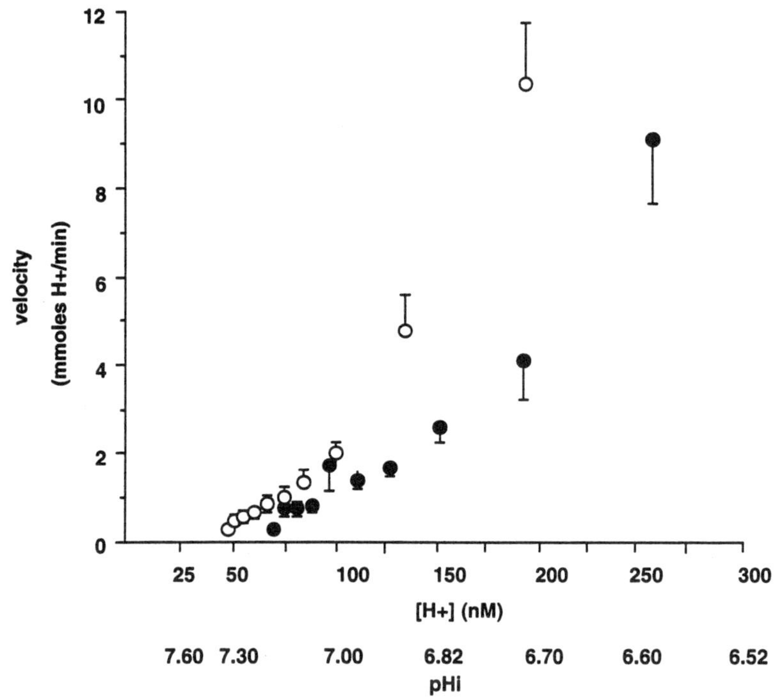

Fig. 5. Na^+/H^+ exchange activity as a function of intracellular H^+. Cells were acutely acidified in the absence of HCO_3^-/CO_2 and the pH_i recovery was measured over time. The pH_i recovery rates at each interval were converted to H^+ efflux rates (ΔpH_i x B) and plotted against the intracellular H^+ concentration. These data were then used to determine the V_{max} and Hill coefficients for SHR (○) and WKY cells (●). Data from ref. *39* with permission.

or internal H^+ kinetics *(73)*. This is different from the mechanism whereby growth factors such as serum or PDGF stimulate NHE, in which the antiporter is activated through modification of internal H^+ kinetics *(72)*.

Stimulation of the Na^+/H^+ antiporter may take on two separate forms. Short-term stimulation appears to be mediated through phosphorylation of the antiporter via PKC *(52)* or other kinase pathways. Long-term stimulation of the antiporter may involve increases in the expression of NHE-1 mRNA and subsequently an increase in the synthesis of new antiporter units *(43)*. Serum, PDGF, and fibroblast growth factor (FGF) each stimulate the expression of NHE-1 mRNA levels in rat aortic VSMC *(43)*. AII causes an acute increase in pH_i, but does not induce either an increase in NHE-1 mRNA levels or an increase in pH_i after chronic exposure (24 h) *(43)*. In fact, long-term AII stimulation causes a decrease in pH_i *(43,77)*. In contrast, after 24-h incubation with serum or PDGF, pH_i is increased by about 0.1 pH units *(43,77)*. After 24 h of AII exposure, the rate of NHE-dependent pH_i recovery from an acute acid load is enhanced, whereas serum exposure for 24 h decreases the NHE activity *(77)*. These differing effects of AII and other mitogens on NHE activity, pH_i, and steady-state mRNA levels may partly account for the finding that AII is hypertrophic but does not cause hyperplasia after 24 h of exposure *(43,78,79)*, although there is a delayed hyperplastic response to AII in VSMC (about 48 h) *(80)*.

OTHER H+ TRANSPORT PROTEINS

Na^+-Independent Cl^-/HCO_3^- and N^+-Dependent Cl/HCO_3 Exchange

Under normal physiologic conditions, i.e., in the presence of HCO_3/CO_2, there are two additional major membrane transporters that help to maintain the steady-state pH_i. These are the Na^+-independent Cl^-/HCO_3^- exchanger and the Na^+-dependent Cl^-/HCO_3^- exchanger *(3,81,82)*. A functional Na^+-independent Cl^-/HCO_3^- exchanger exists in VSMC *(83,84)*, and cultured mesangial cells *(81)*. Immunoreactivity of VSMC to antibodies against the erythrocyte band 3 protein has also been demonstrated *(85)*. Na^+-independent Cl^-/HCO_3^- exchange consists of a family of proteins derived from related genes. Three Na^+-independent Cl^-/HCO_3^- exchange genes have been identified to date. In addition, the genes generate alternative mRNA that can lead to different protein transcripts *(86,87)*. Thus, there may be a large number of closely related Na^+-independent Cl^-/HCO_3^- exchange proteins in a variety of cells. The proteins have been given the name AE (anion exchanger) and a number. AE1 is the band 3 protein that was originally characterized in erythrocytes *(88)*. Immunological identification of the specific AE genes being expressed is extremely difficult, if not impossible, because there is a high degree of homology between the different Na^+-independent Cl^-/HCO_3^- exchangers, and the fact that multiple polypeptides can be generated from a single gene *(86,87)*.

The Na^+ independent Cl-/HCO_3- exchanger translocates intracellular HCO_3^- in exchange for extracellular Cl^-. It is an electroneutral exchanger that is nearly inactive at steady-state pH_i, and it is activated by high intracellular pH and reduces the pH_i by the removal of HCO_3^-. The Na^+-independent Cl^-/HCO_3^- exchanger is a symmetric transporter and is freely reversible. Removal of external Cl^- causes an increase in the pH_i by reversal of this exchanger, as well as through the stimulation of another Cl^-/HCO_3^- exchanger, the Na^+-dependent Cl^-/HCO_3^- exchanger *(3)*. The Na^+-independent Cl^-/HCO_3^- exchanger may act in conjunction with NHE during hyperosmotic stress to bring Na^+ and Cl^- into the cell. Under this condition, stimulation of NHE increases Na^+ influx into the cell in exchange for intracellular H^+, which would result in an increase in the pH_i if it was not coupled to the removal of base, or influx of acid equivalents. Coupling of NHE with Na^+-independent Cl^-/HCO_3^- exchange therefore helps to maintain a constant pH_i during hypertonic stress *(16)*. The Na^+-dependent Cl^-/HCO_3^- exchanger is an electroneutral exchanger that transports 1 Na^+ and 2 Cl^- for every 2 H^+ equivalents in the cell *(89)*. The Na^+-dependent Cl^-/HCO_3^- exchanger is relatively active at steady-state pH_i as opposed to NHE and Na^+-independent Cl^-/HCO_3^- exchange, which are stimulated by extremes of pH_i and are less active near steady-state pH_i *(3)*. During the recovery from an acute acid load, the Na^+-dependent Cl^--/HCO_3^- exchanger may account for nearly half the pH_i recovery *(81,82)*.

Na^+–HCO_3^- Symport in VSMC

Evidence for a Na^+–HCO_3^- symport in VSMC comes from studies examining the recovery from an acute acid load in cells depleted of intracellular Cl^- *(38,81,90–92)*. A component of pH_i recovery that was apparently electroneutral, Na^+-, and HCO_3^--dependent, but Cl^--independent, and SITS inhibitable has been identified *(90)*. This component of pH_i recovery accounts for about 25% of the recovery in these cells in the presence of HCO_3^--/CO_2. An EIPA-insensitive Na^+–HCO_3^- cotransporter in cultured VSMC from human mammary arteries and rat aorta has been reported *(91,92)*. We examined the Na^+–HCO_3^- symport in VSMC by measuring pH_i recovery in the presence of HCO_3^-/CO_2 in control cells and in cells that had undergone Cl^- depletion for 60 min and then maintained in a Cl^- free solution throughout the experiment *(38)*. Compared to controls, NHE inhibition with EIPA reduced the pH_i recovery from an experimentally induced cellular acidification (about 40% inhibition). Anion exchange inhibition by addition of SITS also blocked pH_i recovery by about 40%. Addition of EIPA and SITS together or Na^+ removal (not shown) decreased the pH_i recovery by about 75%. Cl^- depletion, on the other hand, had little effect on the pH_i recovery. Addition of SITS to Cl^- depleted cells, significantly reduced the pH_i recovery compared to Cl^-- depleted cells that had not been exposed to SITS. Taken together, these data suggest that in the presence of HCO_3^-/CO_2, a SITS sensitive, Cl^--independent, but Na^+-dependent mechanism of pH_i regulation exists in cultured VSMC.

H^+-ATPase in VSMC

Evidence for the existence of an H^+–ATPase in the plasma membrane of VSMC is based on functional studies using inhibitors of H^+–ATPase and immunohistochemistry studies *(93)*. Inhibition of H^+–ATPase A1 results in a decline in pH_i. The effect of N-ethylmaleimide (NEM) on steady-state pH_i is additive to inhibition of NHE by removal of Na^+ from the media or the addition of EIPA *(93)*. During recovery from an acute acid load, removal of external Na^+, or addition of EIPA, in the absence of HCO_3^--/CO_2, results in an almost complete inhibition of pH_i recovery. There is, however, a slight, but significant recovery that remains, and this residual pH_i recovery is inhibited by addition of NEM along with Na^+ removal or addition of NEM and EIPA together. Immunohistochemistry of intact VSMC with antibodies against H^+–ATPase reveals staining of the cell *(93)*. These data favor the possibility that an H^+–ATPase is present on the plasma membrane of VSMC. The extent that this H^+–ATPase contributes to the maintenance of pH_i homeostasis is, however, at the present time unknown.

H^+/K^+–ATPase in VSMC

Evidence for the presence of an H^+/K^+–ATPase in VSMC is based on functional studies using known H^+/K^+–ATPase inhibitors. Inhibition of H^+/K^+–ATPase by incubation with inhibitors reduce Rb^+ uptake by about 25% in cultures of aortic and canine coronary VSMC *(94)*. Addition of NC-1300B or omeprazole is also associated with a decline of the pH_i of 0.14 and 0.20 pH units, respectively *(94)*. Cytosolic alkalization decreases the effect of NC-1300B on Rb^+ uptake, whereas cytosolic acidification increases the effect of NC-1300B on Rb^+ uptake, consistent with the inhibition and stimulation of H^+/K^+–ATPase, respectively. These findings suggest the presence of an H^+/K^+–ATPase in VSMC. Additional studies are needed to characterize the properties of this transporter in VSMC.

INTERACTIONS BETWEEN H^+ AND OTHER IONS

Free Cytosolic Na^+ (Na^+_i)

Under normal steady-state conditions, inhibition of NHE with EIPA reduces the rate of Na^+ uptake by 80% in both cultured VSMC and aortic strips, thus demonstrating that NHE is the major mechanism of Na^+ entry in VSMC *(35)*. Na^+ influx through the antiporter is stimulated by intracellular acidification or extracellular alkalization and inhibited by extracellular acidification *(57)*. Changes in NHE activity via alterations in extracellular

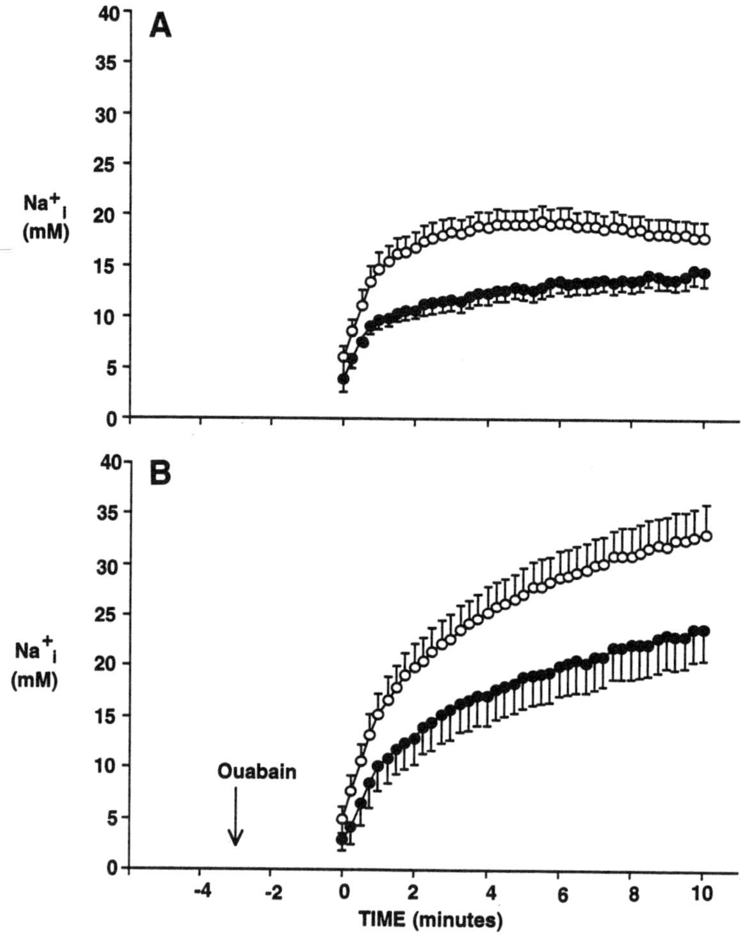

Fig. 6. Na^+_i accumulation during the recovery from cell acidification assayed in the nominal absence of HCO_3^-/CO_2 (HEPES buffer). Na^+_i was monitored after cells were acutely acidified to a pH_i of about 6.5 (time 0) by removal of NH_4Cl. **(A)** The initial increase in Na^+_i was greater in cells from the SHR (○, $n = 19$) than in those from WKY rats (●, $n = 18$). **(B)** Ouabain (2 m*M*) was added 3 min prior to cell acidification (at the arrow). During the recovery from acute cell acidification, Na^+_i accumulation was significantly greater in cells from the SHR (○, $n = 8$) than in those from WKY rats (●, $n = 7$). Addition of ouabain to the superfusate resulted in a greater increase in Na^+_i than in cells not exposed to ouabain in cells from both SHR and WKY rats (compare A and B). Data from ref. *39* with permission.

pH alters the Na^+ influx into the cells, but have no effect on cell $[Na^+]_i$ owing to parallel changes in Na^+/K^+–ATPase activity *(35)*. $[Na^+]_i$ is markedly higher in control cells than in VSMC preincubated with EIPA for only 5 min (control 11 m*M* vs EIPA 5 m*M*) *(69)*. Stimulation of these cells with AII leads to a rapid rise in $[Na^+]_i$, which is due to the activation of the Na^+/H^+ antiporter *(69)*. pH_i recovery from an acute acid load is associated with an increase in $[Na^+]_i$ *(39)*. Because the concentration of $[Na^+]_i$ represents the balance of Na^+ entry and Na^+ extrusion (largely via Na^+/K^+–ATPase) from cells, Na^+ entry has been assessed during recovery from cell acidification after the inhibition of Na^+/K^+–ATPase with ouabain. The increase in $[Na^+]_i$ over time is greatly augmented by ouabain (Fig. 6).

Preincubation of the cells with EIPA completely blocks the initial rise in $[Na^+]_i$ triggered by cell acidification indicating that the rise in $[Na^+]_i$ is caused by stimulation of Na^+/H^+ exchange. In the presence of HCO_3/CO_2, preincubation with EIPA greatly, but incompletely, inhibits the initial rate of Na^+_i accumulation thus demonstrating the presence of an EIPA-insensitive mechanism of $[Na^+]_i$ accumulation in the presence of HCO_3/CO_2 *(39)*.

The concerted activities of the Na^+/H^+ antiporter and the Na^+/K^+–ATPase would be expected to result in Na^+ cycling. An increase in NHE activity increases Na^+ entry into the cell and secondarily stimulates the electrogenic Na^+ pump *(33,35)*. An increase in the Na^+/K^+–ATPase activity results in an increase in K^+ entry into the cell *(35)* and, because of its electrogenic nature, an increase in the membrane potential. Increased Na^+ influx through the antiporter could also cause an increase in $[Ca^{2+}]_i$ by stimulating Na^+/Ca^{2+} exchange. Thus, any factor that stimulates NHE could cause an increase in the pH_i of the cell as well as an increase in Na^+, K^+, and Ca^{2+} influxes, and alter the cell's membrane potential.

Free Cytosolic Ca^{2+}

Stimulation of VSMC with AII results in a rapid increase in $[Ca^{2+}]_i$ (Fig. 7). In the absence of HCO_3^-/CO_2, after an initial cell acidification, pH_i and $[Na^+]_i$ increase as well (Fig. 7). The delayed increases in pH_i and $[Na^+]_i$ are caused by stimulation of the Na^+/H^+ antiporter, since they are blocked by amiloride and its analogs *(68,69,96,97)*. Blockade of the $[Ca^{2+}]_i$ increase with BAPTA prevents initial cell acidification, but does not prevent the delayed increase in pH_i, which reflects stimulation of the Na^+/H^+ antiporter *(95)*. These data suggest that the antiporter can be stimulated by AII, in a Ca^{2+}-independent manner. The pathway through which the Ca^{2+}-independent activation of the Na^+/H^+ antiporter works may involve direct activation of PKC or by activation of G-protein-coupled tyrosine kinases such as the MAP kinase cascade *(60)*.

Agonists that increase $[Ca^{2+}]_i$ in VSMC cause a brief cell acidification that is followed by a marked alkalization when HCO_3^--/CO_2 is absent from the medium *(59,67,68,75,96)*. In a HCO_3^-/CO_2-containing media, the initial cell acidification still occurs, but the fall in pH_i is not followed by a subsequent cell alkalization *(67,68,75,96)*. Agonists may simultaneously activate three major transmembrane H^+ transporter systems: NHE, Na^+-dependent Cl^--/HCO_3^- exchange, and Na^+-independent Cl^-/HCO_3^- exchange *(35)*. In the absence of HCO_3^-/CO_2, net alkalization occurs because of stimulation of NHE. When HCO_3^-/CO_2 is present in the media, the Na^+-independent Cl^-/HCO_3^- exchanger is predominantly stimulated. This leads to the net removal of HCO_3^- from the cell and thus a fall in pH_i. However, treatment of VSMC with DIDS (and EIPA) to block the Na^+-independent Cl^-/HCO_3^- exchanger, does not prevent the rapid fall in pH_i when the cells are stimulated with AII *(97)*. This suggests that net acidification in the presence of HCO_3^-/CO_2 is the result of a mechanism other than HCO_3^- exit via stimulation of the Cl^-/HCO_3^- exchanger. We noted that the rise in $[Ca^{2+}]_i$ elicited by AII is associated with a fall in pH_i, which coincides with the recovery from the $[Ca^{2+}]_i$ surge *(97)*. That cell acidification does not occur when the increase in $[Ca^{2+}]_i$ is prevented using the Ca^{2+} chelator, BAPTA suggests that changes in $[Ca^{2+}]_i$ are responsible for the initial fall in pH_i *(97)*.

Inhibition of Ca^{2+} exit via the plasma membrane Ca^{2+}–ATPase using cadmium at very low concentrations also blocks cell acidification *(97)*. This suggests that this cell acidification is a result of entry of acid equivalents into the cell via the plasma membrane

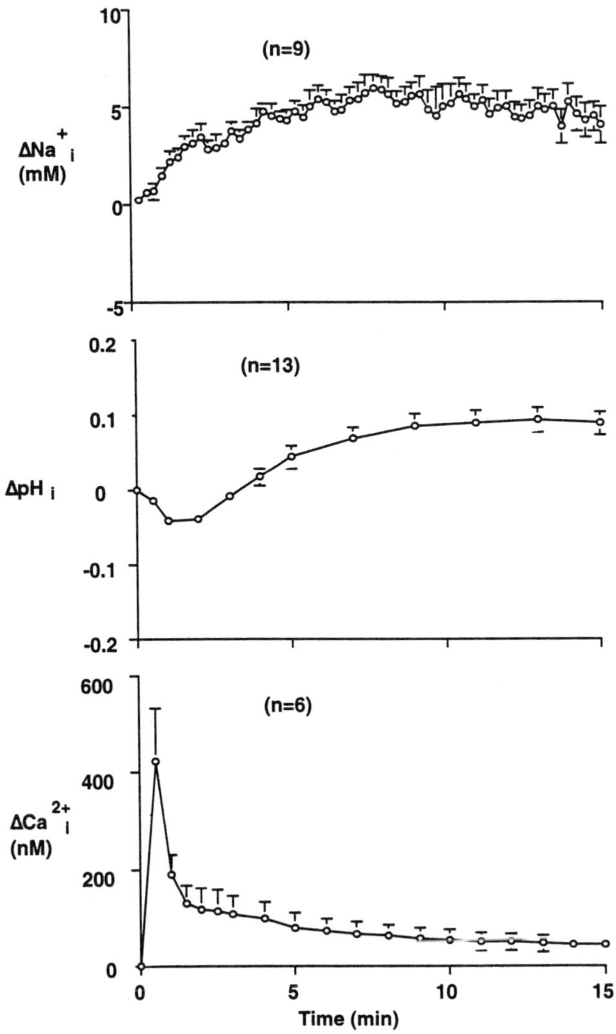

Fig. 7. Effect of AII on intracellular (i) Na^+_i, pH_i, and Ca^{2+}_i in the absence of HCO_3^-/CO_2. Addition of AII caused an immediate increase in Ca^{2+}_i that rapidly returned to control values (bottom panel). The fall in Ca^{2+}_i was associated with a decline in pH_i that was followed by a rise in pH_i above basal values (middle panel). This delayed increase in pH_i was accompanied by an increase in Na^+_i. Data from ref. *95* with permission.

Ca^{2+}–ATPase acting as a Ca^{2+}/H^+ exchanger. Although the plasma membrane Ca^{2+}–ATPase subserves a primary role in the regulation of $[Ca^{2+}]_i$, our data also suggest that it may modify pH_i in the process of extruding Ca^{2+}, particularly when activated by agonists that increase $[Ca^{2+}]_i$ such as AII *(97)*.

Effect of Rapid Fluctuations of pH_i on $[Ca^{2+}]_i$

In VSMC lines and primary cultures of aortic VSMC, intracellular alkalization *(98–100)* or acidification increases $[Ca^{2+}]_i$ *(100)*. Both cell alkalization and acidification result in a rise in $[Ca^{2+}]_i$, owing to mobilization from internal stores. The amplitude of the $[Ca^{2+}]_i$

increase is unaffected by either the removal of external Ca^{2+} or the inhibition of Ca^{2+} entry via Ca^{2+} channels and via the Na^+/Ca^{2+} exchanger *(100,101)*. Cell alkalization increases $[Ca^{2+}]_i$ by promoting its release from an intracellular store that is inhibited by depletion of sarcoplasmic reticulum (SR) Ca^{2+} stores, suggesting that acute intracellular alkalization likely triggers the release of $[Ca^{2+}]_i$ by the SR. Cell acidification, on the other hand, increases $[Ca^{2+}]_i$ from an intracellular store(s) *(100)*. The increase in $[Ca^{2+}]_i$ produced by cell acidification may be caused by displacement of $[Ca^{2+}]_i$ from internal buffers with similar affinities for Ca^{2+} and H^+, and as cytosolic H^+ levels increase, there may be a preferential binding of H^+ to these buffers in place of Ca^{2+}, simply owing to the mass action effect *(100)*. Intracellular acidification may also affect $[Ca^{2+}]_i$ by reducing uptake of Ca^{2+} by the SR *(24,25,42,102,103)*. Indeed, cell acidification induced by propionic acid reduces Ca^{2+} entry into VSMC via Ca^{2+} channels *(100)*. This effect of propionic acid on Ca^{2+} channels may be the result of acidification of the extracellular compartment. Extracellular acidification decreases the probability of channel opening, whereas extracellular alkalization increases the open probability of the channel *(105)*.

In cardiac cells, cell acidification induced by ischemia has little effect on $[Ca^{2+}]_i$ levels *(5)*. During reperfusion, however, enhanced Na^+ influx via the NHE, activated as a result of intracellular acidosis, augments Ca^{2+} influx via the Na^+/Ca^{2+} exchanger *(5)*. In contrast, in cultured aortic VSMC, blockade of external Ca^{2+} entry through Na^+/Ca^{2+} exchange and Ca^{2+} channels by the addition of $NiCl_2$ or the removal of external Ca^{2+} has no effect on the acidification-induced Ca^{2+} transient *(100)*. Differences in myocardium and VSMC are likely caused by differences in the levels of Na^+/Ca^{2+} exchange activity between the different cell types. The level of Na^+/Ca^{2+} activity is extremely high in cardiac cells, and Na^+/Ca^{2+} exchange is responsible for a large portion of Ca^{2+} entry during cell depolarization (reverse mode of operation) and in the efflux of $[Ca^{2+}]_i$ during muscle relaxation (forward mode of operation) *(101,106)*. In cultured VSMC, the level of activity appears to be relatively low under normal resting physiologic conditions, whereas it is greatly stimulated when $[Ca^{2+}]_i$ is increased by agonists such as AII *(107–109)*, and under this condition contributes to the extrusion of $[Ca^{2+}]_i$ from the cells *(101,106)*.

The mechanism whereby a rapid increase in pH_i results in Ca^{2+} mobilization may involve increased IP_3 formation, or enhancement of the sensitivity of the SR to IP_3, as shown in platelets *(110)*. It is possible that cytoplasmic alkalization could sensitize the IP_3 receptor to endogenous levels of IP_3 as shown for sulfhydryl reagents *(111)*. Another possibility is that pH_i may affect IP_3 binding. Binding of IP3 to cerebellar membranes shows a dependence on pH with the highest binding levels occurring between pH 8.0 and 9.0 *(112)*. In addition, the presence of pH-regulated Ca^{2+} channels in intracellular Ca^{2+} pools has been proposed *(113)*.

After the initial rise in $[Ca^{2+}]_i$ produced by cell alkalization, $[Ca^{2+}]_i$ rapidly recovers toward normal values despite the continued presence of a high intracellular pH (Fig. 8). $[Ca^{2+}]_i$ recovery is caused by stimulation of the plasma membrane Ca^{2+} pump, stimulation of internal reuptake by a Ca^{2+}/H^+ exchanging ATPase in the SR, and possibly by stimulation of calcium efflux via Na^+/Ca^{2+} exchange. These processes are all simultaneously stimulated whenever $[Ca^{2+}]_i$ increases rapidly. Cell alkalization per se, however, could enhance any or all of these various mechanisms of $[Ca^{2+}]_i$ recovery. The pH optimum of the plasma membrane Ca^{2+}–ATPase has been reported to be between 7.0 and 7.5, and therefore, cell alkalization may enhance the activity of

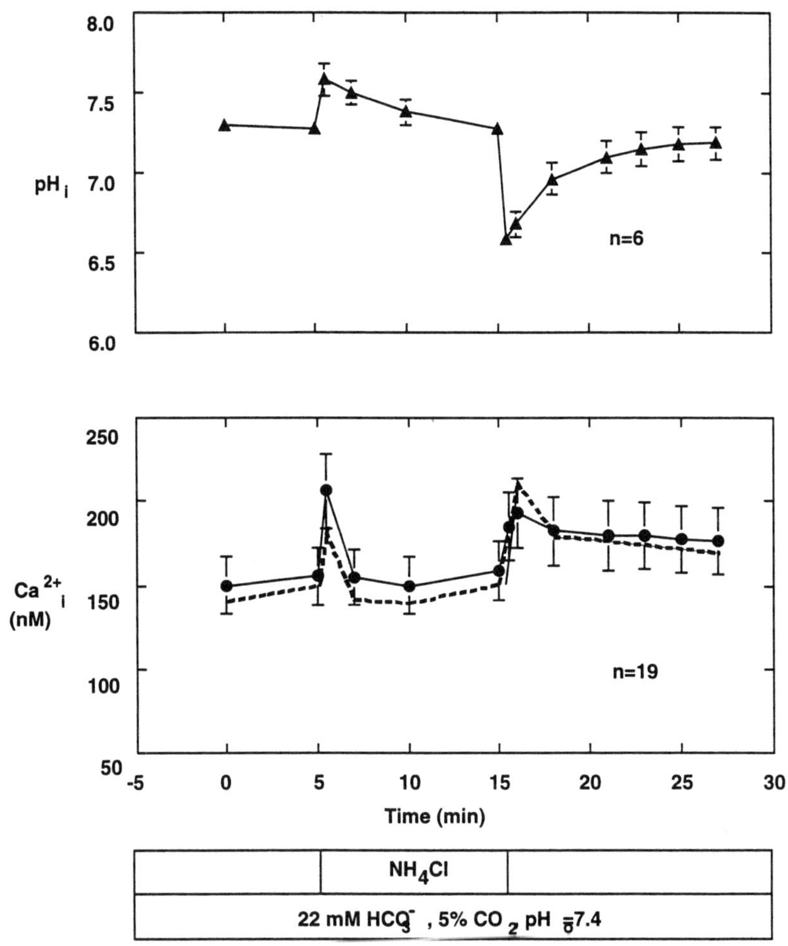

Fig. 8. Cell alkalinization, recovery, and acidification using the NH_4Cl technique. The top panel represents experiments measuring pH_i using BCECF, and the bottom panel represents parallel experiments measuring $Ca^{2+}{}_i$ using fura-2. In both experiments, NH_4Cl was introduced into the perfusate at 5 min, causing rapid cell alkalinization. Despite the continued presence of NH_4Cl, pH_i returned to normal in about 10 min. At this point (15 min), washout of NH_4Cl resulted in rapid cell acidification, followed by spontaneous pH_i recovery. In the bottom panel, the solid circles represent computed $Ca^{2+}{}_i$ values without correcting for pH_i effects on the fura-2 kDa for calcium. The broken line represents values after correction of the fura-2 kDa for alterations in pH_i. $Ca^{2+}{}_i$ increased after both alkalinization and acidification in every experiment performed. Data from ref. *100* with permission.

the plasma membrane Ca^{2+} pump that transports Ca^{2+} to the extracellular space. Intracellular Ca^{2+} reuptake also occurs by the SR via a Ca^{2+}/H^+-exchanging ATPase *(1,114,115)*. Accordingly, a reduction in the concentration of cytosolic H^+ (i.e., a rise in pH_i) would be expected to increase the driving force for Ca^{2+}/H^+ exchange and thereby facilitate $[Ca^{2+}]_i$ recovery. Thus, acute intracellular alkalization triggers the rapid release of Ca^{2+} from the SR, while at the same time, it facilitates the removal of Ca^{2+} from the cytosol via the plasma membrane and SR Ca^{2+}–ATPase, which act as Ca^{2+}/H^+ exchangers *(97,100)*.

REFERENCES

1. Roos A, Boron W. Intracellular pH. Physiol Rev 1981;61:296–434.
2. Saleh A, Batlle D. Basic mechanisms of intracellular pH homeostasis in lymphocytes. Sem Nephrol 1991;11:3–15.
3. Redon J, Batlle D. Regulation of intracellular pH in the spontaneously hypertensive rat. Role of bicarbonate-dependent transporters. Hypertension 1994;23:503–512.
4. Frelin C, Vigne P, Ladoux A, Lazdunski M. The regulation of the intracellular pH in cells from vertebrates. Eur J Biochem 1988;174:3–14.
5. Fliegel L, Frohlich O. The Na^+/H^+ exchanger: an update on structure, regulation and cardiac physiology. Biochem J 1993;296:273–285.
6. Saleh A, Rombola G, Batlle D. Intracellular buffering power and its dependency on intracellular pH. Kidney Int 1991;39:282–288.
7. Aronson P, Nee J, Suhm M. Modifier role of internal H^+ in activating the Na^+–H^+ exchanger in renal microvillus membrane vesicles. Nature 1982;299:161–163.
8. Franchi A, Cragoe E, PouyssÄgur J. Isolation and properties of fibroblast mutants overexpressing an altered Na^+/H^+ antiporter. J Biol Chem 1986;261:14,614–14,620.
9. Franchi A, Perruca-Lostanen D, PouyssÄgur J. Functional expression of a transfected Na^+/H^+ antiporter human gene into antiporter-deficient mouse L cells. Proc Natl Acad Sci USA 1986;83:9388–9392.
10. PouyssÄgur J, Sardet C, Franchi A, L'Allemain G, Paris S. A specific mutation abolishing Na^+/H^+ antiport activity in hamster fibroblasts precludes growth at neutral and acidic pH. Proc Natl Acad Sci USA 1984;81:4833–4837.
11. Sardet C, Franchi A, PouyssÄgur J. Molecular cloning, primary structure, and expression of the human growth factor-activatable Na^+/H^+ antiporter. Cell 1989;56:271–280.
12. Noel J, Pouyssegur J. Hormonal regulation, pharmacology, and membrane sorting of vertebrate Na^+/H^+ exchanger isoforms. Am J Physiol 1995;268:C283–C296.
13. Fliegel L, Dyck JR. Molecular biology of the cardiac sodium/hydrogen exchanger. Cardiovas Res 1995;29:155–159.
14. LaPointe MS, Batlle DC. Na^+/H^+ exchange and vascular smooth muscle proliferation. Am J Med Sci 1994;307(Suppl. 1):S9–S16.
15. Wakabayashi S, Sardet C, Fafournoux P, Counillon L, Meloche S, PagÄs G, PouyssÄgur J. Structure function of the growth factor-activatable Na^+/H^+ exchanger (NHE1). Rev Physiol Biochem Pharmacol 1992;119:157–185.
16. Grinstein S, Rotin D, Mason M. Na^+/H^+ exchange and growth factor-induced cytosolic pH changes. Role in cellular proliferation. Biochem Biophys Acta 1989;988:73–97.
17. Tse M, Levine S, Yun C, Brant S, Counillon L, Pouyssegur J, Donowitz M. Structure/function studies of the epithelial isoform of the mammalian Na^+/H^+ exchanger gene family. J Mem Biol 1993;135:93–108.
18. Tse C-M, Levine SA, Yun CHC, Montrose MH, Littles PJ, Pouyssegur J, Donowitz M. Cloning and expression of a rabbit cDNA encoding a serum-activated ethylisopropylamiloride-resistant epithelial Na^+/H^+ exchanger isoform (NHE-2). J Biol Chem 1993;268:11,917–11,924.
19. Tse CM, Watson AJM, Ma AI, Pouyssegur J, Donowitz M. Cloning and functional expression of a second novel rabbit ileal villus epithelial cell Na^+/H^+ exchanger (NHE-2). Gastroenterology 1992;100:A258.
20. Tse C-M, Brant SR, Walker MS, Pouyssegur J, Donowitz M. Cloning and sequencing of a rabbit cDNA encoding an intestinal and kidney-specific Na^+/H^+ exchanger isoform (NHE-3). J Biol Chem 1992;267:9340–9346.
21. Tse CM, Ma AI, Yang VW, Watson AJM, Levine S, Montrose MH, Potter J, Sardet C, Pouyssegur J, Donowitz M. Molecular cloning and expression of a cDNA encoding the rabbit ileal villus cell basolateral membrane Na^+/H^+ exchanger. EMBO J 1991;10:1957–1967.
22. Wakabayashi S, Fafournoux P, Sardet C, PouyssÄgur J. The Na^+/H^+ antiporter cytoplasmic domain mediates growth factor signals and controls "H^+-sensing." Proc Natl Acad Sci USA 1992;89:2424–2428.
23. Borgese F, Sardet C, Cappadoro M, Pouyssegor J, Motais R. Cloning and expression of a cAMP-activated Na^+/H^+ exchanger: Evidence that the cytoplasmic domain mediates hormonal regulation. Proc Natl Acad Sci USA 1992;89:6765–6769.
24. Baird N, Menon A, Wang Z, Meneton P, Su Y, Orlowski J, Shull G. Identification and cloning of a fifth member of the Na^+/H^+ exchanger gene family. J Am Soc Nephrol 1994;5:246.
25. Orlowski J, Kandasamy RA, Shull GE. Molecular cloning of putative members of the Na/H exchanger gene family. J Biol Chem 1992;267:9331–9339.

26. Mattei M, Sardet C, Franchi A, Pouyssegur J. The human amiloride-sensitive Na^+/H^+ antiporter is localized to chromosome 1 by in situ hybridization. Cytogenet Cell Genet 1988;48:6–8.
27. Kolyada A, Madias N. Proximal regulatory elements and nuclear activities for transcription of the human Na^+/H^+ exchanger (NHE-1) gene. Biochem Biophys Acta 1994;1217:54–64.
28. Kolyada A, Madias N. Transcriptional regulation of the human Na^+/H^+ exchanger (NHE-1) gene. In: DeSanto NG, Campaso G, eds. Acid-Base and Electrolyte Balance. Molecular, Cellular, and Clinical Aspects. Instituto Italiano per gli Studi Filosofici, Naples, Italy, 1995, pp. 19–28.
29. Szpirer C, Szpirer J, Riviere M, Levan G, Orlowski J. Chromosomal assignment of four genes encoding Na/H exchanger isoforms in human and rat. Mammalian Genome 1994;5:153–159.
30. Fafournoux P, Noel J, Pouyssegur J. Evidence that Na^+/H^+ exchanger isoforms NHE1 and NHE3 exist as stable dimers in membranes with a high degree of specificity for homodimers. J Biol Chem 1994;269:2589–2596.
31. Counillon L, Pouyssegur J. Structure-function studies and molecular regulation of the growth factor activatable sodium-hydrogen exchanger (NHE-1). Cardiovasc Res 1995;29:147–154.
32. Brock T, Lewis L, Smith J. Angiotensin increases Na^+ entry and Na^+/K^+ transport in cultures of smooth muscle from rat aorta. Proc Natl Acad Sci USA 1982;79:1438–1442.
33. Smith J, Brock T. Analysis of angiotensin-stimulated sodium transport in cultured smooth muscle cells from rat aorta. J Cell Physiol 1983;114:284–290.
34. Owen N. Platelet-derived growth factor stimulates Na^+ influx in VSMCs. Am J Physiol 1984;247: C501–C505.
35. Little PJ, Edward J, Cragoe J, Bobik A. Na-H exchange is a major pathway for Na influx in rat vascular smooth muscle. Am J Physiol 1986;251:C707–C712.
36. Bobik A, Grooms A, Little P, Cragoe E, Grinpukel S. Ethylisopropyl-amiloride-sensitive pH control mechanisms modulate VSMC growth. Am J Physiol 1991;255:C581–C588.
37. Weissberg P, Little P, Cragoe E, Bobik A. Na-H antiport in cultured rat aortic smooth muscle: its role in cytoplasmic pH regulation. Am J Physiol 1987;253:C193–C198.
38. LaPointe MS, Batlle DC. Na-dependent, HCO_3—dependent acid extrusion in vascular smooth muscle. Clin Res 1991;39:362A (abstract).
39. LaPointe M, Ye M, Moe O, Alpern R, Batlle D. Na^+/H^+ antiporter (NHE-1 isoform) in cultured vascular smooth muscle from the spontaneously hypertensive rat. Kidney Intern 1995;47:78–87.
40. Moolenaar W, Tertoolen L, de Laat S. Na^+/H^+ exchange and cytosolic pH in the action of growth factors in human fibroblasts. Nature 1983;304:645–648.
41. Moolenaar W, Tertoolen L, de Laat S. The regulation of cytoplasmic pH in human fibroblasts. J Biol Chem 1984;259:7563–7569.
42. LaPointe M, Batlle D. Control of steady state intracellular pH (pH_i) in VSMCs (vsmc). Am J Hypertens 1989;2:69A.
43. Rao G, Sardet C, PouyssÄgur J, Berk B. Differential regulation of Na^+/H^+ antiporter gene expression in VSMCs by hypertrophic and hyperplastic stimuli. J Biol Chem 1990;265:19,393–19,396.
44. Lucchesi PA, DeRoux N, Berk BC. Na(+)-H^+ exchanger expression in vascular smooth muscle of spontaneously hypertensive and Wistar-Kyoto rats. Hypertension 1994;24:734–738.
45. Balkovetz D, Wang D, Warnock D. The cytosolic tail influences H^+-affinity and maximal velocity of the human Na^+/H^+ exchanger (NHE-1). J Am Soc Nephrol 1994;5:265.
46. Otsu K, Kinesella J, Sacktor B, Froelich J. Transient state kinetic evidence for an oligomer in the mechanism of Na^+–H^+ exchange. Proc Natl Acad Sci USA 1989;86:4818–4822.
47. Otsu K, Kinesella J, Heller P, Froelich J. Sodium dependence of the Na(+)–H^+ exchanger in the pre-steady state. Implications for the exchange mechanism. J Biol Chem 1993;268:3184–3193.
48. Clark J, Limbird L. Na(+)–H^+ exchanger subtypes: a predictive review. Am J Physiol 1991;261: C945–C953.
49. Counillon L, Franchi A, Pouyssegur J. A point mutation of the Na^+/H^+ exchange gene (NHE-1) and amplification of the mutated allele confer amiloride resistance upon chronic acidosis. Proc Natl Acad Sci USA 1993;90:4508–4512.
50. Goss G, Woodside M, Wakabayashi S, Pouyssegur J, Waddell T, Downey G, Grinstein S. ATP dependence of NHE-1, the ubiquitous isoform of the Na^+/H^+ antiporter. J Biol Chem 1994;269:8741–8748.
51. Grinstein S, Rothstein A. Mechanisms of regulation of the Na^+/H^+ exchanger. J Mem Biol 1986;90:1–12.
52. Sardet C, Counillon L, Franchi A, PouyssÄgur J. Growth factors induce phosphorylation of the Na^+/H^+ antiporter, glycoprotein of 110 kD. Science 1990;247:723–726.
53. Sardet C, Fafournoux P, PouyssÄgur J. A-thrombin, EGF and okadaic acid activate the Na^+/H^+ exchanger, NHE-1, by phosphorylating a set of common sites. J Biol Chem 1991;266:1916,1917.

54. Wakabayashi S, Bertrand B, Shigekawa M, Fafournoux P, Pouyssegur J. Growth factor activation and "H(+)-sensing" of the Na^+/H^+ exchanger isoform 1 (NHE1). Evidence for an additional mechanism not requiring direct phosphorylation. J Biol Chem 1994;269:5583–5588.
55. Bertrand B, Wakabayashi S, Ikeda T, Pouyssegur J, Shigekawa M. The Na^+/H^+ exchanger isoform 1 (NHE1) is a novel member of the calmodulin-binding proteins. Identification and characterization of calmodulin-binding sites. J Biol Chem 1994;269:13,703–13,709.
56. Wakabayashi S, Bertrand B, Ikeda T, Pouyssegur J, Shigekawa M. Mutation of calmodulin-binding site renders the Na^+/H^+ exchanger (NHE1) highly H(+)-sensitive and Ca^{2+} regulation-defective. J Biol Chem 1994;269:13,710–13,715.
57. Aronson P. Kinetic properties of the plasma membrane Na^+–H^+ exchanger. Annu Rev Physiol 1985;47:545–560.
58. Saleh A, Batlle D. Kinetic properties of the Na^+/H^+ antiporter of lympocytes from the spontaneously hypertensive rat. J Clin Invest 1990;85:1734–1739.
59. Berk BC, Aronow MS, Brock TA, Edward Cragoe J, Michael A, Gimbrone J, Alexander RW. Angiotensin II-stimulated Na^+/H^+ exchanger in cultured VSMCs. J Biol Chem 1987;262:5057–5064.
60. Lucchesi PA, Berk BC. Regulation of sodium-hydrogen exchange in vascular smooth muscle. Cardiovasc Res 1995;29:172–177.
61. Batlle D, Redon J, Gutterman C, LaPointe M, Saleh A, Rombola G, Ye M, Gomez L, Sobrero M. Acid-base status and intracellular pH regulation in lymphocytes from rats with genetic hypertension. J Am Soc Nephrol 1994;5:S6–S11.
62. LaPointe M, Bacallao R, Batlle D. Differential expression of the NHE-1 isoform of the Na^+/H^+ antiporter in lymphocytes and cultured VSMCs from the spontaneously hypertensive rat. J Am Soc Nephrol 1994;5:543.
63. Moolenaar W, Boonstra J, van der Saag P, de Laat S. Sodium/proton exchange in mouse neuroblastoma cells. J Biol Chem 1981;256:12,883–12,887.
64. Moolenaar W, Mummery C, van der Saag P, de Laat S. Rapid ionic events and the initiation of growth in serum-stimulated neuroblastoma cells. Cell 1982;23:789–798.
65. Moolenaar W, Tertoolen L, de Laat S. Phorbol ester and diacylglycerol mimic growth factors in raising cytoplasmic pH. Nature 1984;312:371–374.
66. Okada K, Ishikawa S, Saito T. Mechanisms of vasopressin-induced increase in intracellular Na^+ in VSMCs. Am J Physiol 1991;261:F1007–F1011.
67. Kikeri D, Zeidel M, Ballermann B, Brenner B, Hebert S. pH regulation and response to AVP in A10 cells differ markedly in the presence vs. absence of CO_2-HCO_3^-. Am J Physiol 1990;259:C471–C483.
68. Ganz M, Boyarsky G, Boron W, Sterzel R. Effects of angiotensin II and vasopressin on intracellular pH of glomerular mesangial cells. Am J Physiol 1988;254:F787–F794.
69. Ye M, Flores G, Batlle D. Angiotensin II and angiotensin 1-7 effects on free cytosolic sodium and intracellular pH and the Na^+/H^+ antiporter in vascular smooth muscle. Hypertension 1996;27:72–78.
70. Johnson E, Theler J, Capponi A, Vallotton M. Characterization of oscillations in cytosolic free Ca^{2+} concentration and measurement of cytosolic Na^+ concentration changes evoked by angiotensin II and vasopressin in individual rat aortic smooth muscle cells. Use of microfluorometry and digital imaging. J Biol Chem 1991;266:12,618–12,626.
71. Mene P, Dubyak G, Scarpa A, Dunn M. Regulation of cytosolic pH of cultured mesangial cells by prostaglandin F2 alpha and thromboxane A2. Am J Physiol 1991;260:C159–C166.
72. Paris S, PouyssÄgur J. Growth factors activate the Na^+–H^+ antiporter in quiescent fibroblasts by increasing its affinity for intracellular H^+. J Biol Chem 1984;259:10,989 10,994.
73. Vallega G, Canessa M, Berk B, Brock T, Alexander W. Vascular smooth muscle Na^+-H^+ exchanger kinetics and its activation by angiotensin II. Am J Physiol 1988;254: C751–C758.
74. Krug L, Berk B. Na^+,K^+-adenosine triphosphate regulation in hypertrophied VSMCs. Hypertension 1992;20:138–143.
75. Hatori N, Fine B, Nakamura A, Cragoe E, Aviv A. Angiotensin II effect on cytosolic pH in cultured VSMCs. J Biol Chem 1987;262:5073–5078.
76. Taubman M, Berk B, Izumo S, Tsuda T, Alexander R, Nadal-Ginard B. Angiotensin II induces c-fos mRNA in aortic smooth muscle. Role of Ca^{2+} mobilization and PKC activation. J Biol Chem 1989;264:526–530.
77. Lyall F, Morton JJ, Lever AF, Cragoe EJ. Angiotensin II activates Na^+-H^+ exchange and stimulates growth in cultured VSMCs. J Hypertens 1988;6:S438–S441.
78. Geisterfer AA, Peach MJ, Owens GK. Angiotensin II induces hypertrophy, not hyperplasia, of cultured rat aortic smooth muscle cells. Circ Res 1988;62:749–756.

79. Campbell-Boswell M, Robertson AL, Jr. Effects of angiotensin II and vasopressin on human smooth muscle cells in vitro. Exp Mol Pathol 1981;35:265–276.
80. Weber H, Taylor DS, Molloy CJ. Angiotensin II induces delayed mitogenesis and cellular proliferation in rat aortic smooth muscle cells. Correlation with the expression of specific endogenous growth factors and reversal by suramin. J Clin Invest 1994;93:788–798.
81. Boyarsky G, Ganz M, Sterzel R, Boron W. pH regulation in single glomerular mesangial cells II. Na-dependent and -independent Cl^--HCO_3^--exchangers. Am J Physiol: Cell 1988;255:C857–C869.
82. Boyarsky G, Ganz M, Sterzel R, Boron W. pH regulation in single glomerular mesangial cells I. Acid extrusion in absence and presence of HCO_3^--. Am J Physiol: Cell 1988;255:C844–C856.
83. Korbmacher C, Helbig H, Stahl F, Wiederholt M. Evidence for Na/H exchange and Cl^-/HCO_3^- exchange in A10 VSMCs. Pflugers Arch 1988;412:29–36.
84. Vigne P, Breittmayer J, Frelin C, Lazdunski M. Dual control of the intracellular pH in aortic smooth muscle cells by a cAMP-sensitive HCO_3^-/Cl^- antiporter and a protein kinase c-sensitive Na^+/H^+ antiporter. J Biol Chem 1988;263:18,023–18,029.
85. Drenckhahn D, Zinke K, Schauer U, Appell K, Low P. Identification of immunoreactive forms of human erythrocyte band 3 in nonerythroid cells. Eur J Cell Biol 1984;34:144–150.
86. Alper SL. The band 3-related anion exchanger (AE) gene family. Annu Rev Physiol 1991;53:549–564.
87. Kopito RR. Molecular biology of the anion exchanger gene family. Intern Rev Cytol 1990;123:177–199.
88. Kopito R, HF L. Primary structure and transmembrane orientation of the murine anion exchange protein. Nature 1985;316:234–238.
89. Boron W. Intracellular pH regulation in epithelial cells. Annu Rev Physiol 1986;48:377–388.
90. Putnam R. pH regulatory transport systems in a smooth muscle-like cell line. Am J Physiol 1990;258:C470–C479.
91. Neylon CB, Little PJ, Cragoe EJ Jr, Bobik A. Intracellular pH in Human Arterial Smooth Muscle. Circ Res 1990;67:814–825.
92. Little PJ, Neylon CB, Farrelly CA, Weissberg PL, Cragoe EJ, Jr, Bobik A. Intracellular pH in vascular smooth muscle: regulation by sodium-hydrogen exchange and multiple sodium dependent HCO_3^- mechanisms. Cardiovasc Res 1995;29:239–246.
93. LaPointe M, Batlle D. A NEM-sensitive, ATP dependent mechanism of Na-independent intracellular pH regulation in VSMCs (VSMC). J Am Soc Nephrol 1990;1:474.
94. McCabe RD, Young DB. Evidence of a K(+)–H(+)-ATPase in VSMCs. Am J Physiol 1992;262:H1955–H1958.
95. Flores G, Ye M, LaPointe M, Batlle D. Ionic effects of angiotensin II and their role in the activation of the Na^+/H^+ antiporter. Kidney Int 1996;49(Suppl. 55), in press.
96. Ganz M, Boyarsky G, Sterzel R, Boron W. Arginine vasopressin enhances pH_i regulation in the presence of HCO_3^- by stimulating three acid-base transport systems. Nature 1989;337:648–651.
97. Daugirdas JT, Arrieta J, Ye M, Flores G, Batlle D. Intracellular acidification associated with changes in free cytosolic calcium. J Clin Invest 1995;95:1480–1489.
98. Siskind M, McCoy C, Chobanian A, Schwartz J. Regulation of intracellular calcium by cell pH in VSMCs. Am J Physiol 1989;256:C234–C240.
99. Putnam R, Douglass P. Effect of changes of pH_i on intracellular calcium in a smooth muscle-like cell line. Mol Cell Biochem 1990;99:89–95.
100. Batlle DC, Peces R, LaPointe MS, Ye M, Daugirdas JT. Cytosolic free calcium regulation in response to acute changes in intracellular pH in vascular smooth muscle. Am J Physiol 1993;264:C932–C943.
101. Batlle D, Godinich M, LaPointe M, Munoz E, Carone F, Mehring N. Extracellular Na^+ dependency of free cytosolic Ca^{2+} regulation in aortic VSMCs. Am J Physiol 1991;261:C845–C856.
102. Dunnett J, Nayler W. Effect of pH on calcium accumulation and release by isolated fragments of cardiac and skeletal muscle sarcoplasmic reticulum. Arch Biochem Biophys 1979;198:434–438.
103. Fabiato A, Fabiato F. Effects of pH on the myofilaments and the sarcoplasmic reticulum of skinned cells from cardiac and skeletal muscles. J Physiol (Lond) 1978;276:233–255.
104. Iino S, Hayashi H, Saito H, Tokuno H, Tomita T. Effects of intracellular pH on calcium currents and intracellular calcium ions in the smooth muscle of rabbit portal vein. Exp Physiol 1994;79:669–680.
105. Root MJ, Mackinnon R. Two identical noninteracting sites in an ion channel revealed by proton transfer. Science 1994;265:1852–1856.
106. Godinich M, LaPointe M, Batlle D. Free cytosolic calcium regulation via Na^+/Ca^{2+} exchange in VSMCs. Ann NY Acad Sci 1991;639:561–565.
107. Smith J. Angiotensin-receptor signalling in cultured VSMCs. Am J Physiol 1986;250:F759–F769.

108. Smith J, Smith L. Extracellular Na^+ dependence of changes in free Ca^{2+}, $45Ca^{2+}$ efflux, and total cell Ca^{2+} produced by angiotensin II in cultured arterial muscle cells. J Biol Chem 1987;262:17,455–17,460.
109. Nabel E, Berk B, Brock T, TW S. Na^+–Ca^{2+} exchange in cultured VSMCs. Circ Res 1988;62:486–493.
110. Brass L, Joseph S. A role for inositol triphosphate in intracellular Ca^{2+} mobilization and granule secretion in platelets. J Biol Chem 1985;260:15,172–15,179.
111. Missiaen L, Taylor C, Berridge M. Spontaneous calcium release from inositol triphosphate sensitive calcium stores. Nature 1991;352:241–244.
112. Snyder S, Suppatapone S. Isolation and functional characterization of an inositol triphosphate receptor from brain. Cell Calcium 1989;10:337–342.
113. Schulz I, Thevenod F, Dehlinger-Kremer M. Modulation of intracellular free Ca^{2+} concentration by IP_3-sensitive and IP_3-insensitive nonmitochondrial Ca^{2+} pools. Cell Calcium 1989;10:325–336.
114. Smith J, Dwyer S, Smith L. Decreasing extracellular Na^+ concentration triggers inositol polyphosphate production and Ca^{2+} mobilization. J Biol Chem 1989;264:831–837.
115. Cobbold P, Rink T. Fluorescence and bioluminescence measurement of cytoplasmic free calcium. Biochem J 1987;248:313–328.

23 Endocrine Regulation of Vascular Smooth Muscle Intermediary Metabolism

Ligia J. Dominguez, MD, *Jacob D. Peuler,* PHD, *and James R. Sowers,* MD

CONTENTS

INTRODUCTION

Vascular smooth muscle (VSM) is uniquely suited to its role as a regulator of blood flow to various tissues. VSM is able to maintain tension for prolonged periods under conditions that would rapidly fatigue skeletal muscle *(1)*. Its relatively slow mechanical properties and high economy of tension maintenance allow for tight coupling between energy supply via intermediary metabolism and energy demand needed for contractile processes *(2)*. Metabolism of VSM cells (VSMC) is characterized by substantial production of lactic acid even under fully oxygenated conditions *(3–6)*. An important physiological role for VSMC aerobic lactate production is to provide energy for membrane sodium–potassium (Na^+–K^+)–adenosine triphosphatase (ATPase) pump activity in basal tonic conditions *(7–9)*. Carbohydrate (CHO) metabolism in VSMC is compartmented and utilizes two functionally independent Embden-Meyerhof pathways *(10,11)*. One pathway is involved in catabolism of extracellular glucose to lactate, and the other involves oxidative metabolism of glycosyl units derived from glycogen. That VSMC produce considerable lactic acid even under fully oxygenated conditions underlies the

From: *Contemporary Endocrinology: Endocrinology of the Vasculature*
Edited by: J. R. Sowers Humana Press Inc., Totowa, NJ

importance of CHO as energy substrate for these cells. However, other data suggest that the primary oxidative substrate in quiescent vascular segments are fatty acid (FA) derived from endogenous VSMC lipid stores *(12–14)*. Alterations in substrate supply and utilization at the vasculature may occur in diseases linked to decreased insulin action, such as type II diabetes mellitus (NIDDM), essential hypertension, and atherosclerosis *(15)*. Furthermore, drugs with effects on carbohydrate and lipid metabolism of vascular tissues, such as biguanides and thiazolidinediones, via changes in substrate utilization, can modify vascular tension maintenance. This chapter reviews intermediary VSMC metabolism and associated effects of drugs that have an impact on this phenomenon.

DIFFERENCES IN ENERGETIC STRATEGY IN SKELETAL VS SMOOTH MUSCLE

VSMC have very low energy demands compared to skeletal muscle *(16,17)*. Skeletal and VSM rely on different mechanisms for provision of ATP to meet contractile energy demands. VSM relies on energy metabolism for the maintenance of its normal function and requires a tight coordination between energy utilization and energy production (Fig. 1A) *(16–18)*. Skeletal muscle contains up to 30 times the amount of phosphocreatine (PC) and preformed ATP compared to that stored in VSM. Thus, normal contractile activity of VSM can be supported for a substantial period of time before metabolic resynthesis is required *(16)*. For example, during contraction frog sartorius skeletal muscle utilizes ATP approx 100 times faster than its aerobic metabolism can resynthesize ATP. This large increase in energy demand is met primarily by the 15–30 µmol/g pool of preformed high-energy phosphate (PO_4) in the form of PC. This store is rapidly decreased during contraction, limiting the ability to maintain force, and is replenished on a time scale much longer than that required for VSMC contractile events *(19)*.

VSMC have a PC pool in the order of magnitude of 1–3 µmol/g, similar to the pool of preformed ATP. Thus, the concept of a pool of PC as a buffer for ATP is less meaningful in VSMC. In contrast to skeletal muscle, tonic contraction of VSM is associated with only a two- to threefold increase in ATP utilization. Essentially no change in the ATP + PC content of the VSM occurs as the ATP breakdown can be matched by the rate of its aerobic resynthesis. VSMC cannot attain the peak of an isometric contraction if solely dependent on the preformed high-energy PO_4 *(20)*.

There are several theories to explain the mechanism underlying the ability of VSM to maintain high levels of force with low rates of PO_4 utilization. The specific actomyosin ATPase activity of VSMC is very low relative to that of skeletal muscle *(21)*. Low actomyosin ATPase and consequently low tension may result from the relatively low rate of dissociation of the actin–myosin complex in VSMC *(22,23)*. Also, an alteration of the kinetics of the actin–myosin interaction during the catch phase results in the formation of attached, noncycling cross-bridges in porcine carotid artery *(24)*. Several types of smooth muscle exhibit myosin light-chain phosphorylation-dependent changes in cross-bridge cycling rates for a given load *(25,26)*. Thus, formation of dephosphorylated, slowly cycling or noncycling latch bridges may act as an internal load on remaining phosphorylated cross-bridges, decrease shortening velocity, with an initial high rate of PO_4 utilization during tension development and a low steady-state level during tension maintenance in parallel with myosin light-chain phosphorylation. Cross-bridges in smooth muscle modified by phosphorylation and dephosphorylation can yield four, rather

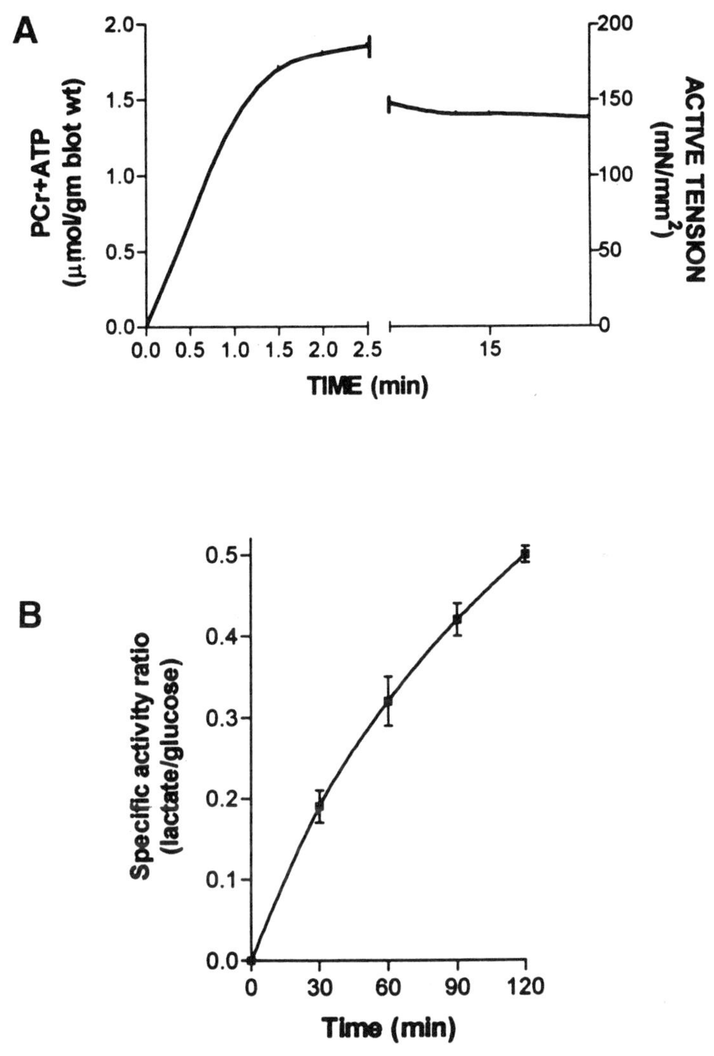

Fig. 1. (A) Relation between phosphagen content (phosphocreatine + ATP) and active isometric tension at 37°C as a function of time after initiation of contraction by addition of 50 mM KCl to the bath medium. Adapted from ref. *2*. **(B)** Equilibration of ^{14}C from media glucose into the lactic acid pool and the effect of K^+ depolarization on the steady state lactate specific activity ratio under aerobic conditions. Reprinted with permission from ref. *10*. Copyright 1983 American Association for the Advancement of Science.

than two, cross-bridge states *(26)*. Ionic calcium (Ca^{2+})-dependent force maintenance without detectable elevations in phosphorylation has been termed latch contraction *(27)*, latch contraction depends on a state of reduced cross-bridge cycling rates that are dependent on low levels of Ca^{2+}-dependent cross-bridge phosphorylation *(28)*. VSMC have regulated cross-bridge cycling rates with variable shortening velocities and ATP consumption rates *(29,30)*.

In early studies, the approach of VSM energetics was phenomenological and involved quantitation of muscle heat production and mechanical output. With the development of techniques for the direct assessment of ATP breakdown during contraction, the emphasis has recently shifted to kinetic studies of the actomyosin ATPase *in situ*. The focus is on how mechanical force affect this reaction, in order to understand the mechanochemical transduction events at the cross-bridge level. In parallel with these studies, VSM energetics now encompasses metabolism particularly energy metabolism, which focuses on mechanisms underlying the coordination of metabolism and contractility.

COMPARTMENTALIZATION OF GLYCOLYTIC AND OXIDATIVE METABOLISM

Early investigations into the coupling between energy transduction and metabolism in VSMC *(31,32)* suggested that specific metabolic pathways could independently supply energy for ion transport and actin–myosin interactions. Indeed, oxidative phosphorylation is coupled to tension generation/maintenance *(33,34)*, and aerobic glycolysis, vital in VSMC metabolism, is independently coupled to Na^+–K^+ transport *(7,35)*. Further, glycolytic and oxidative metabolism can independently supply energy for VSMC metabolism and glycolysis, and lactate production occurs under fully oxygenated conditions in VSMC (Fig. 1B) *(3–6)*.

Diversion of glucose metabolism from lactate production to glucose oxidation has an unfavorable effect on high-energy PO_4 metabolism in resting VSMC *(3)*. Also, in microvascular endothelial cells the primary end product of glucose metabolism is lactate, with relatively small CO_2 and pyruvate production *(36)*. However, there appear to be an increased aerobic lactate production with aging, hypertension, and atherosclerosis *(37,38)*. Under resting conditions, the rate of oxygen consumption and lactate production usually equals approx 30% of the ATP supply coming from aerobic glycolysis. However, at least 90% of glucose metabolism involves glycolysis resulting in considerable lactate production *(39)*. Compartmentation of VSMC metabolism and function is never absolute, and normal ionic gradients can be maintained in VSMC by oxidative metabolism in the absence of glucose, or by glycolysis in the absence of oxygen *(40–42)*.

Evidence for compartmentalized carbohydrate metabolism in VSMC include several studies *(43,44)* showing that the rate of lactate production under aerobic conditions increases in response to stimulation by pharmacological agents as well as by high K^+. However, when there is substitution of K^+ for Na^+, lactate production does not increase during contraction; rather, there is usually a decrease in production rate compared to resting conditions *(8,45)*. Ouabain and other procedures that inhibit Na^+–K^+ transport also result in a decrease in VSMC aerobic lactate production with an increase in oxygen consumption proportional to the active force production. Thus, under fully oxygenated conditions, glycolysis with lactate formation provides the ATP required for Na^+ and K^+ transport. In intact carotid arteries, aerobic lactate production is stoichiometrically linked to K^+ uptake, and glucose is the preferred substrate under physiological conditions *(7)*. Coupling of these independent metabolic pathways with specific energy utilization constitutes a process by which energy production and transduction can be closely and efficiently regulated (Fig. 2).

Coupling between aerobic glycolysis and Na^+–K^+ transport is a sensitive and efficient means of coordinating energy metabolism with VSMC ion transport at the membrane. Additionally, regulation of substrate supply (i.e., glucose transport) also may be closely coordinated with changes in ion transport. Thus, alterations in the microenvironment of

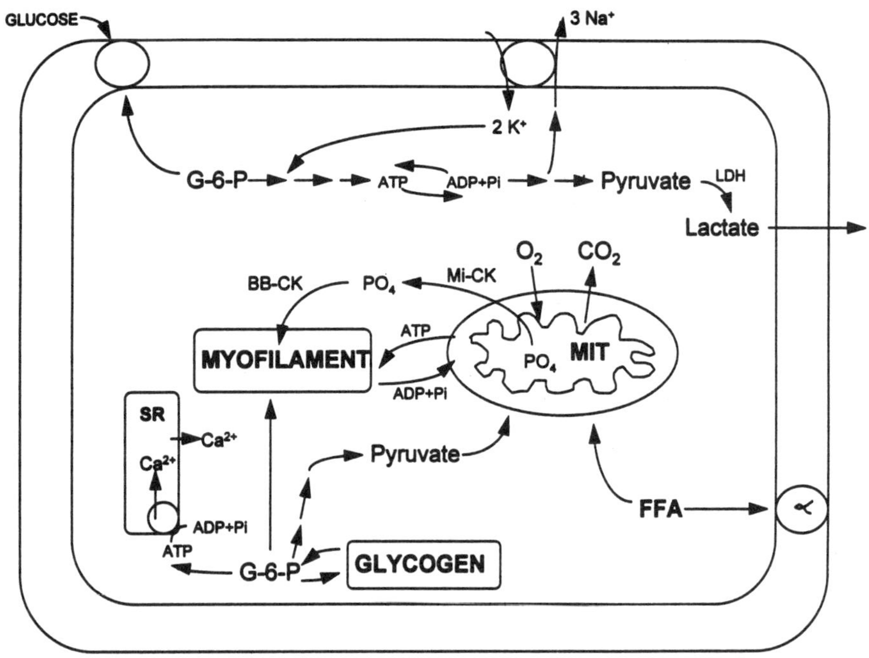

Fig. 2. Compartmentation of energetic metabolism in VCM. This scheme summarizes the coupling of aerobic glycolysis and membrane energy requirements, whereas oxidative metabolism is more strongly correlated with the level of isometric force. FA are oxidated in VSMC and they may enhance α-adrenoreceptor responsiveness. α, α-adrenergic receptor; BB-CK, cytosolic creatine kinase; LDH, lactic dehydrogenase; Mi-CK, mitochondrial creatine kinase; SR, smooth endoplasmic reticulum.

each compartment may independently regulate intermediate metabolism and therefore allow VSMC to quickly and efficiently respond to localized stimuli. Thus, stimulation of Na^+–K^+ transport could effectively regulate energy production at the VSMC membrane level without mobilizing or competing with the energy transduction of other cellular processes. This compartmentation of energy utilization may be highly advantageous, since oxidative metabolism is closely coordinated with mechanical VSM activity and therefore regulation of blood flow.

Glycolysis and VSMC $[Ca^{2+}]_i$ Metabolism

Aerobic glycolysis is also the preferred source for normal $[Ca^{2+}]_i$ homeostasis (Fig. 2) *(46)*. As such, glucose deprivation lead to a number of changes in porcine carotid artery that reflect altered $[Ca^{2+}]_i$ homeostasis:

1. Glucose is required for normal excitation-contraction coupling.
2. It is required for an efficient maintenance of VSMC $[Ca^{2+}]_i$ stores.
3. Basal VSM tension is increased in the absence of glucose, and this effect can be reversed by glucose or a calcium channel blocker, but not by β-hydroxybutyrate.

Alterations of glycolysis can occur under a number of pathological circumstances, such as ischemia or hypoxia that might increase vascular sensitivity via alterations of glycolytic metabolism affecting VSMC $[Ca^{2+}]_i$ homeostasis *(47)*.

VSMC Creatine Kinase (CK)

The small amount of PC found in various smooth muscle tissue is linearly related to its CK activity *(48)*. CK isoenzymes are compartmentalized in VSMC providing evidence of a model where PO_4 is transferred from mitochondria (Mi) to the cytoplasm via Mi-CK at mitochondrial sites and via cytosolic CK (BB-CK) at myofibrillar sites (Fig. 2) *(49)*. This compartmentalized CK activity is associated with subcellular high-energy turnover and takes on a dual role in enzymatic reactions and structural integrity of myofilaments and organelles *(41)*.

Glycogen

Although membrane cation transport function is dependent on aerobic glycolytic metabolism, energy requirements of VSMC contractile proteins may be fulfilled by oxidative metabolism *(10,11,50–53)*. The vascular wall is richly endowed with endogenous stores of fats and glycogen *(12)*, and in steady-state low-tension-generating conditions, lipids appear to be utilized as the primary substrate for Mi oxidative metabolism *(12–14)*. However, glycogen phosphorylase is activated during transitions to higher tension states, implying that glycogen is utilized under these conditions *(54–56)*. Coupling of glycogenolysis to Mi respiration may have evolved as a direct response to VSMC energy needs. Specifically, the large glycogenolytic response in initial contractile stimulation may be necessary to maximize the cellular production of ATP during the pre-steady-state. This is supported by radiolabeled studies showing that glycogen is utilized as a primary oxidative substrate during active tension generation *(56,57)*. However, only 50–60% of the VSMC glycogen content can be mobilized during active contraction *(12,56)*. Furthermore, tension can be maintained at elevated levels even after glycogenolysis has decreased *(51,58)*. Thus, a close coordination of glycogenolysis with rapid increases in Mi respiration (increases in Mi redox potential) may be important for maintenance of stable cellular phosphorylation potential.

VSMC LIPID METABOLISM

A physiological role of CHO in energy metabolism in VSMC is evidenced by the observation of lactic acid production in VSMC, even under oxygenated conditions *(3–6)*. Further, vascular contraction is associated with substantial glycogenolysis, reinforcing the notion that CHO are the primary substrate for VSMC *(12–14)*. However, non-CHO substrates, including certain FA, can restore contractile responses to substrate-depleted rabbit aorta *(58)*. Also VSMC can oxidize FA *(12–14)*. Indeed, the primary oxidative substrate in quiescent vascular segments may be FA-derived from endogenous VSMC lipid stores (Fig. 2) *(12)*. FA can alter glucose and glycogen metabolism in both resting and contracting VSM. Incubation of arterial segments with FA suppress glycolysis and decrease lactate content of porcine carotid arteries *(59)*. Glycogenolysis that accompanies contractile activation of vascular segments by K^+ depolarization is not demonstrable in the presence of FA *(60)*. Further, FA have been shown to stimulate glycogen phosphorylase, phosphorylase kinase, and phosphorylase phosphatase activities in VSMC *(61)*. FA of varying lengths may affect CHO metabolism differently. This is extensively reviewed in Chapter 12.

Recently it has been observed that linoleic acid and its metabolic products are potential mitogens in VSMC *(62)*. Conditions such as oxidative stress and lipid peroxidation, which stimulate production of these substances, may alter VSMC growth. Energy ordinarily generated by the aerobic glycolysis of extracellular glucose to lactate can be provided by the oxidation of FA. Further, activity of the glycolytic pathway accounting for aerobic lactate production can be regulated by feedback of products of FA oxidation *(59)*. These results suggest that functional compartmentation is not absolute or not constantly operative in VSMC, and it can be affected by the availability of different substrates. FA may enhance vascular α-adrenergic tone by various pathways, including direct mechanisms such as increase in sympathetic drive *(63)* and α-adrenoreceptor responsiveness *(64)* as well as indirect routes such as impaired endothelium-dependent vasodilation *(65)* and vascular remodeling *(66,67)*.

Abnormalities in FA as well as glucose metabolism occur in type II diabetes mellitus. Hyperglycemia leads to the production of diacylglycerol, an important regulator of protein kinase C (PKC), which might have an important role in the pathogenesis of diabetic complications *(15,68,69)*. The combined effects of altered FA and CHO metabolism may produce an even greater activation of PKC and worsening of the cardiovascular injury risk than either defect alone. Altered CHO and lipid homeostasis could also change the availability of metabolic substrates, thereby modifying compartmentation of metabolic pathways, leading to increases in VSM contractility and/or proliferation. Indeed, diabetic hypertensive hearts have a marked reduction in the rate of glucose oxidation and relatively greater palmitate oxidation *(70)*. These observations may have relevance in the pathogenesis of cardiomyopathy associated with diabetes mellitus.

PHARMACOLOGIC AGENTS THAT COULD ALTER VSM ENERGETIC METABOLISM

In the clinical setting, drugs that may alter carbohydrate and lipid metabolism of VSMC could alter the substrate availability, transport, and/or metabolic pathway, consequently changing PKC and vascular contractility or ionic handling *(15)*. These drugs include the biguanide metformin which increases peripheral insulin action *(71–73)*, and enhances glucose transport in VSMC, independent of the presence of insulin or IGF-I (Fig. 3) *(74)*. As such, metformin in vitro attenuates KCl^- and norepinephrine (NE)-induced contraction of rat tail artery rings *(75,76)*, attenuates platelet-derived growth factor (PDGF)-, angiotensin II (AII)- *(77)*, and thrombin-induced increases in VSMC $[Ca^{2+}]_i$ responses *(74)*. Metformin also decreases VSMC growth *(77)* and improves cardiac performance in diabetic rats *(78)*. Since metformin also affects lipid metabolism *(79,80)*, it may change the substrate availability for VSMC metabolism.

Another class of insulin-sensitizing agents, the thiazolidinediones, lower blood glucose, plasma triglycerides, plasma insulin concentrations, and blood pressure in insulin-resistant rodent models of diabetes *(81–84)* and in obese patients *(85)*. Treatment of insulin-resistant animals with these compounds results in enhancement of insulin action in vitro in the three major target tissues of insulin action: stimulation of glucose uptake, glucose oxidation, and lipogenesis in adipose and muscle as well as stimulation of lipogenesis and inhibition of glucose output by the liver *(86–88)*. They also prevent hyperglycemia-induced insulin resistant in rat fibroblasts *(89)*. Additionally, these compounds may affect critical steps in the intracellular insulin signaling, such as PI 3-kinase *(90)* and also, may block the effect of tumor necrosis factor-α *(91)*, which may have a

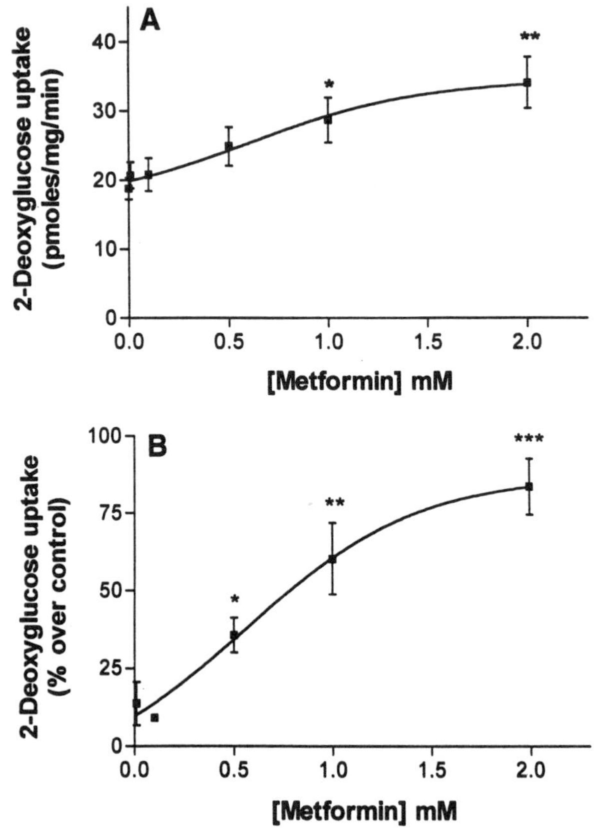

Fig. 3. Effect of metformin on 2-DOG uptake in VSMC. VSMC from Sprague-Dawley rat aortas were isolated and cultured. Cells were incubated with the indicated concentrations for 24 h at 37°C before $[^3H]$2-DOG uptake. **(A)** Results expressed as pmol/mg/min 2-DOG uptake. **(B)** Same results as in A expressed as a percentage change over transport in untreated cells. $*p < 0.05$; $**p < 0.01$; $***p < 0.001$.

direct role in obesity-linked insulin resistance and type II diabetes *(92,93)*. Effects of these compounds on lipid metabolism include normalization of fructose-induced hypertriglyceridemia in rats *(94)* and reduction in total cholesterol and triglycerides in NIDDM patients *(95)*.

There is increasing evidence that the hypotensive effects of the thiazoladinediones may be related to direct vascular metabolic effects. In this regard, both augmented vasoconstriction and impaired vasodilation have been associated with insulin resistance *(15)*. One of these compounds improves the action of insulin in liver, skeletal muscle, and adipose tissue directly *(96)*, and reduces elevated plasma glucose and insulin concentrations in diabetic animals with hyperinsulinemia *(96)*. Troglitazone is currently being studied in humans, and has been shown to improve both fasting and postprandial hyperglycemia and insulinemia in type II diabetics *(81)*, and decrease insulin resistance, improve lipid profiles, and lower blood pressure in obese women *(85)*. Preliminary studies in our laboratory suggest that this agent has both direct and indirect effects to promote vascular relaxation independently of nitric oxide production.

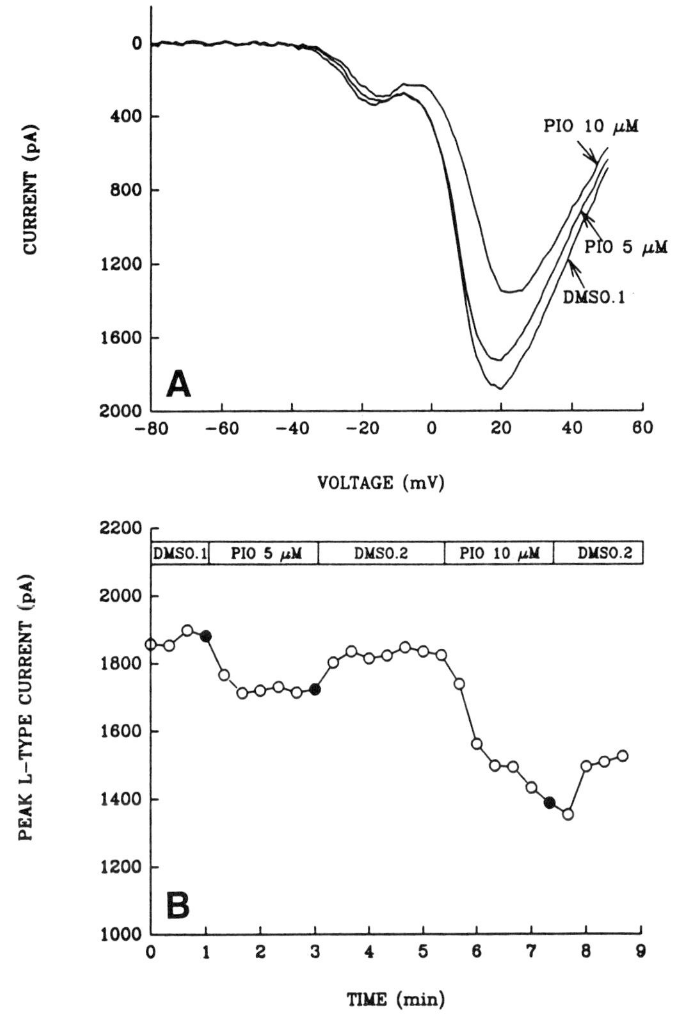

Fig. 4. Effect of pioglitazone on L-type current in tail artery VSMC. **(A)** Currents recorded in 5 and 10 μmol/L pioglitazone and 0.1% DMSO solutions at the solid circles in B. **(B)** representative time course of changes in peak L-type current. Control current was recorded in 0.1% DMSO solution.

The thiazoladinedione, pioglitazone, blocks voltage-dependent calcium channels *(97)* and decreases agonist-stimulated increases in $[Ca^{2+}]_i$ (Fig. 4) *(98)*. Troglitazone also decreases VSM contraction by inhibiting voltage-operated Ca^{2+} channels and by enhancing insulin-stimulated signal transduction *(99)*. Interestingly, metformin and pioglitazone, insulin-sensitizing agents from different groups, attenuate receptor (NE) and nonreceptor (KCl)-mediated contraction in tail arterial rings *(75,76)*, and this attenuation (especially for metformin) is enhanced in the presence of insulin *(75)*. Glyburide and other sulphonylureas (which do not lower blood pressure in animals and humans) close ATP-sensitive K^+ channels in arterial tissue *(100,101)*. Since these K^+ channels are responsible for vascular relaxation, this may account for increases in vascular tone associated with glyburide treatment *(75)*. Indeed, long-term administration of glyburide aggravates hypertension in female stroke-prone spontaneously hypertensive rats, probably related

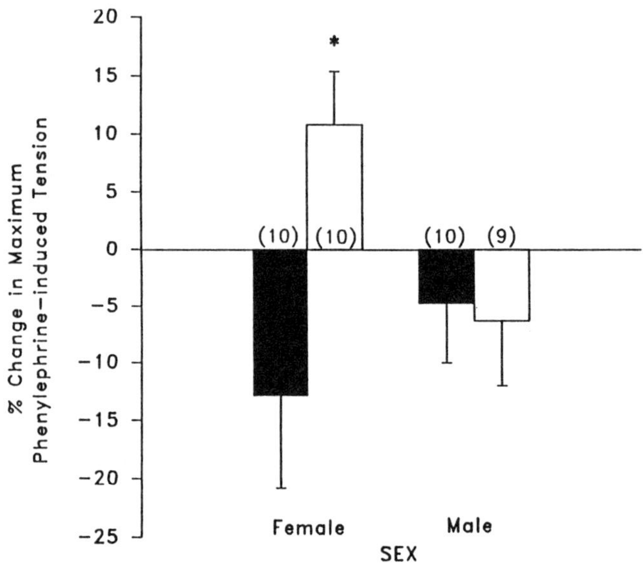

Fig. 5. Changes produced by insulin in vitro in maximum phenylephrine-induced contraction of aortic rings from glyburide-treated and from control male and female stroke-prone hypertensive rats. □, Glyburide-treated rats; ■, control rats; (n), number of rats; $^*p < 0.05$ vs control rats and vs zero changes.

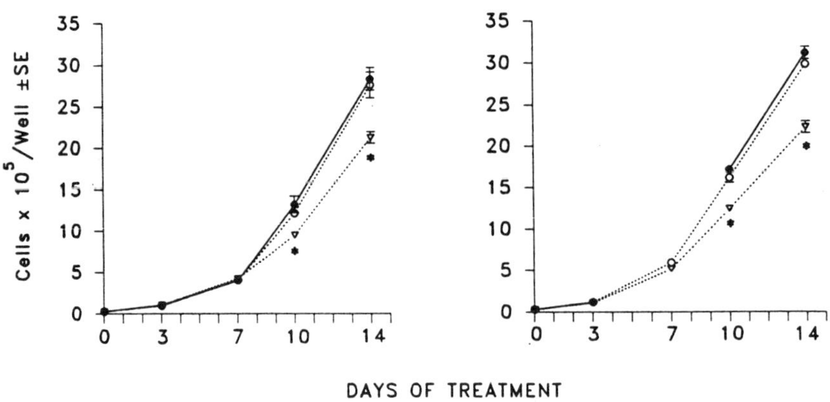

Fig. 6. Effects of glyburide and pioglitazone on proliferative growth of Dahl S rat aortic VSMC in normal culture medium (5% FBS; 6 wells/point cells in pass 7) **(A)** and medium with 5% FBS + 10 mU/mL insulin **(B)** *(103)*. ○, Glyburide (1 μg/mL); ▽, pioglitazone (1 μg/mL); ●, control (vehicle); $^*p < 0.05$ vs control.

to a sustained elevation in circulating insulin and emergence of a paradoxical enhancing effect of insulin on adrenergic contractility (Fig. 5) *(102)*. Pioglitazone also attenuates proliferation of cultured VSMC in response to insulin and other growth factors compared to neutral effects attained with glyburide (Fig. 6) *(103)*. Accordingly, future research should help elucidate mechanisms by which these insulin-sensitizing agents affect VSMC intermediary metabolism, cation metabolism, contractility, and growth.

SUMMARY

Many energy-dependent VSMC functions are differentially regulated and cannot be simply extrapolated from those in skeletal muscle, because of the important differences in their function. VSM clearly differs from skeletal muscle in its independent regulation of cross-bridge number and cycle rate. This has wide ranging consequences with respect to the understanding of the high economy and relatively low efficiency of VSMC. Compartmentation of energy metabolism with specific functions also characterizes VSMC. FA play a prominent regulatory role in VSMC metabolism modulating the availability and utilization of different energetic substrates in this tissue, and consequently the final physiological responses. Manipulation of the intermediary metabolism in VSM with drugs that also have metabolic effects in other type of tissues, can alter the function of VSMC, causing changes in VSMC contractility and proliferation.

REFERENCES

1. Krisanda JM, Paul RJ. Energetics of isometric contraction in porcine carotid artery. Am J Physiol 1984;246:C510–C519.
2. Krisanda JM, Paul RJ. Phosphagen and metabolite content during contraction in porcine carotid artery. Am J Physiol 1983;244:C385–C390.
3. Barron JT, Parrillo JE. Production of lactic acid and energy metabolism in vascular smooth muscle: effect of dichloroacetate. Am J Physiol 1995;268:H713–H719.
4. Hardin CD, Wiseman RW, Kushmerick MJ. Vascular oxidative metabolism under different metabolic conditions. Biochem Biophys 1992;1133:133–141.
5. Lundholm L, Pettersson G, Anderson RGG, Mohme-Lundholm E. Regulation of the carbohydrate metabolism of smooth muscle: some current problems. In: Stephens NL, ed. The Biochemistry of Smooth Muscle, vol. II. University Park, Baltimore, MD, 1985, pp. 85–108.
6. Somlyo AP, Somlyo AV. Vascular smooth muscle: I. Normal structure, pathology, biochemistry, and biophysics. Pharmacol Rev 1968;20:197–272.
7. Campbell JD, Paul RJ. The nature of fuel provision for the Na^+,K^+–ATPase in porcine vascular smooth muscle. J Physiol 1992;447:67–82.
8. Paul RJ, Bauer M, Pease W. Vascular smooth muscle: aerobic glycolysis linked to sodium and potassium transport processes. Science 1979;206:1414–1416.
9. Lynch RM, Paul RJ. Glucose uptake in porcine carotid artery: relation to alterations in active Na^+–K^+ transport. Am J Physiol 1984;247:C433–C440.
10. Lynch RM, Paul RJ. Compartmentation of glycolytic and glycogenolytic metabolism in vascular smooth muscle. Science 1983;222:1344–1346.
11. Lynch RM, Paul RJ. Compartmentation of carbohydrate metabolism in vascular smooth muscle: evidence for at least two functionally independent pools of glucose-6-phosphate. Biochem Biophys Acta 1986;887:315–318.
12. Odessey R, Chace KV. Utilization of endogenous lipid, glycogen and protein by rabbit aorta. Am J Physiol 1982;243:H128–H132.
13. Chace KV, Odessy R. The utilization by rabbit aorta of carbohydrates, fats, ketone bodies, and amino acids as substrates for energy production. Circ Res 1983;52:683–690.
14. Hashimoto S, Dayton S. Utilization of medium and long chain fatty acids by normal rat aorta and the effect of dl-carnitine and their utilization. Atherosclerosis 1971;13:345–354.
15. Epstein M, Sowers JR. Diabetes mellitus and associated, vascular disease, and nephropathy. An update. Hypertension 1995;26(1):869–879.
16. Paul RJ, Krisanda JM, Lynch RM. Vascular smooth muscle energetics. J Cardiovasc Pharm 1984;6:S320–S327.
17. Butler TM, Siegman MJ. High-energy phosphate metabolism in vascular smooth muscle. Annu Rev Physiol 1985;47:629–643.
18. Solaro RJ, DiSalvo J, Paul RJ. Coordination of metabolism and contractility by phosphorylation in cardiac, skeletal and smooth muscle. Fec Proc 1983;42:7,8.

19. Hellstrand P, Paul RJ. Phosphagen content, breakdown during contraction and oxygen consumption in rat portal vein. Am J Physiol 1983;244:C250–C258.
20. Paul RJ. Dependence of ATP consumption on cross-bridge phosphorylation in swine carotid smooth muscle. J Physiol 1994;481:111–117.
21. Murphy RA. Arterial actomyosin: effects of pH and temperature on solubility and ATPase activity. Am J Physiol 1971;220:1494–1500.
22. Krisanda JM, Murphy RA. Tight binding of arterial myosin to skeletal F-actin. J Biol Chem 1980;255:10,771–10,776.
23. Krisanda JM, Breese SS, Murphy RA. High affinity of various smooth muscle myosins for skeletal F-actin demonstrated by enzyme kinetics and electron microscopy. Biochem Biophys Acta 1982;702:125–132.
24. Dillon PF, Murphy RA. Tonic force maintenance with reduced shortening velocity in arterial smooth muscle. Am J Physiol 1982;242:C102–C108.
25. Aksoy MO, Murphy RA, Kamm KE. Role of Ca^{2+} and myosin light chain phosphorylation in regulation of smooth muscle. Am J Physiol 1982;242:C109–C116.
26. Murphy RA. What is special about smooth muscle? The significance of covalent cross-bridge regulation. FASEB J 1994;8:311–318.
27. Dillon PF, Aksoy MO, Driska SP, Murphy RA. Miosin phosphorylation and the cross-bridge cycle in arterial smooth muscle. Science 1981;211:464–466.
28. Ratz PH, Hai CM, Murphy RA. Dependence of stress on cross-bridge phosphorylation in vascular smooth muscle. Am J Physiol 1989;256:C96–C100.
29. Singer HA, Kamm KE, Murphy RA. Estimates of activation in arterial smooth muscle. Am J Physiol 1986;251:C465–C473.
30. Wingard CJ, Paul RJ, Murphy RA. Dependence of ATP consumption on cross-bridge phosphorylation in swine carotid smooth muscle. J Physiol 1994;481:111–117.
31. Bulbring E. Measurements of oxygen consumption in smooth muscle. J Physiol 1953;122:11–134.
32. Lundholm L, Mohme-Lundholm E. Contraction and glycogenolysis of smooth muscle. Acta Physiol Scand 1963;56:125–129.
33. Born GVR. The relation between the tension and the high energy phosphate content of smooth muscle. J Physiol 1956;131:704–711.
34. Lynch RM, Paul RJ. Compartmentation of carbohydrate metabolism in vascular smooth muscle: effects of different energy loading conditions. Am J Physiol 1987;252:C328–C334.
35. Balaban RS, Bader JP. Studies on the relationship between glycolysis and (Na^+–K^+) ATPase in cultured cells. Biochem Biophys Acta 1984;804:419–426.
36. Wu G, Majumdar S, Zhang J, Lee H, Meininger CJ. Insulin stimulates glycolysis and pentose cycle activity in bovine microvascular endothelial cells. Comp Biochem Physiol 1994;108C:179–185.
37. Daley MM. Effect of age and hypertension on utilization of glucose by rat aorta. Am J Physiol 1976;230:30–33.
38. Morrison ES, Scott RF, Kroms M, Frick J. Glucose degradation in normal and atherosclerotic aortic intima-media. Atherosclerosis 1972;16:175–184.
39. Paul RJ. Smooth muscle energetics. Annu Rev Physiol 1989;51:331–349.
40. Campbell, JD, Agubosim S, Paul RJ. Compartmentation of metabolism and function in vascular smooth muscle: quantitation of Na-pump activity and aerobic glycolysis. FASEB J 1988;2:A755.
41. Ishida Y, Riesinger I, Walliman T, Paul RJ. Compartmentation of ATP synthesis and utilization in smooth muscle: roles of aerobic glycolysis and creatine kinase. Mol Cel Biochem 1994;133/134:39–50.
42. Coburn RF, Moreland S, Moreland RS, Baron CB. Rate-limiting energy-dependent steps controlling oxidative metabolism-contraction coupling in rabbit aorta. J Physiol 1992;448:473–492.
43. Gluck E, Paul RJ. The aerobic metabolism or porcine carotid artery and its relationship to isometric force. Pflugers Arch 1977;370:9–18.
44. Hellstrand P. Mechanical and metabolic properties related to contraction in smooth muscle. Acta Physiol Scand 1979;464:1–54.
45. Paul RJ. Functional compartmentalization of oxidative and glycolytic metabolism in vascular smooth muscle. Am J Physiol 1983;244:C399–C409.
46. Chong Z, Paul RJ. Excitation-contraction coupling and relaxation in porcine carotid arteries are specifically dependent on glucose. Am J Physiol 1994;267:H1996–H2004.
47. Ishida Y, Paul RJ. Effects of hypoxia on high-energy phosphagen content, energy metabolism and isometric force in guinea-pig taenia caeci. J Physiol 1990;424:41–56.

48. Iyengar MR. Creatine kinase as an intracellular regulator. J Muscle Res 1984;5:527–534.
49. Wallimann T, Schnyder T, Schlegel J, Wyss M, Wegmann G, Rossi AM, Hemmer W, Eppenberger HM, Quest AFG. Subcellular compartmentation of creatine kinase isoenzymes of CK and octameric structure of mitochondrial CK: important aspects of the phosphoryl-creatine circuit. Prog Clin Biol Res 1989;315:159–176.
50. Davidheiser S, Joseph J, Davies RE. Separation of aerobic glycolysis from oxidative metabolism and contractility in rat anococcygeus muscle. Am J Physiol 1984;247:C335–C341.
51. Lynch RM, Kuettner CP, Paul RJ. Glycogen metabolism during tension generation and maintenance in vascular smooth muscle. Am J Physiol 1989;257:C736–C742.
52. Hellstrand P, Jorup C, Lydrup M. O_2 consumption aerobic glycolysis and tissue phosphagen content during activation of the Na^+/K^+ pump in rat portal vein. Pflugers Arch-Eur J Physiol 1984;401: 119–124.
53. Butler TM, Siegman MJ. High-energy phosphate metabolism in vascular smooth muscle. Annu Rev Physiol 1985;47:629–643.
54. Namm DH. Activation of glycogen phosphorylase in arterial smooth muscle. J Pharmacol Exp Ther 1971;178:299–310.
55. Paul RJ. The effect of isoproterenol and ouabain on oxygen consumption, lactate production and the activation of phosphorylase in coronary artery smooth muscle. Circ Res 1983;52:683–690.
56. Lynch RM, Paul RJ. Compartmentation of carbohydrate metabolism in vascular smooth muscle. Am J Physiol 1987;252:C328–C334.
57. Lundholm L, Mohme-Lundholm E. The carbohydrate metabolism and tone of smooth muscle. Acta Pharmacol 1960;16:374–388.
58. Coe J, Detar R, Bohr DF. Substrates and vascular smooth muscle contraction. Am J Physiol 1968;214:245–250.
59. Barron JT, Kopp SJ, Tow JP, Parrillo JE. Differential effects of fatty acids on glycolysis and glycogen metabolism in vascular smooth muscle. Biochem Biophys Acta 1991;1093:125–134.
60. Barron JT, Kopp SJ, Tow J, Parrillo JE. Fatty acid, tricarboxylic acid cycle metabolites, and energy metabolism in vascular smooth muscle. Biochem Biophys Acta 1994;1012:69–73.
61. Barron JT, Kopp SJ. Phosphorylase b kinase and phosphorylase a phosphatase activities in contracting vascular smooth muscle: stimulation by fatty acid. Biochem Biophys Acta 1991;1973: 550–554.
62. Rao GN, Alexander RW, Runge MS. Linoleic acid and its metabolites, hydroperoxyoctadecadienoic acids, stimulate c-Fos, c-Jun, and c-Myc mRNA expression, mitogen-activated protein kinase activation, and growth in rat aortic smooth muscle cells. J Clin Invest 1995;96:842–847.
63. Grekin RJ, Vollmer AP, Sider RS. Pressor effects of portal venous oleate infusion: a proposed mechanism for obesity hypertension. Hypertension 1995;26:193–198.
64. Stepniakowski KT, Goodfriend TL, Egan BM. Fatty acids enhance vascular α-adrenergic sensitivity. Hypertension 1995;25:774–778.
65. Gonzalez C, Martin C, Hamel E. Endothelial cells inhibit the vascular response to adrenergic nerve stimulation by a receptor-mediated mechanism. Can J Physiol Pharmacol 1990;68:104–109.
66. Egan BM, Schork N, Panis R, Hinderliter A. Vascular structure enhances regional resistance responses in mild hypertension. J Hypertens 1988;6:41–48.
67. Gibbons GH, Dzau VJ. The emerging concept of vascular remodeling. N Engl J Med 1994;330:1431–1438.
68. William B. Glucose-induced vascular smooth muscle dysfunction: the role of protein kinase C. J Hypertens 1995;13:477–486.
69. Barbagallo M, Shan J, Pang PKT, Resnick LM. Glucose-induced alterations of cytosolic free calcium in cultured rat tail artery vascular smooth muscle cells. J Clin Invest 1995:95:763–767.
70. Rodgers RL, Christe ME. Cardiac glucose and fatty acid oxidation in the streptozotocin-induced diabetic spontaneously hypertensive rat. Hypertension 1995:25:235–241.
71. Stumvoll M, Nurjhan N, Perriello G, Dailey G, Gerich JE. Metabolic effects of metformin in non-insulin-dependent diabetes mellitus. N Engl J Med 1995;333:550–554.
72. DeFronzo RA, Goodman AM, Multicenter Metformin Study Group. Efficacy of metformin in patients with non-insulin-dependent diabetes mellitus. N Engl J Med 1995;333:541–549.
73. Klip A, Leiter LA. Cellular mechanism of action of metformin. Diabetes Care 1990;13:696–704.
74. Dominguez LJ, Davidoff AJ, Srinivas PR, Standley PR, Walsh MF, Sowers JR. Effects of metformin on tyrosine kinase activity, glucose transport and intracellular calcium in rat vascular smooth muscle. Endocrinology 1996;137:113–121.

75. Peuler JD, Zamman HY, Stowe MP, Sowers JR, Soltis EE. Inhibition of arterial contractility by non-sulfonylurea insulin-sensitizing drugs. Program of the 76th Annual Meeting of the Endocrine Society, Anaheim, CA, 1994, p. 414 (abstract).
76. Zammam HY, Soltis EE, Sowers JR, Peuler JD. Effects of insulin-sensitizing drugs on arterial contractile responses. Hypertension 1994;24:403.
77. Sharma RV, Bhalla RC. Metformin attenuates agonist-stimulated calcium transients in vascular smooth muscle cells. Clin Exp Hypertens 1995;17:913–929.
78. Verma S, McNeill JH. Metformin improves cardiac function in isolated streptozotocin-diabetic rat hearts. Am J Physiol 1994;266:H714–H719.
79. Wu M-S, Johnston P, Sheu WH-H, Hollenbeck CB, Jeng C-Y, Goldfine ID, Chen Y-DI, Reaven GM. Effect of metformin on carbohydrate and lipoprotein metabolism in NIDDM patients. Diabetes Care 1990;13:1–8.
80. Rains SG, Wilson GA, Richmond W, Elkeles RS. The effects of glibenclamide and metformin on serum lipoproteins in type II diabetes. Diabetic Med 1988;5:653–658.
81. Suter SL, Nolan JJ, Wallace P, Gumbiner B, Olefsky JM. Metabolic effects of new oral hypoglycemic agent CS-045 in NIDDM subjects. Diabetes Care 1992;15:193–203.
82. Petty RG, Pearson JD. The influence of hypoglycemic agents on growth and metabolism of human endothelial cells. Diabetic Med 1992;9:30–37.
83. Dubey RK, Zhang HY, Reddy SR, Boegehold MA, Kotchen TA. Pioglitazone attenuates hypertension and inhibits growth of renal arteriolar smooth muscle in rats. Am J Physiol 1991;265:R726–R732.
84. Fujiwara T, Yoshioka S, Yoshioka T, Ushiyama I, Horikoshi H. Characterization of new oral antidiabetic agent CS-045, a new antidiabetic agent. Metabolism 1990;39:1056–1062.
85. Nolan JJ, Ludnik B, Beerdsen P, Joyce M, Olefsky J. Improvement in glucose tolerance and insulin resistance in obese subjects treated with troglitazone. N Engl J Med 1994;331:1188–1193.
86. Iwamoto Y, Kuzuya T, Matsuda A. Effects of new oral antidiabetic agent CS-045 on glucose tolerance and insulin secretion in patients with NIDDM. Diabetes Care 1991;14:1083–1086.
87. Ciaraldi TP, Gilmore A, Olefsky JM, Goldberg M, Heidenreich KA. In vitro studies on the action of CS-045, a new antidiabetic agent. Metabolism 1990;39:1056–1062.
88. Kobayashi M, Iwanishi M, Egawa K, Shigeta Y. Pioglitazone increases insulin sensitivity by activating insulin receptor kinase. Diabetes 1992;41:476–483.
89. Kellerer M, Kroder G, Tippmer S, Berti L, Kiehn R, Mosthaf L, Häring H. Troglitazone prevents glucose-induced insulin resistant of insulin receptor in rat-1 fibroblasts. Diabetes 1994;43:447–453.
90. Zhang B, Szalkowski D, Dias E, Hayes N, Smith R, Berger J. Potentiation of insulin stimulation of phosphatidylinositol 3-kinase by thiazolidinedione-derived antidiabetic agents in chinese hamster ovary cells expressing human insulin receptors and L6 myotubes. J Biol Chem 1994;269:25,735–25,741.
91. Szalkowski D, White-Carrington S, Berger J, Zhang B. Antidiabetic thiazolidinediones block the inhibitory effect of tumor necrosis factor-α on differentiation, insulin-stimulated glucose uptake, and gene expression in 3T3-L1 cells. Endocrinology 1995;136:1474–1481.
92. Hotamisligil GS, Shargill NS, Spiegelman BM. Adipose expression of tumor necrosis factor-α: direct role in obesity-linked insulin resistance. Science 1993;259:87–90.
93. Hofmann C, Lorenz K, Braithwaite SS, Colca JR, Palazuk BJ, Hotamisligil GS, Spiegelman BM. Altered gene expression for tumor necrosis factor-α and its receptor during drug and dietary modulation of insulin resistance. Endocrinology 1994;134:264–270.
94. Lee M, Philip DG, Khoursheed M, Gao K, Moossa AR, Olefsky JM. Metabolic effects of troglitazone on fructose-induced insulin resistance in the rat. Diabetes 1994;43:1435–1439.
95. Mimura K, Umeda F, Hiramatsu S, Taniguchi S, Ono Y, Nakashima N, Kobayashi K, Masakado M, Sako Y, Nawata H. Effects of a new oral hypoglycaemic agent (CS-045) on metabolic abnormalities and insulin resistance in type 2 diabetes. Diabetic Med 1994;11:685–691.
96. Fujiwara T, Yoshioka S, Yoshioka T, Ushiyama I, Horikoshi H. Characterization of new oral antidiabetic agent CS-045: studies in KK and ob/ob mice and Zucker fatty rats. Diabetes 1988;37:1549–1558.
97. Zhang F, Sowers JR, Ram JL, Standley PR, Peuler JD. Effects of pioglitazone on calcium channels in vascular smooth muscle. Hypertension 1994;24:170–175.
98. Buchanan TA, Meehan WP, Jeng YY, Yang D, Chan TM, Nadler JL, Scott S, Rude RK, Hsueh WA. Blood pressure lowering by pioglitazone. Evidence for a direct vascular effect. J Clin Invest 1995;96:354–360.
99. Goud C, Webb RC. The insulin-sensitizing agent CS-045 inhibits contraction of rat vascular smooth muscle. Hypertension 1995;26:553, (abstract).

100. Meisheri KD, Kahn SA, Martin JL. Vascular pharmacology of ATP-sensitive K^+ channels: interactions between glyburide and K^+ channels openers. J Vasc Res 1993;30:2–12.
101. Inagaki N, Gonoi T, Clement JP IV, Namba N, Inazawa J, Gonzalez G, Aguilar-Bryan L, Susumo S, Bryan J. Reconstitution of I_{KATP}: an inward rectifier subunit plus the sulphonylurea receptor. Science 1995;270:1166–1170.
102. Peuler JD, Johnson BAB, Phare SM, Sowers JR. Sex-specific effects of an insulin secretagogue in stroke-prone hypertensive rats. Hypertension 1993;22:214–220.
103. Sowers JR, Sowers PS, Peuler JD. Role of insulin resistance and hyperinsulinemia in development of hypertension and atherosclerosis. J Lab Clin Med 1994;123:647–652.

24 Analogy Between Endothelial/Mesangial Cell and Endothelial/Vascular Smooth Muscle Cell Interactions

Role of Growth Factors and Mechanotransduction

George L. Bakris, MD, *Paul R. Standley,* PHD, *Carlos E. Palant,* MD, *Mary F. Walsh,* PHD, *and James R. Sowers,* MD

CONTENTS

INTRODUCTION

There are many parallels between renal glomerular and vascular structure and function. Endothelial cells line both glomeruli and vessels, and mesangial cells are modified vascular smooth muscle cells (VSMC) *(1–3)*. Endothelial and mesangial cells together account for about 85% of the total number of cells that make up the glomerulus *(1–2)*, and these cells are distinguished by their biological characteristics and function *(1–4)*. Both produce a variety of mitogens and cytokines known to have autocrine and paracrine activity. Their ability to produce growth factors is relevant given the anatomic relationship of the cells to each other. Anatomically, the glomerular basement membrane incompletely surrounds the endothelial wall, leaving an area of direct contact between the

From: *Contemporary Endocrinology: Endocrinology of the Vasculature*
Edited by: J. R. Sowers Humana Press Inc., Totowa, NJ

Table 1
Factors that Affect IGF-1 Synthesis in the Kidney[a]

Increased	*Decreased*
Growth hormone	Fasting (calorie restriction)
Epidermal growth factor	
Acute ischemia	
Diabetes (hyperglycemia)	
Normal tissue adjacent to infarcted tissue	
Unilateral nephrectomy	

[a]Note that IGF-1 increases are age dependent; the older the individual, the less of an increase in IGF-1.

mesangial cells and the endothelium *(2)*. This simulates the anatomical and functional relationship between endothelial cells and VSMC in the vasculature *(3,4)*.

Abnormalities in both endothelial and mesangial cell function have been described in diabetes mellitus *(3)*. Specifically, there is decreased production and release of endothelial-derived relaxing factor or nitric oxide (NO) and prostaglandins (PGs) in diabetic states *(5–6)*. Both these endothelial-derived factors are known to attenuate the effects of various mitogens such as insulin-like growth factor-1 (IGF-1) whereas IGF-1 directly affects growth of both endothelial and mesangial cells in normal and hyperglycemic states *(3,7–9)*. Consequently, IGF-1, along with other growth factors, interacts with these cells to change their fundamental biologic responses to a variety of stimuli in health and disease *(9)*.

This chapter reviews interactions between the endothelium and mesangium as well as the endothelium and VSMC particularly as related to IGF-1 and other growth factors. These interactions are discussed in the context of both normal and abnormal physiologic conditions such as hyperglycemia. We review the basic anatomy and physiology of each cell type including their biological function. This is followed by a discussion of IGF-1 interactions between endothelial and mesangial cells/VSMC and the potential role of mechanotransduction in diabetic glomerular/vascular disease. Finally, the role of IGF-1 on the regulation of vascular endothelial and VSMC metabolism is reviewed.

IGF

Regulation of cell growth and function that occurs during development and differentiated cell homeostasis is determined by two distinct classes of trophic factors: classic endocrine hormones and growth factors with paracrine and/or autocrine properties. IGFs, produced both in the arterial vasculature and the glomerulus, are such paracrine/autocrine factors *(9)*. In the developing human fetus, IGF-2 is first expressed shortly after implantation *(10)*, and late in the first and early in the second trimester, IGF-1 and IGF-2 mRNA are found in various embryonic mesodermal-derived tissues *(10)*.

IGF-1 is a proinsulin-like peptide, 70 amino acids in length. Its production in the liver supports a predominately endocrine function. However, IGF-1 generated in extrahepatic tissues such as the kidney and vasculature has both autocrine and paracrine actions *(9,11)*. Renal IGF-1 has full biologic activity and its expression is regulated by growth hormone and other factors *(12)* summarized in Table 1. The wide-spread expression of IGF receptors seen in development is further evidence for a paracrine and/or autocrine role for IGF-1.

Table 2
Characteristics of Mesangial Cells

Anatomic	*Immunochemical*
Located between the capillaries	Fail to stain for factor VIII and cytokeratins
Multiple extracellular processes	Positive surface antigens for fibronectin
Regular nucleus with less dense cytoplasm	Positive staining for actin and myosin
	Lack of angiotensin-converting enzyme activity
	Lack of Ia positive cells
	Lack of Weibel-Palade bodies

IGFs in blood or tissues are always found in association with specific binding proteins. The affinity of these binding proteins for IGF-1 is equal to or greater than that for high-affinity type I receptors *(10–12)*. There are at least six different IGF-1 binding proteins, each of which is 200–300 amino acids in length *(11–14)*. In the kidney these binding proteins are primarily localized in the papillary and cortical collecting ducts as well as the thick ascending limbs of Henle's loop *(12–14)*. Synthesis of binding proteins occurs primarily in the liver and is growth hormone dependent *(10)*. Paracrine/autocrine actions of IGFs in renal/vascular tissues are dependent on interactions with these binding proteins.

MESANGIAL CELLS

The concept of the mesangium as a structural entity of a glomerular tuft was introduced several decades ago *(15)*. The mesangium is an intercapillary array of mononucleated stellate cells embedded in extracellular amorphous matrix surrounded by the capillary loops. Despite close contact and marked similarities with endothelial cells, mesangial cells can be identified by specific characteristics summarized in Table 2. Mesangial cells share many properties with VSMC such as contraction in response to agonists such as vasopressin, angiotensin II (AII) and endothelin-1 *(3,9)*. This is an important feature as the mesangium binds together capillary loops; contraction of the mesangium can thus alter glomerular capillary flow.

A number of factors affect mesangial cell growth and homeostasis. These include glucose concentration, IGF-1, endothelin, and other related mitogens. These mitogens act, in part, through activation of one of three signaling mechanisms: cyclic guanylate monophosphate (cGMP), cyclic adenylate monophosphate (cAMP), and/or inositol phosphates-calcium-diacylglycerol. All three systems share a similar sequence of activation that involves breakdown of a phosphorylated precursor by enzymes activated by receptor occupancy. A discussion of each of these mitogens is beyond the scope of this chapter, but the subject is thoroughly reviewed elsewhere *(2–4)*.

Mesangial cells are generally quiescent under in vivo conditions. This concept is supported by autoradiographic analysis of DNA turnover in rat glomeruli where it has been noted that mesangial cells have a slower turnover rate than epithelial or endothelial cells *(16)*. Under normal conditions, mesangial cell turnover rate is estimated to be between 50 and 100 d *(3)*. There is a marked slowing of mesangial cell turnover under hyperglycemic conditions in the absence of insulin or IGF-1 *(17)*. Addition of insulin with concomitant hyperglycemia further slows proliferation of mesangial cells in response to mitogens such as vasopressin and endothelin *(18,19)*. Conversely, mesangial matrix production is increased by IGF-1 under hyperglycemic conditions *(20–22)*.

The effects of insulin may be the result, in part, of activation of IGF-1 receptors located on mesangial cells *(14)*. The mechanisms by which IGF-1 receptor activation may alter cell and matrix turnover under hyperglycemic conditions is unclear although there are increases in both IGF and insulin receptor protein levels under these conditions *(14)*. In addition, IGF-1 and insulin attenuate increases in cell calcium $[Ca^{2+}]_i$ in response to various growth and vasoactive factors *(3,7,9,23,24)*. Interestingly, extracellular protein matrix also contains an abundance of IGF binding proteins which may potentiate the action of IGF-1 *(22)*. Taken together, these findings may account for the clinical observation of a marked expansion in matrix without mesangial cell proliferation in diabetes.

Cultured mesangial cells release IGF-1 which displays a high affinity for mesangial cell IGF-1 receptors *(25,26)*. IGF-1 binding is over 200 times greater than that of insulin in these cells *(13)*. IGF-1 production occurs at an especially high rate in diabetic mice, and mesangial cells isolated from these mice exhibit higher levels of IGF-1 receptors suggesting that the mesangial cell autocrine/paracrine functions of the IGF-1 system are enhanced in the diabetic state *(14)*. IGF-1 released from mesangial cells may also have paracrine activity. Endothelial cells contain IGF receptors which, when stimulated, increase proteoglycan production *(27)*. Thus, given the close proximity of these cells to the endothelium it is plausible that paracrine as well as autocrine effects of IGFs released from mesangial cells are important in glomerular physiology.

GLOMERULAR ENDOTHELIAL CELLS

The endothelium is a single layer of cells lining the capillary network within the glomerulus as well as the systemic vasculature. Control of growth of the endothelium is unique since these cells are normally monolayered and static. The usual turnover time of the endothelium is very slow, approx 10,000 d *(28)*, but, under certain culture conditions the cells will rapidly divide and become mitogenic. Specifically, exposure to endothelial cell mitogens, such as fibroblast growth factor (FGF) and IGFs in plasma, may stimulate growth and proliferation of endothelial cells *(29)*. Experiments in our laboratory demonstrate that IGF-1 alone does not stimulate mitogenesis of endothelial cells (unpublished data). Conversely, in the presence of both FGF and epidermal growth factor, IGF-1 potentiates endothelial growth effects *(29)*.

Glomerular endothelial cells synthesize vasoconstricting growth factors such as platelet-derived growth factor (PDGF) and endothelin-1 necessary for regulation of tone and cellular homeostasis *(4,5)*. Endothelin-1, produced by mesangial cells, as well as endothelial cells, has both autocrine and paracrine effects *(18,19,30)*. Glomerular endothelial cells also produce IGF-1 and have an unusually high number of type I IGF-1 receptors *(31)*. Given the anatomical location of the endothelium relative to the capillary lumen and mesangium, the endothelium is exposed to the contents of plasma in the capillary area. This occurs through the area of direct contact between the endothelium and mesangium defined as the juxtamesangial portion of the capillary wall *(30)*. Therefore, a number of growth factors found in the plasma and expressed under certain circumstances, most notably diabetes, can potentially affect mesangial cell function *(9)*.

ENDOTHELIAL/MESANGIAL CELL INTERACTIONS

An extensive literature examining the in vitro interactions of mesangial and endothelial cells does not exist. Studies are largely limited to those that seek to develop a model by which these interactions can be assessed. One such study examined the effects of endothelial cell culture supernatant on mesangial cell proliferation *(32)*. In crossover experiments, supernatant from endothelial cells exposed to increased laminar flow inhibit proliferation of mesangial cells *(32)*. These results are consistent with the hypothesis that increased arterial pressure causes substances to be released from endothelial cells that directly inhibit mitogenesis of mesangial cells. Others have examined the effects of endothelial cells on mesangial cell proliferation in a coculture model *(33)*. When placed in direct contact with endothelial cells treated with mitomycin C, growth of mesangial cells was inhibited during the first 72 h, but a high level of proliferation was observed in the ensuing 2 d. This biphasic growth pattern is not seen when similar experiments with mesangial cells and fibroblasts are performed. Consequently, these studies are consistent with the notion that endothelial cells control proliferation of mesangial cells through paracrine factors.

Most published studies that examine the interaction of glomerular endothelial cells with the mesangium have done so in the context of changes in extracellular mesangial matrix synthesis of proteins. Recent studies indicate that IGF-1 increases fibronectin levels in the culture media of both VSMC and mesangial cells and this is regulated transcriptionally *(20)*. Modulation of fibronectin synthesis by insulin is similar to that seen with IGF-1, but insulin does not induce an increase in fibronectin synthesis in the mesangial cells themselves. However, there is no additive effect on fibronectin synthesis when IGF-1 is added to insulin.

One of the major homeostatic mechanisms regulating increased mitogenic activity by both endothelial and mesangial cells is production of PGs by the cells themselves. Recently, coculture experiments with glomerular endothelial cells and mesangial cells were performed to assess whether coculturing would alter mesangial cell prostaglandin E (PGE_2) production by mesangial cells *(34)*. Mesangial cells were found to have a much higher rate of PGE_2 synthesis when cocultured with endothelial cells, an affect that is owing to endothelin stimulation of mesangial PGE_2 production. Thus, these cells, which anatomically abut each other, can regulate their own function and impact adjacent cells.

MESANGIAL MECHANOTRANSDUCTION

Increases in renal glomeruli capillary wall tension, as exist in diabetes mellitus, may lead to enhanced extracellular matrix (ECM) synthesis and deposition, leading to progression of glomerulosclerosis *(35)*. In this regard, mechanical stimulation of cultured rat mesangial cells increases ionic currents and expression of early response proto-oncogenes such as c-*fos* that encode mesangial cell hypertrophy and proliferation *(36–38)*. These processes appear to be linked since stretch-induced proto-oncogene expression is partially dependent on the presence of extracellular Ca^{2+}. Palant and colleagues *(38)* studied stretch-activated ion currents in rat mesangial cells which possess at least two stretch-activated ion channels (SACs) *(39,40)*. One, a divalent cation-selective SACs or Ca^{2+}-SAC has been recently described *(38)*. Similar to SACs, Ca^{2+}-SACs can be activated by both an applied membrane stretch or by hyposmolar solutions. Ca^{2+} influx through the Ca^{2+}-SAC may play an important role in a mechanotransduction ensemble that may involve ECM proteins, integrin receptors, and cytoskeletal microfilaments *(37,38)*. Further, the nature of the ECM appears to dictate the functionality of SACs. Indeed, mesangial cells cultured in fibronectin exhibit greater SAC sensitivity to mechanical stimulation when compared

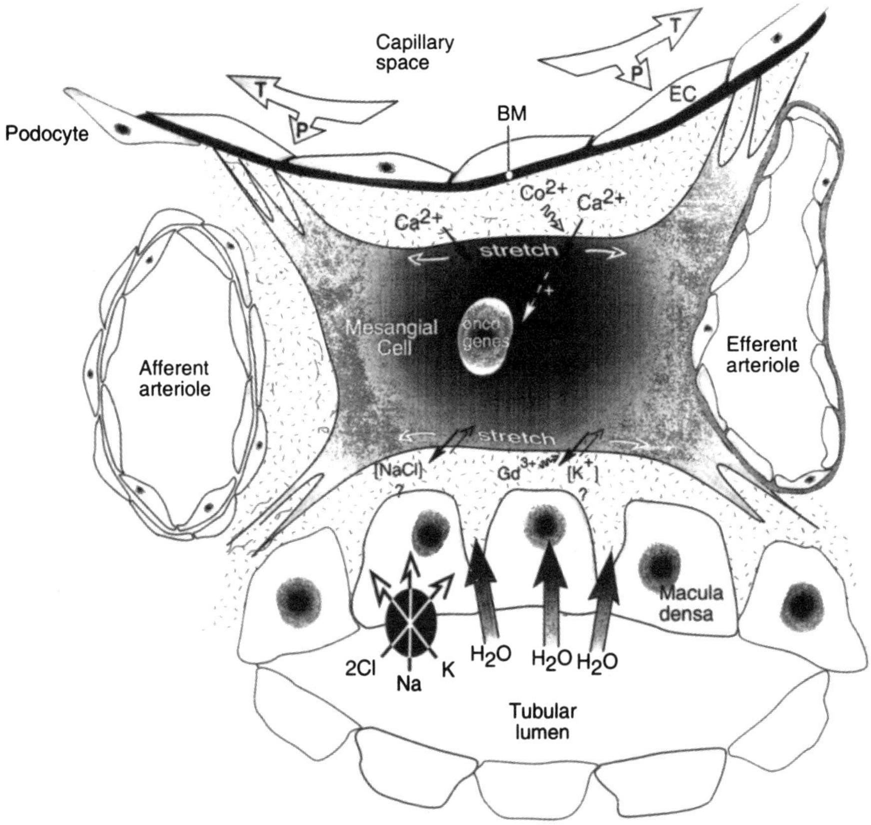

Fig. 1. Schematic representation of structural–functional relationships between mesangial and other glomerular cells. BM, basement membrane; EC, endothelial cell; [K], intracellular K; P, pressure; T, tension.

to SACs of mesangial cells grown on collagen type IV. Since Ca^{2+}-SAC may regulate mesangial cell osmoregulation and tone *(37,38)*, Palant and colleagues *(38)* proposed that an optimal mix of glycoproteins in the mesangium is necessary for appropriate transmission of mechanical impulses to mesangial cells in order to insure regulation of cell osmolality and tone through stretch-induced ion currents. It is quite possible that in states such as aging and diabetes where glomerular collagen deposition is increased *(39)*, inability to generate appropriate mechanosensitive currents may impair mesangial cell-structural and functional regulation of glomerular filtration.

The mesangial cell mechanotransduction ensemble is illustrated in Fig. 1. In the region closest to the glomerular capillary, mesangial cells emit cytoplasmic projections that insert into the glomerular basement membrane in a manner that resembles microscopic tendons *(40)*. As a result of this intimate anatomical relationship, mesangial cells likely experience significant mechanical stress resulting from transmission of pressures and tension across endothelial fenestrations. As illustrated in Fig. 1, in contrast to the afferent arteriole which is enveloped by a well-defined layer of both granular and nongranular smooth muscle, the efferent arteriole has a significant intraglomerular segment that is mostly surrounded by mesangial cells *(41)*. Micropuncture experiments show that mesangial cells regulate the glomerular ultrafiltration coefficient, efferent arteriolar resistance, and glomerular capillary hydrostatic pressure *(42)*. Glomerular hydrodynamic forces depicted in Fig. 1 (P = blood pressure and T = capillary wall tension) could exert significant mechanical stimulation of the mesangial cell membrane transmitted through microinsertions in the glomerular basement membrane *(40)*.

Thus, Ca^{2+}-SACs may regulate mesangial cell tone in response to intraglomerular mechanical forces *(38)*. Accordingly, increases in mesangial cell tone induced by glomerular capillary stretch-induced Ca^{2+} influx would strengthen structural support of the filtration barrier when glomerular pressures and flows are augmented and preserve the efferent arteriolar lumen diameter when afferent arteriolar hydrostatic pressures, transmitted across the mesangium tend to collapse them *(41,42)*. According to this notion, Ca^{2+}-SACs act as cellular baroreceptors that modulate mesangial cell tone in response to prevailing intraglomerular forces. In the region closest to the macula densa, the juxtaglomerular cleft, mesangial cells encounter varying osmotic gradients that result from uncoupled transport of NaCl and H_2O across the macula densa epithelial cell (lower region of Fig. 1). Thus, mesangial cell SACs and Ca^{2+}-SACs function as osmostats and maintain appropriate cell volumes in the face of substantial osmotic gradients *(38,43)*.

Mesangial cells, like VSMC, when cultured under pulsatile stretch conditions, undergo significant metabolic, phenotypic, and functional changes. For example, they increase their synthesis of total protein and of important components of the ECM, such as collagen I and IV, laminin, and fibronectin *(44)*. In response to pulsatile stretch, there appears to be a role for both activation of protein kinase C *(36)* and Ca^{2+} influx through a SAC *(45)* in stimulation of gene induction and ECM protein synthesis. As previously noted, mesangial cells project cytoplasmic insertions into the glomerular basement membrane coming in direct contact with the glomerular capillary lumen across endothelial fenestrations *(40)*. These microscopic attachments to the glomerular basement membrane (GBM) are composed of fibronectin and/or other adhesive glycoproteins that appear contiguous with the mesangial cell cytoskeleton. Connections between the ECM and the cell membrane-cytoskeleton may provide structural support to the glomerular capillary and additionally act as a sensory pathway whereby mesangial cells receive incoming mechanical signals. Normally, ECM appears to have a well-balanced mix of elastic and nonelastic glycoproteins which vary in their capacity to transmit capillary wall tension to the mesangial cell *(46,47)*. Although collagen fibrils stiffen the ECM in response to increased stretch *(46)*, fibronectins are primarily adhesive glycoproteins that facilitate force transmission *(47)*. Fibronectin production is stimulated by growth factors *(20)* and Ca^{2+} *(12–14)* through activation of the inositol-phosphate cascade, gene transcription/transduction, and protein production *(48)*. Thus, capillary wall tension and the ECM are part of a complex, subtly regulated system whose derangement may lead to both structural changes and physiological dysfunction.

IGF-1 AND THE VASCULATURE

IGF-1 and insulin have effects on the systemic vasculature similar to those noted in the renal glomerulus *(7–9,49–65)*. VSMC and vascular endothelial cells, like skeletal muscle and adipose tissue, have receptors for IGF-1 and insulin and are sensitive to the metabolic effects of both of these hormones *(9,49–65)*. In this regard, studies have confirmed that insulin and IGF-1 regulate endothelial cell and VSMC glucose and cation metabolism *(9,62)*. Both IGF-1 and insulin stimulate glucose transport *(3,9,63–65)*, and the consti-

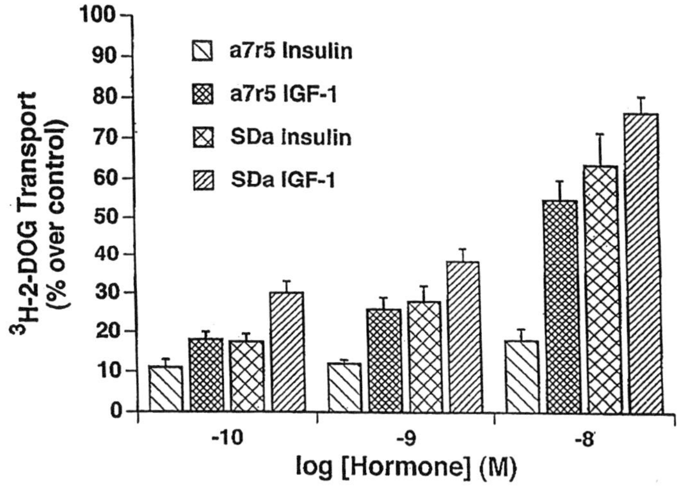

Fig. 2. The effects of insulin and IGF-1 on glucose transport in freshly prepared Sprague-Dawley aortic (SDa) and a7r5 VSMC.

tutive NO synthase (cNOS) in endothelial cells *(5,58)*. Both IGF-1 and insulin also stimulate glucose transport in VSMC *(52,63–65)* (IGF-1 is more potent), clearly establishing VSMC as an IGF-1 and insulin-sensitive tissue in the "classical sense" (Fig. 2). Recent data from our laboratory indicate that IGF-1 stimulates VSMC synthesis of NO, presumably by activating inducible NOS (iNOS), because this requires at least 1 h and is inhibited by aminoguanidine *(58)*. Furthermore, preliminary data from our laboratory indicates that IGF-1 may also stimulate cNOS in VSMC as well as in endothelial cells. Unlike insulin, which must traverse the endothelium before acting on VSMC, IGF-1 is synthesized by VSMC and is more likely to act in an autocrine and paracrine fashion *(9,60,61)*.

IGF-1, like insulin, attenuates vasoconstriction and increases blood flow in regional vascular beds *(53–58)*, including the renal vasculature *(55,56–58)*. As previously noted, the vasodilatory effects of IGF-1 as well as insulin, are mediated partly through the stimulation of endothelial cell release of NO *(58)*. However, IGF-1 may modulate vascular responses through alterations in VSMC $[Ca^{2+}]_i$ *(3,7,9)*. Studies in our laboratory have demonstrated that IGF-1 attenuates $[Ca^{2+}]_i$ responses to vasoconstrictors such as serotonin (Fig. 3). IGF-1, like insulin *(62)*, increases VSMC sodium–potassium ATPase (Na^+–K^+–ATPase) activity. This is a potentially important vascular function for IGF-1, because decreased Na^+–K^+–ATPase activity leads to an accumulation of Na^+, and owing to subsequent changes in Na^+–Ca^{2+} exchange, an increase in VSMC $[Ca^{2+}]_i$ as well *(9)*.

Immunofluorescent and mRNA detection techniques have shown the presence of the insulin-sensitive glucose transporter (GLUT-4) in arterial vasculature *(3,9,52,63)*. IGF-1 and insulin appear to regulate VSMC glucose transport by increasing expression/translocation of the insulin-sensitive glucose transporter, GLUT-4 *(3,9,52,63–65)*. Elevated VSMC $[Ca^{2+}]_i$ is associated with decreased insulin-stimulated glucose transport in several insulin-sensitive tissues *(3,66–68)*. It was recently observed that the V_{max} for glucose transport is altered in VSMC from insulin-resistant Zucker obese rats *(6)* in association with increased VSMC $[Ca^{2+}]_i$ responses *(67)*. Glucose transport in VSMC appears to be critical for the regulation of both vascular tone *(69,70)* and cation transport *(71)*. That

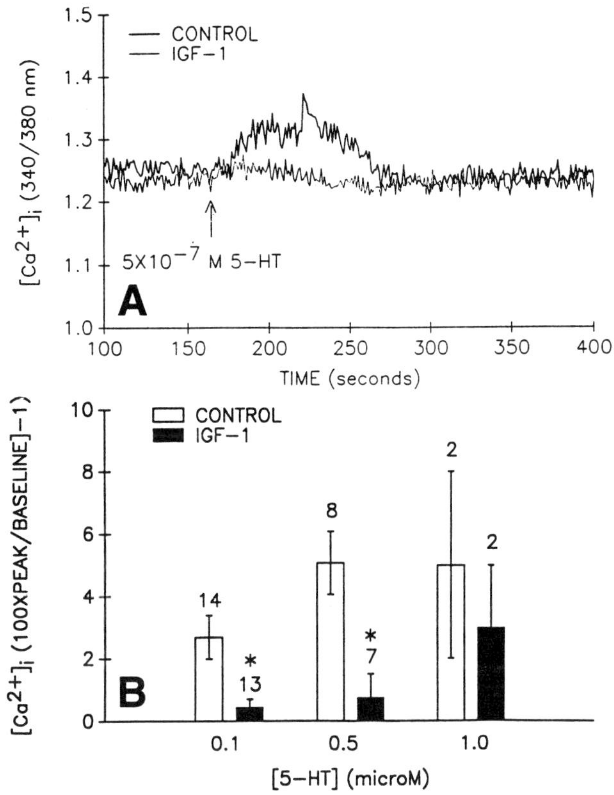

Fig. 3. The effects of IGF-1 on VSMC $[Ca^{2+}]_i$ responses to serotonin. **(A)** Effects of 60-min treatment with 10 n*M* IGF-1 on 5-HT-induced in VSMC $[Ca]_i$; **(B)** summary of IGF-1 effects on 5-HT-induced rises in VSMC $[Ca]_i$.

glucose transport is altered in VSMC in hypertension accompanying insulin resistance suggests that a disordered energy balance may play an important role in the altered cation transport *(9,49,65)* and enhanced vascular contractility *(3,9,67,72)* seen in the disease.

ROLE OF IGF-1 IN VASCULAR GROWTH

IGF-1 may exert atherogenic effects through influences on both vascular endothelial cells and VSMC *(9,50,51)*. Both insulin and IGF-1 increase mitogenic signaling pathways and thymidine incorporation into DNA in endothelial and VSMC (Fig. 4) and function as progression factors or cofactors to promote the proliferative properties of several cytokines, including tumor necrosis factor *(73)*. Indeed, insulin and IGF-1 appear to act synergistically with respect to those effects *(50)*. Recently IGF-1 and insulin have been shown to enhance cholesterol ester accumulation in VSMC by decreasing arterial cholesterol hydrolysis *(74)*. Thus, there are a number of mechanisms (some discussed in this chapter) by which the IGFs and insulin may cause vascular proliferation and remodeling and contribute to the development of atherosclerosis.

There is accumulating evidence that the IGF-1 produced by VSMC plays a significant role in postinjury (i.e., restenosis) related vascular growth and remodeling *(75–82)*. Medial thickening (i.e., VSMC growth) of the vessel wall is a hallmark of restenotic

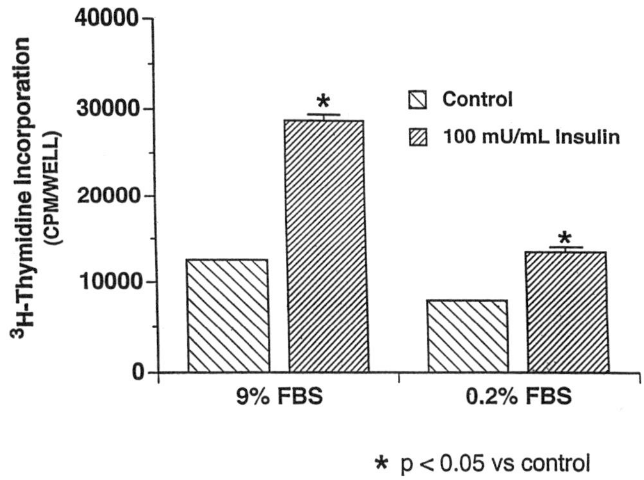

Fig. 4. Insulin-stimulated DNA thymidine incorporation into VSMC. (Large dose of insulin indicates action through an IGF-1 receptor.)

lesions in humans and animals. A preliminary event in this process is platelet adherence and degranulation but the mechanism of hyperplastic/hypertrophic medial VSMC growth has not been fully established. Aortic IGF-1 mRNA and protein content is increased in rat aortae after balloon angioplasty; this effect peaks 7 d after injury and continues past 3 wk *(83)*, long after disappearance of platelets from the injured site. The site of IGF-1 induction has been demonstrated to be the VSMC of the injured vessel. Thus, VSMC expression of IGF-1 and its potential autocrine effect that may account for increased arterial thickening in essential hypertension and postinjury cases.

VSMC cultures constitutively transcribe IGF-1 and secrete it into culture medium *(61,79,84)*. Although pharmacological quantities of insulin are required, physiological concentrations of IGF-1 increase thymidine uptake in VSMC *(85)*. Additive effects are seen with low levels of serum supplementation suggesting that IGF-1 (a progression factor) is permissive for serum-derived competence factors (such as PDGF), which when combined, induce VSMC DNA synthesis *(85)*. That VSMC secrete IGF-1, suggests that IGF-1 may act in an autocrine fashion via a positive feedback loop mechanism to regulate mitogen-induced VSMC growth *(86)*. For example, IGF-1 and high levels of insulin, known to act via IGF-1 receptors, induce VSMC IGF-1 mRNA *(79)*. The mitogens AII and PDGF are also potent stimuli for transcription and secretion of VSMC IGF-1 *(61,79,84)*. Interestingly, both PDGF *(80,84)* and AII *(61)* are also produced by VSMC, leading to the conclusion that on appropriate stimulation, VSMC produce a variety of mitogens, both progression and competence factors, which most likely act in an autocrine fashion to regulate growth. Whether expression of these factors depend on one another is an area requiring further investigation.

Arterial blood vessels respond to an elevation in luminal pressure with active force development (the myogenic response). Demonstration of Ca-SAC in VSMC suggests a mechanism by which stretch increases VSMC $[Ca^{2+}]_i$, the primary event in excitation–contraction coupling. Since balloon angioplasty necessarily evokes a stretch stimulus, the role of stretch in VSMC proliferation has also been investigated *(87)*. Cultured VSMC

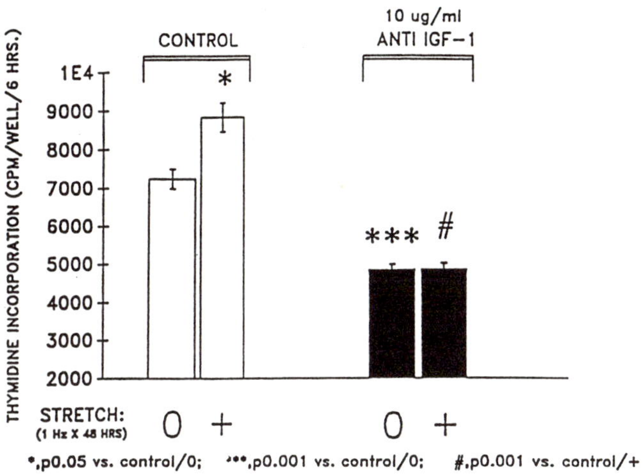

Fig. 5. Effects of IGF-1 antibody (anti-IGF-1) on stretched-induced increases in DNA synthesis rate.

when stretched display increased rates of thymidine uptake and collagen synthesis *(87)*. Pulsatile stretch similar to what VSMC encounter in normal physiology also was investigated *(88)*. When stretched to 125% of initial length at 60 cycles/min, cultured VSMC increased thymidine uptake and cell number after 24 h *(89)*. Similar studies using increase ambient pressure (40–120 mmHg) (rather than direct stretch) also resulted in a stimulation of VSMC thymidine incorporation and cell division *(90)*. Stretch- and pressure-induced increases in thymidine incorporation and cell division are blocked by an inhibitor of tyrosine kinase activity *(90)*. Since IGF-1 receptors possess an intrinsic tyrosine kinase domain, it is plausible that IGF-1 may be implicated in this response.

We have investigated the role of stretch in VSMC IGF-1 expression. Preliminary experiments show that cyclic stretch increases VSMC thymidine uptake and IGF-1 secretion. Interestingly, addition of IGF-1 antibodies to the growth medium inhibited stretch-induced growth (Fig. 5). However, the role of PDGF in VSMC autocrine growth cannot be overlooked since other investigators have demonstrated that similar stretch paradigms induced PDGF expression/secretion. Blocking PDGF action with anti-PDGF antibodies attenuates, but does not abolish, stretch-induced growth. Given that PDGF increases VSMC IGF-1 expression *(81)*, it is becoming increasingly clear that autocrine VSMC growth is under the control of several locally produced factors.

In vivo studies are consistent with stretch/pressure-induced regulation of IGF-1-mediated VSMC growth. Increased transmural pressure following portal vein ligation results in a fourfold increase in VSMC IGF-1 mRNA after 7 d *(91)*. VSMC IGF-1 mRNA increased ninefold 1 wk postballoon catheterization; the involvement of growth hormone was ruled out since results were similar in hypophysectomized rats suggesting that a local IGF-1 system was responsible. VSMC proliferation was greatest at sites with the least re-endothelialization indicating that VSMC under the greatest impact of pulsatile blood pressure respond with greater increases in IGF-1 production or that endothelial cells produce inhibitors of VSMC proliferation. Clearly, mechanical as well as hormonal stimuli regulate VSMC expression of IGF-1 in a manner analogous to that seen for control of mesangial cell function.

REFERENCES

1. Olivetti G, Anversa P, Melissari M, Loud A. Morphometry of the renal corpuscle during postnatal growth and compensatory hypertrophy. Kidney Int 1980;17:438–454.
2. Mene P, Simonson MS, Dunn MJ. Physiology of the mesangial cell. Physiol Rev 1989;69:1347–1424.
3. Standley PR, Bakir MH, Sowers JR. Vascular insulin abnormalities, hypertension, and accelerated atherosclerosis. Am J Kidney Dis 1993;21:6:39–46.
4. Gryglewski RJ, Botting RM, Vane JR. Mediators produced by the endothelial cell. Hypertension 1988;12:530–548.
5. Tsukahara H, Gordienko DV, Tonshiff B, Gelato MC, Goligorsky MS. Direct demonstration of insulin-like growth factor induced nitric oxide production by endothelial cells. Kidney Int 1994;45:598–604.
6. Doni MC, Whittle DJ, Palmer RM, Moncada S. Actions of nitric oxide on the release of prostacyclin from bovine endothelial cells in culture. Eur J Pharmacol 1988;151:19–25.
7. Epstein M, Sowers JR. Diabetes mellitus and hypertension. Hypertension 1992;19:403–418.
8. Bakris GL, Bhandaru S. Effects of IGF-1 on proliferation of human mesangial cells in culture under hyperglycemic conditions. J Invest Med (in press).
9. Sowers JR, Epstein M. Diabetes mellitus and associated hypertension, vascular disease and nephropathy: an update. Hypertension 1995;26:869–879.
10. Logan A, Hill DJ. Bioavailability: is this a key event in regulating the actions of peptide growth factors? J Endocrinol 1992;134:157–161.
11. Cohick WS, Clemmons DR. The insulin like growth factors. Annu Rev Physiol 1993;55:131–153.
12. Hammerman MR, Miller SB. The growth hormone insulin-like growth factor axis in kidney revisited. Am J Physiol 1993;265:F1–F14.
13. Arnquist HJ, Ballerman BJ, King GL. Receptors for and effects of insulin and IGF-1 in glomerular mesangial cells. Am J Physiol 1988;254:C411–C416.
14. Oemar BS, Foellmer HG, Hodgdon-Anandant L, Rosenzweig SA. Regulation of insulin like growth factor-I receptors in diabetic mesangial cells. J Biol Chem 1991;226:2369–2373.
15. Zimmermann KW. Uber den bau des glomerulus der saugerniere: weitare mitteilunger. Z Mikrosk Anat Frosch 1933;32:176–278.
16. Pabst R, Sterzel RB. Cell renewal of glomerular cell types in normal rats. An autoradiographic analysis. Kidney Int 1983;24:626–631.
17. Bakris GL. An approach to the hypertensive diabetic patient: emphasis on renal preservation. In: Epstein M, ed. Calcium Antagonists in Clinical Medicine. Hanley and Belfus, Philadelphia, PA, 1992, pp. 326–352.
18. Bakris GL, Fairbanks RF, Traish A, Akerstrom V, Kern S. Arginine vasopressin stimulates human mesangial cell production of endothelin. J Clin Invest 1991;87:1158–1164.
19. Bakris GL, Re RN, Bhandaru S. Endothelin modulates angiotensin II-induced mitogenesis of human mesangial cells. Am J Physiol 1993;264(Renal and Electrolyte Physiol. 33):F937–F942.
20. Tamaroglio TA, Lo CS. Regulation of fibronectin by insulin-like growth factor-1 in cultured rat thoracic aortic smooth muscle cells and glomerular mesangial cells. Exp Cell Res 1994;215:338–346.
21. Wakisaka M, Spiro MJ, Spiro RG. Synthesis of type VI collagen by cultured glomerular cells and comparison of its regulation by glucose and other factors with that of type IV collagen. Diabetes 1994;43:95–103.
22. Jones JI, Gockerman A, Busby WH, Camacho-Hubner C, Clemmons DR. Extracellular matrix contains insulin like growth factor binding protein-5: potentiation of the effects of IGF-1. J Cell Biol 1993;121:679–687.
23. Inishi Y, Okuda T, Arakama T, Kurokawa K. Insulin attenuates intracellular calcium responses and cell contraction caused by vasoactive agents. Kidney Int 1994;45:1318–1325.
24. Kikkawa R, Haneda M, Togawa M, Koya D, Kajiwara N, Shigeta Y. Differential modulation of mitogenic and metabolic actions of insulin like growth factor-I in rat glomerular mesangial cells in high glucose culture. Diabetologia 1993;36:276–281.
25. Conti FG, Striker LJ, Elliott SJ, Andreani D, Striker GE. Synthesis and release of insulin-like growth factor I by mesangial cells in culture. Am J Physiol 1988;255(Renal Fluid Electrolyte Physiol 24): F1214–F1219.
26. Aron DC, Rosenswerg JL, Abboud HE. Synthesis and binding of insulin-like growth factor I by human glomerular mesangial cells. J Clin Endocrinol Metab 1989;68:585–591.
27. Bar RS, Dake BL, Stueck S. Stimulation of proteoglycans by IGF-1 and II in microvessel and large vessel endothelial cells. Am J Physiol 1987;253:E21–E27.

28. Hobson B, Denekamp J. Endothelial proliferation in tumors and normal tissues: continuous labelling studies. Br J Cancer 1984;49:405–413.
29. Joseph-Silverstein J, Rifkin DB. Endothelial cell growth factors and the vessel wall. Sem Thromb Hemost 1987;13(4):504–513.
30. Marsden PA, Dorfman DM, Collins T, Brenner BM, Orkin SH, Ballerman BJ. Regulated expression of endothelin-1 in glomerular capillary endothelial cells. Am J Physiol 1991;261:F117–F125.
31. Ohashi H, Rosen KM, Smith FE, Villa-Komaroff L, Nayak RC, King GL. Characterization of type I IGF receptor and IGF-1 mRNA expression in cultured human and bovine glomerular cells. Regul Peptides 1993;48:9–20.
32. Morigi M, Zoja C, Figliuzzi M, Remuzzi G, Remuzzi A. Supernatant of endothelial cells exposed to laminar flow inhibits mesangial cell proliferation. Am J Physiol 1993;264:C1080–C1083.
33. Saeki T, Morioka T, Arakaura M, Shimizu F, Oile T. Modulation of mesangial cell proliferation by endothelial cells in co-culture. Am J Pathol 1991;139:949–957.
34. Uchida K, Ballerman BJ. Sustained activation of PGE2 synthesis in mesangial cells co-cultured with glomerular endothelial cells. Am J Physiol 1992;263:C200–C209.
35. Daniels BS, Hostetter TH. Adverse effects of growth in the glomerular microcirculation. Am J Physiol 1990;258(Renal Fluid Electrolyte Physiol 27):F1409–F1416.
36. Akai Y, Homma T, Burns KD, Yasuda T, Badr KF, Harris RC. Mechanical stretch/relaxation of cultured rat mesangial cells induces protooncogenes and cyclooxygenase. Am J Physiol 1994;267(Cell Physiol 26):C482–C490.
37. Craelius W, Ross MJ, Harris DR, Chen VK, Palant CE. Membrane currents controlled by physical forces in cultured mesangial cells. Kidney 1993;43:535–543.
38. Chen V, Guber H, Palant CE. Mechanosensitive single channel calcium currents in rat mesangial cells. Biochem Biophys Res Comm 1994;203:773–779.
39. Kartunnen T, Risteli J, Autio-Harmainen H, Risteli L. Effect of age and diabetes on type IV collagen and laminin in human kidney cortex. Kidney Int 1986;30:586–591.
40. Sakai T, Kriz W. The structural relationship between mesangial cells and basement membrane of the renal glomerulus. Anat Embryol 1987;176:373–386.
41. Elger M, Sakai T, Winkler D, Kriz W. Structure of the outflow segment of the efferent arteriole in rat superficial glomeruli. Contrib Nephrol 1991;95:1–12.
42. Blantz RC, Gabbai FB, Tucker BJ, Yamamoto T, Wilson CB. Role of mesangial cell in glomerular response to volume and angiotensin II. Am J Physiol 1993;264(Renal Fluid Electrolyte Physiol 33):F158–F165.
43. Rich A, Moore LC. Transport-coupling hypothesis of tubuloglomerular feedback signal transmission. Am J Physiol 1989;257:F882–F892.
44. Riser BL, Cortes P, Zhao X, Berstein J, Dumler F, Narins RG. Intraglomerular pressure and mesangial stretching stimulate extracellular matrix formation in the rat. J Clin Invest 1992;90:1932–1943.
45. Kent RL, Cooper G IV. Load-accelerated protein synthesis of stretched adult cardiocytes depends upon stretch-activated calcium (Ca) influx. Physiologist 1994;37:10–13 (abstract).
46. Alberts B, Bray D, Lewis J, Raff M, Roberts K, Watson JD. Cell adhesion, cell junctions and extracellular matrix. In: Alberts B, ed. Molecular Biology of the Cell, 2nd ed. Garland, New York, 1989, pp. 791–836.
47. Wang N, Butler JP, Ingber DE. Mechanotransduction across the cell surface and through the cytoskeleton. Science 1993;260:1124–1127.
48. McNamee HP, Ingber DE, Schwartz MA. Adhesion to fibronectin stimulates inostal lipid synthesis and enhances PDGF-induced inositol lipid breakdown. J Cell Biol 1993;121:673–678.
49. Sowers JR, Sowers PS, Peuler JD. Role of insulin resistance and hyperinsulinemia in development of hypertension and atherosclerosis. J Lab Clin Metab 1994;123:647–652.
50. King GL, Goodman AD, Buzrey S, Masis A, Kahn CR. Receptors and growth-promoting effects of insulin and insulin-like growth factors on cells from bovine retinal capillaries and aorta. J Clin Invest 1985;75:1028–1036.
51. Inoguchi T, Xia P, Kunisaki M, Higashi S, Feener EP, King GL. Insulin's effect on protein kinase C and diacylglycerol induced by diabetes and glucose in vascular tissues. Am J Physiol 1994;267:E369–E379.
52. Kaiser N, Sasson S, Feener EP, Bonkalja-Varoli N, Hagashi S, Moller DE, Davidheiser S, Przybylski RJ, King GL. Differential regulation of glucose transport and transporters by glucose in vascular endothelial and smooth muscle cells. Diabetes 1993;42:80–89.
53. Hirschberg R, Kopple JD. Evidence that insulin-like growth factor 1 increases renal plasma flow and glomerular filtration rate in fasted rats. J Clin Invest 1989;83:326–330.

54. Elahi D, McAloon-Dyke M, Fukagawa NK. Hemodynamic and metabolic responses to human insulin-like growth factor-1 in men. In: Spencer EM, ed. Modern Concepts in Insulin-Like Growth Factors. Elsevier, New York, 1991, pp. 219–224.
55. Hirschberg R, Brunori G, Kopple JD, Guler HP. Effects of insulin-like growth factor-1 on renal function in normal men. Kidney Int 1993;43:387–397.
56. Diez J, Ruilope LM, Rodicio JL. Is insulin-like growth factor-1 determinant of renal hemodynamics in obesity hypertension. J Hypertens 1993;11:5192–5193.
57. Copeland KC, Sreekuran K. Recombinant human insulin-like growth factor-1 increases forearm blood flow. J Clin Endocrinol Metab 1994;79:230–232.
58. Walsh MF, Barazi M, Pete G, Muniyappa R, Dunbar JC, Sowers JR. IGF-1 diminishes vascular contractility when administered in vivo, and in vitro. Endocrinology (in press).
59. Sarzani R, Brecher P, Chobanian AV. Growth factor expression in aorta of normotensive and hypertensive rats. J Clin Invest 1989;83:1404–1408.
60. Murphy LJ, Ghahary A, Chakrabarti S. Insulin regulation of IGF-1 expression in rat aorta. Diabetes 1990;39:657–661.
61. Delafontaine P, Bernstein KE, Alexander RW. Insulin-like growth factor 1 gene expression in vascular cells. Hypertension 1991;17:693–699.
62. Tirupattur PR, Ram JL, Standley PR, Sowers JR. Regulation of Na^+,K^+–ATPase gene expression by insulin in vascular smooth muscle cells. Am J Hypertens 1993;6:626–629.
63. Standley PR, Rose KA. Insulin and insulin-like growth factor-1 modulation of glucose transport in arterial smooth muscle cells: implication of GLUT-4 in the vasculature. Am J Hypertens 1994;7:357–362.
64. Brosius PC, Briggs JP, Marcus RG, Barac-Nieto M, Charron MJ. Insulin-responsive glucose transporter expression in renal microvessels and glomeruli. Kidney Int 1992;42:1086–1092.
65. Dominguez LJ, Davidoff A, Srinivas PR, Standley PR, Walsh MF, Sowers JR. Effects of metformin on tyrosine kinase activity, glucose transport and intracellular calcium in rat vascular smooth muscle. Endocrinology 1996;137:113–121.
66. Begum N, Leitner W, Reusch JE-B, Sussman KE, Draznin B. GLUT-4 phosphorylation and its intrinsic activity: mechanism of Ca^{2+}-induced inhibition of insulin-stimulated glucose transport. J Biol Chem 1993;268:3352–3356.
67. Standley PR, Ram JL, Sowers JR. Insulin attenuation of vascular smooth muscle calcium responses in Zucker lean and obese rats. Endocrinology 1993;133:1693–1699.
68. Standley PR, Rose KA, Sowers JR. Increased basal arterial smooth muscle glucose transport in the Zucker rat. Am J Hypertens 1995;8:48–52.
69. Barron JT, Kapp SJ, Tow JP, Messer JV. Effect of altering carbohydrate metabolism on energy status and contractile function of vascular smooth muscle. Biochem Biophys Acta 1989;976:42–52.
70. Hardin CD, Wiseman RW, Kushmerich MJ. Vascular oxidative metabolism under different metabolic conditions. Biochem Biophys Acta 1992;1133:133–141.
71. Sussman I, Schultz V, Gupta S, Grady C, Ruderman NB, Tornheim K. Differential effect of metabolic fuels on the energy state of the Na^+,K^+–ATPase in isolated cerebral microvessels. Am J Physiol 1993;265:E777–E782.
72. Lorenzi M, Cagliero E, Toledo S. Glucose toxicity for human endothelial cells in culture: delayed replication, disturbed cell cycle and accelerated death. Diabetes 1985;34:621–627.
73. Hotamisligil GS, Murray DL, Choy LN, Spiegelman BM. Tumor necrosis factor α inhibits signaling from the insulin receptor. Proc Natl Acad Sci 1994;91:4854–4858.
74. Fujiwara R, Shimada A, Tamai T, Nakai T, Miyabo S. Effects of insulin, insulin-like growth factor-1, and phorbol esters on neutral cholesterol esterase activity in cultured rat vascular smooth muscle cells. J Lab Clin Med 1995;126:240–249.
75. Chen Y, Bornfeldt KE, Arner A, Jennische E, Malmqvist U, Uvelius B, Arnqvist HJ. Increase in insulin-like growth factor I in hypertrophying smooth muscle. Am J Physiol 1994;266:E224–E229.
76. Cercek B, Sharifi B, Barath P, Bailey L, Forester JS. Growth factors in pathogenesis of coronary arterial restenosis. Am J Cardiol 1991;68:24C–33C.
77. Kulik TJ, Alvarado, SP. Effect of stretch on growth and collagen synthesis in cultured rat and lamb pulmonary arterial smooth muscle cells. J Cell Phys 1993;157:615–624.
78. Yang Z, Nol G, Luscher TF. Calcium antagonists differently inhibit proliferation of human coronary-smooth muscle cells in response to pulsatile stretch and platelet-derived growth factor. Circulation 1993;88:832–836.
79. Bornfeldt KE, Arnqvist HJ, Norstedt G. Regulation of insulin-like growth factor-I gene expression by growth factors in cultured vascular smooth muscle cells. J Endocrinol 1990;125:381–386.

80. Wilson E, Mai Q, Krishnankutty S, Weiss RH, Ives HI. Mechanical stretch induces growth of vascular smooth muscle cells via autocrine action of PDGF. J Cell Biol 1993;123:741–747.
81. Rubini M, Werner H, Gandini E, Roberts CT, LeRoith D, Baserga R. Platelet-derived growth factor increases the activity of the insulin-like growth factor receptor gene. Exp Cell Res 1994;211:374–379.
82. LeRoith D, Werner H, Beitner-Johnson D, Roberts CT. Molecular and cellular aspects of the insulin-like growth factor I receptor. Endocrin Rev 1995;16:143–163.
83. Khorsandi MJ, Fagin JA, Giannella-Neto D, Forrester JS, Cercek B. Regulation of insulin-like growth factor-1 and its receptor in rat aorta after balloon denudation. Evidence for local bioactivity. J Clin Invest 1992;90:1926–1931.
84. Delafontaine P, Lou H. Angiotensin II regulates insulin-like growth factor 1 gene expression in vascular smooth muscle cells. J Biol Chem 1993;268:16,866–16,870.
85. Cascieri MA, Chicchi GG, Hayes NS, Slater EE. Stimulation of DNA synthesis in rat A10 vascular smooth muscle cells by threonine-59 insulin-like growth factor I. Circ Res 1986;59:171–177.
86. Clemmons DR. Exposure to platelet-derived growth factor modulates the porcine aortic smooth muscle cell response to somatomedin-C. Endocrine 1985;117:77–83.
87. Kuklik TJ, Alvarado SP. Effect of stretch on growth and collagen synthesis in cultured rat and lamb pulmonary arterial smooth muscle cells. J Cell Physiol 1993;157:615–624.
88. Yang Z, Noll G, Luscher TF. Calcium antagonists differently inhibit proliferation of human coronary smooth muscle cells in response to pulsatile stretch and platelet-derived growth factor. Circulation 1993;88:832–836.
89. Predel HG, Yang Z, von Segesser L, Turina M, Buhler FR, Luscher TF. Implications of pulsatile stretch on growth of saphenous vein and mammary artery smooth muscle. Lancet 1992;340:878,879.
90. Hishikawa K, Nakaki T, Marumo T, Hayashi M, Suzuki H, Kato R, Saruta T. Pressure promotes DNA synthesis in rat cultured vascular smooth muscle cells. J Clin Invest 1994;93:1975–1980.
91. Chen Y, Bornfeldt KE, Arner A, Jennische E, Malmqvist U, Uvelius B, Arnqvist HJ. Increase in insulin-like growth factor 1 in hypertrophying smooth muscle. Am J Physiol 1994;266(2 Pt 1):E224–E229.

25 Arachidonic Acid Metabolites in the Vasculature

Michael S. Golub, MD, *Mark T. Hori,* BS, *and Michael L. Tuck,* MD

Contents

INTRODUCTION

Early evidence that prostaglandins (PGs) or other arachidonic acid (AA) metabolites might play a role in blood vessels and blood pressure regulation focused on the kidney *(1)*. Hypertension accompanying the removal of the kidneys could not be attributed to alterations in fluid and electrolyte function alone, for ureteral implantation into the vena cava created the same degree of renal failure but substantially less elevation of blood pressure *(1)*. Subsequent identification of the PGs as vasodilatory lipids present in the medullary interstitial cells suggested that these compounds might be the renal vasodilatory hormones that prevented renoprival hypertension. The first PGs identified in the kidney, PGE_2 and PGA_2, were vasodilatory and promoted sodium excretion when they were infused into the renal artery. However, PGE_2 was metabolized by one pass through the pulmonary circulation in animals *(2)*, and in humans, a high degree of extraction of PGE_2 by the lung was demonstrated *(3)*. Although PGA_2 escaped pulmonary degradation it was

From: *Contemporary Endocrinology: Endocrinology of the Vasculature*
Edited by: J. R. Sowers Humana Press Inc., Totowa, NJ

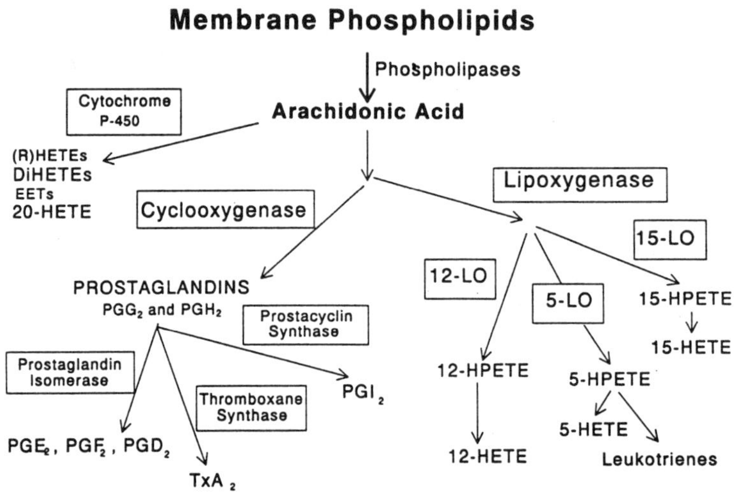

Fig. 1. Enzyme pathways of AA metabolism. AA is released from membrane phospholipids via the actions of phospholipases. Subsequent conversions by the cytochrome P-450 family of enzymes, CO, and/or LO yields biologically active metabolites summarized in this diagram.

rapidly cleared from the circulation *(3)*. Subsequent studies indicated that PGs of the A family probably do not exist in vivo and most likely are dehydration products of PGE produced in extraction procedures. Within the kidney, PGE_2 has been shown to be the principal PG and may have significant effects on renal blood flow (especially in reduced flow states), glomerular function, renal renin release, and water reabsorption *(4)*.

Recent advances in the chemistry of the eicosanoids have revealed that there are multiple metabolic pathways for these substances and regulation of their production is still poorly understood. AA, the principal substrate for these products, is a 20 carbon fatty acid (FA) that is incorporated in the phospholipids of cellular plasma membranes and is released by the action of stimulus-coupled phospholipase enzymes. Activation of the phospholipase is a critical step that can be triggered by various physical or hormonal stimuli. In several tissues *(5–7)*, phospholipase A_2 is activated by a calcium (Ca^{2+})-calmodulin complex which is sensitive to changes in intracellular Ca^{2+} ($[Ca^{2+}]_i$) concentration. An alternative source of AA is through the action of phospholipase C (PLC), a hormone-sensitive enzyme that produces the important intracellular messengers, inositol triphosphate (IP_3) and diacylglycerol (DAG) *(8)*. DAG is acted on by lipases to release AA.

Release of AA from the plasma membrane appears to be the major rate-limiting step in the generation of eicosanoid products. However, the specific compounds formed are tissue specific. AA can be re-esterified or metabolized by one of several enzyme systems (Fig. 1). The cyclo-oxygenase (CO) enzyme complex generates the classic PGs and thromboxanes. Lipoxygenase (LO) enzymes add an oxygen molecule at specific sites to form the hydroperoxyeicosatetraenoic acids (HPETEs) which generate the more stable hydroxyeicosatetraenoic acids (HETEs). Various cytochrome P-450 enzyme systems can utilize AA as a substrate to form HETEs, epoxides, and dihydroxy-HETEs. Many other pathways and FA substrates may also contribute to the local cellular environment that regulates vascular contractility.

CO PRODUCTS

A major pathway, the synthesis of PGs, is initiated by the CO enzyme complex acting on the AA substrate. Incorporation of oxygen into the AA molecule results in unstable, but biologically active endoperoxide intermediates. The discovery *(9)* that aspirin and other nonsteroidal antiinflammatory drugs inhibit the CO enzyme has been instrumental in studying this pathway. Blocking PG synthesis does not allow us to completely understand the role of this pathway however, as several PGs with differing biologic potencies can be blocked by these drugs. Tissue factors, cofactors, and specific enzymes may play a part in determining which PG is formed in a given tissue. Endoperoxides are intermediates for the formation of PGE_2, PGF_2, PGI_2 and thromboxane A_2. In some circumstances it appears that a tissue can change the pattern of its PG products. For example, the hydronephrotic kidney produces large amounts of thromboxanes instead of PGE_2 *(10)*, and this change in metabolism may contribute to the renal vasoconstriction in this model.

In blood vessels, particularly larger arteries, the predominant PG is prostacyclin or PGI_2, which is enzymatically converted from an endoperoxide intermediate *(11)*. There again was speculation that this PG might be a circulating vasodilatory and natriuretic hormone, for it escaped pulmonary metabolism *(12)*, but this PG cannot be measured in the blood by chromatography techniques because production of this very short-lived PG is not sufficient to maintain a circulating blood level *(13)*. The major metabolite of PGI_2 is 6-keto-$PGF_{1\alpha}$ which has a longer half-life but little or no biological activity. In addition to its vascular smooth muscle cell (VSMC) relaxing properties, PGI_2 is a potent natural inhibitor of platelet aggregation.

Thus, the eicosanoid pathways should be regarded as local, or paracrine, modulators within the blood vessel, where PGI_2 is the principal PG. Although the endothelial cell appears to be the major source of this material in vivo *(14)*, VSMC also produce PGI_2 *(15)*. Despite the lower synthetic rate in VSMC, their relatively large vascular mass may contribute to substantial production of PGI_2. In vitro, the de-endothelialized rat tail artery produces substantial amounts of PGI_2 *(16)*.

Thromboxanes are another vascular tissue product of CO activity *(17)*, and the vascular receptor for thromboxane/endoperoxides responds differently to antagonists than the platelet receptor *(18)*. In cerebral arterial tissue, endothelium-dependent contractions are blocked by thromboxane synthetase inhibition *(19)*, but in other studies thromboxane antagonists are more effective than thromboxane synthetase inhibitors *(20)*. Indeed, the short-lived CO endoperoxide intermediate, PGH_2, may activate the same receptor as thromboxane A_2. A thromboxane antagonist can lower blood pressure in coarctation hypertension in rats, a renin-dependent model *(21)*, and in a genetic model of hypertension, the Lyon rat, elevated thromboxane levels in the urine are decreased by thromboxane antagonists and synthesis inhibitors *(22)*. In these studies the pressure is lowered gradually after 3 wk, suggesting a mechanism separate from the direct vasoconstriction of thromboxane/endoperoxide receptor activation. $PGF_{2\alpha}$ is another CO product that has vasoconstrictive properties. Its actions appear to be mediated by a membrane receptor distinguishable from the endoperoxide/thromboxane receptor *(23)*.

CO PRODUCT EFFECTS ON CONTRACTILITY AND HYPERTENSION

If CO products contribute in some way to contractility how would this be mediated? A deficiency of vasodilatory PGs would be anticipated to augment vasoconstrictor responses. The classic example is that of an increased intrarenal vascular response to angiotensin II (AII) following CO inhibition *(24)*. CO inhibitors tend to counteract the effectiveness of antihypertensive medications *(25,26)*. Literature on the effects of CO inhibitors on vascular contractility is conflicting, perhaps owing to the nonspecific nature of the inhibitors and interspecies and intervessel differences *(27)*. Adrenergic responses are increased in rabbit celiac, ear, and pulmonary arteries; are not affected in aortic and carotid strips; and are reduced in the femoral artery following administration of CO inhibitors *(28)*. Further, flow-dependent changes in peripheral resistance in skeletal muscle arterioles are markedly decreased by CO inhibition *(29)*.

Differences in CO products between normotensive and hypertensive animals or subjects have been reported, but a causative link to hypertension has not been established. In humans a few reports of decreased urinary vasodilatory PGs in low-renin hypertension have been reported *(30,31)*. In Dahl salt-sensitive rats there is increased aortic production of PGI_2 along with decreased renomedullary PGE production in response to a high salt intake *(32)*. Increased vascular thromboxane production occurs in this model *(33)*, and increased basal PGI_2 production is seen in the mesenteric circulation of New Zealand hypertensive rats *(34)*. Although increased thromboxane production has been reported in the kidney of SHR *(35)* and DOCA-salt models *(32)*, and marked reductions in mesenteric vascular responses to nerve stimulation and AII occur after administration of thromboxane synthesis inhibitors *(36)*, not all studies of thromboxane inhibitors or antagonists have shown an effect on blood pressure *(37)*.

P-450 METABOLITES

Other oxygenated derivatives of AA may have important biologic functions. Inhibition of the P-450-dependent mixed function oxidase, which converts AA to epoxides in leukocytes and renal medullary cells, prevents development of hypertension in young SHR *(38,39)*. Paradoxically, this enzyme system appears to produce vasodilatory materials when AA is injected into the preconstricted perfused kidney *(40)*, since the vasodilatory response is enhanced by inducers of the enzyme and decreased by inhibitors. Epoxyeicosatrienoic acids (EETs) produced by P-450 have direct activity on potassium (K) channel opening *(41)*, and P-450 products may be responsible for the endothelial-dependent hyperpolarizing factor elicited by stimulation with bradykinin *(42)*. There is production of EETs by VSMC *(43)* suggesting an autocrine/paracrine function of these substances in the vasculature.

Some P-450 isoforms can produce 20-hydroxyeicosatetraenoic acid (20-HETE) in cat cerebral microvessels *(44)* and in rat kidney. Inhibition of production of this material with 17-octadecenoic acid (17-ODYA) suggests that 20-HETE is vasoconstrictive and may play a role in autoregulation of renal blood flow *(45)* and in afferent arteriolar responses to increased pressure *(46)*. A greater vasodilatory response to the use of P-450 inhibitors has been observed in preglomerular blood vessels of SHR than in normotensive controls *(47)*.

LO PRODUCTS

Another series of AA metabolites that may influence vascular responses are oxygenated derivatives of the LO enzymes, which are found in inflammatory cells and may play an important role in modulating bronchial smooth muscle tone. Products of 5-LO, the leukotrienes, are thought to explain the biologic effects of the material previously identified as slow reacting substance of anaphylaxis. Although leukotrienes may be important in the vascular collapse of anaphylaxis, they may have vasoconstrictive effects in isolated blood vessels. Leukotrienes may be produced in the adventitia of the vasculature by macrophages and mast cells in response to antigenic challenge *(48)*. Studies have demonstrated LO products in the blood vessel, independent of immunologic stimulation, although there is controversy regarding levels and biosynthetic origin of these materials. Canine and human coronary arteries generate 5-HETE, 12-HETE, and 15-HETE in addition to leukotrienes C4, D4, and E4 *(49)*, and HETEs (11-, 12- and 15-HETE) are in incubates of calf aorta and ductus arteriosus particulate fractions *(50)*. All three of these products are in endothelial cells from coronary arteries *(51)* and 15-HETE has been identified in human umbilical vein endothelial cell cultures *(52)*. Only minute amounts of LO pathway products are found in vascular tissue, and production of 11- and 15-HETE in VSMC has been attributed to the CO rather than the LO pathway *(53)*. In contrast, others *(54)* showed LO activity in freshly prepared rabbit aortic rings and found that HETE production could be reduced by LO pathway inhibitors. In rabbit aortic VSMC 5-, 12- and 15-LO activity has been noted with the predominate production of 12-HETE *(55)*. 12-HETE production in de-endothelialized aortic tissue that is reduced by LO pathway inhibitors *(56)*. 5-,12-, and 15-HETE also have been detected in endothelial cells from bovine coronary arteries *(57)*. There is LO activity in brain microvessels which produce 12(S)-HETE when stimulated with exogenous AA or the Ca^{2+} ionophore A23187 *(58)*. Two separate 12-LO enzymes are expressed in different tissues, a platelet enzyme and a newly identified enzyme found in mononuclear white cells and adrenal glomerulosa *(59)*. This form of the enzyme is found in VSMC and appears to correlate with the hypertrophic response to AII *(60)*. In human endothelial and VSMC the 12-LO enzyme is of the leukocyte type and is upregulated by AII *(61)*.

VASCULAR ACTIONS OF LO PRODUCTS AND INHIBITORS

LO products may exert a positive effect on Ca^{2+} entry into VSMC *(62)*. 15-HETE and 15-HPETE have vasoconstrictor activity, but Ca^{2+} blockers do not influence this constriction *(63)*. LO metabolites can mediate hormonal signals in several systems, such as the effect of glucose on insulin secretion *(64)* and AII's effect on renin suppression *(65)* and aldosterone secretion *(50)*. In rats pretreatment with LO pathway blockers such as phenidone, baicalein, and esculetin attenuate pressor responses to AII, but not to norepinephrine (NE) *(56)*, suggesting that the LO system specifically interacts with AII in various tissues. In addition to mediating vasoconstrictive responses, vasodilatory activity of 15-LO products in the rat aorta has also been reported *(66)*. Indeed, 15-hydroperoxyeicosatetraenoic (15-HPETE) and 15-HETE have endothelium-dependent and independent vasodilatory and vasoconstrictive activities depending on the species, the vessel, the dose, or the use of other vasoregulators *(67)*. Data with the specific LO inhibitor 5,8,11-eicosatriynoic acid (ETI) also suggest that LO products may have differing effects dependent on the contractile agonist (Fig. 2). In the femoral artery preparation, ETI markedly decreases contractile responses to certain agonists (U46619, AII, vasopressin, and NE), has little effect on others (KCl, serotonin), and potentiates endothelin-1 responses. AII responses are also inhibited in this vessel by two other LO inhibitors, esculetin and baicalein *(56)*. In the rat tail artery the KCl responses are markedly potentiated by ETI pretreatment *(68)*, demonstrating variability of responses depending on the

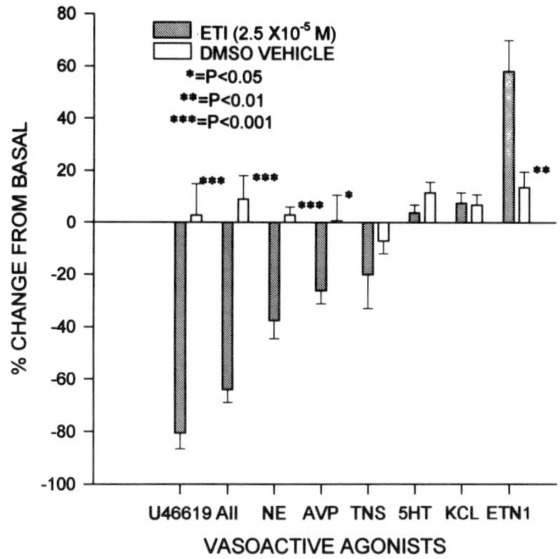

Fig. 2. Effect of the suicide substrate LO inhibitor, ETI, on contractile responses of rat femoral artery rings. Isolated segments of rat femoral arteries were contracted in vitro with various agonists prior to a 30-min exposure to ETI ($2 \times 10^{-5} M$) or dimethyl sulfoxide (DMSO) vehicle, after which they were exposed again to the following agonists: U46619 (thromboxane mimetic), AII; NE; AVP; TNS (transmural electrical nerve stimulation); 5HT; KCL; and ETN1 (endothelin 1).

particular vessel. Using detergent bile acids to remove the endothelium, we have performed preliminary studies that have demonstrated that the de-endothelialized tail artery contraction with NE is very sensitive to the effects of LO inhibition with ETI. This suggests that the endothelium is not critical to the effect of LO inhibition on contraction.

LO AND HYPERTENSION

We have shown the contribution of LO activity in the development of AII-dependent renovascular hypertension in the rat *(69,70)*. The nonspecific LO/CO pathway blocker, phenidone, attenuates the development of hypertension in the Goldblatt two-kidney, one-clip renovascular rat model *(69,70)*, but does not affect pressure in the DOCA-salt model *(69)*. LO inhibition also lowers pressure in SHR more than in WKY rats. Chronic treatment with a LO inhibitor arrests the evolution of hypertension in SHR *(71)*. There are elevated levels of plasma 12-HETE in prehypertensive SHR versus age-matched WKY rats *(72)*, and in WKY, 12-HETE plasma levels decline with age, whereas they remain elevated in SHR. 12-HETE production from de-endothelialized aortic tissue is also elevated in SHR, and there is increased LO activity in platelets from SHR compared to WKY *(73)*. In acute and chronic studies in the SHR, administration of LO inhibitors produces major reductions in systolic blood pressure (SBP) *(74)*. These data suggest an early abnormality in 12-LO activity in this genetic model of hypertension.

Elevated $[Ca^{2+}]_i$ and PLC activity in VSMC and other cells from SHR *(75,76)* suggest enhanced postreceptor signaling in tissues that regulate blood pressure. These reports also support the notion that LO products are determinants of AII-related blood pressure control. In the vasculature the LO pathway products may serve either as obligatory mediators, or regulatory modulators (cofactors) for the pressor-induced intracellular signals that culminate in VSMC contraction. This notion is based on the observations cited, that LO inhibitors can markedly reduce vascular contractility in vitro and blood pressure in vivo.

INTERACTION OF EICOSANOIDS AND OTHER PARACRINE FACTORS

In considering the vascular effects of eicosanoids, it should be recognized that there is shunting of substrate between the several pathways and that inhibitors have limited specificity. In a study in platelets, aspirin, indomethacin, and sodium salicylate were all found to interfere with the conversion of 12-HPETE to 12-HETE *(77)*. Another CO inhibitor, meclofenamate, may also inhibit the 5-LO enzyme *(78)*. Both 12-HETE *(79)* and 15-HETE *(80)* can inhibit the CO enzyme complex, and inhibition of CO can, in turn, increase LO products *(81)*. P-450 metabolites in the kidney can be further metabolized by CO to vasoactive compounds *(82)*, suggesting that AA compounds generated by the kidney tubules can then be metabolized to compounds affecting regional blood flow.

Eicosanoids are not the only potential paracrine modulators of vascular contractility. There are a host of relaxing and contracting factors, many of endothelial cell origin *(83)*. Endothelial-derived relaxing factor (EDRF)/nitric oxide (NO) induces relaxation and decreases platelet aggregation secondary to stimulation of cyclic guanosine monophosphate (cGMP) *(83)*. Although LO products were implicated as possible EDRF-like materials, the evidence was based on the use of inhibitors that also interfere with cGMP generation *(84)*. Similarly, studies aimed at linking AA release or metabolites to EDRF release have not been fruitful *(84)*, although AA may produce other relaxing materials in addition to PGI_2.

The biological importance of a number of endothelial-derived vasoconstrictors has also become evident. In addition to the generation of endoperoxide/thromboxane materials, the CO, as well as the LO pathway *(85)*, can generate superoxide anions. Indeed, in the cerebral circulation these materials, inhibitable by superoxide dismutase, may be responsible for endothelium-dependent contractions *(86)*. LO inhibitors affect the cGMP system, and antioxidants may produce superoxide anions which impair EDRF action as well *(87)*.

MECHANISM OF VASCULAR ACTION OF AA PRODUCTS

Many of the actions of PGs and thromboxanes on tissues are mediated by a family of membrane receptors, and progress is being made in cloning and characterizing these receptors *(88)*. A single agonist may activate more than one of the receptors and produce biphasic dose-response curves. For example, carbacylin, a PGI_2 analog, has vasorelaxant effects at low concentrations but vasoconstrictive effects at high concentrations, compatible with stimulation of a PGI–PGE vasorelaxant receptor at low doses and a TxA_2–PGH receptor at higher doses *(89)*. Receptor-mediated effects can involve several intracellular and membrane pathways. Vasodilatory responses probably involve the stimulation of cyclic adenosine monophosphate (cAMP). Although cGMP is stimulated by NO, this pathway is not involved directly with AA-derived products. However, some inhibitors of AA pathways may also influence cGMP formation. Stimulus-receptor interactions in VSMC activate G-protein-coupled reactions that result in activation of PLC or membrane

Ca^{2+} channels. A single receptor may activate more than one pathway. For example, the human IP_3 receptor is coupled to both cAMP and $[Ca^{2+}]_i$ changes *(88)*. PGs *(90)* and P-450 epoxide products *(82)* have effects on enzymatic systems such as the sodium–potassium (Na^+–K^+)–ATPase pump that can alter $[Ca^{2+}]_i$ and thus affect basal tone and vascular reactivity. AA itself, as well as AA metabolites and other fatty acids (FA), have direct effects on membrane channels, particularly K channels *(90)*. Membrane stretch and several FA, including AA, directly activate large conductance VSMC Ca^{2+}-activated K channels *(90)*. In cardiac myocytes AA and endothelin inhibit K channels through a protein kinase-dependent pathway *(91)*, suggesting that AA metabolism has complex effects on VSMC cation metabolism.

LO AND STIMULUS-COUPLED SIGNAL TRANSDUCTION

Pharmacologic experiments utilizing structurally dissimilar LO antagonists, baicalein, and ETI have demonstrated that LO inhibition attenuates AII-induced $[Ca^{2+}]_i$ transients in VSMC *(92)*. This attenuation can be reversed by preincubating the cells with exogenously added 12(S)-HETE, suggesting that 12(S)-HETE may play a role in modulating AII-mediated increases in VSMC $[Ca^{2+}]_i$ and contraction. Although in vitro treatment with 12(S)-HETE alone has no effect on basal VSMC $[Ca^{2+}]_i$, subsequent stimulation with AII results in augmented $[Ca^{2+}]_i$ responses *(72)*.

LO pathway products may also participate in other second messenger events for signal transduction. In endothelial cells, AII-induced chemoattractant generation is blocked by LO inhibition, and AII-dependent feedback inhibition of renin secretion is also prevented by LO inhibitors *(65)*. Direct addition of 12- and 15-HETE inhibits renal renin secretion, emulating the actions of AII *(93)*. 12- and 15-HETE increase thrombin-induced platelet aggregation and 15-HETE stimulates platelet IP_3 production *(94)*. LO products also have a role in stimulus-response coupling in other endocrine cells.

A mechanism of hormone-induced VSMC contraction is the receptor-linked activation of PLC, resulting in the hydrolysis of phosphatidylinositol biphosphate (PIP_2) and the liberation of IP_3 and DAG. IP_3 increases $[Ca^{2+}]_i$ release from the sarcoplasmic reticulum, and DAG activates protein kinase C (PKC), which, in turn, stimulates Ca^{2+} influx from extracellular spaces (Fig. 3). Vascular contractions are mediated by increases in $[Ca^{+2}]_i$, either by release from intracellular stores, or as a result of influx from the extracellular space. Changes in $[Ca^{2+}]_i$ affect intracellular AII action, and $[Ca^{+2}]_i$ can be altered by LO products. In VSMC, LO products, specifically 12-HETE, can mediate AII-induced $[Ca^{2+}]_i$ increases *(92)*. However, the mechanism by which LO products affect mobilization varies with different agonists and tissues. LO products are the major intermediates of AA-induced contraction of canine cerebral arteries *(95)*. In rat VSMC, AII, and vasopressin- and endothelin-induced increases in $[Ca^{+2}]_i$ are inhibited by ETI *(96)*. The inhibitory effect of ETI on Ca^{2+} transients induced by pressor agonists suggests that LO inhibition alters the mobilization of $[Ca^{+2}]_i$ from intracellular sites. That addition of the LO pathway product 12-HETE can restore the initial AII-induced VSMC $[Ca^{+2}]_i$ responses following LO blockade suggests that this LO product modulates AII-dependent Ca^{2+} transients in VSMC. The lack of an effect with 5-HETE and 15-HETE demonstrate the specificity of LO products in the vascular action of AII. That direct addition of 12-HETE to VSMC does not affect $[Ca^{2+}]_i$ suggests that this LO product may act more as a cofactor or intermediate in the action of AII in vascular tissue.

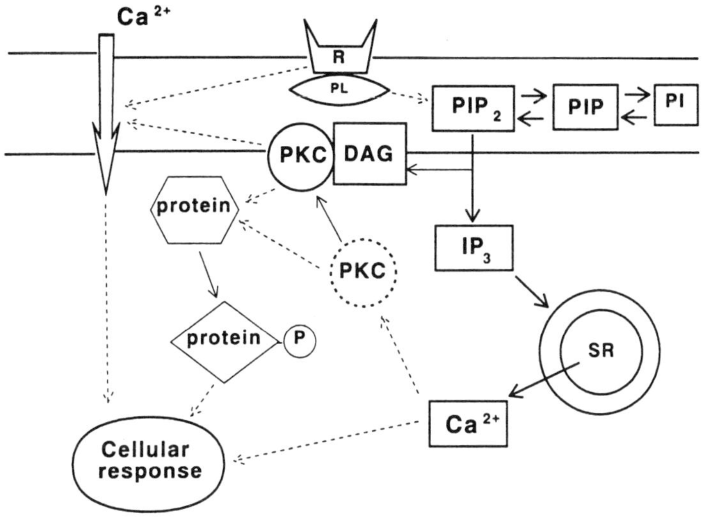

Fig. 3. Receptor-activated PLC messenger system. Activation of the receptor (R) opens Ca^{2+} channels and induces hydrolysis of PIP_2 by PLC, generating DAG and IP_3. Water soluble IP_3 bind to specific receptors on the sarcoplasmic reticulum (SR) effecting the release of stored Ca^{2+}. Increasing $[Ca^{2+}]_i$ invokes multiple cellular responses including translocation and activation of PKC, which in turn mediates other physiologic pathways via phosphorylation of serine and threonine residues on cellular proteins.

MECHANISMS OF HETE ACTION

There are two potential mechanisms by which LO products might participate in cellular-effector mechanisms in the vasculature. First, LO products such as 12- and 15-HETEs may act as obligate intermediates of the pressor effects of these agonists through direct stimulation of signal transduction pathways such as the phosphoinositide/Ca^{2+}/PKC messenger system. Secondly, variations in the FA components of DAG, owing to the action of LO activity, could influence intracellular effector pathways. Indeed, eicosanoids, such as HETEs, substitute for AA at the sn-2 position of DAG. These changes occur through constant, ongoing acylation/deacylation reactions, and are concentration and time dependent. Variations in the FA content of DAG may change the tertiary structure of these substrates (Fig. 4). This modification could indirectly alter the kinetics of enzymes, such as PLC and PKC, which act on these substrates. Thus, although no direct biological effects of these exchanges may be noted, they can be expected to influence responses elicited by stimulation.

LO products are likely important mediators for the agonist-induced mobilization of intracellular Ca^{2+}. Potential sites for 12-HETE increases in $[Ca^{2+}]_i$ in response to agonists include intracellular Ca^{2+} mobilization, Ca^{2+} fluxes, Na^+–Ca^{2+} exchange, and the Ca-ATPase pump. 12-HETE can induce VSMC migration via changes in Ca^{2+} flux *(97)*, and IP_3-mediated mobilization of Ca^{2+} stores is impaired by LO inhibitors. Pretreatment of VSMC with ETI inhibits thapsigargin-sensitive increments in $[Ca^{2+}]_i$, and attenuates AII-induced Ca^{2+} influx *(98)*. There is potentiation of thrombin-induced platelet aggregation and nucleotide release by 15-HETE and 12-HETE as well as potentiation of thrombin-induced DAG, IP_3, $[Ca^{2+}]_i$, and 47kDa-protein production by 15-HETE *(94,99)*.

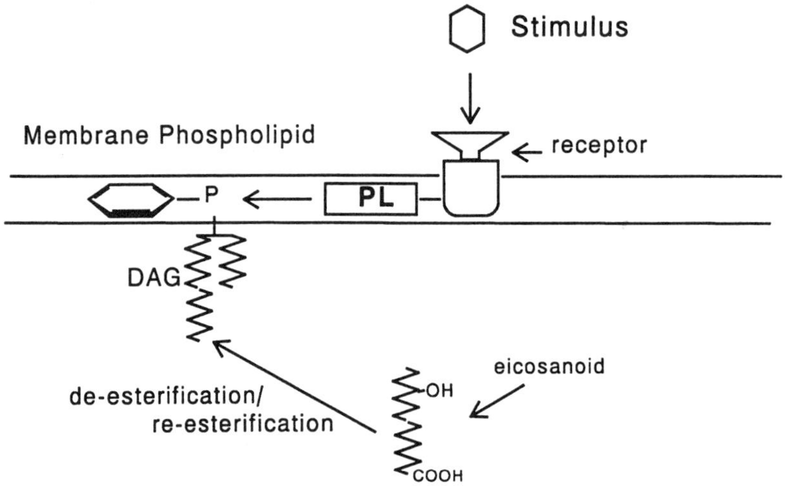

Fig. 4. Diagram of a possible mechanism of eicosanoid modulation of cell signaling pathways. Remodeling of membrane phospholipids via substitution of specific FA residues (i.e., HETEs) for AA at the sn-2 position of DAG may change the activity of subsequent enzymatic activation by altering kinetics of enzyme–substrate interaction.

12-HETE potentiates thrombin-induced platelet aggregation, presumably by preventing cAMP production *(100)*. There is evidence for eicosinoid incorporation (including HETEs) into the cellular membrane phospholipid pools *(101,102)*. There is specific incorporation of 5-HETE into endothelial phosphatidylcholine *(101)*, and 15-HETE can be incorporated into phosphatidylinositides with subsequent hydrolysis resulting in a structurally altered DAG messenger *(102)*.

Variation in FA content of DAG affects the activation of PKC isomers *(103)*, and ETI dose dependently inhibits AII-induced PLC activity, illustrating an effect of LO inhibition on phosphoinositide metabolism. Thus, VSMC changes in the FA content of DAG through HETE incorporation may alter the kinetics of phosphoinositide metabolism and PKC activation, suggesting a novel control point for agonist action, i.e., FA substitutions on membrane phospholipids. Thus, remodeling of membrane phospholipids via HETE substitution for AA may modulate agonist-induced signal transduction by changing the activity of enzymes that subsequently act on these substrates (i.e., PLC affinity for PIP_2, PKC activation). These data provide a compelling impetus for further investigation of 12-HETE regulation of phospholipases, IP_3 sensitivity, phosphoinositide turnover, and DAG and PKC.

CONCLUSION

In summary, LO products, particularly 12-HETE, may play an important role in modulating vascular responsiveness to agonists and in the development of hypertension. Specifically, we hypothesize that 12-HETE, by enhancing pressor-induced cytosolic Ca^{2+} and PLC-linked responses in vascular tissue, may modulate pressor-induced vascular reactivity. LO inhibitors modulate the actions of a variety of pressor-stimulated Ca^{2+} signals, suggesting that LO products might be involved in effector mechanisms of many systems which utilize the Ca^{2+}–DAG messenger system. The precise mechanism of 12-LO action in the vasculature, however, remains to be elucidated.

REFERENCES

1. Grollman A, Muirhead E, Vanatta J. Role of the kidney in pathogenesis of hypertension as determined by a study of the effects of bilateral nephrectomy and other experimental procedures on the blood pressure of the dog. Am J Physiol 1949;157:21–30.
2. Ferreira SH, Vane JR. Prostaglandins: their disappearance from and release into the circulation. Nature 1967;216:868–873.
3. Golub M, Zia P, Matsumoto M, Horton R. Metabolism of prostaglandins A1 and E1 in man. J Clin Invest 1975;56:1404–1410.
4. Dunn MJ. Renal prostaglandins. In: Dunn MJ, ed. Renal Endocrinology. Williams and Wilkins, Baltimore, MD, 1983, pp. 1–74.
5. Scharschmidt LA, Dunn MJ. Prostaglandin synthesis by rat glomerular mesangial cells in culture. J Clin Invest 1983;71:1756–1764.
6. Whorton AR, Young SL, Data JL, Barchowsky A, Kent RS. Mechanism of bradykinin-stimulated prostacyclin synthesis in porcine aortic endothelial cells. Biochem Biophys Acta 1982;712:79–87.
7. Seid JM, MacNeil S, Tomlinson S. Calcium, calmodulin, and the production of prostacyclin by cultured vascular endothelial cells. Biosci Rep 1983;3:1007–1015.
8. Majeras PW, Connoly T, Deckmyn H, Ross T, Ishii H, Bansal V, Wilson D. The metabolism of phosphoinositide-derived messenger molecules. Science 1986;234:1519–1526.
9. Vane JR. Inhibition of prostaglandin synthesis as a mechanism of action for aspirin-like drugs. Nature-N Biol 1971;231:232–235.
10. Morrison AR, Nishikawa K, Needleman P. Thromboxane A2 biosynthesis in the ureter obstructed isolated perfused kidney of the rabbit. J Pharmacol Exp Ther 1978;205:1–8.
11. Moncada S, Gryglewski JP, Bunting S, Vane JR. An enzyme isolated from arteries transforms prostaglandin endoperoxides to an unstable substance that inhibits platelet aggregation. Nature 1976;263:663–665.
12. Moncada S, Korbut R, Bunting S, Vane JR. Prostacyclin is a circulating hormone. Nature 1978;273:767–768.
13. Christ-Hazelhof E, Nugteren DH. Prostacyclin is not a circulating hormone. Prostaglandins 1981;22:739–746.
14. Eldor A, Falcone DJ, Hajjar DP, Minick CR, Weksler BB. Recovery of prostacyclin production by deendothelialized rabbit aorta. J Clin Invest 1981;679:735–744.
15. Baenziger NL, Becherer PR, Majerus PW. Characterization of prostacyclin synthesis in cultured human arterial smooth muscle cells, venous endothelial cells and skin fibroblasts. Cell 1979;16:967–974.
16. Golub MS, Berger ME, Powell M. Adrenergic stimulation of prostacyclin production in the rat tail artery. I. Response to agonists and antagonists. Prostaglandins Leukotrienes Med 1985;20: 299–311.
17. Ally AI, Horrobin DF. Thromboxane A2 in blood vessel walls and its physiological significance: relevance to thrombosis and hypertension. Prostaglandins Leukotrienes Med 1980;4:431.
18. Mais DE, Saussy DL, Chaikhouni A, Kochel PJ, Knapp DR, Hamanaka N, Halushka PV. Pharmacologic characterization of human and canine thromboxane A2/prostaglandin H2 receptors in platelets and blood vessels: evidence for different receptors. J Pharmacol Exp Ther 1985;233:418–424.
19. Katusic ZS, Shepherd JT, Vanhoutte PM. Endothelium-dependent contractions to calcium ionophore A23187, arachidonic acid and acetylcholine in canine basilar arteries. Stroke 1988;19:476–479.
20. Toda N, Inoue S, Bian K, Okamura T. Endothelium-dependent and independent responses to prostaglandin H2 and arachidonic acid in isolated dog cerebral arteries. J Pharmacol Exp Ther 1988;244:297.
21. Lin L, Mistry M, Stier CT, Nasjletti A. Role of prostanoids in renin-dependent and renin-independent hypertension. Hypertension 1991;17:517.
22. Geoffroy J, Benzoni D, Vincent M, Sassard J. Thromboxane A2 and development of genetic hypertension in the Lyon rat strain. Hypertension 1990;16:655.
23. Dorn GW II, Becker MW, Davis MG. Dissociation of the contractile and hypertrophic effects of vasoconstrictor prostanoids in vascular smooth muscle. J Biol Chem 1992;267:24,897–24,905.
24. Aiken JW, Vane JR. Intrarenal prostaglandin release attenuates the renal vasoconstrictor activity of angiotensin. J Pharmacol Exp Ther 1973;184:678–687.
25. Moore TJ, Crantz FR, Hollenberg NK, Koletsky RJ, Leboff MS, Swartz SL, Levine LL, Podolsky S, Dluhy RG, Williams GH. Contribution of prostaglandins to the antihypertensive action of captopril in essential hypertension. Hypertension 1981;3:168–173.

26. Golub MS, Berger ME, Vlachakis ND, Eggena P, Sambhi MP. The role of prostaglandins on the renin, catecholamine, and blood pressure responses to hemorrhage and captopril in conscious rabbits. Prostaglandins Leukotrienes Med 1982;9:445–457.
27. Hadhazy P, Malomvolgyi B, Magyar K. Endogenous prostanoids and arterial contractility. Prostaglandins Leukotrienes Essential Fatty Acids 1988;32:175–185.
28. Hadhazy P, Malomvolgyi B, Magyar K. Differential contractile responsiveness of isolated rabbit arteries from different vascular beds to cyclooxygenase inhibitors and PGI2. Eur J Pharmacol 1984;98:323–330.
29. Koller A, Kaley G. A new role for prostaglandins in the regulation of peripheral resistance. Prostaglandins Thromboxane Leukotriene Res 1990;21:595–598.
30. Tan SY, Sweet P, Mulrow PJ. Impaired renal production of prostaglandin E2: a newly identified lesion in human essential hypertension. Prostaglandins 1978;15:139–150.
31. Campbell WB, Holland OB, Adams BV, Gomez-Sanchez CE. Urinary excretion of prostaglandin E2, prostaglandin F2 and thromboxane B2 in normotensive and hypertensive subjects on varying sodium intakes. Hypertension 1982;4:735–741.
32. Limas C, Goldman P, Limas CJ, Iwai J. Effect of salt on prostaglandin metabolism in hypertension-prone and resistant Dahl rats. Hypertension 1981;3:219–224.
33. Uehara Y, Tobian L, Iwai J, Ishii M, Sugamoto T. Alterations of vascular prostacyclin and thromboxane A2 in a Dahl genetic strain susceptible to salt-induced hypertension. Prostaglandins 1987;33:727–738.
34. Pipili E, Poyser NL. Release of prostaglandins I2 and E2 from the mesenteric arterial bed in spontaneously hypertensive rats. Effects of sympathetic nerve stimulation and norepinephrine administration. Prostaglandins 1982;23:543–549.
35. Roman RJ, Kaldunski ML, Mattson DL, Mistry M, Nasjletti A. Influence of eicosanoids on renal function of DOCA-salt hypertensive rats. Hypertension 1988;12:287–294.
36. Jackson EK. Effects of thromboxane synthase inhibition on vascular responsiveness in the in vivo rat mesentery. J Clin Invest 1985;76:2286–2295.
37. Grone HJ, Grippo RS, Arendshorst WJ, Dunn MJ. Role of thromboxane in control of arterial pressure and renal function in young spontaneously hypertensive rats. Am J Physiol 1986;250:F488–F496.
38. Ferreri NR, Schwartzman M, Ibraham NG, Chander PN, McGiff JC. Arachidonic acid metabolism in a cell suspension isolated from rabbit renal outer medulla. J Pharmacol Exp Ther 1984;231:441.
39. Sacerdoti D, Escalante B, Abraham NG, McGiff JC, Levere RD, Schwartzman ML. Treatment with tin prevents the development of hypertension in spontaneously hypertensive rats. Science 1989; 243:388.
40. Oyekan AO, McGiff JC, Quilley J. Cytochrome P-450-dependent vasodilation of rat kidney by arachidonic acid. Am J Physiol 1991;261:H714–H719.
41. Hu S, Kim HS. Activation of K^+ channel in vascular smooth muscles by cytochrome P450 metabolites of arachidonic acid. Eur J Pharmacol 1993;230:215–221.
42. Hecker M, Bara AT, Bauersachs J, Busse R. Characterization of endothelium-derived hyperpolarizing factor as a cytochrome P450-derived arachidonic acid metabolite in mammals. J Physiol 1994;481: 407–414.
43. Hasunuma K, Terano T, Tamura Y, Yoshida S. Formation of epoxyeicosatrienoic acids from aracidonic acid by cultured rat aortic smooth muscle cell microsomes. Prostaglandins Leukotrienes Essential Fatty Acids 1991;42:171–175.
44. Harder DR, Gebremedhin D, Narayanan J, Jefcoat C, Falck JR, Campbell WB, Roman R. Formation and action of a P-450 metabolite of arachidonic acid in cat cerebral microvessels. Am J Physiol 1994;266:H2098–H2107.
45. Zou AP, Imig JD, Kaldunski M, Ortiz de Montellano PR, Sui Z, Roman RJ. Inhibition of renal vascular 20-HETE production impairs autoregulation of renal blood flow. Am J Physiol 1994;266:F272–F282.
46. Imig JD, Zou AP, Ortiz de Montellano PR, Sui Z, Roman RJ. Cytochrome P-450 inhibitors alter afferent arteriolar responses to elevations in pressure. Am J Physiol 1994;266:H1879–H1885.
47. Gebremedhin D, Ma YH, Imig JD, Harder DR, Roman RJ. Role of cytochrome P-450 in elevating renal vascular tone in spontaneously hypertensive rats. J Vasc Res 1993;30:53–60.
48. Feurstein G. Leukotrienes and the cardiovascular system. Prostaglandins 1984;27:781–802.
49. Piomelli D, Feinmark SJ, Cannon PJ. Leukotriene biosynthesis by canine human coronary arteries. J Pharmacol Exp Ther 1987;241:763.
50. Nadler J, Natarajan R, Stern N. Specific action of the lipoxygenase pathway in mediating angiotensin II induced aldosterone synthesis in isolated adrenal glomerulosa cells. J Clin Invest 1987;80:1763–1769.

51. Revtyak GE, Johnson AR, Campbell WB. Cultured bovine coronary arterial endothelial cells synthesize HETEs and prostacyclin. Am J Physiol 1988;254:C8–C19.
52. Hopkins NK, Oglesby TD, Bundy GL, Gorman RR. Biosynthesis and metabolism of 15-hydroperoxy-5,8,11,13-eicosatetranoic acid by human umbilical vein endothelial. J Biol Chem 1984;259:14,048–14,053.
53. Takayama H, Gimbrone MAJ, Schafer AI. Vascular lipoxygenase activity: synthesis of 15-hydroxyeicos-atetranoic acid from arachidonic acid by blood vessels and cultured endothelial cells. Throm Res 1987;45:803–816.
54. Greenwald JE, Bianchine JR, Wong L. The production of the arachidonate metabolite HETE in vascular tissue. Nature 1979;281:588,589.
55. Larrue J, Rigand M, Razaka G, Daret D, Demond-Henri J, Bricaud H. Formation of monohydroxy-eicosatetranoic acids from arachidonic acids by cultured rabbit smooth muscle cells. Biochem Biophys Res Comm 1983;112:242–249.
56. Stern N, Golub M, Nozawa K, Berger M, Knoll E, Yanagawa N, Natarajan R, Nadler JL, Tuck ML. Selective inhibition of angiotensin II mediated vasoconstriction by lipoxygenase blockade. Am J Physiol 1989;257:H434–H443.
57. Revtyak GE, Hughes MJ, Johnson AR, Campbell WB. Histamine stimulation of prostaglandin and HETE synthesis in human endothelial cells. Am J Physiol 1988;255:C214–C225.
58. Moore SA, Figard PH, Spector AA, Hart MN. Brain microvessels produce 12-hydroxyeicosatetraenoic acid. J Neurochem 1989;53:376–382.
59. Gu J, Natarajan R, Ben-Ezra J, Valente G, Scott S, Yoshimoto S, Yamamoto S, Rossi JJ, Nadler J. Evidence that a leukocyte type of 12-lipoxygenase is expressed and regulated by angiotensin in human adrenal glomerulosa cells. Endocrinology 1994;134:70–75.
60. Natarajan R, Gonzales N, Lanting L, Nadler J. Role of the lipoxygenase pathway in angiotensin II-induced vascular smooth muscle cell hypertrophy. Hypertension 1994;23:142–147.
61. Kim JA, Gu J, Natarajan R, Berliner JA, Nadler JL. A leukocyte type of 12-lipoxygenase is expressed in human vascular and mononuclear cells. Throm Vasc Biol 1995;15:942–948.
62. Vanhoutte PM, Rimele TJ, Flavahan NA. Lipoxygenase and calcium entry in vascular smooth muscle. J Cardiovasc Pharmacol 1985;7(Suppl. 6):S47.
63. Van Diest MJ, Verbeuren TJ, Herman AG. Cyclo-oxygenase blockers influence the effect of 15-lipoxygenase metabolites of arachidonic acid in isolated canine blood vessels. Prostaglandins 1986;32:97–100.
64. Metz SA. Lipoxygenase inhibitors reduce insulin secretion without impairing calcium mobilization. Endocrinology 1987;120:2534–2546.
65. Antonopillai I, Nadler JL, Horton R. Angiotensin feedback inhibition on renin release is expressed via the lipoxygenase pathway. Endocrinology 1988;122:1277–1281.
66. Uotila P, Vargas R, Wroblewska B, d'Alarcao M, Matsula SP, Corey EJ, Cunard CM, Ramwell PW. Relaxing effect of 15-lipoxygenase products of arachidonic acid on rat aorta. J Pharmacol Exp Ther 1987;242:945–949.
67. Matsuda H, Miyatake K, Dahlen S. Phamacodynamics of 15(S)-hydroperoxyeicosatetraenoic acid (15HPETE) and 15(S)-hydroxyeicosatetraenoic acid (15HETE) in isolated arteries from guinea pig, rabbit, rat and human. J Pharmacol Exp Ther 1995;273:1182–1189.
68. Golub M, Ormsby B, Berger M. Suicide substrate lipoxygenase inhibitors potentiate contractions to K chloride in the rat tail artery. FASEB J 1993;7:287 (abstract).
69. Nozawa K, Tuck ML, Golub MS, Eggena P, Nadler JL, Stern N. Inhibition of the lipoxygenase pathway reduces blood pressure in renovascular hypertensive rats. Am J Physiol 1990;259:H1774–H1780.
70. Nozawa K, Tuck ML, Golub M, Eggena P, Nadler JL, Stern N. Hypotensive effects of lipoxygenase inhibition phenidone in two-kidney, one clip Goldblatt hypertension. Am J Hypertens 1989;2:853–855.
71. Stern N, Nozawa K, Golub M, Eggena P, Knoll E, Tuck ML. The lipoxygenase inhibitor phenidone is a potent hypotensive agent in the spontaneously hypertensive rat. Am J Hypertens 1993;6:52–58.
72. Sasaki M, Hori MT, Hino T, Tuck ML. Elevated 12-lipoxygenase activity in the spontaneously hypertensive rat. Hypertens Res Clin Exp (submitted).
73. Gecse A, Sonkondi S, Mezei Z, Telegdy G. Arachidonate cascade in mesenteric blood vessels and platelets of spontaneously hypertensive rats. Agents Actions, Supplements 1987;22:43–48.
74. Stern N, Nozawa K, Golub M, Eggena P, Knoll E, Tuck ML. The lipoxygenase inhibitor phenidone is a potent hypotensive agent in the spontaneously hypertensive rat. Am J Hypertens 1993;6:52–58.
75. Oshima T, Young EW, Bukoski RD, McCarron DA. Abnormal calcium handling by platelets of spontaneously hypertensive rats. Hypertension 1990;15:606–611.

76. Osanai T, Dunn MJ. Phospholipase C responses in cells from spontaneously hypertensive rats. Hypertension 1992;19:446–455.
77. Siegel MI, McConnell RT, Cuatrecasas P. Aspirin-like drugs interfere with aracidonate metabolism by inhibition of the 12-hydroperoxy-5,8,10,14-eicosatetraenoic acid peroxidase activity of the lipoxygenase pathway. Proc Natl Acad Sci 1979;76:3774.
78. Boctor AM, Eickholt M, Puglsye TA. Meclofenamate sodium is an inhibitor of both the 5-lipoxygenase and cyclooxygenase pathways of the arachidonic acid cascade in vitro. Prostaglandins Leukotrienes Med 1986;23:229.
79. Hadjiagapiou C, Spector AA. 12-hydroxyeicosatetraenoic acid reduces prostacyclin production by endothelial cells. Prostaglandins 1986;31:1135.
80. Setty BNY, Stuart MJ. 15-hydroxy-5,8,11,13-eicosatetraenoic acid inhibits human vascular cyclooxygenase. J Clin Invest 1986;77:202–207.
81. Docherty JC, Wilson TW. Indomethacin increases the formation of lipoxygenase products in calcium ionophore stimulated human neutrophils. Biochem Biophys Res Commun 1987;148:534–538.
82. McGiff JC, Carroll, Escalante B, Ferreri NR. Pieces in the puzzle: novel arachidonate metabolites. Adv Prostaglandin Thromboxane Leukotriene Res 1995;23:187–192.
83. Shepherd JT, Katusic ZS. Endothelium-derived vasoactive factors: I. Endothelium-dependent relaxation. Hypertension 1991;18:III76–III85.
84. Milner PG, Izzo NJ Jr, Saye J, Loeb AL, Johns RA, Peach MJ. Endothelium-dependent relaxation is independent of arachidonic acid release. J Clin Invest 1988;81:1795–1803.
85. Kukreja RC, Kontos HA, Hess ML, Ellis EF. PGH synthase and lipoxygenase generate superoxide in the presence of NADH or NADPH. Circ Res 1986;59:612–619.
86. Katusic ZS, Vanhoutte PM. Superoxide anion is an endothelium-derived contracting factor. Am J Physiol 1989;257:H33–H37.
87. Ignarro LJ, Byrns RE, Buga GM, Wood KS, Chaudhuri G. Pharmacological evidence that endothelium-derived relaxing factor is nitric oxide: use of pyrogallol and superoxide dismutase to study endothelium-dependent and nitric oxide-elicited vascular smooth muscle relaxation. J Pharmacol Exp Ther 1988;244:181–189.
88. Abramovitz M, Adam M, Boie Y, Grygorczyk R, Rushmore TH, Nguyen T, Funk CD, Bastien L, Rochette C, Slipetz DM, Metters KM. Human prostanoid receptors: cloning and characterization. Adv Prostaglandin Thromboxane Leukotriene Res 1995;23:499–504.
89. Williams SP, Dorn GW II, Rapoport RM. Prostaglandin I_2 mediates contraction and relaxation of vascular smooth muscle. Am J Physiol 1994;267:H796–H803.
90. Kirber MT, Ordway RW, Clapp LH, Walsh JVJ, Singer JJ. Both membrane stretch and fatty acids activate large conductance Ca^{2+}-activated K^+ channels in vascular smooth muscle cells. FEBS Lett 1992;297:24–30.
91. Damron DS, Van Wagoner DR, Moravec CS, Bond M. Arachidonic acid and endothelin potentiate Ca^{2+} transients in rat cardiac myocytes via inhibition of distinct K^+ channels. J Biol Chem 1993;263:27,335–27,342.
92. Saito F, Hori MT, Ideguchi Y, Berger M, Golub M, Stern N, Tuck ML. 12-lipoxygenase products modulate calcium signals in vascular smooth muscle cells. Hypertension 1992;20:32–41.
93. Antonopilai I, Nadler JL, Robin EC, Horton R. The inhibitory role of 12- and 15-lipoxygenase products on renin release. Hypertension 1987;10:61–66.
94. Setty BNY, Werner MH, Hannun YA, Stuart MJ. 15-hydroxyeicosatetraenoic acid-mediated potentiation of thrombin-induced platelet functions occurs via enhanced production of phosphoinositide-derived second messengers -sn-1,2-diacylglycerol and inositol-1,4,5-trisphosphate. Blood 1992;80:2765–2773.
95. Jancar S, Shultz R, Krueger C, Cook DA. Mechanisms of arachidonic acid-induced contractions of canine cerebral arteries. Eur J Clin Pharmacol 1987;136:345–352.
96. Blomgren H, Hammarstrom S, Wasserman J. Synergistic enhancement of mitogen response of human lymphocytes by inhibitors of cyclo-oxygenase and 5,8,11-eicosatriynoic acid, an inhibitor of 12-lipoxygenase and leukotriene biosynthesis. Int Arch Allergy Appl Immun 1987;83:247–255.
97. Nakao J, Ito H, Chang W, Koshihara Y, Murota S. Aortic smooth muscle cell migration caused by platelet-derived growth factor is mediated by lipoxygenase product(s) of arachidonic acid. Biochem Biophys Res Comm 1983;112:866–871.
98. Kanda H, Hori MT, Tuck ML. Pathways of arachidonic acid metabolism differentially mediate angiotensin II-induced signaling pathways in cultured vascular smooth muscle cells. Hypertension 1995;26:565(abstract).

99. Setty BNY, Graeber JE, Stuart MJ. The mitogenic effect of 15- and 12-hydroxyeicosatetraenoic acid on endothelial cells may be mediated via diacylglycerol kinase inhibition. J Biol Chem 1987; 262:17,613–17,622.
100. Sekiya F, Takagi J, Usui T, Kawajiri K, Kobayashi Y, Sato F, Saito Y. 12-hydroxyeicosatetraenoic acid plays a central role in the regulation of platelet activation. Biochem Biophys Res Comm 1991;179:345–351.
101. Richards CF, Campbell WB. Incorporation of hydroxyeicosatetraenoic acids into cellular lipids of adrenal glomerulosa cells: inhibition of aldosterone release by 5-HETE. Prostaglandins 1989;38:565–580.
102. Legrand AB, Lawson JA, Meyrick BO, Blair IA, Oates JA. Substitution of 15-hydroxyeicosatetraenoic acid in the phosphoinositide signaling pathway. J Biol Chem 1991;266:7570–7577.
103. Nishizuka Y. Intracellular signalling by hydrolysis of phospholipids and activation of protein kinase C. Science 1992;258:607–614.

26 Arachidonic Acid Metabolites on Renin and Vascular Smooth Muscle Cell Growth

Rama Natarajan, PhD, *Naftali Stern*, MD, *and Jerry Nadler*, MD

Contents

GROWTH FACTOR ACTION AND METABOLISM OF ARACHIDONIC ACID (AA)

The interaction of hormones, growth factors, or cytokines to their specific cell surface receptors can lead to the stimulation of a cascade of biochemical events including the activation of several phospholipases which in turn can result in the release of several lipid second messengers *(1)* as outlined in Fig. 1. Thus, the action of angiotensin II (AII) or other vascular smooth muscle cell (VSMC) growth factors can activate one or more phospholipases, phosphoinositide phospholipase C (PI-PLC), phosphatidylcholine-specific PLC (PC-PLC), or phospholipase D (PLD). This process results in the formation of the second messengers inositol trisphosphate (IP_3), which leads to calcium (Ca^{2+}) mobilization from intracellular stores, as well as diacylglycerol (DAG) which in turn can activate the Ca^{2+}- and phospholipid-sensitive protein kinase C (PKC) *(2–5)*. It has been suggested that the cellular response to AII is obtained by the temporal integration of the IP_3/Ca^{2+}-calmodulin branch responsible for the initial transient response and the DAG/

From: *Contemporary Endocrinology: Endocrinology of the Vasculature*
Edited by: J. R. Sowers Humana Press Inc., Totowa, NJ

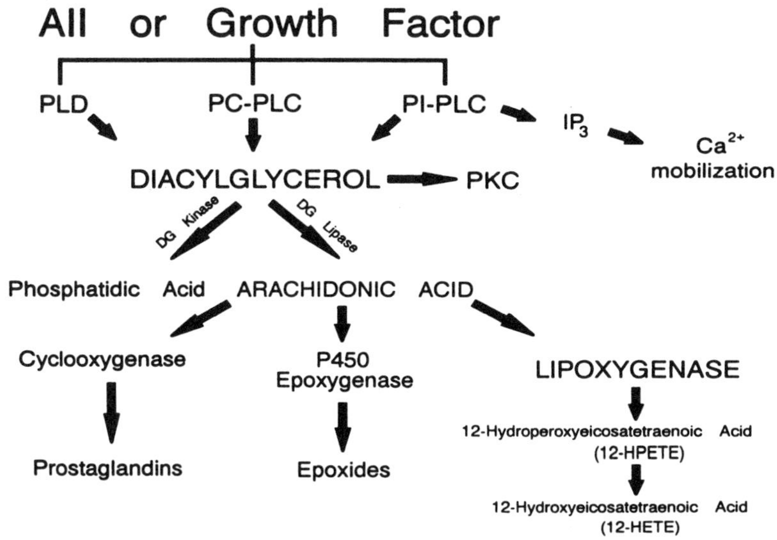

Fig. 1. Pathways of AA metabolism by growth factors.

PKC branch responsible for the sustained phase of AII action *(6)*. DAG is also a rich source of AA that can be released by the action of the enzyme DAG lipase *(7)*, whereas the enzyme DAG-kinase can convert DAG to phosphatidic acid (Fig. 1) *(8)*.

AA can be directly released from membrane phospholipids by the activation of phospholipase A2 (PLA_2) *(1)*. It has been suggested that AA release from the *sn*-2 position of membrane phospholipids may be one of the signals leading to cell proliferation *(9)*. AII can lead to release of AA in VSMC *(10)* and AA is further metabolized by three major pathways, the cyclo-oxygenase (CO) pathway, which leads to the formation of prostaglandins and thromboxane, the lipoxygenase (LO) pathway, which forms hydroperoxyeicosatetraenoic acids (HPETEs), hydroxyeicosatetraenoic acids (HETEs), and leukotrienes; and the cytochrome P-450 mono-oxygenase pathway, which leads to the formation of epoxides such as epoxyeicosatrienoic acids as well as HETEs (Fig. 1) *(11)*. A distinction between cytochrome P-450 mono-oxygenase and LO-derived HETEs can be found in the stereoselectivity of product formation with the former yielding (R)-HETEs and the latter yielding (S)-HETEs *(12)*. The LOs, mainly called 5-, 12- and 15-LOs, are named for their ability to insert molecular oxygen at the 5, 12, or 15 carbon atom of AA *(13)*. The 5-LO pathway leads to the formation of 5-HETE and leukotrienes whereas the 12- and 15-LOs can form 12- and 15-HETEs. The production of 12- and 15-HETE has been shown in several vascular tissues including cultured VSMC, endothelial cells, aorta, and coronary arteries. Various lines of evidence indicate that the LO products exhibit cellular growth-related effects. This chapter is mainly dedicated to reviewing the role of the LO pathway of AA metabolism on basal and growth factor-mediated growth of VSMC. Other references support the role of the LO pathway in renin-aldosterone regulation and in adrenal cell growth *(14–18)*.

There are at least two major isoforms of 12-LOs *(19–21)*. The platelet-type has been cloned from human platelets and the megakaryocytic cell line, HEL *(22,23)*. The other 12-LO, namely the leukocyte-type, has been detected in porcine leukocytes *(24)*, pituitary *(25)*, VSMC *(26)*, and also in human adrenal glomerulosa cells *(27)*, human monocytes, endothelial, and VSMC *(28)*. The cDNA for porcine leukocyte 12-LO *(24)* and murine leukocyte 12-LO *(29)* have been cloned. Porcine leukocyte 12-LO is only 65% homologous to the human platelet 12-LO *(22–24)* whereas it is 87% homologous to human 15-LO *(24,30)*. A bovine-trachea epithelial-cell 12-LO cDNA has also been cloned which is 86% identical to the human 15-LO and 89% identical to the porcine 12-LO *(31)*. The two distinct 12-LO cDNAs have recently been cloned from the same species, namely the mouse *(29)*. 15-LO has been cloned from human reticulocytes *(30)*.

THE LO PATHWAY IN ATHEROSCLEROSIS AND DIABETES

Increasing evidence has implicated the LO enzymes and their products namely HETEs (from AA) and hydroxyoctadecadienoic acids (HODEs) (from linoleic acid) in the pathogenesis of atherosclerosis. The oxidation of low-density lipoprotein (LDL) renders it more atherogenic than native LDL *(32)* and oxidized LDL plays a key role in the pathogenesis of atherosclerosis *(33)*. The LO enzyme has been suggested to mediate the oxidative modification of LDL since LO inhibitors, but not CO inhibitors, can reduce LDL oxidation by endothelial cells *(34)* and purified LO can oxidize LDL in vitro *(35)*. Furthermore, it has been shown that 15-LO mRNA and protein are expressed in macrophage-rich areas of rabbit atherosclerotic lesions and that the expression colocalizes with the epitopes characteristic for oxidized LDL *(36)*. Similar findings in human fatty streaks as well as in more advanced atherosclerotic lesions have been reported *(37)*. Atherosclerotic lesions of rabbit and human aorta also show higher levels of 15-LO enzymatic activity than corresponding normal arteries *(38,39)* and increased levels of HETEs have been found in the aortas of atherosclerotic rabbits *(40)*.

Increased amounts of LO products have been shown to be present in early atherosclerotic lesions *(41)* but not in later lesions where nonenzymatic oxidation reactions related to lipid peroxidation predominate. Recent studies support the involvement of the LO pathway in the atherogenic process since analysis of the lipid oxidation products in human atherosclerotic lesions reveal that the oxidation of polyunsaturated fatty acids therein is mainly mediated by the LO enzyme *(42)*. LDL incubated with fibroblasts overexpressing 15-LO have enhanced levels of lipid hydroperoxides further implicating the LO enzyme in the oxidative modification of LDL *(43)*. We also have new evidence supporting the presence of a leukocyte-type of 12-LO in human and porcine atherosclerotic lesions (unpublished observations).

Abnormal VSMC proliferation and growth are key features in the development of atherosclerosis and hypertension. A close examination of the signal transducing mechanisms of action of certain key VSMC growth factors may provide valuable information on the mechanism of VSMC growth which, in turn, would lead to potential therapeutic modalities to interfere with abnormal cellular growth. Diabetes mellitus is associated with the development of several vascular complications as well as a substantially increased prevalence of atherosclerotic disease and cardiovascular mortality. However, the mechanisms underlying the accelerated atherosclerotic disease associated with diabetes are not very clear. Prolonged hyperglycemia is considered to be a key factor in leading to diabetic vascular complications since it can alter several key biochemical pathways related to glucose metabolism *(44)*. Studies examining VSMC growth in response to various growth factors under hyperglycemic conditions may provide valu-

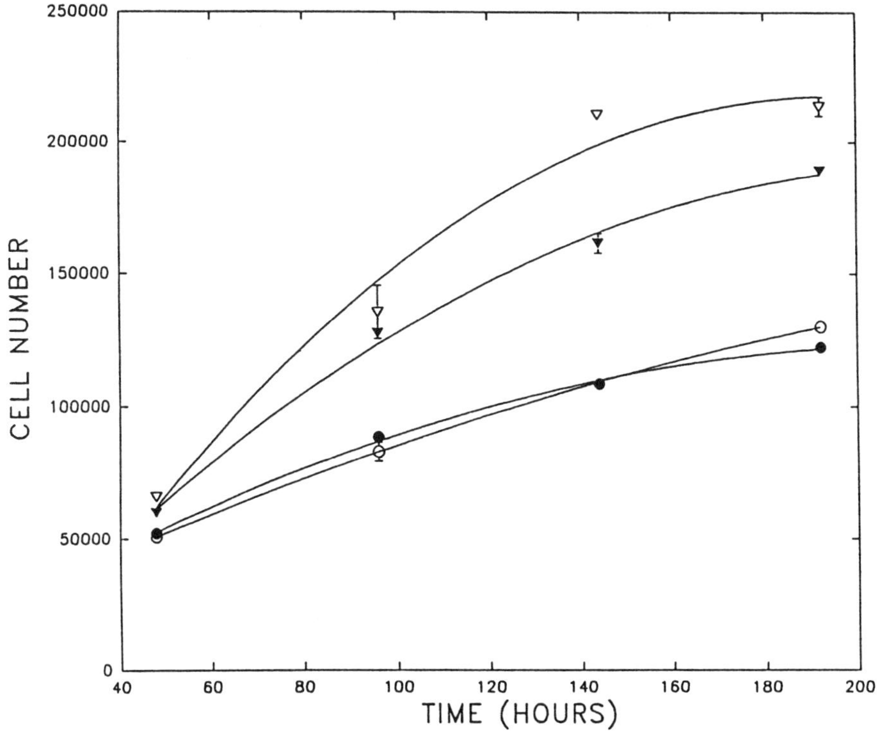

Fig. 2. Effect of the LO inhibitor, baicalein, on serum-induced proliferation of porcine VSMC cultured under normal glucose (5.5 m*M*, ○, ●) or high glucose (25 m*M*, ▽,▼) conditions. Cells growing in regular growth medium containing 10% fetal calf serum in normal glucose (○) or in high glucose medium (▽) for at least two passages were treated with vehicle alone (0.1% dimethyl sulfoxide) or with baicalein ($10^{-6}M$) (●, ▼) and cell counts obtained every 48 h.

able information on the signals responsible for the increased risk of cardiovascular disease in diabetes. It has been observed that porcine VSMC cultured under high glucose conditions (25 m*M*, ▽) (Fig. 2) for at least two passages to simulate chronic hyperglycemia exhibit an increased rate of proliferation in response to 10% fetal calf serum when compared to cells cultured under normal glucose conditions (5.5 m*M*, ○) (Fig. 2) *(45)*. The increased growth rates in high glucose are not the result of changes in osmolality since cells cultured under high mannose conditions grow slower than those in high glucose. Furthermore, fetal calf serum-induced protein synthesis as well as DNA synthesis ([^{3}H]thymidine incorporation) are both elevated in high glucose. The increases in protein synthesis are accompanied by increases in cell volume *(45)*. In addition, it is seen in the same Fig. 2 that treatment with a specific LO inhibitor, baicalein ($10^{-6}M$), has no significant effect on the rate of serum-induced growth of the cells in normal glucose (●). However, baicalein has a marked inhibitory effect on the proliferation of the cells in high glucose (▼) and reduces the excess growth rate in high glucose toward the rate observed in normal glucose. This suggests that the LO pathway may play a role in the accelerated proliferation of porcine VSMC under hyperglycemic conditions.

Elevated glucose can enhance LO pathway activation and expression. Porcine VSMC which have been cultured under hyperglycemic conditions also synthesize significantly

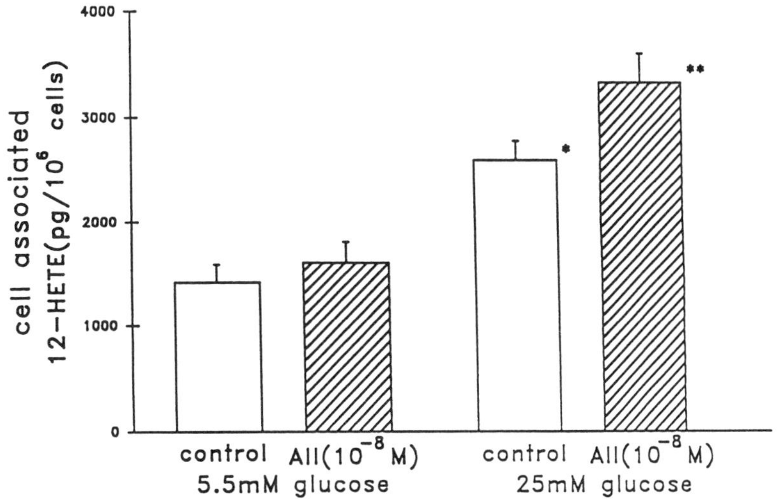

Fig. 3. Effect of high glucose (25 m*M*) and AII on cell-associated 12-HETE levels in porcine aortic VSMC. Control 12-HETE levels in high glucose were significantly greater than in normal glucose (5.5 mM) (*$p < 0.01$); AII increased 12-HETE levels over control only in high glucose (**$p < 0.05$). Reprinted from ref. *26* with permission.

greater amounts of cell-associated 12-LO product, 12-HETE, than those cultured under normal glucose conditions (Fig. 3) *(26)*. 12-HETE in the cells was measured by a specific radioimmunoassay after hydrolysis and extraction. Cell-associated 12-HETE levels in mannose-grown cells are not different from those in normal glucose. Furthermore, treatment with AII increases cell-associated 12-HETE levels only in cells cultured under high-glucose conditions (Fig. 3) *(26)*. In addition, the cells in high glucose display much higher intracellular 12-LO enzyme activity levels than cells in normal glucose (Fig. 4) *(26)*. A distinct peak with the same retention time as 12-HETE is seen in the basal state in the cells cultured under both normal as well as high glucose conditions (panels 3 and 5) indicating the presence of 12-LO activity in these VSMC. A 35% increase in the activity (12-HETE formation) is seen in the high-glucose control cells as compared to that in normal glucose control cells. AII (100 n*M*) causes a further increase (38%) in 12-LO activity in normal glucose (panel 4) and an additional 60% increase in high glucose (panel 6).

Other studies implicating HETEs in the pathogenesis of diabetic vascular disease include the observation that vessels from the infants of diabetic mothers have significantly elevated levels of 15-HETE and decreased formation of the vasodilatory prostanoid, prostacyclin *(46)*, and endothelial cells cultured under hyperglycemic conditions produce increased amounts of HETEs *(47)*. HETEs have also been shown to have direct mitogenic effects in endothelial and adrenal cells *(48,18)*. They also have potent chemotactic effects in VSMC, inducing migration at concentrations as low as 1 p*M (49)*. Human adrenal glomerulosa cells express a leukocyte-type 12-LO whose activity and expression is upregulated by AII *(27)*. Furthermore, the mitogenic effects of AII in adrenal cortical cells is attenuated by LO inhibitors *(18)*. In diabetic subjects urinary excretion of the 12-LO product, 12-HETE is markedly increased compared to matched nondiabetic controls *(50)*. Therefore, substantial in vitro and in vivo evidence support the hypothesis that elevated glucose and diabetes can augment LO pathway activation.

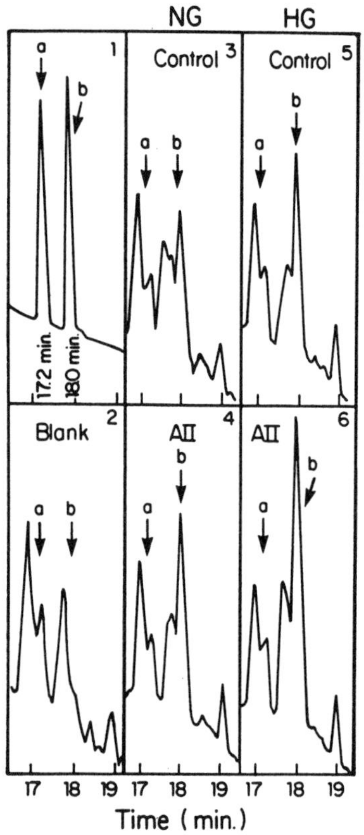

Fig. 4. Reverse-phase HPLC analysis of products of cold arachidonate metabolism by sonicated porcine VSMC grown in normal glucose (NG) (panels 3 and 4) or high glucose (HG) (panels 5 and 6). Detection was at 237 nm. Arrows a and b indicate positions of 15- and 12-HETE respectively. Panel 1 shows the retention times of authentic cold 15- and 12-HETE (17.2 and 18.0 min, respectively). Panel 2 depicts tracing of enzyme blank. Panels 3 and 5 show basal (control) activity in NG and HG respectively. Panels 4 and 6 show activity with 10-min AII ($10^{-7}M$) treatment in NG and HG, respectively. Reprinted from ref. *26* with permission.

REGULATION OF THE LEUKOCYTE-TYPE 12-LO EXPRESSION BY VSMC GROWTH FACTORS, AII, AND PLATELET-DERIVED GROWTH FACTOR (PDGF)

A leukocyte-type of 12-LO has been identified in porcine VSMC using a combination of molecular and immunological approaches *(26)*. A specific polyclonal antibody to the porcine leukocyte-type 12-LO can detect a protein with a molecular mass of about 72 kDa, similar to the reported molecular mass of porcine leukocyte 12-LO (Fig. 5) *(24)*. Furthermore, using a specific 15-LO antibody, no band is detected around 70 kDa. In addition, antibody-blocking studies have been performed to confirm the identity of the band. Thus immunoprecipitation of the 72-kDa band obtained with authentic porcine leukocyte 12-LO enzyme as well as porcine VSMC cytosols can be completely prevented by using antibody that had been preadsorbed with partially purified porcine leukocyte 12-LO enzyme.

Basal 12-LO protein expression is increased nearly fivefold in the VSMC cultured in high glucose compared to those in normal glucose (Fig. 5). Treatment of the cells

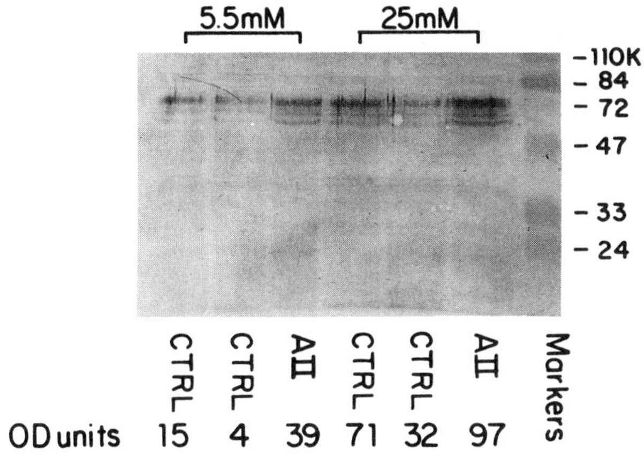

Fig. 5. The expression of porcine leukocyte type 12-LO (72 kDa) in porcine VSMC cultured in normal glucose (5.5 m*M*) or high glucose (25 m*M*) and after AII (10^{-7}*M*) treatment for 45 h. Equal amounts of protein were electrophoresed and blots probed with a specific antibody to porcine leukocyte 12-LO. Intensities of the bands are expressed as arbitrary optical density (OD) units obtained by densitometry. Reprinted from ref. *26* with permission.

with AII (100 n*M*) causes a marked stimulation (two- to threefold) in normal glucose as well in high glucose (Fig. 5) *(26)*. A leukocyte-type 12-LO has been reported in human VSMC, endothelial cells, and monocytes *(28)*. VSMC 12-LO can be induced by AII *(28)*, whereas monocyte 15-LO expression is increased by interleukin-4 (IL-4) or IL-13 *(51,52)*.

Regulation of 12-LO mRNA in porcine and human VSMC has been studied by a specific reverse-transcriptase polymerase chain reaction (RT-PCR) method *(26,28)*. The size of the PCR-amplified fragment is 333 bp for both 12- and 15-LO. Specific conditions were developed to distinguish leukocyte 12-LO from the human 15-LO. Figure 6 is a Southern blot analysis of the RT-PCR (25 cycles)-amplified products from porcine VSMC RNA. The 333-bp-specific amplified products of porcine leukocyte-type 12-LO is detected in the cells cultured in both normal as well as high-glucose conditions. The cells cultured in high glucose have a much greater expression of the 333-bp 12-LO PCR-amplified product than those cultured in normal glucose, with actually very little basal expression seen in normal glucose (Fig. 6A) *(26)*. Regulation of 12-LO mRNA expression by AII (10^{-7}*M*) at 24 h was also studied and the results are also depicted in Fig. 6A. AII causes a three- to fourfold increase in expression of the 333-bp PCR product in both normal and high-glucose cultured cells after correction for the expression of the internal control for PCR, namely glyceraldehyde-3-phosphate dehydrogenase (GAPDH) expression (280 bp) seen in Fig. 6B. However, in these cells, using specific primers and probes for 15-LO PCR, no amplified products of 15-LO were detected, suggesting that the VSMC do not express a 15-LO *(26)*.

12-LO activity and expression also can be potently upregulated by another VSMC growth factor, namely, PDGF. A 4-h treatment of VSMC with PDGF leads to a dose-dependent increase in the formation of the 12-LO product, 12-HETE, as well as an increase in intracellular 12-LO enzyme activity *(53)*. In addition, a 24-h treatment lead to an increase in the expression of both the leukocyte-type 12-LO mRNA as well

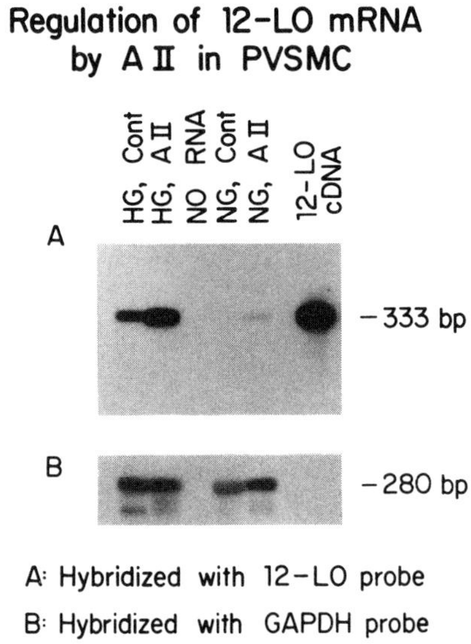

Fig. 6. Identification of porcine leukocyte type 12-LO mRNA in porcine VSMC by RT-PCR and its regulation by high glucose (HG) and AII ($10^{-7}M$ for 24 h). mRNA samples (0.5 μg each) were amplified for 25 cycles with porcine leukocyte 12-LO primers. The positive control for PCR, 12-LO (12-LO) cDNA amplification, is seen on the far right lane. **(A)** Hybridized with 12-LO oligonucleotide probe. **(B)** Same membrane hybridized with GAPDH probe. Reprinted from ref. *26* with permission.

as protein. Studies have indicated that the LO pathway may mediate the proliferative effects of not only PDGF but also that of fibroblast growth factor (FGF) in VSMC *(54)*. Further, it has been suggested that 12-HETE may mediate the chemotactic effects of PDGF *(55)*. New studies also suggest that cytokines such as IL-1, -4, and -8 can increase 12-LO activity and expression in porcine and human aortic VSMC *(56,57)*. These results indicate that LO in vascular and mononuclear cells can be induced by growth factors and cytokines and may contribute to their growth and chemotactic effects and thereby play a role in the formation of the atherosclerotic plaque.

THE LO PATHWAY HAS DIRECT GROWTH EFFECTS AND CAN ALSO MEDIATE THE HYPERTROPHIC EFFECTS OF AII IN VSMC

Evidence suggests that 12-LO products have direct mitogenic effects and also can mediate the mitogenic effects of AII in adrenal cortical cells *(18)*. To examine their potential growth effects in VSMC, it was determined that LO products have hypertrophic effects in these cells *(58)*. AII-induced increases in total cellular protein content of porcine aortic VSMC are attenuated by a specific LO inhibitor, baicalein, whereas, in contrast, a CO inhibitor, ibuprofen, has no effect (Fig. 7). Neither inhibitor alone alters basal cellular protein levels. Furthermore, direct addition of the 12-LO product, 12-HETE at 10^{-7} and $10^{-6}M$, increases total cell protein content in cells cultured under normal glucose conditions (5.5 m*M*) (Fig. 8). 15-HETE has no effect under these conditions. Interest-

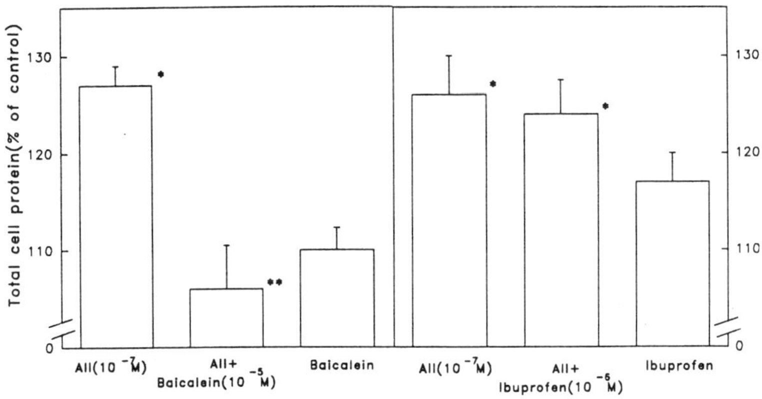

Fig. 7. Effect of a specific LO inhibitor (baicalein) and a CO inhibitor (ibuprofen) on AII-induced protein synthesis as evaluated by total cell protein content. $*p < 0.01$ vs basal; $**p < 0.03$ vs AII. Reprinted from ref. *58* with permission.

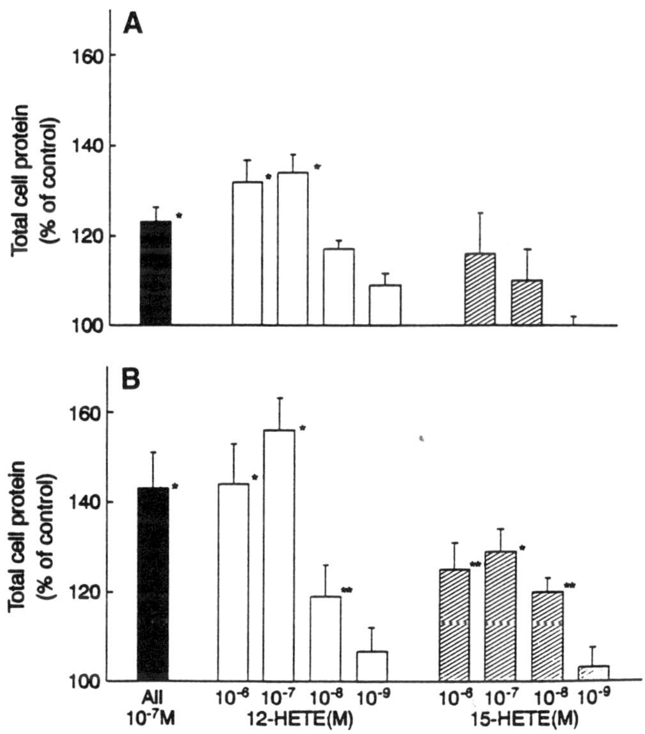

Fig. 8. The effects of AII and of HETEs on total cell protein content in porcine VSMC cultured in **(A)** normal glucose ($*p < 0.02$ vs basal) or in **(B)** high glucose ($*p < 0.01$ vs basal; $**p < 0.05$ vs basal). Reprinted from ref. *58* with permission.

ingly, the stimulatory effects of 12-HETE are markedly enhanced in cells cultured under high-glucose (25 m*M*) conditions (Fig. 8B) with 12-HETE at $10^{-8}M$ also showing a response. The effects of 15-HETE also were potentiated by the high-glucose culture

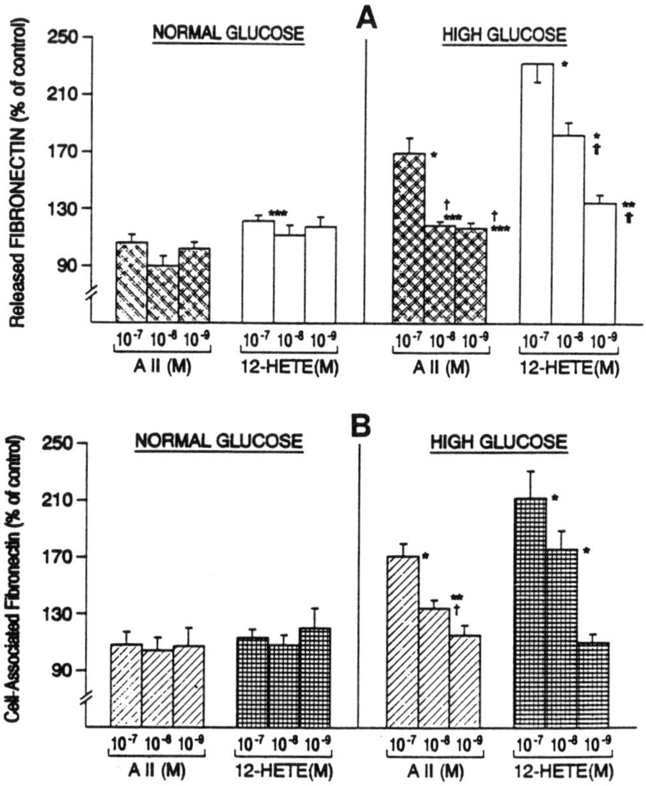

Fig. 9. The effect of AII or 12-HETE treatment on the levels of released fibronectin **(A)** and cell-associated fibronectin **(B)** in porcine VSMC. (A) Released fibronectin: $*p < 0.001$, $**p < 0.01$, $***p < 0.05$ vs basal, respectively; $^{\dagger}p < 0.03$ vs AII $10^{-7}M$; $^{\dagger\dagger}p < 0.02$ vs 12-HETE $10^{-7}M$. (B) Cell-associated fibronectin: $*p < 0.001$, $**p < 0.01$ vs basal respectively; $^{\dagger}p < 0.01$ vs AII $10^{-7}M$. In addition, AII and 12-HETE effects were greater in high glucose ($p < 0.01$). Reprinted from ref. *58* with permission.

conditions, although it is less potent than 12-HETE. In the same study, it was also shown that the hypertrophic effects of AII are also potentiated by high-glucose culture conditions (Fig. 8A,B) and the effects of 12-HETE were comparable to that of AII under both normal and high-glucose conditions *(58)*.

The study also examined the effects of AII and 12-HETE on the levels of the matrix protein fibronectin as measured by a specific enzyme-linked immunosorbent assay *(58)*. Figure 9A (left panel) shows that neither AII nor 12-HETE have any effect on released fibronectin levels in porcine VSMC cultured under normal glucose conditions. In contrast, both agents lead to increases in released fibronectin levels in the cells cultured under high-glucose conditions (Fig. 9A, right panel). Levels of cell-associated fibronectin are similarly increased by both 12-HETE and AII only in high-glucose cultured cells (Fig. 9B). Since AII as well as elevated glucose can increase the formation of LO products in these VSMC *(26)*, it is attractive to speculate that the enhanced growth-promoting effects of the LO products in high glucose may represent a potential mechanism for the accelerated VSMC growth and for the enhanced hypertrophic effects of AII under hyperglycemic conditions.

POTENTIAL MECHANISMS BY WHICH LO PRODUCTS MAY MEDIATE THE VSMC GROWTH

There are several mechanisms by which LO products may mediate cellular growth. They activate several oncogenes including, c-*fos* as well as *ras (59,60)*. HETEs also can activate PKC directly *(18,61,62)* or indirectly by incorporating into membrane phospholipids which then generate HETE-containing DAG species to activate PKC *(63)*. Activation of the leukocyte-type of 12-LO may cause structural modification of membrane phospholipids since it can oxidize both free fatty acids and those esterified to phospholipids, unlike the platelet form of 12-LO *(64)*. Studies have also shown that LO products can modulate intracellular Ca^{2+} ($[Ca^{2+}]_i$) levels in VSMC *(65)*. Thus, LO inhibitors can attenuate AII-stimulated increases in $[Ca^{2+}]_i$, and the addition of 12-HETE, but not 5- or 15-HETE, restores the initial $[Ca^{2+}]_i$ response to AII in rat VSMC. This suggests that LO products such as 12-HETE in particular may act as mediators of the intracellular actions of AII and also other growth factors *(65)*. Furthermore, a receptor-mediated mechanism of action with high-affinity binding sites for 12-HETE also has been demonstrated in certain cells *(66)*. In VSMC, LO products of AA (HETEs) and linoleic acid (HODEs) can directly activate mitogen-activated protein kinases *(67,68)*. Since mitogen-activated protein kinases are key components in the signaling pathways initiated by several growth factors and hormones *(69)*, AA and its LO metabolites may mediate growth factor-induced activation of mitogen-activated protein kinases and hence play a key role in the aberrant growth of VSMC observed in atherosclerosis and restenosis. Further studies will be needed to determine the role of LO products in activating other key signals including tyrosine kinase and other growth-related kinases.

There appears to be inhibition of renin release by products of the CO and LO pathways *(16,70)*. However, there is evidence that AA, prostaglandin I (PGI), and PGE_2 may all stimulate renin secretion *(16,71–73)*. Most data suggest the prostaglandins (PGs) which stimulate renin secretion function as first messengers, perhaps via activation of adenylate cyclase *(74)* and lowering of juxtaglomerular cell (modified VSMC) $[Ca^{2+}]_i$ *(73,74)*. PGI appears to stimulate renin release directly at the afferent arteriole, whereas PGE_2 stimulates release via the macula densa *(75)*. Indeed, PGs may play an integral role in renin gene expression in response to certain stimuli, such as lowering of renal perfusion pressure *(76)*. Products of the LO pathway play a modulatory role, inhibiting PG stimulation of renin secretion *(16,77–79)* and in both AII *(17,80)* and high dietary salt-induced *(80)* renin expression. Thus, AA products may indirectly affect vascular tone and growth via their role in modulating renin–angiotensin system which has a major impact on vascular biology.

In summary, LO enzymes in human vascular, inflammatory, and adrenal cells can form products that have several physiological and pathological effects. These include potent growth-promoting effects which therefore implicate them in the pathogenesis of diseases such as atherosclerosis, hypertension, and diabetic vascular complications. There are currently no clinically available safe and selective inhibitors of LO enzymes. One approach could be to use gene therapy to block these LO enzymes. We have developed a novel ribozyme or catalytic RNA directed against the porcine leukocyte 12-LO *(81)*. We showed that this ribozyme can efficiently cleave 12-LO mRNA in vitro and can also dose-dependently decrease 12-LO mRNA and protein expression when transfected into porcine VSMC *(81)*. Hence, therapeutic modalities and novel ribozyme technology approaches to effectively block these pathways may provide new ways to combat cardiovascular diseases.

ACKNOWLEDGMENTS

This work was supported by grants from the National Institutes of Health, R29 HL48920 and PO1 HL55798 (to R. Natarajan), RO1 DK39721 and PO1 HL55798 (to J. Nadler), and a Grant-in-Aid from the American Heart Association (to R. Natarajan).

REFERENCES

1. Liscovitch M. Crosstalk among multiple signal-activated phospholipases. Trends Biochem Sci 1992;17:393–399.
2. Berridge MJ. Inositol trisphosphate and diacylglycerol as second messengers. Biochem J 1984;220: 345–360.
3. Nishizuka Y. Role of protein kinase C in cell surface signal transduction and tumor promotion. Nature 1984;308:693–698.
4. Alexander RW, Brock T, Gimbrone MA, Rittenhouse SE. AII increases inositol trisphosphate and Ca^{2+} in vascular smooth muscle. Hypertension 1985;7:447–451.
5. Griendling KK, Rittenhouse SE, Brock TA, Ekstein LS, Gimbrone MA Jr. Sustained diacylglycerol formation from inositol phospholipids in AII-stimulated VSMC. J Biol Chem 1986;261:5901–5906.
6. Kojima, I, Kojima K, Kreutter D, Rasmussen H. The temporal integration of the aldosterone secretory response to AII occurs via two intracellular pathways. J Biol Chem 1984;259:14,448–14,457.
7. Bell RL, Kennerly DA, Stanford N, Majerus PW. Diglyceride lipase: a pathway for arachidonate release from human platelets. Proc Natl Acad Sci USA 1979;76:3238–3241.
8. Berridge MJ, Irvine RF. Inositol trisphosphate, a novel second messenger in cellular signal transduction. Nature 1984;312:315–321.
9. Millar JBA, Rozengurt E. AA release by bombesin. A novel postreceptor target for heterologous mitogenic desensitization. J Biol Chem 1990;265:19,973–19,979.
10. Rao GN, Lasseue B, Alexander RW, Griendling KK. AII stimulates phosphorylation of high-molecular-mass phospholipase A2 in VSMC. Biochem J 1994;299:197–201.
11. Smith WL. The eicosanoids and their biochemical mechanisms of action. Biochem J 1989;259:315–324.
12. Fitzpatrick FA, Murphy RC. Cytochrome P-450 metabolism of AA: formation and biological actions of "epoxygenase"-derived eicosanoids. Pharmacol Rev 1989;40:229–241.
13. Yamamoto S. "Enzymatic" lipid peroxidation: reactions of mammalian LOs. Free Radical Biol Med 1991;10:149–159.
14. Nadler J, Natarajan R, Stern N. Specific action of the LO pathway in mediating AII-induced aldosterone synthesis in isolated adrenal glomerulosa cells. J Clin Invest 1987;80:1763–1769.
15. Natarajan R, Stern N, Hseuh W, Do Y, Nadler J. Role of the LO pathway in mediating AII-induced aldosterone biosynthesis in human adrenal glomerulosa cells. J Clin Endocrinol Metab 1988;67:584–591.
16. Antonipillai I, Nadler J, Robin EC, Horton R. The inhibitory role of 12- and 15-LO products on renin release. Hypertension 1987;10:61–66.
17. Antonipillai I, Horton R, Natarajan R, Nadler J. A 12-LO product of arachidonate metabolism is involved in angiotensin action on renin release. Endocrinology 1989;125:2028–2034.
18. Natarajan R, Gonzales N, Hornsby PJ, Nadler J. Mechanism of AII-induced proliferation in bovine adrenal cortical cells. Endocrinology 1992;131:1174–1180.
19. Yamamoto S. Mammalian LOs: molecular structures and functions. Biochem Biophys Acta 1992;1128:117–131.
20. Funk CD. Molecular biology in the eicosanoid field. In: Cohn WE, Moldave K, eds. Progress in Nucleic acid Research and Molecular Biology. Academic, New York, 1993;45:67–98.
21. Sigal E. The molecular biology of mammalian AA metabolism. Am J Physiol(Lung Cell Mol Physiol) 1991;260:L13–L28.
22. Funk CD, Furci L, FitzGerald GA. Molecular cloning, primary structure and expression of the human platelet/erythroleukemia cell 12-LO. Proc Natl Acad Sci USA 1990;87:5638–5642.
23. Izumi T, Hoshiko S, Radmark O, Samuelsson S. Cloning of the cDNA for human 12-LO. Proc Natl Acad Sci USA 1990;87:7477–7481.

24. Yoshimoto T, Suzuki H, Yamamoto S, Takai T, Yokoyama C, Tanabe T. Cloning and sequence analysis of the cDNA for arachidonate 12-LO of porcine leukocytes. Proc Natl Acad Sci USA 1990;87:2142–2146.
25. Ueda N, Hiroshima A, Natsui K, Shinjo F, Yoshimoto T, Yamamoto S, Ii K, Gerozissis K, Dray F. Localization of arachidonate 12-LO in parenchymal cells of porcine anterior pituitary. J Biol Chem 1990;265:2311–2316.
26. Natarajan R, Gu JL, Rossi J, Gonzales N, Lanting L, Xu L, Nadler J. Elevated glucose and AII increase 12-LO activity and expression in porcine aortic smooth muscle cells Proc Natl Acad Sci USA 1993;90:4947–4951.
27. Gu JL, Natarajan R, Ben-Ezra J, Valente G, Scott S, Yoshimoto T, Yamamoto S, Rossi JJ, Nadler J. Evidence that a leukocyte-type of 12-LO is expressed and regulated by AII in human adrenal glomerulosa cells. Endocrinology 1994;134:70–77.
28. Kim JA, Gu JL, Natarajan R, Esteban J, Berliner JA, Nadler J. A leukocyte-type of 12-LO is expressed in human vascular and mononuclear cells: evidence for upregulation by AII. Arteriosclerosis Throm Vasc Biol 1995;15:942–948.
29. Chen X, Kurre U, Jenkins NA, Copeland NG, Funk CD. cDNA cloning, expression, mutagenesis c-terminal iso-leucine, genomic structure, and chromosomal localizations of murine 12-LOs. J Biol Chem 1994;269:13,979–13,987.
30. Sigal E, Craik CS, Highland E, Grunberger D, Costelo LL, Dixon RAF, Nadel JA. Molecular cloning and primary structure of human 15-LO. Biochem Biophys Res Commun 1988;157:457–464.
31. DeMarzo, N, Sloane DL, Dicharry L, Highland E, Sigal E. Molecular cloning and expression of an airway 12-LO. Am J Physiol 1992;262:L198–L207.
32. Steinberg D, Parthasarathy S, Carew TE, Khoo JC, Witztum JL. Beyond cholesterol. Modifications of low density lipoprotein that increase its atherogenecity. New Engl J Med 1989;320:915–924.
33. Parthasarathy S, Steinberg D, Witztum JL. The role of oxidized low density lipoproteins in the pathogenesis of atherosclerosis. Annu Rev Med 1992;43:219–225.
34. Parthasarathy S, Wieland E, Steinberg D. A role for endothelial cell LO in the oxidative modification of low density lipoprotein. Proc Natl Acad Sci USA 1989;86:1046–1050.
35. Sparrow CP, Parthasarathy S, Steinberg D. Enzymatic modification of low density lipoprotein by purified LO plus phospholipase A2 mimics cell-mediated oxidative modification. J Lipid Res 1988;29:745–753.
36. Yla-Hertualla, S, Rosenfeld ME, Parthasarathy S, Glass CK, Sigal E, Witztum JL, Steinberg D. Colocalization of 15-LO mRNA and protein with epitopes of oxidized low density lipoprotein in macrophage-rich areas of atherosclerotic lesions. Proc Natl Acad Sci USA 1990;87:6959–6963.
37. Yla-Herttuala S, Rosenfeld M, Parthasarathy S, Sigal E, Sarkioja T, Witztum JL, Steinberg D. Gene expression in macrophage-rich human atherosclerotic lesions. LO and acetyl low density lipoprotein receptor messenger RNA colocalize with oxidation-specific lipid-protein adducts. J Clin Invest 1991;87:1146–1152.
38. Henricksson P, Hamberg M, Diczfalusy U. Formation of 15-HETE as a major hydroxyeicosatetraenoic acid in the atherosclerotic vessel wall. Biochem Biophys Acta 1985;834:272–274.
39. Simon TC, Makheja AN, Bailey JM. Formation of 15-hydroxyeicosa-tetraenoic acid (15-HETE) as the predominant eicosanoid from Watanabe heritable hyperlipidemic and cholesterol-fed rabbits. Atherosclerosis 1989;75:31–38.
40. Wang T, Powell W. Increased levels of monohydroxy metabolites of arachidonic and linoleic acids in LDL and aorta from atherosclerotic rabbits. Biochem Biophys Acta 1991;1084:129–138.
41. Kuhn H, Belkner J, Zaiss S, Fahrenklemper T, Wohlfeil S. Involvement of 15-LO in early stages of atherogenesis. J Exp Med 1994;179:1903–1911.
42. Folcik VA, Nivar-Aristy RA, Krajewski LP, Cathcart MA. LO contributes to the oxidation of lipids in human atherosclerotic plaques. J Clin Invest 1995;96:504–510.
43. Benz DJ, Mol M, Ezaki M, Mori-Ito N, Zelan I, Miyanohara A, Friedmann T, Parthasarathy S, Steinberg D, Witztum JL. Enhanced levels of lipoperoxides in low density lipoprotein incubated with murine fibroblasts expressing high levels of human 15-LO. J Biol Chem 1995;270:5191–5197.
44. Ruderman NB, Williamson JR, Brownlee M. Glucose and diabetic vascular disease. FASEB J 1992;6:2905–2914.
45. Natarajan R, Gonzales N, Xu L, Nadler J. VSMC exhibit increased growth in response to elevated glucose. Biochem Biophys Res Commun 1992;187:552–560.
46. Setty BNY, Stuart MJ. 15-Hydroxy-5,8,11,13,-eicosatetraenoic acid inhibits human vascular CO. J Clin Invest 1986;77:202–211.

47. Brown ML, Jakubowski JA, Leventis LL, Deykin D. Elevated glucose alters eicosanoid release from porcine aortic endothelial cells. J Clin Invest 1988;82:2136–2141.
48. Setty BNY, Graeber JE, Stuart MJ. The mitogenic effects of 15- and 12-hydroxyeicosatetraenoic acids on endothelial cells may be mediated via diacylglycerol kinase inhibition. J Biol Chem 1987;262: 17,613–17,622.
49. Nakao J, Ooyama T, Ito H, Chang WC, Murota S. Comparative effects of LO products of AA on rat aortic smooth muscle cell migration. Atherosclerosis 1982;44:339–342.
50. Antonipillai I, Nadler J, Jost-Vu E, Bughi S, Natarajan R, Horton R. Progressive changes in eicosanoids occur in diabetic renal vascular disease. J Invest Med 1995;43:229A.
51. Conrad DJ, Kuhn H, Mulkins M, Highland E, Sigal E. Specific inflammatory cytokines regulate the expression of human monocyte 15-LO. Proc Natl Acad Sci USA 1992;89:217–222.
52. Nasser GM, Morrow JD, Robert LJ II, Lakkis FJ, Badr KF. Induction of 15-LO by IL-13 in human blood monocytes. J Biol Chem 1994;269:27,631–27,634.
53. Natarajan R, Bai W, Gu JL, Rangarajan V, Nadler J. Regulation of 12-LO by platelet-derived growth factor in VSMC. In: Samuelsson B, Paoletti R, Ramwell PW, eds. Advances in Prostaglandin, Thromboxane and Leukotriene Research. Raven, New York, 1995, pp. 435–437.
54. Dethlefsen SM, Sheprod D, D'Amore PA. AA metabolites in bFGF-, PDGF- and serum-stimulated vascular cell growth. Exp Cell Res 1994;212:262–273.
55. Nakao J, Ito H, Chang WC, Koshihara Y, Murota S. Aortic smooth muscle cell migration caused by PDGF is mediated by LO products of AA. Biochem Biophys Res Commun 1983;112:866–871.
56. Natarajan R, Rosdahl J, Gonzales N, Bai W. The regulation of vascular smooth muscle cell 12-LO by inflammatory cytokines. J Invest Med 1995;43:309A.
57. Kim JA, Gu JL, Berliner JA, Natarajan R, Nadler J. Inflammatory cytokines regulate 12-LO expression in human vascular smooth muscle and endothelial cells. Circulation 1995;92(Suppl. I):I160.
58. Natarajan R, Gonzales N, Lanting L, Nadler J. Role of the LO pathway in AII-induced vascular smooth muscle cell hypertrophy. Hypertension 1994;23(Suppl. I):I142–I147.
59. Haliday E, Ramesha C, Ringold G. TNF induces c-fos via a novel pathway requiring the conversion of AA to a LO metabolite. EMBO J 1991;10:109–115.
60. Yu CL, Tsai M, Stacey DW. Serum stimulation of NIH 3T3 cells induces the production of lipids able to inhibit GTPase-activating protein activity. Mol Cell Biol 1990;10:6683–6689.
61. Shearman MS, Naor Z, Segikuchi K, Kishimoto A, Nishizuka Y. Selective activation of the γ-subspecies of protein kinase C from bovine cerebellum by AA and its LO metabolites. FEBS Lett 1989;243:177–182.
62. Natarajan R, Lanting L, Xu L, Nadler JL. Role of specific isoforms of protein kinase C in AII and LO action in rat adrenal glomerulosa cells. Mol Cell Endocrinol 1994;101:59–66.
63. Legrand AB, Lawson JA, Meyrick BO, Blair IA, Oates JA. Substitution of 15-hydroxyeicosatetraenoic acid in the phosphoinositide signaling pathway. J Biol Chem 1991;266:7570–7577.
64. Takahashi Y, Glasgow WC, Suzuki H, Taketani Y, Yamamoto S, Anton M, Kuhn H, Brash A. Investigation of the oxygenation of phospholipids by the porcine leukocyte and human platelet arachidonate 12-LOs. Eur J Biochem 1993;218:165–171.
65. Saito F, Hori MT, Ideguchi Y, Berger M, Golub M, Stern N, Tuck ML. 12-LO products modulate Ca^{2+} signals in VSMC. Hypertension 1992;20:138–143.
66. Liu B, Khan WA, Hannun YA, Timar J, Taylor JD, Lundy S, Butovich, I, Honn, KV. 12(S)-Hydroxyeicosatetraenoic acid and 13(S)-hydroxyoctadecadienoic acid regulation of protein kinase C-α in melanoma cells: role of receptor-mediated hydrolysis of inositol phospholipids. Proc Natl Acad Sci USA 1995;92:9323–9327.
67. Rao G, Baas AS, Glasgow WC, Eling TE, Runge MS, Alexander RW. Activation of MAP kinases by AA and its metabolites in VSMC. J Biol Chem 1994;269:32,586–32,591.
68. Rao GN, Alexander RW, Runge MS. Linoleic acid and its metabolites, hydroperoxyocatadecadienoic acids, stimulate c-fos, c-jun, and c-myc mRNA expression, mitogen-activated protein kinase activation, and growth in rat aortic smooth muscle cells. J Clin Invest 1995;96:842–847.
69. Davis RJ. The mitogen-activated protein kinase signal transduction pathway. J Biol Chem 1993; 268:14,553–14,556.
70. Sedor JR, Davidson EW, Dunn MJ. Effects of nonsteroidal anti-inflammatory drugs in healthy subjects. Am J Med 1986;81(Suppl. 28):S8–S70.
71. Churchill PC. Second messengers in renin release. Am J Physiol 1985;249:F175–F183.
72. Lee FO, Nadler JL, Hsueh WA. Effect of a synthetic prostacyclin analogue on renin release in man. J Hypertens 1986;4(Suppl.):S10–S13.

73. McGiff JC, Quilley CP, Carrol A. The contribution of cytochrome P450 dependent arachidonic metabolites to integrated renal function. Steroids 1993;58:573–579.
74. Keeton TK, Campbell WB. The pharmacologic alteration of renin release. Pharmacol Rev 1980;32:81–227.
75. Ito S, Carretero OA, Abe K, Beierwalters WH, Yoshinaga K. Effect of prostanoids on renin release from rabbit afferent arterioles with and without macula densa. Kidney Int 1989;35:1138–1144.
76. Schricker K, Hamann M, Kaissling B, Kurtz A. Renal autacoids are involved in the stimulation of renin gene expression by low perfusion pressure. Kidney Int 1994;46:1330–1336.
77. Antonopillai I, Nadler J, Horton R. Angiotensin feedback inhibition on renin is expressed via the lipoxygenase pathway. Endocrine 1988;122:1277–1281.
78. Antonopillai I. 12 lipoxygenase products are potent inhibitors of prostacyclin induced renin release. Proc Soc Exp Biol Med 1990;194:224–230.
79. Henrich WL, Falck JR, Campbell WB. Inhibition of renin secretion from rat renal cortical slices by (R)-12-HETE. Am J Physiol 1992;263:F665–F670.
80. Stern N, Knoll E, Gilad S, Kisch E. Specific role of lipoxygenase products in renin suppression during high salt intake. 21st International Aldosterone Conference, p. 11, 1995 (abstract).
81. Gu JL, Veerapanane D, Rossi J, Natarajan R, Thomas L, Nadler J. Ribozyme-mediated inhibition of expression of leukocyte-type 12-LO in porcine aortic VSMC. Circ Res 1995;77:14–20.

INDEX